Thorsons Encyclopaedic Dictionary of Homoeopathy

Thorsons Encyclopaedic Dictionary of Homoeopathy

The Definitive Reference to All Aspects of Homoeopathy

Harald C. Gaier, DHomM, ND, DO, DipAc,
Fellow SA Homoeopathic Association
Member of the Register of Osteopaths (UK)
Member of the Register of Naturopaths (UK)

Thorsons
An Imprint of HarperCollins*Publishers*

Thorsons
An Imprint of HarperCollins*Publishers*
77–85 Fulham Palace Road,
Hammersmith, London W6 8JB

Published by Thorsons 1991
10 9 8 7 6 5 4 3 2

© Harald C Gaier 1991

Harald Gaier asserts the moral right to
be identified as the author of this work

A catalogue record for this book
is available from the British Library

ISBN 0 7225 1823 4

Printed in Great Britain by
Mackays of Chatham, Kent

This volume is dedicated to
Sabine in admiration,
and affectionately to
Rainer, Hermann, Lucien and Florian
as well as to
their children
in the certainty of an imminent
vigorous resurgence of homoeopathy – to become
ever more widely available to them and
their children's children

Möglicherweise wird diese Einschätzung
nicht mehrheitlich akzeptiert,
was jedoch nicht bedeutet, dass sie
deshalb falsch sein muss; denn es gehört
zu den unauflöslichen Widersprüchen
einer pluralistisch tolerierten Ideenvielfalt,
dass die Wahrheit bei der Minderheit,
der Irrtum aber bei der Mehrheit angesiedelt sein kann.

Professor Dr med vet Günther Harisch
and Dr rer nat Michael Kretschmer

Hannover,
April 1990.

Introduction

This *Encyclopaedic Dictionary of Homoeopathy* will, I hope, fill the evident need for such a general reference volume. It is intended for use by homoeopaths and by their antagonists, by pharmacists, scientists, medical historians, educators and philosophers, by professional people of many other kinds – and by the enquiring lay person who wishes to stay abreast of developments in medicine and science.

This book attempts to explain in some detail those technical and other terms that are encountered in reading or during conversation about, as well as in the study and practice of, homoeopathy. It is an alphabetically arranged vocabulary of this entire subject and the fields closely allied to it. In the more complex entries the non-specialist has been borne in mind by providing an introductory summary of the entry in which technical terms are almost entirely avoided.

I have aimed to satisfy the following objectives.

a) In order to allow the user to locate particular material easily, I have provided ample internal cross-references, creating a thesaurus-like logical network of conceptual affinities, that invites the reader to select the most promising onward reference.

b) I have tried for comprehensiveness and to achieve an absence of notable omissions of pertinent material.

c) Sources were diligently checked to eliminate factual errors as far as possible, and the influence of unsubstantiated opinions has sedulously been kept to a minimum.

d) I have given prominent representation to a great deal of material I believe to be relevant, which cannot readily be looked up elsewhere.

e) Motivated by the desire to produce a balanced work of reference, I have allotted proportionately more space to the issues and topics which, in my view, seem to matter more, though that choice remains, despite my efforts at impartiality, I suppose, a matter of my personal opinion. Yet it is equally a matter of the personal opinion of the reader. Let me just say, though, that I attempted to strike as reasonable a balance as seemed possible for as large a spectrum of the readership I anticipated as possible. The reader must judge for him- or herself to what extent I have succeeded in this.

f) To make browsing an attractive prospect I have aimed to offer pleasant surprises to the reader by presenting an assembly of interesting and perhaps unfamiliar facts, often in quasi-paradoxical juxtaposition to each other.

g) To create a sense of what the prime focus of homoeopathy always has to be, I have included a wide selection of medicines (both commonplace and obscure) under a handful of incidental entries covering symptoms (e.g. chilliness, discharges from the body, fever, headache, inflammation, irritability, jaundice, peculiar taste in mouth, etc.). In homoeopathy, obviously, such a list cannot ever claim to be fully exhaustive, as there will always be patients whose semiology will be matched by yet another medicine not listed which will provide the necessary curative homoeopathic impulse. The lists, where they occur, are primarily intended to convey to the reader the immense richness of homoeopathy. Finally, I must emphasize that it is the syndetic pointers which provide the homoeopath with the *aide-mémoire* effect of collective drug characteristics that could lead the successful prescriber to the 'Gestalt' of the one medicine which matches the patient's picture among the manifestly many that can be accessed repertorially, or via exceedingly well-programmed information technology.

h) Material either tangential or central to homoeopathy in the following categories was taken by me to be potentially pertinent to the volume's subject and, therefore, used in the text:

Scientific
Historical and Political
Paradigmatic and Conceptual
Veterinary and Phytopathological
Relating to Research or to Experimental Designs
Comparable with, Contrasting from, or Interrelating with other Medical Schools
Biographical
Philosophical, and specifically Epistemological
Pathological
Generally Informative but not of a 'Vade-Mecum' nature, except to illustrate some other aspect.

i) I have broadly integrated the subject material with the corresponding opinions and perceptions as currently held by the majority in the natural sciences outside of homoeopathy. Occasionally, particularly interesting historical contrasts or antagonisms are recorded too.

I am aware that more, much more, could have been included. For example, there might, perhaps, have been biographical entries for the USA's researching homoeopath J Stephenson, for the nineteenth century's trailblazing pharmacist Willmar Schwabe of Leipzig, for Mathias Dorcsi, the homoeopathic Primarius of Austria's Boltzmann Institute, for the philosopher-doctor Herbert A Roberts of Derby, Connecticut, for the AIH's first woman president, the brilliant Elizabeth Wright Hubbard of Boston, Massachusetts, for Alberto Soler-Medina of the influential Hispanic tradition of Tomas P Paschero, for the innovative researching pharmacist Jean Boiron and his twin brother Henri of Lyon, for three other giants in homoeopathic research, the biophysicist Fritz-Albert Popp, veterinarian Günther Harisch and the biochemist and physiologist Michael Kretschmer, for India's front-ranking homoeopaths, like Diwan Harish Chand, Jugal Kishore and Kailash Narayan Mathur, for some other outstanding French and German homoeopaths, such as M Aubin, A Cier, Othon André Julian, E A Maury, G Netien, Max Tétau, Léon Vannier, Henri Voisin, Lise Wurmser, Horst Barthel, August Bier, E Heintz, Kurt Hochstetter, Gerhard Köhler, Will Klunker, J Künzli, Otto Leeser, J Mezger and Hans Wolter, for some distinguished contemporary British homoeopaths, like Peter Fisher, Robin and Sheila Gibson, and David Taylor Reilly, or a great many more of many other nationalities. Events of special significance, such as the astonishingly successful political manoeuvring in the 1970s and early 1980s by homoeopaths in the Republic of South Africa, which produced a unique educational breakthrough for homoeopathy at full academic level, might have been mentioned; so might institutions like the National College of Naturopathic Medicine in Portland, Oregon, USA, the Bastyr College of Natural Health Sciences in Seattle, Washington, USA, or the Glasgow Medical School, where homoeopathy is beginning to take root again, or the Ludwig Boltzmann Institute for Homoeopathy in Vienna. Such omissions are regrettable. Yet I had to draw the line somewhere. A few may even say that I have included too much material.

I am sure, moreover, that there are aspects that I have missed altogether, or presented incompletely, or inadequately. I should welcome all constructive criticisms and suggestions concerning improvements to any future edition of this reference book. These are to be addressed to me care of the Publishers.

The publication of this *Encyclopaedic Dictionary of Homoeopathy* practically coincides with homoeopathy's bicentenary. It seems incredible that for all that time no such comprehensive reference work was available on the vast, vibrant subject of homoeopathy. I do not subscribe to the cynical opinion held by some that this task was never tackled because so many in positions of influence in homoeopathy were (and still are) contaminated by one or other non-homoeopathic medical model. It is said that to them homoeopathy is a mere 'complementary' adjunct, and such people prefer to pursue the 'soft option' of keeping undefined homoeopathy's discommodious scientific position. I do not subscribe to this, because even if this were so, there would always have been enough homoeopathic purists to produce such a reference work. Nonetheless, this was not done and it would have remained that way, but for the prompting of Dr George Lewith, MA, MRCGP, MRCP, director of the Centre for the Study of Complementary Medicine and editor of Complementary Medical Research.

In 1983 I had written a semi-official homoeopathic manual of 112 pages for the SA Homoeopathic Association entitled *Code of Good Practice for the Prescription, Preparation, Storing, Packing, Labelling and Dispensing of Medicines*. He read it, and later suggested that I might try to write a comprehensive reference volume on the entire subject of homoeopathy and I felt that I might like to do just that. Unsolicited, he contacted the publishers for which I am very grateful. They, in turn, wrote to me in Vienna, where I was living from 1985.

My prior experience stood me in good stead for the task at hand. I had been in homoeopathic practice at the Eastgate Centre, on the outskirts of Johannesburg, RSA, for more than five years immediately prior to my departure for Vienna in 1985. This complex, which, for much of that time, was said to be the largest in the southern hemisphere, officially recorded the numbers of employees and visitors present within it on any given day and the figures peaked on some days at an incredible 70 000 individuals. The experience there was valuable because no orthodox medical practitioner, nor any other medical practitioner for that matter, was in the complex nor within ready access in the surrounding area. That meant for the full period of those five years I was the only registered practitioner who could attend to the emergencies that were a regular occurrence among such an enormous throng of people: the infarcts, the diabetic comas, the anaphylactic shocks, the syncopes, the haemorrhages, the scalds (from the restaurants), the poisonings, the asthmatic attacks and many other acute emergency conditions were a regular feature. I was on duty from 08.00 to 18.00 on weekdays without any break and half-day on alternate Saturdays. Although I was extremely busy and often hard pressed for time there was never once, in nearly six years, any discontent expressed about my treatment or its effectiveness, which can not always be said for some casualty departments which are run in hospitals along non-homoeopathic lines. This has unequivocally pointed to the fact that a qualified and experienced practitioner is able, by entirely non-orthodox means, to attend to all manner of medical (i.e. non-surgical) emergencies promptly, reliably and, above all, extremely effectively. Some of the methods which I used then are described in this volume under 'Emergencies – Homoeopathic Treatment'.

I wish to thank all my teachers as well as the many wise men and women who have written so prolifically on the subject of homoeopathy. I have gathered together what to me is the choicest crop of noetic comments by these Hahnemannian students. Phrases whose authors I knew, and when I could also remember chapter and verse, have been attributed. Yet there will undoubtedly be a *bon mot* here and there that I have appropriated where I am no longer consciously aware of the source. My thanks and acknowledgement goes out to all these original thinkers and seasoned homoeopaths, who – through me – have contributed to this encyclopaedic dictionary.

I also wish to acknowledge my profound indebtedness to Harris Livermore Coulter, Ph.D., the distinguished medical historian. I was inspired by his superlative analysis of the two streams of philosophical thought (*Divided Legacy: A History of the Schism in Medical Thought*, 3 vols, Washington DC: Wehawken Book Co, 1973, 1975 & 1977) the conceptual model of which I have followed and explored further in some of my own forays into historical and philosophical terra incognita in this book.

An author's task is essentially performed alone. So was mine, but there have been two others who have very kindly helped me in my work. One of these is Francis Treuherz, MA, M.Ch., D HT, RSHom, editor of *The Homoeopath*, who, amongst several other constructive suggestions, drew my attention to Edward W Berridge's links with the occult Order of the Golden Dawn and to Vincent van Gogh's connexion with the French homoeopath Gachet.[1] The other is the consultant psychotherapist Irene Lucy, DHP, MIAH, LNCP, who had inherited a fair amount of John Henry Clarke's furniture, library and personal belongings to which she generously offered me access. I am very grateful for their help. I must also thank Biomed International AG of Zurich, Switzerland who had sufficient faith in me and the homoeopathic cause to extend a moderate but nonetheless indispensable financial loan to enable me and my family to live more or less normally during the years I researched and compiled the Dictionary whilst, of necessity, devoting somewhat less time and attention than I ought to my newly established practices in London and Petersfield, where I have made my home since September 1987.

I particularly want to thank Mr John Hardaker, former Editor-in-Chief of Thorsons, for his counsel and encouragement in the early stages of this Encyclopaedic Dictionary, and Ms Veronica Simpson, my hard working editor at Thorsons of HarperCollins Publishers Ltd, for so unfailingly applying her technical and linguistic skills, as well as for the abundant empathy she brought to the material she had to wade through.

This is a time of impending minor conceptual changes within homoeopathy and a season of subtle shifts in opinion both by homoeopaths and their detractors. A few of the cherished minor hypotheses long held by either believers or sceptics may, with some probability, soon turn out to have been illusions, to be replaced by other minor hypotheses. This ordeal of change is, in part, propelled by the progressive experimental probes made in homoeopathy in the past twenty-five years. It is as well to have a record of what homoeopathy has stood for during the last two hundred years and of its current experimental initiatives, before any effacing changes, however minor, take effect.

There are also other changes in the air. These are largely outside of homoeopathy. There are now constant inexorable social and technological pressures towards an individualistic libertarian revival, the implications of which no-one will be able to escape. To quote futurist Francis Kinsman's recent wise admonition: 'Woe betide any business, any political party or indeed any individual that does not attempt to come to grips with them. This is the spirit of the new era, even if its substance is not made flesh quite yet.'[2] The changes he warns about are, of course, the altering attitudes of large numbers of individuals by which they have begun to recognize themselves for being just that, namely individuals. The rebellion against collectivism in the Comecon countries in the last year bears eloquent witness to this wave of change. (In the text – the bulk of which was completed by the end of June 1990 – the

[1]Treuherz, Francis. *J Alt and Comp Medicine*, Nov 1990, Vol VIII, No. 11, p 19.
[2]Kinsman, Francis. *Millennium: Towards Tomorrow's Society*, London: W H Allen & Co PLC, 1989, p 49.

distinction between the GDR and the FRG, viz. German Democratic Republic and German Federal Republic respectively, still had to be made; since the third of October 1990 there is now just one unified Germany, and in the editing stage the previous appellations were mostly replaced simply by 'Germany'.)

The same strong anti-collectivist disposition has become universally evident, not just in eastern Europe. It represents a dramatic approximation by the world's society to the stalwart position consistently occupied by homoeopathy, the champion of individualism in medicine, for two hundred years.

There is, moreover, also a revolution in science that is in the offing. The old medical equation:

'Health equals Order and Disease equals Chaos',

which underpins the determinism of the Rationalist tradition in medicine, is being repudiated as too simplistic and downright misleading. The relevance of chaos having been recently discovered as, in a real sense, 'systematic' will soon be forcing this paradigm shift in medicine. The homoeopathic view, that each patient is his own individual complex dynamic system, embedded in the probabiliorism that is its foundation, is fast gathering momentum.

Why do infections affect different people differently and some not at all? Why do epidemics vary from one to the next, even though the initiating contagion may be the same? Why are not all tobacco smokers taken ill at the same time, or in the same way? Determinism has failed to provide the answers to these and the many similar questions which permeate all of medicine, and have shown medicine to be exasperatingly inexact as long as the vital element of 'the individual response' is not taken into account. The homoeopathic position could be said to be that the equation should read:

'Health equals Order **and** Chaos, patterned by individuals when in Protective Mode,

whereas Chronic Disease equals Rigidly Congealed Order, or non-Systematic Chaos, while

Acute Disease again equals Order **and** Chaos, patterned by individuals when in Defensive Mode'.

There are early signs that this new paradigm may yet come to be widely accepted.

These denouements are very welcome news for homoeopathy, which was seen, until quite recently, by many as an anomaly in science, and by some as having arrived on the stage of science two hundred years too early. Clearly this present cultural change contributes substantially to the rapidly widening appeal experienced by homoeopathy at present. The scientific shift will further strengthen homoeopathy's position.

I hope this book will serve as a source of reference for the old hands in homoeopathy and will help to orientate the newcomers that the wave of change will bring to it.

Harald C Gaier
Petersfield
30th April 1991

Note on 'The Organon'

Unless stated otherwise, all references herein to the 'Organon' are made to the English translation by Prof William Boericke of the sixth edition of Hahnemann's *Organon der rationellen Heilkunde,* originally published in the USA in 1921 under the title *Organon of Medicine,* reprinted New Delhi: B Jain Publishers, 1972.

Abbreviations, Symbols, Weights and Measures

List of abbreviations and symbols used in homoeopathy and very sparingly in this dictionary:

> greater than; whence; decrease; better; amelioration
< less than; derived from; increase; worse; aggravation
= equal to; causes
Rt right
Lt left
Θ (theta) mother tincture
TM tinctura mater; mother tincture; Θ
soln solution
tinct mother tincture; Θ
trit trituration
glob globuli; granules in UK
gran granuli; pillules in UK
pulv powder
liq liquidum; liquid
x decimal potency in UK and USA; microsc. magnification
C centesimal potency; c in UK and USA; Celsius (temp.)
c centesimal potency in UK and USA
CM hundredth millesimal potency, principally in UK & USA
D decimal potency; x in UK and USA
F female; Fahrenheit (temp.)
H prepared by Hahnemannian method of potentization
K prepared by Korsakovian potentization method; Kelvin
LM quinquagenimillesimal potentization scale; 50-milles
M male; millesimal potency, principally in UK and USA
MM thousandth millesimal potency, mostly in UK and USA

Other more general abbreviations and symbols that occasionally are also used in homoeopathy:

+ plus; excess; positive; acidic (acid solution)
− minus; deficiency; negative; alkaline (base solution)
+/− indefinite; approximately
: ratio; 'is to'
:: equality between ratios; 'as'

% per cent
ca. circa; about
& and; also
et al. et alii; and others
bp boiling point
cf conferes; compare
cm centimetre
pd per day
dil dilutio; dilution
excip excipientes; more or less inert vehicle (e.g. syrup)
e.g. exempli gratia; for example
ext extract
fp freezing point
g gram
hr hour
ibid. in the same place; reference from same book or source
ic intracutaneous(ly)
i.e. id est; that is
ir infrared
IU international unit
im intramuscular(ly)
iv intravenous(ly)
k- kilo-; 10^3
l litre
loc. cit. loco citato; in the place cited
max maximum
mo month
mp melting point
m metre
ml millilitre; cubic centimetre; cm^3
mm millimetre
min minute; minimum
NMR nuclear magnetic resonance
op. cit. opere citato; in the work cited
p, pp page, pages
ppm parts per million
qv quod vide; which see
ref refer; reference
s second (time)
sat saturate(d)
sp specific
sg relative density; specific gravity
std standard
sc subcutaneous(ly)
temp temperature

uv ultraviolet
viz. videlicet; namely
vol volume
v/v volume for volume
wk week
wt weight
w/w weight for weight
w/v weight per volume
yr year

Weights and measures in this dictionary and, indeed, in most homoeopathic pharmacies, are generally given in SI Units, i.e. in the agreed nomenclature for metric units of the Système International d'Unites established in 1960. However, when older works are referred to as well, it may help to be reminded that, as an approximation:

1g = 15 grains
4g = 1 drachm
1ml = 15 minims
3.5ml = 1 fl drachm
30ml = 1 fl ounce

Here is a legend for a few other abbreviations occasionally used in this dictionary:

AIH American Institute of Homoeopathy
AMA American Medical Association
CSFR Czechoslovakian Federated Republic
FRG Federal Republic of Germany (West Germany 1945-1990)
GDR German Democratic Republic (East Germany 1945-1990)
RSA Republic of South Africa
UK United Kingdom of Great Britain and Northern Ireland
US(A) United States (of America)
USSR Union of Soviet Socialist Republics
WHO World Health Organization

'The perfecting of our science in this new century is becoming an increasingly sad and gloomy business; without professional liberality and friendliness it will continue to be a science for bunglers for another full century.'

Samuel Hahnemann, 1801, in *View of Professional Liberality at the Commencement of the Nineteenth Century.*

A

Absolute Alcohol

See 'Alcohol'.

Actinotherapy

A naturopathic form of treatment, complementary to homoeopathy, in which light, infra-red, ultra-violet and soft-laser irradiation, as well as radiant heat, are used therapeutically. Cryotherapy, the use of cold in the treatment of disease, belongs here too.

Active Ingredients

Any starting material intended to furnish pharmacological activity in a particular medicine. As homoeopathy proves whole substances, any of these becomes the active ingredient of any of its medicines.

Active Poison

A substance which tends to destroy the living organism, into which it is introduced in ponderal doses.

Active Principle

The potent constituent of a drug.

Acupressure

See 'Acupuncture'.

Acupuncture

● **Treatment where needles are stuck into selected points on the body, sometimes used along with homoeopathy.**

Literally means 'needle-puncture'. It is a method of treating disease, which forms part of the larger system of Oriental Medicine. Thin needles are inserted into the body at specific points, or such points may be stimulated in some other way, thereby affecting the flow of energy that travels round pathways (meridians) in the body. The first written reference to acupuncture that has been found is from 580BC, but many people believe it to be up to 4000 years older than that. This therapy has been found useful by many patients and practitioners when combined with homoeopathy. In fact, under the name 'homoeosiniatry' a hybrid therapy has emerged,[1] in which potentized single remedies are injected intra-dermally at particular acupuncture points for the purpose of enhancing the therapeutic effect (though acupuncture certainly does not recognize Hering's rule nor homoeopathic aggravations). Not all homoeopaths regard acupuncture as a complementary form of therapy, though most seem to. Variations on acupuncture are: acupressure, shiatsu, do-in, soft-laser therapy, reflexology and cupping, where pressure, suction or some other stimulus is applied to the points or meridians. In vol.LXIII no.1, January, 1975 of the *British Homoeopathic Journal* the homoeopath E C Ogden published a paper showing, in some detail, that acupuncture can work harmoniously side by side with homoeopathy. An introduction to the subject of linking the two disciplines is the book *Bioenergetic Medicines: East and West – Acupuncture and Homoeopathy* by Clark A Manning and Louis J Vanrenen (Berkeley, Ca: North Atlantic Books, 1988, 269 pages).

(See also 'Auriculomedicine' and 'Bio-Electronic Regulatory Medicine'.)

Acute Miasma

See 'Miasma'.

Adaptiveness

Individual capacity for appropriate change in the face of alteration in environmental stresses. In homoeopathy the dynamis is often seen to be subject to pressure toward change, in a constructive or formative sense. To the degree that it is able to respond, within constitutional limits and despite other burdens, it is said to have adaptiveness.[2] (See 'Constitutional Type', 'Dynamis', 'Epistemological Assumptions in Homoeopathy' section 4, 'Homoeopathic Laws, Postulates and Precepts', particularly 12, 13 and 15, 'Lamarckism' and 'Miasma'.)

Adeps Lanae

Refined wool-fat (obtained from the wool of the sheep Ovies aries) or anhydrous lanolin; a yellowish-white ointment basis prepared from refined wool-fat 7 and aqua destillata 3, that is partly soluble in alcohol. It is not readily absorbed by the skin, but when mixed with a vegetable oil or Paraffinum mollum flavum (or album), absorption is more rapid and the stickiness greatly

[1] Caba, Theodor, and Marius T. Caba. *Homeosinitria,* Bucharest: Editura Litera, 1983, 508 pages.
[2] Kent, J T. *Lectures on Homoeopathic Philosophy.* Chicago: Ehrhart & Karl, American 'Memorial' Edition of 1929, republished in Calcutta: Roy Publishing House, 1968, p 146.

reduced. Such a mixture can, in turn, be mixed with considerable proportions of aqueous mother tinctures, forming water-in-oil emulsions, the Adeps lanae serving as the emulsifying agent. (See 'Externally Applied Homoeopathic Drugs', 'Ointment' and 'Vehicle'.)

Adolescence, Homoeopathic Remedies During

Adolescence refers to the period in a young person's life around the attainment of complete growth and maturity. Certain disease conditions occur more frequently during that period than at other periods (e.g. acne vulgaris). Donald Foubister in *Tutorials on Homoeopathy* (Beaconsfield: Beaconsfield Publishers Ltd, 1989) devotes chapters 6 to 11 [pp 45-90] to 'Homoeopathy and Paediatrics', where he provides much detailed and valuable advice.

Aetiology

Homoeopathy is often incorrectly described as being a symptomatic and not a causal therapy, since its conception of aetiology differs from that of most other medical philosophies. Homoeopathy, quite on the contrary, regards its approach as truly aetiological. Where its treatment is able to remove the susceptibility to infection, compared with a treatment that applies merely to the pathogen, or when loss of hair due to introspective grieving is cured with the corresponding 'sad and fretful' Muriaticum acidum, rather than by attempts at using any specific hair treatment, such homoeopathic approaches to the problems are more profoundly aetiological than the contraposed treatments.

Aetiotropism

Neologism describing a homoeopathic feature of medicines as these are used on the basis of circumstantial causation, or of particular events, such as the use of Thuja occidentalis in a variety of ailments brought on by the sudden appearance of papulo-vesicular pustules during a past episode of shingles, or the use of Arnica montana in the case of constant headaches since falling from the branch of a tree and having been concussed. (See 'Disease and Drug Action in Homoeopathic Congruity' particularly section 2, 'Drainage', 'Organotropism' and 'Pathotropism'.)

Aggravation

● **Means a worsening and, in homoeopathy, can be seen either as bad organic reaction to a crude chemical substance, or as the signal that the patient is reacting to a homoeopathic medicine, which makes him/her a little worse before very probably improving.**

Chemical Aggravation

Crude substance (undynamized medicine) prescribed according to the law of similars is capable of producing considerable aggravation of the patient's symptoms (see 'Bran', as an instance). Decreasing the chemical quantity present in the dose lessens this form of aggravation but does not diminish the curative effect of the medicine.

Homoeopathic Aggravation

This is the healing 'crisis', which is a slight intensification of the symptoms, brought on because the homoeopathic remedy causes the patient dynamis to react. Though essentially the product of the deep-acting constitutional remedies, it occasionally appears in treatment with 'pathological' remedies (chosen for their more superficial or peripheral reactions, rather than for their deeper actions, which they certainly also possess). It frequently occurs 10 to 14 days after the commencement of constitutional treatment and usually lasts from 2 to 8 days, after which it abates. A homoeopathic aggravation is rare with a pathological remedy. When it does appear it is usually due to too frequent a repetition for too great a period. On such occasions it is of a minor nature and rapidly subsides when the remedy is stopped.

The healing crisis is a beneficial sign, because it heralds the fact that the patient is being taken in the direction of cure. In instances where it would be undesirable to induce such a crisis (in the very old; where a vital organ is grossly diseased; in emergencies; in severe nutritional deficiencies; in those close to death, or in constant great pain) the pathological remedies are substituted in treatment.

Non-interference with the homoeopathic action of the medicine is the rule here, allowing the aggravation to subside and improvement to start. (See 'Constitutional Type' and 'Pathological Remedy'.)

'Aggravation' & 'Amelioration' in Materia Medica

These are contributory signs employed in therapeutics, known as modalities, which feature in Materia Medica, indicating the circumstance(s) making symptoms worse ($<$ = aggravation) or better ($>$ = amelioration). (See 'Aversions and Desires' and 'Disease and Drug Action in Homoeopathic Congruity', particularly section 3.)

Alcohol

● **Is used in homoeopathy, mixed with different amounts of water, (1) to carry or hold medicines, (2) to thin them down, and/or (3) just to ensure that the medicines will keep.**

Ethanol – C_2H_5OH

This reacts with acids to form esters and with alkali metals to form alcoholates. It is used in homoeopathy as a vehicle, as a solvent and as a preservative, relative to internal medicines, and as a rubefacient and disinfectant, externally.

Absolute Alcohol

Anhydrous alcohol, theoretically 100% alcohol. In practice it is dehydrated alcohol, with a minimal admixture of water, at most 1%. Its specific gravity is 0.792.

Alcohol Fortis

Strong alcohol, the alcohol that is used in homoeopathy to make mother tinctures, or to impregnate solid particles medicinally, because it is quick-drying. It is a water-ethanol mixture in the following proportions:

in the USA: water 7.7% and ethanol 92.3% by weight,

which corresponds to

water 5.1% and ethanol 94.9% by volume,

at 15.56 degrees Celsius;

in the UK: water from minimum 7.3% to maximum 8% and ethanol from minimum 92.0% to maximum 92.7% by weight,

which corresponds to

water from minimum 4.8% to maximum 5.3% and ethanol from minimum 94.7% to maximum 95.2% by volume,

at 15.56 degrees Celsius.

In both countries it is casually referred to as '95% v/v alcohol'. Its specific gravity is 0.816.

Dilute Alcohol

In non-homoeopathic pharmacy eight concentrations of dilute alcohol are officially recognized in the UK alone: namely 20, 25, 45, 50, 60, 70, 80 and 90 per cent v/v; and an additional one is official in the USA: namely 48.6% v/v. Yet none of these are the most frequently used dilute alcohol of homoeopathy, which is 30% of ethanol, by volume, to 70% of distilled water. This is used to prepare the final liquid vehicle of the medicine to be administered, as a liquid, say, in drops, to the patient. Its specific gravity is 0.083.

Alcohol Fortis

See 'Alcohol'.

Alexander Technique

A disciplined educational approach, originated by F M Alexander in Tasmania, Australia in the 1920s, aiming to re-create correct postural alignment, thus promoting awareness of balance, posture and movement in normal human activity. By bringing into consciousness previously unnoticed tensions, and by allowing differentiation between appropriate and unnecessary effort and tensions, natural posture is regained. This para-therapeutic approach is complementary to homoeopathy.

Alkaloid

● **A chemical that is part of the make-up of many mother tinctures, or base preparations, which in itself is not usually of great interest to homoeopathy, but is to non-homoeopathic pharmacy.**

Heterocyclic nitrogen-containing plant products that are normal constituents of many homoeopathic mother tinctures. Although they usually contribute only a small part to the overall drug pictures, they have engaged the attention of orthodox pharmacologists who extract them from mother tinctures and use the salts of some alkaloids, and other constituents, as the active principle in certain allopathic, or palliative, medicines, sometimes achieving over-abundant effects. Many examples of this exist (although the following list is not exhaustive, since only the more commonly extracted alkaloids, used by orthodox pharmacy, are shown):

Homoeopathic Drug	Allopathic Alkaloidal Extract
Aconitum napellus	Aconitine
Anhaionium lewinii	Mescaline
Aristolochia clematis	Clematine
Aristolochia serpentaria	Serpentarine
Aspidosperma quebracho	Aspidospermine, Quebrachnine
Astragalus menziesii	Swainsonine
Barosma crenulata (Buchu)	Barosmine
(Atropa) Belladonna	Atropine
Berberis aquifolium	Herbamine, Oxyacanthine, Berberine
Balao fragrans	Boldine
Bryonia alba	Bryonine
Chelidonium majus	Sanguinarine, Chelerythrin, Protopine and Chelidonine
Cicuta virosa	Cicutine
Cinchona officinalis	Quinine, Cichonine, Hydroquinine and Quinidine
Cineraria maritima	Pyrrolizidine
(Erythroxylon) Coca	Cocaine
Coffea cruda	Caffeine
Colchicum autumnale	Colchicine
Conium maculatum	Coniine
Corydalis formosa	Bulbocapnine
Ephedra equisetina	Ephedrine, Nor-ephedrine and Methyl Ephedrine

Euphorbia pilulifera	Homonojirimycine
Gelsemium sempervirens	Sempervirine, Gelsemine
Gentiana lutea	Gentianine
Hydrastis canadensis	Umbellatine, Canadine, Hydrastine
Hyoscyamus niger	Hyoscyamine, Scopalamine, Hyoscine
Ignatia amara	Brucine and Strychnine
(Cephaelis) Ipecacuanha	Emetine
(Cystus) Laburnum	Cytisine
Lobelia inflata	Lobinaline, Isolobinine, Lobeline and Lobelandine
Nux vomica	Strychnine, Vomicine
Oxytropis lamberti	Swainsonine
Opium (Papaver somniferum)	Papaverine and Morphine
Paullinia sorbilis	Guaranine
Petasites offcinalis	Petasine
Physostigma	Eserine and Physostigmine
Pilocarpus microphyllus	Pilocarpine
Rauwolfia Serpentina	Reserpine
Sabadilla	Veratrine
Sanguinaria canadensis	Protopine and Sanguinarine
Sarothamnus scoparius (Cystisus scoparius, Spartium scoparium)	Sparteine, Scoparoside and Tyramine
Sarsaparilla	used as a vehicle for bitter alkaloidal salts, to make these palatable to children; it contains sterols and steroidal saponins
Senecio jacobaea	Pyrrolizidine
Strophanthus hispidus	Strophanthin
Symphytum officinale	Pyrrolizidine
Tabacum	Nicotine
Thea sinensis	Theine
Thuja lobbi & occidentalis	Thujaplicines Alpha, Beta and Gamma
Tussilago farfara & petasites	Pyrrolizidine

Quite a number of these alkaloids have returned to homoeopathy, however. Pathogenetic experiments have been conducted with many of them, so that they now have their own distinct symptomatologies alongside the parent homoeopathic drug. The most complete current listing of homoeopathically proven alkaloids is to be found (with other drugs) in the Addendum to the Homoeopathic Pharmacopoeia of the United States.

An alkaloid, as a small molecule in which nitrogen occurs as part of an identifiable ring structure, may become an important indicator for plant chemists using chemical methods to assist botanists in classifying and naming plants, somewhat like human blood-typing is used to point to the probability of paternity. (See 'Isopathy', section on Sarcodes of Plant Origin.)

Allen, Henry C (1837-1909)

A Canadian homoeopath, writer and researcher, who spent a great deal of time in the USA. He was born in Nilestown, near London, Ontario where he completed his schooling. His medical education was acquired at the Cleveland Homoeopathic College in Ohio, where he graduated in 1861, and later from the College of Physicians and Surgeons of Canada. He joined the Union Army in the US Civil War, serving as surgeon under General Grant. After the war he was offered the professorship in Anatomy at the Cleveland Homoeopathic College. Later he resigned and accepted the same chair in the Hahnemann Medical College of Chicago. In 1868 he was offered the chair of Surgery there, but declined this. From 1880 to 1890 he was professor of Materia Medica at the University of Michigan, while living in Ann Arbour with his wife and two children. Together with Dr Swan, in 1880, he described the original drug test of the nosode Luesinum (Syphilinum, Lueticum), the proving of which was conducted with potentized secretions from syphilitic chancres containing Treponema Pallidum spirochaeta. His contribution to miasmatics was, that, through clinical experience, he had come to maintain that typhoid fever had its origin in the tuberculinic miasma. He was owner and editor of the 'Medical Advance' for many years. His major writings include:

Keynotes of Leading Remedies – this was for a long time on the 'Council List of Books' for use in Canadian Medical Colleges

Boenninghausen's Slip Repertory – the official revision

Materia Medica of the Nosodes

The Homoeopathic Therapeutics of Intermittent Fever

The Homoeopathic Therapeutics of Fevers.

He should not be confused with two other North American homoeopaths:

1) John Henry Allen, who was professor of Diseases of the Skin and Miasmatics, at the Hering Medical College, Illinois and author of *Diseases and Therapeutics of the Skin* and *The Chronic Miasms* (two volumes); and

2) Timothy Field Allen, (1837-1902) (see entry.)

(See also 'Isopathy', section on History of Isopathy.)

Allen, John Henry

See the reference to him under his namesake 'Allen, Henry C (1836-1909)'.

Allen, Timothy Field (1837-1902)

Best known for compiling the monumental homoeopathic reference work that became the profession's standard, *The Encyclopedia of Pure Materia Medica* (circa 8000 pages, in 12 volumes). The reference to 'Pure' materia medica means it is derived from provings (pathogenetic experiments) only, without an admixture derived from clinical usage. This eminent US homoeopath was born in Westminster, Vermont, the son of a physician. He was also known as an organist and composer. He was in homoeopathic practice in Brooklyn, New York. In 1867 he became professor of Anatomy at the New York Homoeopathic Medical College. Four years later (1871) he was made professor of Therapeutics and Materia Medica. Simultaneously he worked as co-editor of the prestigious *New York Journal of Homoeopathy*. In 1870 the New York State legislature appropriated $150 000 toward the construction of a Homoeopathic Insane Asylum in Middletown, New York. Dr Timothy F Allen became director of this institution, which, for decades, then remained the centre of research and treatment of mental disease according to scientific homoeopathic principles. Dr Timothy F Allen's major writings include:

The Encyclopedia of Pure Materia Medica: a Record of the Positive Effects of Drugs Upon the Healthy Organism (1874/79)

Ophthalmic Therapeutics (1876)

The Effects of Lead on Healthy Individuals (1878)

A General Symptom Register of Homoeopathic Materia Medica (1880)

Boenninghausen's Therapeutic Pocket Book – an English adaptation (1886)

A Handbook of Materia Medica and Homoeopathic Therapeutics (1889).

He should not be confused with either of the other two North American homoeopaths, with the surname Allen, both given under the entry for 'Allen, Henry C, (1836-1909)'.

Allergy

- **A strong reaction by the body against something in the air, in the food, in drink, or in anything else with which it may come in contact, or which may even be within itself. Homoeopathy can help to lessen, and sometimes to remove, this tendency to react too strongly.**

A pronounced reaction by an individual organism to one or several environmental constituents manifested as nettlerash, hayfever, bronchial asthma, angioneurotic oedema, blepharitis, eczema, migraine, pompholyx, uveitis, perennial rhinitis, anaphylaxis, gastro-intestinal symptoms, or one of many other non-specific conditions, or in the form of an auto-immune syndrome. Often a familial or miasmatic pattern can be discerned.

Most homoeopaths cannot identify with the assertion regularly made by followers of the various non-homoeopathic medical disciplines, that allergic symptoms are simply the end-effect of a disordered and/or overactive immune system. As an example, the mainstream of orthodox medicine has maintained for the past sixty years or so that the immune system in a so-called classic allergic response reacts against protein substances which for the most part are taken to be intrinsically harmless. Such a view implies that what distinguishes these proteins from other antigens would, of necessity, only be a question of faulty biochemical and biological processes in the host organism. By contrast, the homoeopathic concept is that the fault lies not in the dynamic response by the affected living organism, but instead that allergens themselves have a direct effect, resembling in a sense toxic action (except that these are custom-designed) on those who are constitutionally receptive. (See also 'Constitutional Type' and 'Epistemological Assumptions in Homoeopathy', section 4.)

Why would the plant kingdom, for one, not wish to defend itself, or be pre-emptively aggressive, by means of the weapons with which it is so abundantly endowed (like lectins, gliotoxins, alkaloids, etc.)? The question of how assimilation (homoeosis) has made some individuals response-free to a number of these weapons is discussed under 'Foods as Health Problems' and 'Homoeosis'. (See also 'Alkaloids'.)

In the non-homoeopathic conception of allergy it remains unclear where the exact demarcation lies between allergy and an individual's dynamic response. The following may serve to elucidate this problem a little.

It is known since the time of Hippocrates that a rarely reversible neurological disorder, now labelled neurolathyrism (a paralysis of the lower limbs affecting some individuals, predominantly males, under 30 years of age), can be brought on in many, but not in all, who consume a type of chickpea. The homoeopathic materia medica features this particular dynamic response prominently under the entry for that chickpea, viz. Lathyrus sativus. It is clear that the plant exerts a neurotoxic effect on many, but certainly not on all, who consume it. Does this mean neurolathyrism should be referred to as an allergy? Or is it really an individual's dynamic response that is severe only to the extent of that exposed individual's receptivity to disease? (See 'Altered Receptivity in Disease'.)

What of wheat, rye, oats and barley, which induce idiopathic steatorrhoea (morbus coeliacus) in some but not in most people? (See 'Bran'.)

Should one call ovine facial eczema – that appears on some sheep (but not on others of the same stock and in the same herd) from exposure to the spores of the fungus Pithomyces chartarum that grows on grass in wet climates – an allergy or is it simply the dynamic idiosyncratic response seen sporadically in one or other sheep to a 'Pithomycean weapon', the fungal toxin (spordesmin), to which the affected sheep have not yet undergone homoeotic adaptation? (See 'Idiosyncrasy'.)

Homoeopathy dismisses the idea of a faulty dynamic response, since that conflicts with its philosophical tenets based on vitalism. It prefers to view it as an *idiosyncratic* dynamic response of the homoeotically non-adapted. (See 'Vitalism'.)

For the majority of homoeopaths the triad of treatment of what are generally termed as allergies consists in:

1 administering the potentized known antigen, or an appropriate nosode (see 'Isopathy');
2 allergen exclusion, whenever possible (see 'Foods as Health Problems' and 'Nutritional Equipoise'); and, most important of all,
3 prescribing a homoeopathically well-indicated constitutional remedy (see 'Constitutional Type'). The patient's idiosyncratic hypersensitivity is most significant in guiding the homoeopath to the choice of a matching medicine. (See 'Individualization'.)

There are those homoeopaths, however, who begin with a pathotropic approach, realizing that the patient who may be suffering from, say, seasonal hayfever will first want relief and a permanent cure later. In such event, s/he will select a pathological remedy, along the lines indicated in the few examples given, for some outstanding pathology (in certain hayfever sufferers) he may wish to target.

Example (in hayfever cases):

Homoeopathic Medicine	Pathology to be Relieved
Aranea tela	Nervous asthma & sleeplessness;
Arundo mauritanica	Itching in nostrils, roof of mouth, Eustachian tubes and ears, sneezing;
Euphrasia officinalis	Allergic conjunctivitis;
Histaminum hydrochloricum	Allergic myalgia and skin/mucous membrane irritations;
Phaseolus nana	Angst, frontal headaches, dilated pupils without photophobia and rapid pulse;
Sabadilla	Sneezing bouts with all the classical hayfever symptoms;
Sambucus nigra	Oppressed chest, hoarseness and suffocative coughing spells;
Sanguinaria canadensis	Burning eyes, nose and throat, watery discharge from nose, tickling cough;
Teucrium marum	Eyelids red and puffy, ringing otalgia, mucous polyps, coryza with blocked nostrils, lachrymation and sneezing attacks.

Experimental Evidence

Two separate, statistically significant, controlled studies conducted in the United Kingdom were published. One involved the effects of dynamized house dust mite on the corresponding mite sensitivity, with attempts at allergen exclusion, accompanied by the constitutional homoeopathic remedy. This experiment extended over seven years and was published in July, 1980. Treated with a potency of house dust mite 200 79.6% of adults and 85.2% of children experienced clinical improvement which was maintained at follow-ups.[1] The other was a double blind, placebo-controlled design, comparing a 30C potency of mixed grass pollens with a look-alike placebo. This experiment, published in April, 1985, showed that whereas 82% of patients were helped by the treatment to achieve a significant decrease in symptoms, only 36% experienced

[1]Gibson, Robin G, and Sheila L M Gibson. 'A New Aspect of Psora – The Recognition and Treatment of House Dust Mite Allergy.' Department of Clinical Pharmacognosy, Glasgow Homoeopathic Hospital. *The British Homoeopathic Journal*, vol.LXIX, no.3, July, 1980.

a relative decrease on the placebo.[1] [Some homoeopaths question whether these can truly be referred to as experiments in homoeopathy, since the possibility of individualization is compromised in them.]

(See also 'Auto-Immune Syndrome', 'Detoxication' and 'Migraine'.)

Allopathy

● **A term, loosely, and not always correctly, applied to the practice of mainstream (orthodox) medicine.**

A therapeutic system, occasionally also known as auxotherapy,[1] in which disease is treated by producing a morbid reaction of another kind or in another part, the prime intention of which is to suppress symptoms. The term is composed of the Greek words 'other (auxiliary) suffering' and, according to *The Shorter Oxford English Dictionary*,[2] was coined by Hahnemann as a label for the dominant medical tradition of his time. He referred to it, for example, in footnote 12 to section 22 of the *Organon* and elsewhere on many occasions. Examples in more recent times of the application of this principle are electroconvulsive therapy, or insulin shock treatment, each used as treatment of mental disorders in which convulsions are produced; or the treatment of syphilitic or other infections by inoculation with malarial organisms; or the injection of a strong solution of silver nitrate early in the course of gonorrhoea in order to excite non-specific inflammation, are all procedures that employ the principle of allopathy. Hahnemann describes the allopathic method as the third possible mode of employing medicines. The other two are:

1 the homoeopathic method, in which medicines are administered which yield symptoms similar to those of the diseased state; and
2 the antipathic, or enantiopathic, or palliative, method, in which symptoms are confronted with their opposites in order to suppress them (section 23 of the *Organon of Medicine*).

(Hahnemann vacillated whether or not to recognize the isopathic method as another true mode of employing medicines. See 'Isopathy' for details.)

In the note referred to above (in the *Organon of Medicine*) Hahnemann says: 'The other possible mode of employing medicines for disease besides these two is the allopathic method, in which medicines are given, whose symptoms have no direct pathological relation to the morbid state, neither similar nor opposite, but quite heterogeneous to the symptoms of the disease. This procedure plays,

---

[1] Reilly, David Taylor, MRCP, MRCGP, Medical Registrar and Morag Anne Taylor, B.Sc.(Hons), Honorary Researcher, Glasgow Homoeopathic Hospital. 'Potent Placebo or Potency?' *The British Homoeopathic Journal*, vol.LXXIV no.2, April, 1985.
[2] *Stedman's Medical Dictionary*, XXIInd edition, Baltimore, Maryland: The Williams & Wilkins Co, 1973, p 132.
[3] *The Shorter Oxford English Dictionary*, third edition, 2 vols, vol I, p 46.

as I have shown elsewhere, an irresponsible murderous game with the life of the patient by means of dangerous, violent medicines, whose action is unknown and which are chosen on mere conjectures.' It may well have been that the heteronomous use of medicines whose action is unknown, alongside those having a contrary or palliative effect, by non-homoeopathic medical practitioners, has led to the erroneous but generally accepted blanket description of the methods employed by all such practitioners as 'allopathic'. Examples of procedures that employ a purgative for constipation, a hypnotic for insomnia, an anti-pyretic for fever, an analgesic for pain, a tranquilizer for agitation, or examples of categories of drugs labelled as 'metabolic antagonists', or as 'blocking agents', or as 'antibiotics', are not really allopathic at all, despite having been quoted as such countless times in homoeopathic literature. As all these follow the antagonistic mode of action, propounded as 'contraria contrariis curantur', in terms of their primary drug symptoms, they should correctly be described as antipathic, enantiopathic or palliative procedures. Hahnemann speaks of just such procedures in section 23 of the *Organon of Medicine*, where he says: 'All pure experience . . . and all accurate research convince us that persistent symptoms of disease are far from removed and annihilated by opposite symptoms of medicine (as in the antipathic, enantiopathic or palliative method), that, on the contrary, after transient, apparent alleviation, they break forth again, only with increased intensity, and become manifestly aggravated.' He appends, as an afterthought, in section 53: '. . . although the ordinary physician is in the habit of giving his patient another explanation of this subsequent aggravation.'

Current usage of the phrase has come to describe the non-homoeopathic practice of mainstream medicine as 'allopathic medicine', implying, as it [inaccurately] does, the prescribing of direct opposites in all cases. This is firmly entrenched and is the more unfortunate because it is inaccurate from the point of view of orthodox medicine as well, since by no definition are either the correcting of biochemical or physiological changes, or the replacing of missing substances (e.g. in iron deficiency), or the balancing of defective systems (e.g. a short-term physiological dose of Digitalis in congestive heart failure), or certain other compensation procedures (e.g. immunostimulation), that are all in standard medical use today, to be described as allopathic. Some homoeopaths include enantiopathic and/or allopathic medical procedures in their practices, claiming these to be complementary to homoeopathy. This is an obvious contradiction in terms. (See 'Auto-Immune Syndrome', 'Detoxication', 'Drainage', 'Homoeopathized Allopathica', 'Homoeopathy', 'Isopathy', 'Miasma' and 'Phytotherapy'.)

Almond Oil

See 'Oleum Amygdalae'.

Altered Receptivity in Disease

Refers to the exquisite responsiveness (sensitivity), that always arises in disease states from a latent pre-existing constitutional or acquired susceptibility, to homoeopathically indicated medicinal agents; the greater the homoeopathicity, the more pronounced the receptivity. For a brief description of how this concept was developed, and by whom, as well as of the relevant experimental evidence, refer to the final paragraph of the entry under 'Isopathy'. (See also 'Allergy', 'Aversions and Desires', 'Constitutional Type', section on Experimental Evidence, 'Heterostasis', 'Homoeopathic Laws, Postulates and Precepts', section 5, 'Homoeopathy' and 'Homoeosis'.)

Amelioration

● **Means a betterment.**

See 'Aggravation' and 'Disease and Drug Action in Congruity', particularly section 3. The subject of assessing and interpreting the homoeopathic aggravation and amelioration is discussed in some depth by George Vithoulkas in *The Science of Homoeopathy* (Wellingborough: Thorsons Publishing Group, 1986) particularly on pages 227 to 232.

Anamnesis

The history of a patient; that which is noted down about a patient during case-taking. Hence, 'anamnestic' – relating to this.

Anaphylaxis

Anaphylactic shock; see 'Allergy' and 'Emergencies – Homoeopathic Treatment'.

Anhydrous

A term applied to a substance when it is absolutely free from water. Some homoeopaths maintain that all homoeopathic medicines must carry some water content to enable any of them to carry the pharmacological message (see 'Physiological Response in Homoeotherapeutics, Mechanism of' and 'Solvation Structures').

Animal Experiments

These are not used in the pathogenetic experiments (proving) of homoeopathic medicines, which are carried out on healthy, symptom-free volunteers. In fact, homoeopathy, rooted in medicine's Empirical tradition, should have no requirement to conduct any experiments on animals with the specific intention to explore certain questions. Frequently such questions concern either non-homoeopathic disease classification, or are designed to address problems that really belong into ancillary (usually biological) sciences. In France, however, a good deal of so-called 'humane' experimentation on homoeopathic topics has been conducted on animals in recent times, some of which is referred to in this text, although such investigative techniques have been condemned as reprehensible by a minority of homoeopaths, some of whom describe the mind-set behind such experimental work as 'rank speciesism'. Their argument is that the experimenters are ambivalent about animals. On the one hand, the experimenters justify using animals as models for human physiology or disease on the basis of evolutionary kinship or genealogical continuity.

They do so on the evidence that humans share certain features with other species. (Two examples in homoeopathic experimentation are: the Alloxan experiments on mice of 1965 and 1967; and the carbon tetrachloride/phosphorus experiments on rats of 1975; to be found under 'Potency'.) Yet on the other hand, their moral justification for using animals (and not humans) clearly assumes a discontinuity between humans and animals. Experimenters subject animals to their experiments because they deem it unethical to use humans. Therefore, humans are somehow different in this part of their justification.

As long ago as 1861[1] Eugène Curie (the father of Pierre Curie of Radium fame) undertook experiments on animals in the cause of homoeopathy. He chose domestic cats for his experiments because these animals are the least liable to tuberculosis. He found that prolonged use of Drosera rotundifolia in ponderal doses induced tuberculinization in these cats, making 'its use in tuberculous affections absolutely scientific' (in Margaret L Tyler's words [2] – while she momentarily turned a blind eye both to homoeopathy's symptomatology/pathology dispute and to its general antivivisection stance).

Treatment given to animals by veterinary homoeopaths provides an important regular flow of data on drug actions, which is scientifically objective since the therapeutic component contributed by the practitioner, the 'suggestive element', is virtually nonexistent in veterinary homoeopathy. (See also 'Clinical Trials' and 'Veterinary Homoeopathy'.)

Antacid

Homoeopathy discourages the indiscriminate taking of the heavily advertised antacids. Many bacteria (e.g. Brucella melitensis) are highly susceptible to stomach acids by which they are inactivated. Studies have shown that travellers with antacid-induced hypoacidity contracted certain conditions from

[1]Curie, Eugène. 'Recherches Expérimentales sur Drosera', *Bull. de la Soc. Med. Hom. de Paris*, November 1861 [translation of his article as 'Experimental Researches on Drosera' appeared in the *British Journal of Homoeopathy*, vol XX, p 39].
[2]Tyler, Margaret L. *Drosera*, London: John Bale, Sons & Danielsson Ltd, 1927, pp 3 and 4.

unwittingly consuming unpasteurized dairy produce, whereas fellow travellers with normal stomach acid levels did not. The sodium bicarbonate component of antacids may lead to stone formation in the urinary tract, while magnesium can produce circulatory collapse in some cases. Homoeopathy looks for the causes (e.g. food sensitivities) and introduces dietary constraints alongside the indicated drug for the individual.

Antenatal Homoeopathy

Homoeopathic treatment during the period of gestation is described under 'Euthenic (Nosode) Treatment'. Some useful antepartum, intrapartum and immediate postpartum homoeopathic remedies are:

Arnica montana
Caulophyllum thalictroides
Cimicifuga racemosa (Macrotys, Actea racemosa)
Gelsemium sempervirens
Pulsatilla nigricans.

The guiding symptoms from the experimental pathogeneses in the materia medica, which might prompt the use of these homoeopathic remedies, are:

Arnica montana: Movement of foetus is felt painfully during gestation; soreness in genital area and in rectum with severe labour- and violent after-pains; pronounced affinity to the effects of any mechanical injuries; bleeding of both internal and external parts, as it causes (and therefore cures) haemorrhages of many kinds: including dilatation and rupture of smaller blood vessels. Indicated after prolonged exercise.

Caulophyllum thalictroides: Threatened abortion; spasmodic bearing-down; severe pain in back and loins with only feeble uterine contractions; weak labour-pains which are short, irregular, spasmodic, passing off with a shiver; patient very exhausted, irritable, fretful and apprehensive; haemorrhages; after-pains.

Cimicifuga racemosa (Macrotys, Actea racemosa): This medicine shows wide-ranging organotropism for the utero-ovarian anatomical area, particularly for both the smooth and striated musculature; it is indicated for muscular soreness from exertion; this drug also covers the majority of symptoms presenting in obstetrical procedures; the remedy's mental features in pregnant women are characterized by irritability, dejection, tendency to self-injury and apprehension of the impending parturition, followed afterwards by acute puerperal mania.

Gelsemium sempervirens: Mental confusion; great lassitude associated with total prostration and some trembling, interrupted by periods of excitation; worse from travelling; no dilatation, complete atony, inefficient labour-pains, or none at all; violent lancinating pains shooting upward and into the back; venous congestion.

Pulsatilla nigricans: During delivery the contractions of this drug are characterized by their irregularity, weakness and ineffectuality; they appear suddenly and fade gradually; the pains are erratic accompanied by a sensation of chilliness and by lachrymation; modalities that indicate this remedy: worse in a warm room; improved by movement; this drug is indicated in cases of venous congestion with varicose veins on the lower limbs and varicosities on the thorax and thighs.

Apposite reference works are:

Repertory of Pregnancy, Parturition and Puerperium by Alberto Soler-Medina (Heidelberg: Karl F Haug Verlag, 1989, 79 pages)

Homöopathie in Frauenheilkunde und Geburtshilfe by Erwin Schlüren (Heidelberg: Karl F Haug Verlag, 1980, 211 pages)

(See also 'Foubister, Donald (1902-1988)', 'Gynaecology', 'Obstetrics and Homoeopathy' and 'Pregnancy'.)

Anthropology and Homoeopathy

Anthropology, the systematic study of mankind, is divided into two sections. Physical anthropology studies man, the animal, whereas cultural anthropology is concerned with the origins and history of man's cultures, their evolution and development, and the structure and functioning of human cultures in every place and time. That also includes the homoeopathic setting in the present time, wherever it happens to be.

Anyone's perception of illness and of health is the end result of an imperceptible process of enculturation. Education, identification with a sub-culture, the adoption of a particular set of mores, customs, values and interpretations, as these pertain to health and therapeutics, provide a lifelong explanatory framework for each individual. Such frameworks, which diversely explain to individuals in different societal settings around the world how the body works and how illness is caused, are the object of study by cultural anthropology. Homoeopaths have their own scientific perception of illness and health, that is usually radically different from those held by their patients anywhere. Furthermore, in each era and in every region the linguistic idiom changes. Symptom descriptions in the homoeopathic literature vary greatly in terms of the period and the language in which they were recorded. They also vary noticeably between patients from different cultures. This idiomatic divergence increases the further apart cultures are from one another. Linguistic anthropology, a subdivision of cultural anthropology, studies the many interrelations between the language as used by a people and the other aspects of their culture, and it compares the linguistic idioms between cultures.

The observation made by H L Teuber suggests itself here:

'Language . . . provides a tool . . . in one's mind . . .Language frees us to a large extent from the tyranny of the senses . . . It gives us access to concepts that combine information from different sensory modalities and are thus intersensory or suprasensory, but the riddle remains as to how this is achieved.'[1]

Homoeopathy maintains that it is the dynamis that is the integrating force – ever central to the healing effort – through which this is done.

Cultural anthropology as it pertains to health ought to be a permanent part of any full homoeopathic educational curriculum in a shrinking multi-ethnic world, in order to produce effective homoeopaths who have a deeper understanding of the semantics in patient-practitioner communications. A text-book on the subject is *Culture, Health and Illness* by Cecil G Helman (London: Wright, 1990 [second edition], 344 pages). Astonishingly, the author placed homoeopathy under the heading 'Folk Medicine', but this does not seriously detract from the overall value of this work. (See 'Homoeopathic Ethnopharmacology', 'Homoeopathic Practice', 'Individualization' and 'Repertory'.)

Anthroposophical Medicines

● **Although these are not quite the same as homoeopathic remedies, they are very similar and, therefore, usually work quite well, although, in practice, they would be selected on the basis of conventional (non-homoeopathic) disease names.**

These medicines are sometimes prescribed as a complementary therapy by some homoeopaths, perhaps because of the similarity of their pharmaceutical production process to that for homoeopathic remedies and because Anthroposophy relies extensively upon the homoeopathic materia medica as its chief source of medicines. The Anthroposophical manufacturing pharmacy operates under the worldwide name of Weleda, which was a druid-priestess of the Celtic warrior aristocracy in Brittany. The term Anthroposophy may be rendered as 'human wisdom', or 'knowledge of the nature of man' (cf I Cor. ii. 5 and 13 – in the New Testament); it has been interpreted much more fully by Francis Treuherz (in the footnote on page 73 of the published paper given at the end of this entry) as 'the divine wisdom (Sophia) found in the knowledge of the true being of man and of his relation to the universe.'

The Anthroposophical basis for the choice of remedy is to be found in the analogy of the cosmic signatures principle, rather than in the law of similars. To prescribe Chelidonium majus in liver and biliary complaints, because the plant's yellow juice recalls bile and the shape of its leaves resembles the exact microscopic shape of liver cells, or to prescribe Cuprum metallicum (copper), the red metal, to someone with asthmatic bronchial spasms merely because the patient's astrological birth sign is ruled by Mars, the red planet, but to

Teuber, H L, 'Lacunae and Research Approaches to Them', in C H Millikan and F L Darley (editors) *Brain Mechanisms Underlying Speech and Language*, London/New York: Grune & Stratton, 1967, p 209.

switch to prescribing Stannum (tin) should his birth sign turn out to be ruled by Jupiter, cannot be considered homoeopathic prescribing. Hahnemann described the doctrine of signatures as being one of the 'suppositions of our superstitious forefathers'. Nonetheless, as Douglas M Gibson pointed out when he published his studies of 100 homoeopathic remedies in 47 instalments in the *British Homoeopathic Journal* (between 1963 and 1977), 'these parallels and correspondences (between the world of nature and symbolism) are sufficiently numerous and striking to deserve mention, as well as being an aid to the understanding and memorizing of the materia medica picture of each remedy'. Francis Treuherz presented a paper in November 1984 to the Scottish Branch of the British Faculty of Homoeopathy in Glasgow entitled 'Steiner and the Similimum – Homoeopathic and Anthroposophic Medicine: the Relationship of the Ideas of Hahnemann, Goethe and Steiner' (subsequently published by the *Journal of the American Institute of Homoeopathy*). In it he showed, *inter alia,* how the ideas of Hahnemann were taken up by Goethe, who in turn influenced Steiner to some considerable extent. (See also 'Antibiotic', footnote 4, and 'Goethe, Johann Wolfgang von (1749-1832)'.)

Antibiotic

● **The widespread use of these in lesser illness, with no thought of what other long-term harm they may do in the end, is frowned upon by homoeopaths. Homoeopathy would welcome an 'antibiotic' that could be used only against those bacteria, viruses and other germs that were associated with the patient's disease picture, since these often make a cure more difficult. At the same time, it would have to leave the patient untouched as well as her/his bacterial flora, so necessary to normal life. A little research has been done in that direction.**

The most overused drug in modern orthodox medical practice, the ill-effects of which stem largely from interference with the balance of the normal alimentary, oesophageal and/or vaginal flora. Moreover, the antibiotics, like all other allopathica, have a much broader and deeper alterative effect as extensive pathogenetic experimentations with the drugs (provings of drugs) such as chloramphenicol (chloromycetin), sodium salt of benzyl-penicillin (penicillin G) and maleate of perhexiline (Pexid) have shown.[1]

Clinical experience has established that a diseased organism's own defence mechanisms are usually adequate to cope with an external onslaught, even one of a debilitating nature, if suitable support, in the form of appropriate homoeopathic stimulation, is provided. A functiotropic homoeopathic approach may be elected by the homoeopath. This type of approach may be used for the general stimulation, say, of atopic patients, or for the prophylaxis

[1]Julian, Othon André. *Materia Medica of New Homoeopathic Remedies,* English Translation. Beaconsfield, Bucks: Beaconsfield Publishers Ltd, 1979, pp 144-150 and 399-414.

against, or treatment of, acute febrile infectious conditions (such as bronchitis with a raised temperature or influenza; not, however, of chronic progressive infections, the so-called chronic miasmata [see 'Miasma'], such as multiple sclerosis, tuberculosis, or syphilis). These acute influenza-like infections are precisely where antibiotics are so frequently used in mainstream medicine. A functiotropic homoeopathic approach, on the other hand, would be designed to bring about non-specific immune stimulation: this more particularly of

a) the defensive activities of the polymorphonuclear leukocytes (white blood cells),
b) the cells in different organs chiefly concerned with phagocytosis (the reticulo-endothelial system), and
c) the natural, selectively bactericidal and cytocidal system, occurring normally in the patient's own plasma, of euglobulins, magnesium ions and the thermolabile complement, sensitized by specific complement-fixing antibodies (the complement-properdin system). Some of the remedies that might be considered by the homoeopath for such a functiotropic approach would be:

> Argentum metallicum[1]
> Arsenicum album
> Baptisia tinctoria (low potency) *(bacillus typhosus)
> (Atropa) Belladonna *(streptococcus pyogenes)
> Bryonia alba (low potency)
> Cadmium metallicum (low potency)
> Chincona officinalis (low potency)
> Cuprum metallicum
> Echinacea angustifolia (mother tincture)
> Eupatorium perfoliatum (low potency)
> Ferrum phosphoricum (tissue salt – low potency)
> Gingko biloba (low potency)
> Hepar sulphuris calcareum *(staphylococcus aureus)
> (Trigonocephalus) Lachesis
> Phosphorus *(tubercle bacillus)
> Rajania subsamarata (low potency) *(stimulates macrophages)
> Silica[2]
> Sulfanilamide
> Thuja occidentalis (low potency)
> Veratrum viride *(pneumococcus [diplococcus pneumoniae])

[1]Anthroposophic pharmacologists have managed to produce Argentum metallicum from specific plants; it is possible to prescribe the 'natural combination remedies':
    Argentum per Thujam (sub-cutaneous injection or 1% orally) to stimulate toxic elimination;
    Argentum per Bryophyllum (sub-cutaneous injection or 1% orally) for suppurative or chronic degenerative processes;
    cf: Julian, Othon André. *op. cit.*, p 78.
[2]Davenas, Elizabeth, *et al.* 'Effect on Mouse Peritoneal Macrophages of Orally Administered Very High Dilutions of Silica', *European Journal of Pharmacology*, April 1987, vol CXXXV, pp 313-319.

*Note: The effects of these medicines in strengthening the defensive capability of the organism relative to the bacteria listed in brackets has been described below under Experimental Evidence.

Experimental Evidence

Charles Edwin Wheeler (1868-1946) developed, within the homoeopathic research context, Sir Almroth Wright's classical discoveries of opsonins.[1,2] Wheeler's pioneering work demonstrated experimentally that Arsenicum album is an almost general stimulant to phagocytosis; that Veratrum viride raises the opsonic index to the pneumococcus; Phosphorus that to the tubercle bacillus; Hepar sulphuris calcareum that to Staphylococcus aureus; (Atropa) Belladonna that to Streptococcus pyogenes and that Baptisia tinctoria increases the agglutinating power to bacillus typhosus.[1,2] (Note: Opsonin is an antibody, present in normal serum, that combines with specific antigen and sensitizes it in such a manner to prepare it for phagocytosis [see also 'Altered Receptivity in Disease']. Agglutinin is antibody causing clumping or agglutination of the bacteria or other cells, which contain immunologically similar and, therefore in terms of the law of similars, reactive material. The effects hereof may be observed in vitro and in vivo, under certain conditions.)

Antidote

● Anything, therefore also a homoeopathic medicine, that would neutralize a poison.

Chemical

A substance that will either unite with a poison to form a less harmful chemical compound, or block the absorption of a poison.

Homoeopathic

Antidoting in the bioenergetic field (dynamic antidoting) requires that the antidotal substance be pathogenically similar to the poison, but opposite in the direction of the reactive effect produced by it. The antidoting effect is exerted directly upon the organism, although it takes place indirectly between drugs by neutralization in accordance with the law of repulsion of similars (analogous to the electro-magnetic laws). Boenninghausen observed that 'medicines producing similar symptoms are related to each other and are mutually antidotal in proportion to the degree of their symptom-similarity'. This is fundamentally in line with the law of similars (see 'Homoeopathic Laws,

[1]Wheeler, Charles Edwin. *An Introduction to the Principles and Practice of Homoeopathy.* Rustington, Sussex: Health Science Press, 1971, pp 35-36.
[2]Blackie, Dame Margery Grace. *The Patient, Not The Cure.* London: Macdonald & Jane's, 1982, pp 160-161.

Postulates and Precepts'). An antidote is, therefore, a substance which, by virtue of its similarity in bioenergetic effects, neutralizes the competing substance's field of influence, cancelling its effects. This, to be sure, is precisely what constitutes cure, only achieved by means of true antidoting. It is the same principle at work in the treatment and cure of disease, as is applied to counteract the effects of poisoning. In the materia medica, where applicable, the word 'antidotes' is followed by the names of different homoeopathic drugs, which largely or even fully antidote the remedy under consideration. If such an entry exists, then the prescribing of two applicable remedies, either concurrently or sequentially, within the active period of the first remedy, is contra-indicated; if there is no antidotal relationship recorded, then such concurrent or sequential prescriptions are not likely to forfeit any medicinal effectiveness, unless the previous medicine is still acting, where there may be an attenuation of its effects. A number of homoeopaths, whilst allowing the veracity of the stated situation between two remedies, deny that this holds true for more than two remedies given concurrently, or practically so, and strenuously object to homoeopathic polypharmacy, saying that it is wrong on historical grounds and that masked inimical or antidotal effects arise in multiple-remedy mixtures (so-called 'complex homoeopathy'). All the same, clinical usage during most of the twentieth century (particularly widespread in the Netherlands, Sweden, the FRG and France) as well as confirmation of efficacy in many recent obligatory clinical trials, has convinced many homoeopaths and their patients that certain mixtures of remedies are therapeutically exceptionally effective, provided no inimical or antidotal effects are recorded between component remedies. Clinical usage has shown that Hering's rule, homoeopathic aggravations preceding ameliorations, etc. generally accompany the observed curative processes. It needs to be said that all the homoeopathic drug components of such mixtures will have had to be separately potentized before the mixing together. (See 'Combinations of Homoeopathic Drugs', 'Prescribing' and 'Usage, Clinical'.)

Antipathic Method

Homoeopathy works to strengthen the body's defences, i.e. in harmony with the symptoms, by using 'similars', but the antipathic method aims to deaden the body's symptomatic reaction by using 'opposites'. (See 'Allopathy' and 'Phytotherapy'.)

Antipraxy

See 'History of Homoeopathy before 1900', section headed United Kingdom.

Antiseptic

Disinfectant; destructive to, or a substance that destroys, the germs of putrefaction, fermentation, contagion and decomposition. Oleum cinnamomi in aqueous solution is the best local disinfectant, to be used as a douche, wherever a germicide and disinfectant is needed (including homoeopathic treatment of dental complaints). Wherever there is foetor, pain and haemorrhage (or capillary bleeding) Cinnamomum Zeylanicum (or Cinnamomum Cassia) is likely to be homoeopathically appropriate.[1] The oil's aqueous solution is prepared either:

1 by repeatedly shaking Oleum cinnamomi with 500 times its volume of water during a period of 15 minutes, setting aside for 12 hours, or overnight, and filtering; or
2 by triturating the oil with a sufficient quantity of talc, or kieselguhr, or pulped filter paper, and 500 times its volume of water, and filtering.

Apparatus

See 'Utensils of Homoeopathic Pharmacy'.

Appropriateness of Remedy and Potency

See 'Homoeopathic Practice'.

Aqua Destillata

Distilled water, one of the most important vehicles in homoeopathic pharmacy, used:

1 As a component of water-ethanol (hydro-alcoholic) mixtures;
2 In the preparation of mother tinctures of those substances that are not soluble in alcohol;
3 For potentization;
4 In the administration of medicine;
5 For rectal or vaginal douches, or enemas; and
6 In hypodermic injections.

(See 'Solvation Structures'.)

Aristotle (ca. 384–322 BC)

See 'Hahnemann, Christian Friedrich Samuel (1755-1843)' under The Rationalist Medical Tradition, 'Humoral Pathology in Prescribing' and 'Dynamis'.

---

[1]Boericke, William. *Pocket Manual of Homoeopathic Materia Medica*, ninth edition, Philadelphia, Pennsylvania: Boericke & Runyon, 1927, p 211.

Arndt-Schulz Law

See 'Homoeopathic Laws, Postulates and Precepts'.

Aromatherapy

See 'Massage Therapy'.

Associational Basis in Prescribing

Creating the link or connexion between drug and disease through the un-homoeopathic intermediacy of ideas or cultural constructs, as exemplified in the following two remedies, for neither of which a Hahnemannian proving has yet been conducted:

1) Dr James Compton Burnett (1840–1901) took Bacillinum testium, a nosode prepared from tuberculous testicle, to have a more direct relation to the lower half of the body than (pulmonary) Bacillinum, even though the former does act in pulmonary cases too, and vice versa for the latter.

2) Folliculinum, a sarcode prepared from the natural hormone folliculin (oestrone) secreted by the ovaries, is almost exclusively used in hyperfolliculoid syndromes (e.g. metropathia haemorrhagica, cystic-glandular hyperplasia of the endometrium), menstrual and menopausal complaints, or in functional hyperfolliculinia, an allergy to oestrogen (may be confirmed by Hirschberg's test), even though it has a very full, established symptomatology following an extensive clinical proving, covering the mind, digestive, circulatory, locomotor and respiratory systems, urinary and genital organs and skin, and might well be ideal for chapping eczema, juvenile acne in boys, chronic B. coli infections or other 'neuter' disease conditions.[1] The reason for this strong preference for Folliculinum as a female remedy lies undoubtedly in its name and in the association of ideas generated by it, reinforced by the large-scale experiment on hyper-oestrogenic rats (using Folliculinum in potency) conducted at Larriboisière Hospital (Paris) from 1952 to 1955 (see details in Experimental Evidence under 'Constitutional Type'). Prescribing on an associational basis is commonplace for Anthroposophical medicines, and in both Isopathy and Organotherapy (see entries under these three headings and 'Aetiotropism').

Asylums for Orphans

See 'History of Homoeopathy before 1900'.

---

[1] De Mattos, L. *Pathogenesie des Oestrogènes: Folliculinum*, Asnières: Les Laboratoires Homéopathiques de France, 1977.

Asylums for the Aged

See 'History of Homoeopathy before 1900'.

Asylums for the Insane

Homoeopathy has an excellent track record in successfully running these, after Hahnemann's unacknowledged pioneering work in psychiatry. Evidence of the fact that homoeopathy has treated psychiatric conditions from its earliest days is to be found in that paragraphs 210 to 230 of the *Organon* are devoted to this subject and also in Jahr's outstanding *Allgemeine und spezielle Therapie der Geisteskrankheiten und Seelenstörungen nach homöopathischen* (General and Specific Treatment of Mental and Emotional Disorders Based upon Homoeopathic Principles) published in 1855. (See 'Jahr, Georg Heinrich Gottlieb (1800-1875)' and 'History of Homoeopathy before 1900'.)

Duke Ernst von Sachsen-Gotha placed part of his hunting castle of Georgenthal at Hahnemann's disposal as a nursing-home for mental patients for one year from June, 1792. The reason that this asylum did not stay open for longer was the cost to the families of patients, at a time when nobody was willing to spend much money on the cure of the insane, who were regarded as an embarrassing social taint (or worse) to be kept well out of view. It was early in Hahnemann's career and his fame had not yet spread very far. Still he attracted one insane patient, the distinguished Klockenbring. As would be expected Hahnemann adopted a completely different method of treatment from the one usually applied at that time.

The cure of this famous mental patient, after many other physicians had failed, not only caused a great sensation, but gave Hahnemann's opponents an opportunity for violent attacks on account of the costs involved in his form of treatment of the insane. Nothing much is known about the remedies he employed; only once is Tartarus emeticus mentioned.

The important changes he was the first to introduce, which caused such great professional consternation and animosity, were his orders that the mental patient was not to be insulted, excited or distracted by other people and that he forbade all acts of violence and brutality then customary towards insane patients (Klockenbring still had the wheals and marks from the ropes used to beat and restrain him, when he came to the Georgenthal Asylum). Hahnemann considered the effect produced by the personality of the physician himself to be of the greatest supportive-curative importance: friendliness and humanity, combined with firmness, he prescribed as the necessary combination. He wrote, in 1796, 'The physician in charge of such unhappy people [the insane] must indeed have at his command an attitude which inspires respect but also creates confidence; he will never feel insulted by them, because a being that cannot reason is incapable of insulting anyone.' (Essay in *Lesser Writings of Samuel Hahnemann* compiled and edited by Dr Ernst Stapf, Dresden and Leipzig, 1829, vol II, pp 239- 246.) These principles established by Hahnemann were entirely new to the psychiatry of his day.

Philippe Pinel, the French psychiatrist (1745-1826), is usually credited with the abolition, at about the same time, of forcible restraint in the treatment of the lunatic, and for removing insane asylums from the prisons and workhouses in which they had previously been housed. Since there was no communication between Hahnemann and Pinel at any time, one cannot honourably pass over the former's original contributions to the advancement of psychiatric treatment methods that have since become the norm. The degree of Hahnemann's dedicated pertinacity in executing his vision for the treatment of the insane would have been immense to overcome solidly entrenched professional opposition. When Klockenbring was discharged as cured, there was no-one else to be admitted and the Georgenthal Asylum stood empty. A topical joke making the rounds among physicians was the question: 'How many mad people has Dr Hahnemann in his asylum?', with the answer: 'One, himself!'

Thereafter he treated insane people by taking them as live-in patients in his own home. There was Privy Councillor Habe of Hanover, who lived in the cramped domestic conditions of the Hahnemanns' house, alternately taking himself for Caesar, Mohammed or Alexander the Great, singing songs or reciting poetry, rousing the children's nervous curiosity, but they behaved well to the 'strange' gentleman. He, too, was cured. Hahnemann had other live-in mental patients after that, who were successfully cured. On record are such home-treatments in 1796 at Brunswick, in 1798 at Königslutter, in 1800 at Altona and Mölln in Lauenburg. Subsequently, there was the schizophrenic poet and author, Wezel, who seemed quite calm at first, but suddenly grew very violent, threatening to murder the Hahnemann family and set the house on fire. Hahnemann was only saved by the intervention of the police, alerted by a neighbour. Such were the beginnings of homoeopathic treatment of psychiatric patients. A century later homoeopathy was in the lead in psychiatric treatment. Selden Talcott, a homoeopathic psychiatrist at the 800-bed State Homoeopathic Asylum for the Insane, Middletown, New York, produced *Mental Diseases and Their Modern Treatment* [American Institute of Homoeopathy, Philadelphia and New York, Boericke and Tafel, 1900]. Of interest in this are the published State statistics covering the preceding ten year period, comparing the results of this homoeopathic asylum with three others run along orthodox medical lines. The recovery rate at Middletown upon the numbers discharged each year during the decade was about 50%; the death rate, upon the whole number treated, about 4%. In the other asylums calculations made on the same basis and for the same period show a recovery rate of less than 30% and a death rate of over 6%.(See also 'Medico-Legal'.)

Asylums for Orphans

See 'History of Homoeopathy before 1900'.

Atom

Defined as the smallest particle of an element which can take part in a chemical reaction. This turns out to be a conundrum: If this be so then homoeopathic pharmacodynamics cannot be part of a chemical reaction. Consequently, the link between homoeopathic pharmacodynamics and related physico-chemical phenomena would need to be scientifically investigated. These phenomena include ionization, intermolecular clustering, nuclear magnetic resonance and solvation structures. (See 'Experimental Research in Homoeopathy', 'Ionization', 'Physiological Response in Homoeotherapeutics, Mechanism of', 'Potency' and 'Solvation Structures'.)

Atomism

The reductionist doctrine that any phenomenon or object is no greater or less than the sum of its parts. It assumes a phenomenon is explained when it has been broken down into its constituent parts. It is contrasted with Holism, which, for instance, views systems as more than the sum of its components. (Homoeopathy's holistic approach is, *inter alia,* referred to under 'Epistemological Assumptions in Homoeopathy', section 7 and 'Totality of Signs and Symptoms'.)

Auricular Therapy

A form of acupuncture in which only points in the outer ear (auricle) are used for a more immediate but more ephemeral effect; regarded by some of the homoeopaths who view acupuncture favourably as a complementary therapy.

Auriculomedicine

Originated in France by Dr Paul F M Nogier. Regarded as a complementary form of therapy by a few of the homoeopaths who favour acupuncture; it is a system of treatment involving aspects of chromotherapy, tuina, moratherapy, a development of auricular therapy as well as some residual elements of the homoeopathic constitutional classification used in France. The centre-piece of auriculomedicine is the monitoring of the feedback response to challenges or their filtration, observable in the patient's pulse, namely the 'vascular autonomic signal' (VAS; previously called the 'auriculo-cardiac response', or ACR), which guides the practitioner in his therapy. (See also 'Acupuncture' and 'Bio-Electronic Regulatory Medicine'.)

Auto-Immune Syndrome

Chronic auto-allergy, where the organism reacts immunologically against its own tissues, cells, hormones, etc. A number of widely different disorders are grouped under this heading, such as: Chronic Thyroiditis (Hashimoto's disease); Allergic Neuritis; Uveitis; Disseminated Lupus Erythematosus; and Acquired Haemolytic Anaemia. Many of these are known to be chronic drug-induced miasmata. For example, the last-named condition may be brought on by the injurious effects of allopathic treatment with aminosalicylic acid, diphenylhydatoin, griseofulvin, mesantion, penicillin, phenacetin, quinidine, sodium taurocholate, stibophen, streptomycin or sulfamethoxypyridine.

An auto-immune syndrome is most commonly treated by homoeopaths as a miasma, because this approach has been shown to be the most successful. (See 'Allergy', 'Isopathy' and 'Miasma'.)

Auto-Isopathic

See 'Isopathy'.

Auxotherapy

See 'Allopathy'.

Aversions and Desires

As characteristics of patients they are signs which frequently point in the direction of certain modalities (amelioration or aggravation) indicative of the homoeopathicity of medicines in particular cases. That homoeopathicity will vary from patient to patient in accordance with the exquisite responsiveness (sensitivity) each one manifests.

An example is remedy individualization from food sensitivity, i.e. through aversions to, or desires for, foods, which point the homoeopath in the direction of the appropriate medicine. The altered receptivity to medicine that always arises in such an exquisite responsiveness in disease states (from a latent pre-existing constitutional or acquired susceptibility) frequently seems to be linked in a very characteristic way to the food aversions and desires. That is to say, commonly the aversions or desires will be tied to a food (sub)family, such as the grass family (wheat, rye, oats, barley), or the bean family (peas, lentils, haricot beans, carob, soya, mung beans, chickpeas, marrowfats, dunn peas, string beans, mangetouts), or the nightshade family (eggplant, potato, tobacco, tomato, Cape gooseberries, paprikas, chillis, sweet peppers, capsicum), or the brassica family (cabbage, kale, kohlrabi, calabrese, broccoli, Brussels sprouts, cauliflower, mustard, rapeseed oil, turnip, swede, cress, horseradish, watercress, radish, Chinese leaves), or any of the other thirty-odd food families. The characteristic link is from such 'collective' aversions and desires to 'groups' of remedies. As John Henry Clarke had pointed out in 1904: 'When this individualizing of remedies has been mastered, the grouping becomes of great importance in practice. Of this both Dr Burnett and Dr Cooper made the most brilliant use. I need only instance the working out of the Lobelias by Dr

Cooper, and of some of the Conifers by Dr Burnett. Those who wish to follow up the successes of these great therapeutists will have a light to guide them in my "Repertory of Natural Relationships".'[1] [In it, amongst other things, Clarke arranges homoeopathic medicines in a list of natural orders, as he says, 'in systematic or evolutionary order'.[2]] (See 'Aggravation', 'Altered Receptivity in Disease', 'Disease and Drug Action in Homoeopathic Congruity' sections 3 and 9(iii), 'Foods and Health Problems' and 'Nutritional Equipoise'.)

Avogadro's Number

The constant number of molecules (atoms, ions, electrons) in a mole of any substance; has the value of $6.02252 \times 10^{23} \text{mol}^{-1}$. Mole is the amount of substance that contains as many atoms (molecules, ions, electrons, photons, etc.) as there are atoms in 12g of ^{12}C, the most abundant isotope of carbon. The Avogadro limit is reached at 12CH or 23DH (see 'Potency') and in dynamizations higher than these not a single molecule of the original base substance or mother tincture is expected to remain.

Outside the Anglo-Saxon area of influence this constant is often referred to as the 'Loschmidt Number' for the historical reasons outlined below.

Amadeo Avogadro (1776-1856), an ecclesiastical barrister, mathematician and physicist of Turin, Italy postulated the following hypothesis published in 1811: 'Equal volumes of different gases at the same temperature and pressure contain the same number of simple and/or compound molecules.' (Today these are called atoms and molecules, respectively.) He, like Hahnemann in medicine, was repudiated in chemistry, being accused of unreality, by most leading scientists of his day. Despite this his hypothesis was ultimately adopted as a law of chemistry four years after his death at the Karlsruhe Convention of 1860. Then another five years after that, in 1865, the physicist Josef Loschmidt (1821-1895) calculated the constant to be 6.065×10^{23}, which has since undergone several minor revisions, which increased its accuracy.

It is not known whether Hahnemann – who took a great interest in chemistry – knew him, or of him. Nor whether Avogadro knew Hahnemann. What is known, however, as a historical aside, is that another celebrated contemporary, the Swedish chemist Jöns Jacob Baron von Berzelius (1779-1848) certainly knew (of) Hahnemann. He had a medical degree from Uppsala University, and is often referred to as the Newton of chemistry because of his outstanding contributions to that science. He is on record as having joked on one occasion: 'That man [Hahnemann] would have made a great chemist, had he not turned out a great quack!'[3] The Baron von Berzelius

---

[1] Clarke, John Henry. *A Clinical Repertory to The Dictionary of Materia*, republished Bradford: Health Science Press, 1979, Preface p ix.
[2] Op. cit., p 325.
[3] Cook, Trevor. *Samuel Hahnemann: The Founder of Homoeopathic Medicine*, Wellingborough: Thorsons Publishers Ltd, 1981, p 42.

established the law of multiple proportions, as well as the law of reciprocal proportions (a modification of John Dalton's earlier version). He successfully pushed for the adoption of the atomic theory, and the electro-dualistic theory [the polar nature of elements in electro-chemistry]. His fame is due to the following pioneering work done by him:

He introduced quantitative analysis; a classification of minerals; and a new classification of compounds and a chemical nomenclature. He also discovered selenium and thorium, as well as isolating calcium, barium, silicon, strontium and tantalum.

Ayurvedic Medicine

Originated in India. It has recently begun to take root in many parts of the world and the effects of some of its medicines on patients, particularly those who have links with India, when subsequently consulting a homoeopath, ought to be taken into anamnestic account. A feature of Ayurveda is the highly developed system of pulse diagnosis to detect any current physiological imbalance or signs of future illness. Ayurveda maintains that medicinal plants growing in any country are the most effective for the health maintenance of the people of that country; it divides the medicinal effects of herbs, which it uses in ponderal doses, broadly speaking, into three categories: (i) active, creating energy; (ii) passive, destroying or resisting energy; and (iii) unifying and preserving energy; it addresses the mind, body, behaviour and the environment in its approach to health recovery and maintenance. An examination of the phytopharmaka in the materia medica of Ayurveda[1] reveals, first of all, that there are vast numbers of herbal drugs (used in ponderal doses) which are identical with those of the homoeopathic materia medica: e.g. less common ones like

Apium graveolens
Calotropis gigantea
Operculina turpethum
Piper nigrum
Zingiber officinalis

or more common ones like

Aconitum napellus
Allium cepa
Croton tiglium
Gentiana lutea
Plumbago littoralis.

In fact, the preponderance of herbal drugs used by Ayurveda have also

---

[1]Dash, Vaidya Bhagwan, and Vaidya Lalitesh Kashyap. *Materia Medica of Ayurveda*, New Delhi: Concept Publishing Co, 1980, pp 12-121.

undergone homoeopathic provings and are known to produce pronounced reactions in patients when administered in substantial doses. But an examination of homoeopathy's materia medica shows that a number of homoeopathic medicines started out as Ayurvedic herbal drugs, then after undergoing provings (pathogenetic experiments), these 'ethnopharmaceuticals' were incorporated into homoeopathy's materia medica. For example:

Acalypha indica
Azadirachta indica
Ficus religiosa
Syzygium jambolanum

(See 'Homoeopathic Ethnopharmacology'.)

B

Bach Flower Remedies

Devised in the early 1930s by the English bacteriologist Edward Bach (1886-1936), who maintained that in medicine the patient's personality, rather than his disease, should be treated. He said, specifically in this regard, 'Take no notice of the disease; think only on the outlook on life of the one in distress'. [1] To this end he introduced a significant group of therapeutic agents called the Bach Flower Remedies, which are regarded by many as compatible with homoeopathy. Practitioners who view the mind as an organ in its own right, look upon these remedies as organotropic, even though the method of their preparation is not within the homoeopathic method, with the result that these remedies do not carry a potency symbol. The dose is three drops sublingually three times daily, or more frequently, if needed. An aspect of this therapeutic approach, that is not within the standard precepts of homoeopathy, is that the physical components of a disease are, as already stated, to be ignored by the practitioner in favour of focusing only on the psyche. Moreover, although Bach had explicitly declared this to be a complete system of healing and the thirty-eight flower remedies to be its entire pharmacopoeia, most practitioners who prescribe from it have found that they need to prescribe other (non-Bach) medication along with it.

The thirty-nine Flower Remedies and their main indications are:

1 Agrimony: Mental torture behind brave face
2 Aspen: Fears of unknown origin
3 Beech: Intolerant and precise
4 Centaury: Timid and weak-willed
5 Cerato: Self-doubt, seeking advice all around
6 Cherry Plum: Fear of losing reason and control
7 Chestnut Bud: Failure to learn from past errors
8 Chicory: Selfish and possessive
9 Clematis: Vacant and indifferent
10 Crab Apple: Feeling unclean and self-dislike
11 Elm: Sense of inadequacy when laden by responsibilities
12 Gentian: Easily discouraged
13 Gorse: Utter despair
14 Heather: Absorbed in total self-interest
15 Holly: Jealous or envious
16 Honeysuckle: Dwelling on the past

---

[1] Bach, Edward. Quoted by Philip M Chancellor in *Illustrated Handbook of the Bach Flower Remedies*, Saffron Walden: The C W Daniel Co Ltd, 1986, p 10.

17 Hornbeam: Fatigue, both mental and physical
18 Impatiens: Nervous and impatient
19 Larch: Lack of self-assurance
20 Mimulus: Fears of unknown things
21 Mustard: Endogenous depression
22 Oak: Overworks, but struggles on relentlessly
23 Olive: Total exhaustion
24 Pine: Guilt complex
25 Red Chestnut: Over-concern for others
26 Rock Rose: Terror or panic attacks, also after nightmares
27 Rock Water: Self-denial and rigidity of outlook
28 Scleranthus: Indecisive
29 Star of Bethlehem: Shock
30 Sweet Chestnut: Great anguish
31 Vervain: Perfectionistic and over-anxious
32 Vine: Ruthless
33 Walnut: Over-sensitive to outside influences
34 Water Violet: Aloof
35 White Chestnut: Persistent, unwanted thoughts
36 Wild Oats: Indecision about future plans
37 Wild Rose: Apathetic resignation
38 Willow: Resentment
39 Rescue Remedy: A mixture of five flower remedies, of proven clinical efficacy in any case of sudden collapse when three drops are given every two minutes directly on to patient's tongue until recovery occurs. It is a combination of 6, 9, 18, 26 and 29.

No pathogenetic experiments have been undertaken with these remedies. They are prepared as macerations of plant material (petals) in brandy with all insoluble material filtered out. The most complete bibliography extant on the flower remedies is that by Francis Treuherz.[1] Julian Barnard has edited a representative collection of Edward Bach's writings wherever the latter is the sole author, i.e. excluding joint publications.[2]

Bad Hygiene

See 'Miasma', 'Sanitation', 'Verdi, Tullio Suzzara (1829-1902)' and 'Worms'.

Baglivi, Giorgio (1668-1707)

See 'Philosophical Premise of Homoeopathy'.

[1]Treuherz, Francis. 'A Bibliography of the Bowel Nosodes of Bach and Paterson and the Flower Remedies of Bach', *British Homoeopathic Journal*, vol LXXVII, April 1988, pp 112-116 [copies available from author: Flat 2, 18 The Avenue, Brondesbury Park, London NW6 7YD].
[2]Barnard, Julian, ed. *Collected Writings of Edward Bach*, Hereford: Bach Educational Programme, 1987, 224 pages.

Balances, Chemical and Physical

See 'Utensils of Homoeopathic Pharmacy'.

Bates' Method of Eyesight Training

William H Bates, a graduate from Cornell University and the College of
Physicians and Surgeons of Columbia University, practised from 1885 as an
ophthalmologist at the New York Eye and Ear Infirmary. One of his
achievements was the improvement of the retinoscope. In 1923 he introduced
the forerunner of today's lie-detector, when he used the retinoscope to measure
minute contractions in the eyeball caused by mental strain associated with
lying. This then became the lie-detection method for the next three decades.
Bates also devised a method of eyesight training for the correction of the
common sight defects, which involves various relaxation and strengthening
exercises aimed at counteracting the developmental oculopathies. This is set
out in detail in his book *Perfect Sight Without Glasses*. R Brooks Simpkins of
Eastbourne, Sussex, England amplified this orthoptic method by saying:

> 'The eyes collect light energy and transmit it to the intra-cranial processes of vision –
> to produce the sense of sight, and also to activate the motor nerves of the external
> and ciliary muscles. It follows that the therapeutic employment of visible rays, in
> imitation of normal light could be made to activate those same motor nerves.'

He wrote four books on this subject, lectured on it and practised what he
preached very successfully for close on thirty years from the mid-1930s.
   This therapeutic approach is not in conflict with homoeopathy.

Beam Therapy

See 'Chromotherapy'.

Benjamin, Alva (1884-1975)

Homoeopath with an abiding interest in dermatology, who obtained his
medical degree from Sydney University, worked at the Royal London
Homoeopathic Hospital from 1923 to 1956 and was treasurer to the Faculty
of Homoeopathy for many years. He also contributed frequently to the *British
Homoeopathic Journal*. In earlier years he had been secretary-general and later
president of the Liga Medicorum Homoeopathica Internationalis. He founded
the Hahnemann Society in 1958. His major address was to the Liga
Medicorum Homoeopathica Internationalis' quinquennial congress in
London in 1956, entitled: 'The World's Present-Day Need of Homoeopathy'.

Berridge, Edward W

UK homoeopath, who obtained his MD (by examination) at the Pennsylvania Homoeopathic College, after he had graduated as an MB Ch.B. from London University. He was resident homoeopathic officer to the Liverpool homoeopathic dispensary in England for some considerable time. In 1869 he published the *Complete Repertory of the Homoeopathic Materia Medica for Diseases of the Eye*. He was a strong proponent of high-potency remedies at a time when the influence of Richard Hughes was on the ascendant and high potencies were out of favour. He managed to convince the antagonistic Thomas Skinner MD (from Edinburgh) of the clear therapeutic merits of homoeopathy, when treating him in Liverpool (with high dynamizations). Thereafter he became Skinner's mentor, on whom he exerted a strong influence.

Berridge, the homoeopath, was also a fervent occultist and as the 'Very Honoured Frater Resurgam', his alter ego, he was the leading member of the Hermetic Order of the Golden Dawn (founded in 1887 in London) who made a major addition to the doctrines of the French ceremonial Magus, Eliphas Levi, by adding a fourth law to his three, namely the law of imagination – without which, Berridge claimed, the will-power in magical matters remained ineffectual.[1] To what extent, if at all, such esoteric interests coloured his tutelage of Skinner, the originator of 'Skinner's continuous fluxion apparatus', is not known. The latter certainly gave no evidence of ever having engaged in such divertissements. Berridge's two other major homoeopathic writings are:

Index to Cases of Poisoning in the Allopathic Journals;
The Pathogenetic Record.

(For details on the influence exerted by Richard Hughes refer to 'History of Homoeopathy before 1900', section headed United Kingdom, and to 'Hughes, Richard (1836-1902)'; reference to Skinner's 'continuous fluxion apparatus' is made under 'Potentizing Methods' section International Distribution of Scales and Methods; see also 'Skinner, Thomas (1825-1906)'.)

'Bioavailability'

Insoluble substances (e.g. metals) only become soluble on dynamization (potentization) once colloidal solubility is reached at the 8DH potency level: only from there on do these remedies become medicinally active. Similarly, 'inert' substances (e.g. Silica [pure flint, silex]) become active upward from the same level of dynamization. (See 'Colloid'.)

Biochemic Medicine System

See 'Tissue Salts'.

[1] King, Francis, ed. *Astral Projection, Magic and Alchemy*, London: Spearman, 1971

Biochemic Remedies
See 'Biochemic Therapy'.

Biochemic Therapy
● **Treatment using only so-called tissue salts in a way originated in the nineteenth century by Schüssler, which is in harmony with his nutritional theory.**

The method of combating disease by restoration of the proper balance of the inorganic salts found in the organism's cells (the tissue). This nutritional theory was originated by Dr Wilhelm H Schüssler in 1873, at first as *An Abridged Homoeopathic Therapy* using the twelve tissue salts. Later he insisted that his Biochemic System of Medicine was separate from homoeopathy and in the 25th edition of his book on the subject he roundly denied all connexion with homoeopathy. He said his method was not based on the law of similars, but upon physiologico-chemical processes taking place within the organism. After his death in 1898, Biochemic Therapy was gradually re-amalgamated with homoeopathy, with the twelve tissue salts retaining a high degree of popularity. Most of the so-called tissue salts, or biochemic remedies, had been proved homoeopathically and were included in the list of standard homoeopathic remedies many years before Schüssler promulgated his Biochemic System of Medicine. Moreover, the tissue salts are administered in potency and are chemically (usually) only one millionth (= 6DH) of the organic salts strength, which would not enable them to act as direct cell nutrients. In recent years there has been a minor revival, under various new names, of Schüssler's ideas underlying Biochemic Therapy. The naturopath Maurice C H Blackmore referred to the tissue salts as 'colloidal minerals' and 'micro-nutrient elements' in his book *Mineral Deficiencies in Human Cells,* originally published in 1954. The trade names 'Celloids' and 'Mineraloids' have been registered for the tissue salts. (See also 'Mineral Remedies', 'Schüssler, Wilhelm Heinrich (1821-1898)' and 'Tissue Salts'.)

Biochemic Tissue Salts
See 'Tissue Salts'.

Biochemistry
Biological chemistry; physiological chemistry; studies the patterns of chemical changes occurring in living organisms. (See 'Physiological Response in Homoeotherapeutics, Mechanism of' and 'Vitalism'.)

Biocybernetics, Ultrafine
See 'Bio-Resonance Therapy'.

Bio-electronic Regulatory Medicine

● **Method for diagnosis and treatment with medicines, that relies heavily on the practitioner's diagnostic interpretation of changes in measurements of the electrical potential at a point on the patient's skin.**

Following upon Boyd's emanometer (see 'Boyd, William Ernest (1891-1955)'), Dr med Reinhold Voll, of the FRG, demonstrated in the 1950s electronically:

(i) that there was, indeed, some relationship between acupuncture meridians and the organs traditionally associated with them in Oriental Medicine;
(ii) that if a meridian was not functioning optimally there was a voltage indicator drop evident; and
(iii) that if appropriate potentized remedies were incorporated into the circuit in series with the patient and the instrument's probe, the readings on the meridian returned to normal.

Though clinically reputed to be effective, this method was laborious, even if it was considerably less cumbersome than Boyd's emanometer, where a healthy human subject was an indispensable part of its circuit. Helmut W Schimmel, MD, DDS, also of the FRG, a pupil of Voll, simplified the method. He introduced electronic measurement at one point only (on a finger or a toe) and used organ attestants (that is, 'proxy' preparations of the tissues of each organ) to replace the measuring of many points in turn on each of the various meridians (representing organs). Any abnormality that was detected during the testing procedure was corrected, as Voll had done, by incorporating a potentized remedy into the circuit in series with the patient and the probe. It is held that the instrument will indicate hidden precipitating factors in disease (e.g. accumulated toxins, hypersensitivities, infected foci or inherited factors) as well as aiding in the selection of the appropriate dynamized medicine. A bio-electronic regulatory technique which is virtually independent of the instrument's operator is the segmental electrogram which indicates areas of electrical disturbance in diverse segments of the patient's body, which, taken together with the anamnesis and the examination results, may determine the organ that is under stress in the indicated segment. This detection method has been taken to provide the earliest indications of a diseased condition, even before overt pathological changes have actually set in. The diagnostic and therapy-support bases contained in bio-electronic regulatory techniques are, in themselves, not inconsistent with homoeopathic principles, but they certainly do not constitute homoeopathic practice. Recent attempts by Schimmel and others to validate the method experimentally have, so far, not produced any confirmation of the claims made for this particular diagnostic/treatment method. (See also 'Acupuncture', 'Auriculomedicine', 'Bio-Resonance Therapy', 'Isopathy', section on Twentieth Century History of Isopathy, 'Psionic Medicine' and 'Regulation Thermography'.)

Bio-resonance Therapy

● Method for diagnosis and treatment, either without medicines or with simulated remedies, that uses a machine to accept and read the many complicated wave patterns sent out by (parts of) the patient, and then to make inversions or other changes of these patterns (e.g. mirror images of the emanating wave patterns) and to send these back into the patient with increased or reduced intensity – thus neutralizing the patient's 'bad vibrations'. Relying to some extent on the old theory of the radiant state of matter these inverted oscillations, or correcting energy waves, may also be transmitted into unmedicated pharmaceutical vehicles in order to 'charge' these with the particular patient's 'individualized remedy' (though not in any homoeopathic sense). Comparably, 'emanations' from medicines may also be sent straight into unmedicated vehicles; this is known as remedy simulation. In a similar manner 'emanations' from crystals, or from a colour, or a sound, etc. may be sent into either a patient, or an unmedicated vehicle that, it is said, may be 'charged' in this manner.

Ultrafine biocybernetics (for which common proprietary terms are 'Bicom-', 'Indumed-', 'Mora-' and 'Multicom-therapy') was developed from Paul F Nogier's auriculomedicine. The idea was conceived by F Morell, and realized by him together with L Mersmann and E Rasche (Mora is a contraction of Mersmann, Morell and Rasche).

In the jargon used by W Ludwig, a doctor of science,[1,2] Bio-Resonance Therapy taps endogenous signals from the patient through skin electrodes and re-transmits them, selectively inverted, filtered and amplified (on one instrument they are also optionally reducible), to other parts of the body. The patient and the instrument form a feedback control system within the therapeutic application which is proper to the method's rationale. An optional possibility is the use of optoreceptors to separate plain low-frequency amplitude modulations of visible light, then to amplify these electronically, and to apply them therapeutically by using skin electrodes. Because an organism lives in a state of resonance with the environment (as exemplified, for instance, by the electron plasma oscillations of trace elements, or the Schumann rays [of wavelengths between 1850 and 1230 angstrom]), such signals may also be passed on to the organism magnetically in the micro-tesla range, through one of the instruments. Another optional extra is the possibility to convert sound therapy and/or crystal therapy into electronic messages to the patient's body. This form of stimulation therapy may, possibly, be compatible with homoeopathy, though it cannot claim to be any direct part of it. Nonetheless

[1] Ludwig, L. 'Bioresonance Diagnosis and Therapy', section 3 of 'Bioenergetic Medicine', *De Natura Rerum*, August 1988, vol II, no 3, pp 118-120.
[2] Ludwig, L. *Diagnose- und Therapieverfahren im ultrafeinen Bioenergie-Bereich*, edited by Hans Brüggemann, Heidelberg: Karl F Haug Verlag, 1984, pp 198-206.

remedy simulation has been an aspect of this medical approach (bio-resonance therapy) since W E Boyd's emanometer of the 1920s and 1930s. This therapy which many homoeopaths dismiss as 'unhomoeopathic' and as belonging more appositely into Psionic Medicine likes to lay claim to kinship with R Voll's, and later H W Schimmel's, remedy 'testing' procedures of Bio-Electronic Regulatory Medicine, though, in fact, it has more in common with neurologist Albert Abrams' oscilloclast, or Ruth Drown's and George de la Warr's 'black boxes'. (See 'Auriculomedicine', 'Bio-electronic Regulatory Medicine', 'Psionic Medicine' and 'Regulation Thermography'.)

Biphasic Drug Action

Hormesis. (See 'Epistemological Assumptions in Homoeopathy', section 10, 'Hahnemann, Christian Friedrich Samuel [1755-1843]', section entitled 'Hahnemann's Contribution to Science and his Impact on the Practice of Medicine', 'Homoeopathic Laws, Postulates and Precepts', section 5 and 'Hormesis'.)

Bites

For animal bites and insect stings (bites) see 'Emergencies – Homoeopathic Treatment'.

Blackie, Dame Margery Grace (1898-1981)

This well known UK homoeopath qualified in medicine in 1923 at the London School of Medicine for Women and obtained her degree from the University of London in 1928. She was the great-niece of James Compton-Burnett (1840-1901) and was physician to the Royal British household for the last fifteen years of her life, succeeding Sir John Weir GCVO, MD (1879-1971). She had been Dean of the Faculty of Homoeopathy from 1965 to two years before her death. This widely respected homoeopath enlivened students, patients and all who came in contact with her by her stimulating presence for more than half a century (she had been at the Royal London Homoeopathic Hospital since 1924). She was an able public speaker and later in life she began to support homoeopathic research. In fact, she established the Blackie Research Trust to continue this support after her death. She was a high-potency prescriber in the Kentian mould, using a single, unrepeated dose.

Most of her lectures were recorded on audio-tapes. Her most important writings include:

The Challenge of Homoeopathy; Macdonald and Jane's, London, 1976, which in countries outside the UK is entitled:

The Patient, Not the Cure; New Delhi: Rupa & Co, 1977.

Posthumously her recorded lectures have been edited and collated by the homoeopaths Charles Elliott and Frank Johnson entitled:

Classical Homoeopathy; Beaconsfield, Bucks: Beaconsfield Publishers Ltd, 1986.

She was a close friend of homoeopath Frank Bodman (1900-1980) since the 1920s when they both served as house-physicians under Douglas Borland (1885-1960). The latter homoeopath had been taught by James Tyler Kent (1849-1916) in Chicago, USA before the first World War, and he had a profound influence upon her high-potency style of homoeopathic practice, which she freely acknowledged. Her other teachers included John Henry Clarke (1853-1931) and Charles Edwin Wheeler (1868-1946), who both employed potencies in the entire spectrum, except for the very high potencies. They did not influence her significantly, though. She seemed to use only two potencies: 6CH for functiotropic and pathotropic prescriptions, and a single 10M dose, frequently divided into three twelve-hourly administrations, for constitutional prescriptions. If an aggravation set in, she would not change the selected remedy but increase the potency to CM. The 3DH, 6DH, 12CH, 30CH, 200CH or 1M dynamizations that were in fairly common use in the UK during the mid-twentieth century she all but ignored. Times were when she would forestall or abort an aggravation by dissolving the 10M potency in drinking water to be taken in little unhurried sips, as required to control such symptoms.[1] During her 57 years at the Royal London Homoeopathic Hospital and later at the Faculty of Homoeopathy her example influenced untold numbers of students of homoeopathy to pursue a similar high-potency approach to therapeutics.

She loved the countryside, was mildly addicted to solving jigsaw puzzles and enjoyed giving excellent supper parties at her Kensington, London home for those whom she felt to be fired by a kindred spirit to her own.

Three salient quotations from this outstanding homoeopath are appended:

'Homoeopathy is "the" alternative medicine' [spoken on several occasions]

'The wholesale destruction of the forests of the Amazon, where so many natural sources of medicine will be lost, is surely one of the great tragedies of our time and for the future health of the world' [1976: *The Patient, Not the Cure,* p 191]

'Homoeopathy, as formulated by Hahnemann, is the most scientific and the most successful system of medical treatment yet devised. Our responsibility for its pure and truthful presentation is great.' [*Classical Homoeopathy,* quotation on frontispiece]

A full biography of Dame Margery entitled *Champion of Homoeopathy,* Life of Dr Margery Blackie was written by Constance Babington Smith (London: John Murray Ltd, 1986).

Bodman, Francis Hervey (1900-1980)

Francis Bodman's father and grandfather had both also been practising

---

[1] Elliott, Charles, and Frank Johnson, eds. *Classical Homoeopathy: Margery Grace Blackie,* Beaconsfield: Beaconsfield Publishers Ltd, 1986, pp iii and iv.

homoeopaths. This unusually gifted student graduated from Bristol University in 1922, having won three gold medals, and was with the Bristol Royal Infirmary until 1925. He studied homoeopathy with Margery Grace Blackie (1898-1981) under Charles Edwin Wheeler (1868-1946) and Douglas Borland (1885-1960), doing his housemanship at the Royal London Homoeopathic Hospital, in obstetrics. Through that he came to see a great deal of domiciliary midwifery at a time when home deliveries were the norm. He also obtained the psychiatric qualification DPM. Later he established his very successful homoeopathic practice in Bristol. He wrote many thought-provoking articles in the *British Homoeopathic Journal,* whose editor he was for a time, and always showed a strong perception of the value of good communication. He was elected president of the Faculty of Homoeopathy in London from 1955 to 1957. In harmony with his psychiatric qualification, he was fully sensible to the high value of homoeopathic 'mentals' in each case. An outstanding tract is: *The Foresight of Hahnemann* (1931).

Bodman's erudition was wide-ranging, lecturing on subjects as disparate as botany and social science, and translating works from French to English, such as *Petite Histoire de l'Organon et de ses Metamorphoses* by J Baur (1975). However, his most original homoeopathic writing was put together as a monograph by Anita Davies and Robin Pinsent under the title *Insights into Homoeopathy* (Beaconsfield: Beaconsfield Publishers Ltd, 1990, 125 pages), featuring homoeopathic approaches to common problems in general practice and psychiatry, as well as featuring an analysis of the extraordinary contribution made by Samuel Hahnemann, and the wider issues of homoeopathy in a present-day setting, concluding with a paper on the rationale underlying homoeopathic research.

Boenninghausen, Clemens Maria Franz Baron von (1785-1864)

After Hahnemann, with Jahr the most important of the early practitioners of homoeopathy, who was born on 12th March, 1785 on the family estate of Heringhaven, in Overyssel, the Netherlands. He was a scion of a family originating from within the oldest military nobility of Westphalia, which traced its lineage back to Austria: to one ancestor who was a field marshal from 1632 under Hapsburg Emperor Ferdinand II (Holy Roman Emperor [1578-1637] who spent his reign in war against the Protestants, opening the Thirty Years' War).

At twelve years he went to a German-medium high school in Münster, from which he matriculated at eighteen, going on to the Dutch University of Groningen, where he simultaneously attended the lectures in three different faculties: law, natural history and medicine. He graduated as 'Doctor utrinque juris' on 30th August, 1806 and was called to the Bar at Deventer thirty-two days later. In 1807 the young advocate, who was also fluent in French, accompanied his father to the Utrecht Royal Court of Louis Bonaparte, the then King of the Netherlands. Baron von Boenninghausen Snr, whose command of French was inadequate for the occasion, was the Representative of the Overyssel Election Committee. The son was admitted as spokesman to audience with the king where his natural charm, eloquence and highly developed mental abilities found immediate favour. The young barrister was made Auditor to the Privy Council and within the short space of a year became Auditor to the king himself. Very soon he advanced to the position of Secretary-General to the king, by virtue of which, ex officio, he held the posts of Royal Librarian and Chief of the Topographical Bureau, amongst other semi-automatic appointments. On 1st July, 1810 when Louis Bonaparte, of whom Boenninghausen had genuinely come to be very fond, abdicated as King of the Netherlands, he retired from the Dutch State service and began to devote his time to agriculture and the study of botany. He married in the Autumn of 1812 and in the Spring of 1814 moved to the ancestral estate at Darup, Westphalia. He published several small botanico-agricultural studies at that time and by precept and example he made a serious attempt to improve the lot of the Westphalian peasantry. To that end he established the Agricultural Society for the District of Münster. This was the first of its kind in what were to become known as the West-Prussian States. In an extended form, but unaltered in the core of its objectives, that society still exists today. In 1816 the Provincial Court of Justice for Westphalia appointed the then thirty-one year old advocate as County Councillor of the Coesfeld district, in which Darup lies. Six years later he was appointed Commissioner-General of the newly created Deeds' Registry (for official real estate conveyancing records) for the Rhineland and Westphalia. On the many extensive travels entailed in the execution of his official duties, he had ample opportunity for studying the indigenous flora. In 1824 he published a book *Prodromus florae monasteriensis* in which he was the first to draw attention to the similarity of the flora in England to that of Westphalia and the Rhineland. Through this and other botanical studies he achieved much distinction, leading firstly to the attachment of his name to two plant families (at the instances of botanists Reichenbach and Sprengel), and secondly to his appointment as Director of the Münster Botanical Gardens.

In the Autumn of 1827 Clemens von Boenninghausen became very seriously ill. Two eminent physicians, who were called in separately, both diagnosed 'purulent tuberculosis'. Efforts were made for half a year to improve his condition, but this only worsened steadily. In the Spring of 1828 all hope of recovery was openly abandoned by the physicians. He then wrote a farewell letter to an old botanical friend, Dr A Weihe in Hervorden. This physician had recently become a homoeopath, though Boenninghausen did not know this. Weihe was very distressed by the news and wrote back asking for a very detailed description of the symptoms. Boenninghausen was told that there was a new scientific form of medicine that had just been developed that could probably help him. He scrupulously complied with Weihe's request and the latter then sent him the homoeopathically corresponding medicine (Pulsatilla nigricans) with dosage regimens. Boenninghausen immediately began to improve and was fully cured by the end of that summer. In this manner homoeopathy gained one of its keenest followers, who, at the same time, was possessed of a lawyer's very nimble mind, was characterized by an enlightened versatility in the natural sciences, enjoyed immense social standing, and was a thoroughly charming gentleman besides.

He immediately revived his academic knowledge of medicine. Because he had not graduated as a physician, he had no licence to practise as such. For this reason he devoted himself to studying, and also writing about, subjects connected with homoeopathy. He made an effort to inspire the Orthodox practitioners of Münster, with whom he was in close contact as a founder-member of their medical society. After several astonishing cures achieved homoeopathically two of these physicians, Drs Tuisting and Lutterbeck, were 'converted' to the new scientific medical system he was advocating. He set to work on carefully studying all of Hahnemann's work, and a lively correspondence sprang up between the system's discoverer and himself that endured until the former's death. He was the favourite and most intimate disciple of Hahnemann. The knowledge he had acquired during his years at university in medicine and natural science afforded him a solid foundation for the study of homoeopathy in greater depth. Then he began to conduct pathogenetic experiments (to prove medicines). Here again his great knowledge of botany served him well. Through his literary labours he became famous in homoeopathy. Physicians from many countries, but particularly from France, the Netherlands and the USA, made special trips to him in Münster for advice concerning matters of health. On his frequent official journeys he was obliged, more and more, to render medical advice, which stirred the antagonism of non-homoeopathic medical practitioners.

From all this he realized that homoeopathy required a materia medica that was as perfect as possible to convey the knowledge of the action of medicines. Yet, if the homoeopath is to fight the disease in any given case successfully, it would be necessary for him or her to be able to find quickly and reliably the characteristics of each individual remedy. To this end he produced and published quite independently of G H G Jahr (who did the same) a series of repertories from 1833 to 1846 (this collectively became the compilation as published and augmented by C M Boger entitled *Boenninghausen's Characteristics and Repertory*, Bombay: Roy & Co, 1937, 1071 pages). Most of his other systematic and lucid work on homoeopathy appeared regularly from 1828 to shortly before his death; apart from this he wrote many essays in the *Archiv für homöopathische Heilkunst*, the *Allgemeine homoeopathische Zeitung* and the *Homoeopathe Belge*, to each of which he was a constant contributor.

In early 1843 he had completed the setting up of the Deeds' Register. Then, on account of his patently wide-ranging medical knowledge and great learning the Cabinet of King Friedrich Wilhelm IV of Prussia granted him the right to practise medicine, quite exceptionally without requiring him to undergo any examination, on 11th July, 1843 (coincidentally on the very day of Hahnemann's burial at Montmartre cemetery). He requested to be allowed to retire from state service. This was granted and he took up the full-time practice of homoeopathy. He built up a very large practice and acquired great fame as a homoeopath in a short time.

He always undertook a very detailed examination of the patient each time, making a complete tabulation of all presenting disease symptoms. The potency he favoured was the 200CH, which he had prepared by Gottfried Lehmann in Schöningen, Duchy of Brunswick (now part of Germany). Veterinary homoeopathy received a strong impetus from Boenninghausen too; he successfully used the remedies in the treatment of animals in the same manner. From 1848 he arranged an annual gathering of homoeopaths of Westphalia and the Rhineland, which continued to take place after his death. The Cleveland Homoeopathic Medical College bestowed an honorary degree of Doctor of Medicine upon him on 1st March, 1854. Emperor Napoleon III created him Knight of the Legion of Honour on 20th April, 1861. Since 1854 the French Empress Eugénie had called upon Boenninghausen of Münster in Westphalia for medical attendance, because he was considered the most celebrated homoeopathic physician alive, although many notable French homoeopaths practised in Paris. As had come to be expected of this man who used the new scientific medical method, he successfully cured this imperial patient of her illness on each occasion.

He had a stroke on 23rd January, 1864 and passed away three days later. Boenninghausen had been a close friend of Adolph Lippe and Carroll Dunham, who both expressed their admiration for his pioneering work in the *American Homoeopathic Review,* vol IV. Lippe mentions particularly his accurate repertorial work (before his there was only one very brief index in Latin by Hahnemann, which lack entailed the study of remedy after remedy for many hours before the simillimum might be found). It seems as though Boenninghausen inspired Lippe's own interest in repertorial work.

His son Karl (1826-1902) married Hahnemann's adopted daughter, Sophie Hahnemann (née Bohrer) (1838-1899), settled in Paris and practised homoeopathy there in conjunction with Hahnemann's widow, Karl's mother-in-law.

His other son Friedrich (1828-1910), like his father first qualified as a lawyer. He had been practically blind for a number of years, and after having been totally cured by the homoeopathic skill of his father, he fervently decided to go back to university to study medicine, in which he graduated 'cum laude'. The effect of this remarkable cure was evident throughout his life: he could read the finest print without spectacles right up to the eighty-third year, his last.

Boenninghausen's fifteen major literary works in the order of their appearance are:

Repertory of the Antipsoric, Antisyphilitic and Antisycotic Medicines 1832

Appendix to the Repertory (sub-titled: *Summary View of the Chief Sphere of Operation of the Antipsoric Remedies and their Characteristic Peculiarities*) 1833

Homoeopathic Therapy of Intermittent Fever: a Trial 1833

Contributions to the Knowledge of the Peculiarities of Homoeopathic Remedies 1833

Homoeopathic Diet and a Complete Image of a Disease 1833

Homoeopathy: Manual for the non-Medical Public 1834

Repertory of non-Antipsoric Medicines 1835

Assay of the Relative Kinship of Homoeopathic Medicines 1836

Therapeutic Manual for Homoeopathic Physicians, for use at the Sickbed and in the Study of the Materia Medica Pura 1846

    Basic Instructions for non-Physicians as to the Prevention and Cure of Cholera 1849

    Laterality of the human body and Consequent Relationships 1853

    The Homoeopathic Domestic Physician in Brief Therapeutic Diagnoses (Submitted for Collegial Consideration) 1853

    The Homoeopathic Treatment of Whooping Cough in its Various Forms 1860

    The Aphorisms of Hippocrates Annotated by a Homoeopath 1863

    Homoeopathic Therapy of Intermittent and other Fevers: a Trial (second, augmented and revised edition), Part I 'The Pyrexy' 1864

Boericke, William (1849-1929)

Eminent US homoeopath. Born in Austria and originally named Wilhelm which he anglicized. He had studied for one year at Vienna Medical School, before settling in Ohio. He became a graduate of the Philadelphia Medical College in 1876. Soon afterwards he moved to San Francisco where he worked as a homoeopath for more than fifty years. It was in the period when he was the editor of the *California Homoeopath* that he travelled (in 1906) to Darup, near Münster, in the Ruhr area of Germany, with Dr Richard Haehl, in an unsuccessful attempt to negotiate with the heirs to the estate of Baron Dr Karl von Boenninghausen, the widower of Samuel Hahnemann's adopted daughter, for the publication rights to Hahnemann's sixth edition of the *Organon*. He founded the prestigious *Pacific Coast Journal of Homoeopathy* in 1880 and remained its editor until 1915. He was co-founder of the Pacific Homoeopathic Medical College and Hahnemann Hospital in 1881. This was incorporated into the University of California, where he became the first professor of Homoeopathic Materia Medica and Therapeutics, which post he held for thirty years. He became the elected President of the California State Homoeopathic Society. In early 1920, only after twenty-three years of written and oral negotiations with Dr Boenninghausen Jnr and later with the executors of his estate, both by Richard Haehl and William Boericke, did the former manage to procure the manuscript of the sixth edition of the *Organon* with the latter's financial support.

Prof William Boericke became the translator of this sixth edition from the German idiom to plain, lucid English. It was finally published in December, 1921 having been completed by Hahnemann almost eighty years earlier (in February, 1842).

His major published works comprise:

The Twelve Tissue Remedies of Schüssler (1888)

A Compendium of the Principles of Homoeopathy (1912)

Pocket Manual of Homoeopathic Materia Medica (Ninth Edition – 1927)

The last-mentioned edition is considered to have ranked as the world's consistent top-selling homoeopathic materia medica for more than sixty years.

This man is not to be confused with either of the following namesakes:

A) Franz (or Francis) E Boericke, MD, born in Glauchau, Saxony, in 1826, who became a lecturer at the Hahnemann Medical College in Philadelphia, where he settled, and where he established what has become the largest US homoeopathic pharmacy as well as a very highly regarded homoeopathic publishing house.

B) Oscar E Boericke, AB, MD, who published a 328-page *Clinical Repertory and Therapeutic Index of Homoeopathic Materia Medica*.[1] He remodelled it and brought it up to date to coincide with the ninth edition of the said *Pocket Manual of Homoeopathic Materia Medica* published by his namesake in June, 1927. It is now always also incorporated into Prof W Boericke's *Pocket Manual*.[2] Oscar E Boericke aptly observed that 'it is only by the persistent use of **one** repertory, that its peculiar and intricate arrangements gradually crystallize . . . in definite outline in the mind of the student of the same, and thus s/he attains the ready ease and practical insight of the collator, thereby' developing 'such a bee-line' technique 'well-nigh indispensable in our day of labour-saving devices'.[3]

Boger, Cyrus M (1861-1935)

There has probably never been a more thorough student of Clemens Maria Franz von Boenninghausen than this US homoeopath. He worked incessantly from early 1933 to his death in September 1935 on the translation, compilation and augmentation of *Boenninghausen's Characteristics and Repertory* (the information was previously scattered in many smaller books; the first edition of a Boenninghausen 'compendium' was commissioned by, and published in Bombay by, Roy & Co, 1937, 1071 pp; they brought out a second edition in 1952 but a third in 1976 was brought out in New Delhi by B Jain Publishers.).

His outstanding contribution to the homoeopathic system was the co-ordination and assembly of significant features of seemingly dissociated symptom groups in his *A Synoptic Key of the Materia Medica* (fourth edition, New Delhi: B Jain Publishers, 1973). He realized that upon these significant features depended almost wholly the homoeopath's final choice of the simillimum. He sought out, as it were, a speaking image of the correctly indicated remedy (the so-called genius of the drug), by focusing on differentiations. He said that

---

[1] Boericke, Oscar E. *Clinical Repertory and Therapeutic Index of Homoeopathic Materia Medica,* last published by Boericke & Runyon, Philadelphia, Pennsylvania, USA in 1927; re-published Calcutta: Roy Publishing House, 1969, 328 pages.

[2] Boericke, William. *Pocket Manual of Homoeopathic Materia Medica Comprising the Characteristics and Guiding Symptoms of All Remedies* [Clinical and Pathogenetic], ninth edition – including Oscar E Boericke's *Repertory,* Philadelphia: Boericke & Runyon, 1927, 1050 pages.

[3] Boericke, Oscar E. op. cit., in 'Prefatory Note to the Repertory', p 8, dated June, 1927.

ultimately his only purpose was 'intended to orient the searcher'. He held that every prescriber was duty-bound to use the utmost care in selecting the curative remedy, because 'the possibilities that inhere in the contact of the simillimum with the disordered vital force can not be foreknown'. His other major writings include:

Additions to Kent's Repertory
A Systematic Alphabetic Repertory of Homoeopathic Remedies
Times of the Remedies and the Moon Phases

Borland, Douglas Morris (1885-1960)

Born in Glasgow, Scotland, and a medical graduate from that city in 1909. He became an outstanding lecturer, who influenced many in Britain to adopt high-potency prescribing in the Kentian tradition of the single dose. He had studied with Sir John Weir, GCVO (1879-1971) under Kent in the USA. From 1913 he was on the staff of the Royal London Homoeopathic Hospital. During World War I he was in charge of a field hospital first in Salonika and then in Upper Armenia. During World War II he was in charge of the Royal London Homoeopathic Hospital and, on one occasion, was flung out of his bed by the bombardment of the Nurses' Home nearby. From 1945 he became governor of that hospital. His monogram on 'Children's Types' has become a classic (discussed in some detail under 'Constitutional Type'). Other major tracts by him are:

Digestive Drugs
Homoeopathy for Mother and Infant
Homoeopathy in Practice
Influenzas
Pneumonias
Treatment of Certain Heart Conditions by Homoeopathy
In 1982 Kathleen Priestman assembled and prepared Borland's hitherto unpublished lectures under the title:
Homoeopathy in Practice (219 pages) (1982)
Sheila Epps compiled a symptom index for this book and it was reprinted, with index, in 1988. In this is to found practical advice not only on the homoeopathic treatment of injuries and minor ailments and their sequelae, but there are also explicit sections on obstetrics and gynaecological conditions, as well as the pre- and post-operative treatment in homoeopathy. In this publication he also deals with the appropriate use of the four major nosodes (Psorinum, Medorrhinum, Lueticum [Syphilinum, Luesinum], Tuberculinum).

Botanical Medicine

See 'Phytotherapy'.

Bottles

In homoeopathic practice bottles of tinted, clear glass are used. These may be round or square, but not usually bulbous. Except for poisonous starting materials, the outer surface should be smooth, since ribbing might be seriously misleading to those handling the homoeopathic medicines, tinctures or solutions. This is due to the fact that convention in pharmacy has it that the outer surface of a bottle, if of a lesser capacity than 1.15 litres, when used for the sale or supply of a liquid poison, must be fluted vertically with ribs or grooves recognisable by touch. For the dispensing of liquid dynamizations amber bottles, and for the storage of mother tinctures green flasks are often used to soften the effects of light rays by means of filtration. Corks are not to be interchanged between bottles. (See 'Cleansing of Utensils and Sterilization'.)

Bowel Nosodes

A special category of nosode which, in turn, is a remedy, homoeopathically prepared from disease products, with its own full distinct drug picture (other nosodes will be found under 'Isopathy'). The major bowel nosodes are Bach's 1 to 5, and Paterson's 8 to 13 of the twenty listed here:

Name of Nosode	Laboratory Classification & Originator	Associated Non-Lactose Fermenting Bacilli, Cocci and/or Viruses
1. E coli (a.k.a. B coli or Colibac)[1]	Bach	Escherichia coli
2. Dys co	Bach	composite of Dysenteriae bacilli
3. Gaertner	Bach	Salmonella enteritidis (a.k.a. Gaertner's bacillus)
4. Mutabile (a.k.a. Colimutab)	Bach	Colibacterium mutabile
5. Froteus co (a.k.a. Proteus polyvalente or Polyvalent bowel vaccine)	Bach	Proteus vulgaris, inconstans, mirabilis, rettgeri and/or iliacus
6. Faecalis (a.k.a. Faecalisalkali	Bach	Faecalis alkaligenes a.k.a. Streptococcus faecalis

[1] Colibacillinum was introduced as one of the 'Isopathic microbic toxin-remedies' by Leon Vannier: *Communication au premier congrès de Thérapeutique*, Paris, October 1933, 'Pathogenesie de Colibacilline', published as 'Colibacilline dans le traitement de la Colibacillose', *L'Homéopathie Francaise*, 1933; Meningotoxinum and Pneumotoxinum are examples of other such microbic toxin-remedies then much in use in the francophone area.

Name of Nosode	Laboratory Classification & Originator	Associated Non-Lactose Fermenting Bacilli, Cocci and/or Viruses
7. Morgan co	Bach	[subdivided into: Paterson's (i) Morgan (pure), and (ii) Morgan-Gaertner, below]
8. Morgan (pure)	Paterson	Proteus morganii
9. Morgan-Gaertner	Paterson	Salmonella enteritidis and Proteus morganii
10. Sycotic co	Paterson	Diplococcus pneumoniae, Neisseriae gonorrhoeae and/or meningitidis that were found in bowel
11. Bac No VII	Paterson	[so named because it was the 7th non-lactose fermenting bacillus observed in laboratory]
12. Bac No X	Paterson	[so named because it was the 10th non-lactose fermenting bacillus observed in laboratory]
13. Coccal co (a.k.a. Sycoccus)	Paterson	polyvalent gram-positive bowel cocci, including Streptococci anginosus, durans, faecalis and other enterococci
14. Skatole	Stephenson	3-Methylindole formed in the intestine by bacterial decomposition of tryptophan
15. Mucolibacteriophagum	Coat	Polyphagum intestinale
16. Flexner	Stearns	Shigella paradysenteriae (a.k.a. Flexner's bacillus)
17. Dysentery bacteriophage	Stearns	virus with specific affinity for Salmonella typhosa
18. Streptococcus rheumaticus	Stearns	Streptococcus viridans cordis rheumatici
19. Streptococcus viridans cardiacus	Stearns	Streptococci faecalis, mitis, and/or sanguis
20. Muco coli pseudomembranosus	Stearns	Staphylococcus aureus in pseudomembranous enterocolitis, as a sequel to orthodox antibiotic therapy or surgery

These homoeopathic remedies were first developed in the 1920s by the bacteriologist Edward Bach, who, later, also became the renowned originator of the Bach Flower Remedies (see entry). From 1928 Drs John and Elizabeth

Paterson of Glasgow, Scotland did very extensive and extremely valuable work on the bowel nosodes, and published their results in the *British Homoeopathic Journal*. John Paterson (1890-1955) was a bacteriologist as well as a homoeopathic physician, his wife, Elizabeth (1907-1963), only the latter. Eight further contributors to the development of bowel nosodes were Drs C W Coat, Guy Beckley Stearns, J Stephenson, William B Griggs, C O Kennedy, Paul S Wyne, Isaac Sossnitz and Rosario Ferrara, who each did considerable work in specific areas of the bowel nosode field. Yet despite this, not one of these nosodes has undergone a traditional homoeopathic proving, that is an experimental assay on healthy human beings.

These nosodes were derived from cultures of stools. In the past the percentage of organisms found in the stool of a patient served as the indicator for which nosode was to be prescribed. With the proliferation of antibiotics and resulting widespread dysbiosis it became quite difficult to cultivate non-lactose fermenting organisms from patients' stools. As a consequence these nosodes were later, and are now, chiefly prescribed on particular clinical indications, or in association with related homoeopathic drugs.

Whenever a homoeopath, at the beginning of a case, finds that the patient's presenting symptoms are insufficiently defined to permit the selection of the simillimum, a single dose of a nosode (generally in a 30CH potency) is frequently prescribed, whose field of action is close to that of a likely group of applicable remedies. This is not repeated in under about 8 to 10 weeks, during which period related remedies are administered. In a somewhat similar manner some of these nosodes may be employed in homoeopathic prophylactic treatment. Low potencies of these nosodes are used in disease conditions with advanced pathology. In such cases the customary potency is 6CH given in a daily dose over a period determined by clinical observation and evidence of reaction. Associated remedies are:

to Dysenteriae Co	Anacardium orientale; Argentum nitricum; Arsenicum album; Cadmium metallicum; Kalmia latifolia; Veratrum album; Veratrum viride.
to Gaertner	Calcarea fluorata; Calcarea hypophosphorosa; Calcarea hypophosphorosa; Calcarea phosphorica; Calcarea silicica; Kali phosphoricum; Mercurius vivus; Natrum phosphoricum; Natrum silicofluoricum; Phosphorus; Phytolacca decandra; Pulsatilla nigricans; Silica; Zincum phosphoricum.
to Morgan (pure)	Alumina; Baryta carbonica; Calcarea carbonica; Calcarea sulphurica; Digitalis purpurea; Ferrum Carbonicum; Graphites; Kali carbonicum; Magnesia carbonica; Natrum carbonicum; Petroleum; Sepia

	officinalis; Sulphur; Medorrhinum; Psorinum; Tuberculinum bovinum.
to Sycotic Co	Antimonium tartaricum; Bacillinum; Calcarea muriatica; Ferrum metallicum; Natrum sulphuricum; Nitricum acidum; Rhus toxicodendron; Sulphur; Thuja occidentalis.
to Bacillus VII	Arsenicum iodatum; Bromium; Ferrum iodatum; Iodium; Kali bichromicum; Kali bromatum; Kali carbonicum; Kali iodatum; Magnesia muriatica; Muriaticum acidum; Natrum muriaticum; Secale cornutum.
to Faecalis Alkaligenes	Sepia officinalis.
to Morgan-Gaertner	Carbo vegetabilis and other carbons; Chelidonium majus; Chenopodium anthelminticum; Helleborus niger; Hepar sulphuris calcareum; (Trigonocephalus) Lachesis; Lycopodium ciavatum; Mercurius sulphuricus; Sanguinaria canadensis; Taraxacum dens leone.
to Mutabile	Ferrum phosphoricum; Kali sulphuricum; Pulsatilla nigricans.

The theoretic development of the bowel nosodes dates from 1912 when it was first suggested that resident bacteria of the lower bowel may contribute to chronic disease. Bach was unable to establish a direct link between chronic disease and these non-lactose fermenting organisms. So he decided to investigate whether a specific type of such organisms might not be linked to a particular set of symptoms, by introducing an auto-vaccine of the particular organism found in the stool of the patient concerned. Of a series of 500 patients thus vaccinated, 95% showed clinical improvement after an initial aggravation. There was also a marked increase in the number of such bacteria, decreasing slowly thereafter. Only from 1921 did Bach potentize the vaccines and administer them as auto-nosodes (isotherapeutics). [1] At this time, until 1928, Bach also potentized and used polyvalent nosodes run up from many of the specimens of bacteria. The Patersons systematized the bowel nosodes after Bach. [2]

[1] Edward Bach's principal publications relative hereto are:
(a) 'The Relation of Vaccine Therapy to Homoeopathy' *British Homoeopathic Journal*, April 1920;
(b) 'Intestinal Toxaemia in its Relation to Cancer' *British Homoeopathic Journal*, October 1924;
(c) *Chronic Disease: a Working Hypothesis*, book written in 1925 jointly with Dr C E Wheeler;
(d) 'The Problem of Chronic Disease' Paper read to the International Homoeopathic Congress, 1927;
(e) 'The Rediscovery of Psora', *British Homoeopathic Journal*, January 1929;
(f) 'An Effective Method of Preparing Vaccines for Oral Administration', *Medical World*, January 1930.

[2] John and/or Elizabeth Paterson's principal publications relative hereto are:
(a) 'Sycosis and Sycotic Co (Paterson)' by JP, *British Homoeopathic Journal*, April 1933;

A minority within the homoeopathic profession have, for a long time, had serious reservations about certain aspects of the bowel nosodes.[1] These rest on the following four points:

1 Their legitimacy is called into question, because use is based, not on provings, but primarily on Bach's theory of intestinal toxaemia;

2 Paterson's theories of bacterial mutation unfortunately cast a long shadow, even over much of his classical work in the bowel nosodes;

3 Imprecise methods resulted in the starting material for bowel nosodes actually being composed of several different bacteria, which meant that many of the nosodes run up from these will have had various bacteria in common, which, in turn, caused the existing lack of distinct definition in drug pictures, i.e. the absence of any clearly differentiated set of symptoms for each bowel nosode;

4 The bowel-nosode nomenclature is such that there is difficulty in identifying the bacterial species involved (see listing above, where the names of the principal related bacilli, etc. appear alongside the name of the bowel nosode), which opacity has adverse repercussions in the area of pharmaceutical manufacture of these nosodes.

The call from this group of homoeopaths is not to jettison the bowel nosodes, which are universally regarded as valuable, despite any such alleged defects, but to conduct separate standard placebo-controlled Hahnemannian provings on all bowel nosodes, which will have had to be previously re-identified, or, alternatively, to undertake controlled clinical research with them, similarly re-identified, to establish distinct, full and reliable symptomatologies for the materia medica.

The most complete bibliography extant on the bowel nosodes of Bach and Paterson is that by Francis Treuherz.[5] Y R Agrawal has written *A Treatise on Bowel Nosodes* in concise and practical form (New Delhi: Vijay Publications,

Footnote [2]continued from previous page.

(b) 'Psora and Sycosis in Relation to Modern Bacteriology' by JP, *Transactions of the XIth Congress of the Liga Medicorum Homoeopathica Internationalis held in Glasgow, Scotland 24th to 29th August 1936;*

(c) 'Lecture-Demonstration showing the Technique in the Preparation of the Non-Lactose Fermenting Nosodes of the Bowel and the Clinical Indications for their Use' by JP, *Transactions of the XIth Congress of the Liga Medicorum Homoeopathica Internationalis held in Glasgow, Scotland 24th to 29th August 1936;*

(d) 'Some Bacteriological and Clinical Aspects of Rheumatism', by JP, *British Homoeopathic Journal,* October 1933;

(e) 'The Role of the Bowel Flora in Chronic Disease', by JP, *British Homoeopathic Journal,* January 1949;

(f) 'The Bowel Nosodes', by JP, *British Homoeopathic Journal,* July 1950;

(g) 'A Survey of the Nosodes', by EP, British Homoeopathic Journal, July 1960.

[1]Neustädter, R. 'Critique of the Bowel Nosodes', *British Homoeopathic Journal,* April 1988, vol LXXVII, pp 108-111.

[2]Treuherz, Francis. 'A Bibliography of the Bowel Nosodes of Bach and Paterson and the Flower Remedies of Bach', *British Homoeopathic Journal,* vol LXXVII, April 1988, pp 112-116 [copies available from author: Flat 2, 18 The Avenue, Brondesbury Park, London NW6 7YD].

1981, 45 pages). Also informative on the principal bowel nosodes is B K Sarkar's compilation *Up-to-Date with Nosodes* (Calcutta: Roy Publishing House, 1971, 191 pages). (Refer also to 'Isopathy'.) Volume LXII of *The British Homoeopathic Journal* in 1973 featured the bowel nosodes prominently: on pp 42-44 'The Bowel Nosodes' by A C Gordon Ross; on pp 69-84 'Role of the Bowel Flora in Chronic Disease' (reprint of January 1949 publication) by John Paterson; and on pp 131-175 'On the Genesis, Nature and Control of Migraine with Particular Reference to the Bowel Nosodes as Expounded by Dr John Paterson' by S J Lambert Mount.

Boyd's Drug Classification

William Ernest Boyd, MA, MD, MBritIRE (1891-1955), an eminent homoeopath and scientist of Glasgow, Scotland was also a research engineer. He broke with the anthropomorphic classification system for drugs traditional in homoeopathy and assembled remedies according to their apparent electro-physical properties, into twelve groups. Boyd discovered that a patient tends to remain 'constitutionally' in his own group throughout life, for so long as the normal balance of health obtains. His analyses have indicated, furthermore, that among the twelve groups of drugs there exist very specific relationships, one to another. Whenever a patient's normal balance of health is disrupted, and that disturbance is not due to acute conditions, the tendency is for the patient to change into a group of a related series of drugs. As Kailash Narayan Mathur puts it, Boyd became convinced 'by experiments that homoeopathic drugs in infinitesimal potencies emanate electrophysical energy which acts on the human body and produces similar symptoms as produced by disease conditions.' He discovered twelve groups on the basis of his emanometric biophysical research according to vibrations or emanations produced by homoeopathic drugs (see 'Bio-Resonance Therapy', 'Psionic Medicine' and 'Radiant State of Matter, Theory of'). Drugs of each group have a complementary or supplementary relationship with each drug of the same group, so that if a drug is found to be the simillimum but does not act vigorously enough another suitable drug of the same group could be chosen as a complementary or supplementary remedy:[1]

Boyd's Groups are:

Group One

Aconitum napellus
Bromium
Calcarea bromata
Chlorinum
Cobaltum metallicum
Cyclamen europaeum

Ferrum bromatum
Ferrum metallicum
Ferrum muriaticum
Glonoinum (Nitro-glycerine)
Guaiacum officinale
Hippomane mancinella

[1] Mathur, Kailash Narayan. *Principles of Prescribing – Collected from Clinical Experiences of Pioneers of Homoeopathy*, New Delhi: B Jain Publishers, 1981, pp 448-449.

Nerium oleander
Oleum animale aetherum (Dippel's oil)
Oleum jecoris aselli

Sepia officinalis (Cuttlefish ink)
Veratrum album
Veratrum viride

Group Two

Aurum bromatum
Aurum metallicum
Aurum muriaticum
Aurum sulphuratum
Bothroips lanceolatus
Calcarea muriatica
Cenchris contortrix
Crotalus horridus
Dasyatis centrura (Sting ray)
Elaps corallinus

Hura brasiliensis
(Trigonocephalus) Lachesis
Loligo pealii (Squid)
Murex purpurea
Naja tripudians
Syzygium jambolanum
Toxicophis pugnax
Trombidium muscae domesticae
Vipera communis

Group Three

Medicago sativa (Alfalfa)

Trinitrotolouene (T.N.T.)

Group Four

Aesculus hippocastanum
Ammonium carbonicum
Ammonium muriaticum
Badiaga
Baryta carbonica
Baryta muriatica
Bryonia alba
Caladium seguinum
Calcarea acetica
Calcarea carbonica
Calcarea chlorinata
Calcarea fluorata
Calcarea hypophosphorosa
Calcarea lactica
Calcarea ovi tostae
Calcarea oxalica
Conium maculatum
Carduus marianus

Corallorhiza
Digitalis purpurea
(Solanum) Dulcamara
Equisetum hyemale
Fluoricum aciudum
Ignatia amara
(Achillea) Millefolium
Moschus tunquinensis
Myosotis symphytifolia
Onosmodium virginianum
Ovariae residuum tuberculinum
Parathyroidinum
Podophyllum peltatum
Sarsaparilla
Sinapsis nigra
Thyroidinum
Tongo (Dipterix odorata)
Viburnum opulus

Group Five

Acidum aceticum
Acidum benzoicum
Acidum carbolicum
Actaea racemosa (Macrotys, Cimicifuga racemosa)

Actaea spicata
Adrenalinum
Agnus castus
Aloe socotrina
Alumina (Argilla)

Aluminium metallicum
Aluminium phosphoricum
Apis mellifica
Argentum metallicum
Argentum nitricum
Arum triphyllum
(Atropa) Belladonna
(Lycoperdon) Bovista
Cadmium lacticum
Cadmium natrum silicea fluoricum
Cadmium phosphoricum
Cadmium silicatum
Cajuputum
Calcarea phosphorica
Cannabis indica
Cannabis sativa
Carcinosinum
Ceanothus americanus
Cinchona officinalis (China)
Chloralum hydratum
Clematis erecta
Chromium metallicum
Cina
Coccus cacti
Condurango
Cupressus lawsoniana
Cuprum metallicum
(Ecballium) Elaterium
Fagopyrum esculentum
Ferrum phosphoricum
Fragaria vesca
Genoscopolamine
Influenzinum
Iris tenax
Iris versicolor
Juglans regia
Kalmia latifolia
Lac caninum
Lactuca sativa
Lactuca virosa
Ledum palustre
Leptandra virginica
Lilium tigrinum
Lobelia inflata
Lycopodium clavatum

Magnesia muriatica
Magnesia phosphorica
Manganum metallicum
Melilotus alba
Muriaticum acidum
Myrica cerifera
Myrtus communis
Natrum benzoicum
Natrum bicarbonicum
Natrum bromatum
Natrum carbonicum
Natrum lacticum
Natrum morrhuicum (Sodium
    oleate, containing fatty acid of
    cod-liver oil)
Natrum muriaticum
Natrum phosphoricum
Natrum salicylicum
Natrum silicofluoricum
Neoarsphenamine
Nux moschata
Orchitinum
Ornithogalum umbellatum
Oxalicum acidum
Palladium metallicum
Phosphoricum acidum
Phosphorus
Phytolacca decandra
Plumbum metallicum
Ranunculus bulbosus
Ranunculus sceleratus
Raphanus sativus
Sabadilla officinarum
Scarlatininum
Scirrhinum (Carcinominum)
Secale cornutum
Senecio aureus
Solanum tuberosum aegrotans
    (diseased potato)
Spigelia anthelmia
(Delphinium) Staphisagria
Strontium carbonicum
Sulphuricum acidum
'S.U.P.36' (British Drug House's
    trade name for Tetrasodium

urea-MN'bis [4"-(8-(4'-
benzamidobenzamido)-1-hydroxy-
naphthalene-3:6-disulphonate)], a
medicinal solution)
(Cortex glandulae) Suprarenalis
(Nicotiana) Tabacum

Theridion curassavicum
Uricum acidum (Lithic acid)
Ustilago maidis
Vespa crabro
Wyethia helenoides

Group Six

Allium cepa
(Semecarpus) Anacardium orientale
Anthracinum
Antimonium arsenicosum
Antimonium crudum
Antimonium tartaricum
Aranea diadema
Arsenicum album
Arsenicum metallicum
Arundo mauritanica
Baptisia tinctoria
Bismuthum metallicum
Cactus grandiflorus
Cadmium arsenicum
Cadmium metallicum
Cadmium muriaticum (Cadmium
  chloride)
Cadmium sulphuratum (Cadmium
  sulphide)
Calcarea arseniaca
Calcarea caustica
Calcarea silicica
Capsicum annuum
Causticum
Cedron simaba
Cocculus indicus
Corallium rubrum
Crataegus oxyacantha
Crocus sativus
Curare
Echinacea angustifolia

Euphrasia officinalis
Ferrum arsenicosum (Ferrous
  arsenate)
Gelsemium sempervirens
Graphites
Gratiola officinalis
Hydrocyanicum acidum
Hypericum perforatum
Kali chloratum (Kali muriaticum)
Kali nitricum
Lapis albus
Lithium carbonateum
Malaria officinalis
Mephitis mephitica Putorius
Natrum Arsenicatum
Neurochypophysis (Pituitarum
  posterium)
Pareira brava
Pituitaria glandula (anterior lobe of
  hypophysis)
Sambucus nigra
Sanguinaria canadensis
Spongia tosta
Squilla maritima (Scilla, Sea onion)
Sticta pulmonaria
Tarentula cubensis
Teucrium marum verum
Verbascum thapsus
Vinca minor
Viola odorata

Group Seven

Arsenicum iodatum
Kali arsenicosum
Kali carbonicum
Lac defloratum

Lachnantes tinctoria
Luesinum (Syphilinum)
Nuphar luteum
Thea sinensis

Group Eight

Agaricus muscarius
Albumen ovi recens (the liquid egg white of Gallus bankiva domesticus)
Aphis chenopodii glauci
Aralia racemosa
Artemisia vulgaris
Bacillinum
Berberis vulgaris
Bowel nosodes of Bach
Bufo rana
Cadmium calcarea iodata
Cadmium iodata
Cantharis vesicatoria
Carbo animalis
Carbo vegetabilis
Carboneum sulphuratum
Caulophyllum thalictroides
(Matricaria) chamomilla
Chelidonium majus
Chenopodium anthelminticum
Chimaphila umbellata
Chinchonininum
Chininum sulphuricum
Cicuta virosa
Coffea cruda
Colchicum autumnale
(Citrullus) colocynthis
Dioscorea villosa
Dirca palustris
Drosera rotundifolia
Eupatorium perfoliatum
Ferrum iodatum
Gnaphalium polycephalum
Hamamelis virginiana
Hydrastis canadensis
Indigo
Iodium
(Cephaelis) Ipecacuanha
Kali bichromicum
Kali bromatum
Kali chloricum
Kali iodatum
Kali muriaticum
Kali sulphuricum
Koch's cancer serum
Kreosotum
Latrodectus mactans
Lyssinum
Magnesia carbonica
Magnesia sulphurica
Malandrinum
Medorrhinum
Menyanthes trifoliata
Mercurius cyanatus
Mercurius dulcis
Mercurius iodatus flavus
Mercurius iodatus ruber
Mercurius solubilis hahnemanni
Mercurius sulphuricus
Mercurius vivus
(Daphne) Mezereum
Morphinum acetatum
Natrum iodatum
Natrum sulphuricum
Nitrum cum sulphuri et carboni
Nux vomica
Oenanthe crocata
Opium
Oxytropis lamberti
Petroleum
(Carum) Petroselinum
Phellandrium aquaticum
Picricum acidum
Platinum metallicum
Prunus spinosa
Psorinum
Pulsatilla nigricans
Pyrogenium (Sepsinum)
Radium bromatum
Rhododendron chrysanthum
Rhus toxicodendron
Ruta graveolens
Sclerosinum
Selenium
(Polygala) Senega
Silicea
Stannum metallicum

(Datura) Stramonium
Sulphur
Sulphur iodatum
(Ferula) Sumbul
Sycotic composita (Bowel nosode
　　according to Paterson)
Symphoricarpus racemosus
Taraxacum dens leonis

Tellurium
Terebinthina oleum
Variolinum
Viscum album
Zincum metallicum
Zincum muriaticum
Zincum sulphuricum

Group Nine
Borax Veneta (Natrum
　　biboracicum)
Galium aparine

Gambogia (Tincture of the resinous
　　gum from Garcinias morella tree)
(Juniperus) Sabina

Group Ten
Arnica montana
Calcarea sulphurica
Chininum arsenicosum
Cistus canadensis
Helleborus niger
Hepar sulphuris calcarea
Hippozaeninum
(Cerasus) Laurocerasus

Nitricum acidum
Osmium
Plantago major
Rheum palmatum
Symphytum officinale
Tuberculinum
Uranium nitricum
Veratrum viride

Group Eleven
(Narthex) Asafoetida
Calotropis gigantea
Helonias dioica
Paeonia officinalis
Solanum nigrum

Stillingia sylvatica
Thallium metallicum
Thallium acetatum
Thuja occidentalis

Group Twelve
Valeriana officinalis

Boyd unfortunately died before he had completed this analytical work on medicines, but his contribution to homoeopathy is of significance, with the result that his groups are given in the better compilations of materia medica published since his demise.

Boyd's Groups
See 'Boyd's Drug Classification'.

Boyd, William Ernest (1891-1955)
This is, perhaps, the most extraordinary homoeopath of the twentieth century.

He lived, worked, studied and practised homoeopathy in Glasgow, Scotland, throughout his entire life. Early on he was impressed by the work of Dr R Gibson Miller (notably the work concerning 'hot and cold remedies' [i.e. predominantly aggravated by cold, or by heat, or sensitive to both extremes of temperature] and that published as *Relationship of Remedies with Approximate Duration of Action)*, which influenced him to become a committed homoeopath. For this he had the right attributes: empathy and an ability for keen observation. Yet he was also a research engineer, alive to concepts concerned with practical functionality and a deep interest in electro-physics. Using these personal qualities, he developed what is now called 'Boyd's Drug Classification' or 'Boyd's Groups' (see entry under former). He also carried out and published extensive scientific physiological and biochemical research. For several years, from 1946 to 1952, he was involved in his major scientific investigation, published in January, 1954 in the *British Homoeopathic Journal*, vol.XLIV, no.1, pp 6–44, under the title 'Biochemical and Biological Evidence of the Activity of High Potencies' (see 'Potency'). Yet, probably the most remarkable episode in his life surrounds the Horder Committee's investigation undertaken by the Royal Society of Medicine. Boyd had designed and constructed an instrument, which he called 'emanometer', capable (i) of demonstrating the measurable force in homoeopathic potencies and (ii) of matching these with the emanations from a patient's tissue-fluids, thereby assisting in selecting the correct, homoeopathically corresponding drug.

The impact of this instrument was such that the Royal Society of Medicine initiated an investigation into this diagnostic method. After some preliminary experiments, which yielded improbably high results in favour of the emanometer's efficacy, tests were conducted under the supervision of a committee appointed by the RSM, whose chairman was Sir Thomas – later, Lord – Horder. Boyd, and those working with him, were asked to identify, with the aid of this instrument, chemicals and tissues presented to them 'indistinguishable by visual or other normal' means; and later to differentiate between bottles of white powder, some of which had had a few drops of homoeopathically prepared water added to them. It must be pointed out that later even Horder and members of his committee undertook to take the place of Boyd and his assistants with the emanometer. The result in a series of twenty-five successive trials was 100% accuracy. The Horder Committee had to report this to the RSM: 'All were successful. The chance of this result being by accident is 1 : 33 554 432.' This, despite the constant assistance given to the investigation by Dr E J Dingwall, acknowledged expert in fraud detection in the area of psychical research for half a century subsequently. The embarrassingly spectacular findings were published in the *British Medical Journal* and the *Lancet* on 24th January, 1925 and have, from that quarter, been passed over in stunned silence ever since, simply because a dynamic concept (rooted in vitalism), that subtle bioenergy fields create their own characteristic, measurable emanations, is irredeemably at odds with the dominant mechanistic paradigm of orthodox medicine, its Cartesian legacy from the seventeenth century. (See 'Bio-electronic Regulatory Medicine', 'Bio-resonance Therapy' and 'Psionic Medicine'.)

Bradford, Thomas Lindsley

This distinguished US homoeopath was professor of Medical History at the Hahnemann Medical College, Philadelphia, Pennsylvania, as well as its Chief Librarian, towards the very end of the nineteenth century. He was also a Senior of the American Institute of Homoeopathy and an officer of the Philadelphia County Homoeopathic Medical Society.

Abounding contradictions and vague statements concerning the exact location of Hahnemann's final resting-place in Montmartre Cemetery, Paris, France provided the impulse for him to have his colleague professor Platt (of the Chemistry department at the Hahnemann Medical College) search for Hahnemann's real grave in that cemetery. Bradford reported in detail in the *Hahnemannian Monthly* of October 1896. The relevant section reads:

> 'Grave no.9 in the 16th section, stated to be Hahnemann's grave, was the grave of Hahnemann's widow. It had the inscription: Marie Melanie d'Hervilly, Vve de Chrétien Frederic Samuel Hahnemann, née le 2 février, 1800, decedée le 27 mai, 1878, – Maman – amour – toujours. (Born 2nd February, 1800, died 27th May, 1878, – Mother – love – forever.)'

More of Platt's report was given: 'The inscription is very weather-beaten. A number of laurel wreaths are deposited on the grave.'

It followed that Hahnemann's grave had to be the adjacent one, no.8, in the same row. On this point Bradford quoted Platt:

> 'Grave no.8 has no inscription, only C.P. (concession perpétuelle) 1832-1834. This block is entered in the cemetery books under the name of Lethière. But on perusal of the books it was found that this is Hahnemann's real resting-place. . . . Your small photograph is a good representation of the grave and that is fortunate; for I did not manage to get a photograph and an attempt to draw a sketch for you resulted in my being threatened with imprisonment if I did not immediately destroy the sketch on the very spot. It is forbidden by [French] law to make any sketch in the cemetery.'

Bradford's report goes on to describe how the municipality of Paris was being owed 110 French francs (= US$22) because the grave occupied somewhat more ground than had originally been paid for, and of how the municipality had lost all trace of any person connected with that grave. Imminent disinterment was threatened. Platt had 'asked the cemetery authorities to have a little patience and to delay the exhumation for a time until' he had 'received a reply from the United States of America.' It was with this article that Bradford set in motion the chain of events that eventually led to Hahnemann's reburial among the famous and the highly honoured, now lying buried in the Père Lachaise cemetery (recorded under 'Hahnemann, Christian Friedrich Samuel (1755-1843)').

Bradford's literary output concerns itself with historical and other reference material pertinent to homoeopathy:

Homoeopathic Bibliography of the United States (1892)

The Life and Letters of Dr Samuel Hahnemann (1895)

The Pioneers of Homoeopathy (1898)

The Logic of Figures (1900)

Index to Homoeopathic Provings (1901)

The last-mentioned is one of only eleven drug source references recognized by the Homoeopathic Pharmacopoeia of the United States for the US Homoeopathic Dispensatory and List of Drugs. In *The Logic of Figures* Bradford carefully compares (in detail) the death rates in orthodox medical hospitals against the death rates in homoeopathic hospitals. In it he established that the overall percentage death rate in homoeopathic hospitals was from one-half to, occasionally, one-eighth that of orthodox medical hospitals; the comparison was particularly significant in the case of epidemics (Asiatic cholera, typhoid fever, etc.).

(See 'Cholera Epidemics', 'Epidemiology' and 'Verdi, Tullio Suzzara (1829-1902)'.)

Bran

A by-product of the milling of certain grains (notably wheat, rye, barley, oats) and of the polishing process of others (particularly rice [Oryza Sativa] and water-rice [Zizania Aquatica]). It contains approximately 20% of indigestible cellulose, and has, for this reason, been indiscriminately prescribed as a bulk cathartic, in the form of special cereal, or bran, products. It is well known that this approach very frequently leads to a notable aggravation of the condition it is intended to cure. Since no substance is homoeopathically inert, and since pathogenetic experiments with various grasses of the natural order Graminaceae have clearly established that these are capable of eliciting a reactive response in provers, and given the patient's 'altered state of receptivity' (refer to this entry) in his disease, it is hardly surprising that substantial doses of such substances will produce an aggravation. Homoeopathic pathogenetic experiments have been carried out on:

Triticum repens (Quitch-grass, very closely related to Triticum aestivum, which is wheat)

Secale cereale (rye)

Avena sativa (oats)

and they form part of the materia medica. (Thomas Lindsley Bradford, *Index to Homoeopathic Provings*, Philadelphia: Boericke & Tafel, 1901.) (See 'Aggravation', 'Dietary Therapy', 'Foods as Health Problems', 'Homoeopathic Practice', section Supportive Diet, 'Nutritional Equipoise' and 'Obesity'.)

Bruise

Contusion without rupture of the skin, that may produce a haematoma. (See 'Emergencies – Homoeopathic Treatment'.)

Burnett, James Compton (1840-1901)

Great-uncle of Dame Margery Blackie and one of the most renowned writers among British homoeopaths of the nineteenth century. He had studied medicine in Vienna, Austria, but returned to take his Glasgow MB in 1872. His ability to expound the principles and clinical efficacy of homoeopathy stimulated much serious interest in this scientific system. He was an 'organotropic' prescriber and a supporter of Johann Gottfried Rademacher's concepts of Paracelsic 'Organopathy'. He also worked with enthusiasm with sarcodes and nosodes, and introduced Bacillinum to homoeopathy. He was the man who originated the concept of 'vaccinosis' – the disease triggered by vaccination – in the mid-1890s and the certainly the first practitioner to study this systematically.

His major literary work is recognized as:

The Prevention of Congenital Malformation Defects (1881)

His other important writings include:

Curability of Cataract with Medicines (1882)

Enlarged Tonsils Cured by Medicines (1883)

Curability of Tumours by Medicine (1884)

Diseases of the Skin from the Organismic Stand-Point (1886)

Ringworm: its Constitutional Nature and Cure (1888)

The Diseases of the Liver (1890)

Fifty Reasons for being a Homoeopath (1892)

Organ Disease of Women (1893)

Gout and Its Cure (1894)

Delicate, Backward, Puny and Stunted Children (1895)

Tumours of the Breast (1896)

Vaccinosis (2nd edn) (1897)

The Change of Life in Women (1898)

C

Calcination

Rendering white like chalk by expelling, through heat, from a chemico-organic compound, such as bones or plant material, all water, carbon dioxide and volatile matter. Calcined material has been added back to the succus when a so-called spagyric mother tincture is made in homoeopathy. (See 'Spagyric'.)

Cancerinic Miasma

Oncotic miasma. (See 'Miasma'.)

Carbonic Constitution

See 'Constitutional Type'.

Carbo-Nitrogenoid Constitution

See 'Constitutional Type'.

Carbo-Phosphoric Constitution

See 'Constitutional Type'.

Causal Similarity in Disease and Drug Action

See 'Disease and Drug Action in Homoeopathic Congruity'.

Causation

● **Origin or source of some change; in illness the body tries to change for the better, which homoeopathy encourages.**

Action of bringing about, by the operation of causal energy; its result is termed 'the effect'. Homoeopathic medicinal action is normally very specifically aimed at the level of operation of causal energy generated by the patient's dynamis. That of other medical systems is always specifically directed elsewhere (e.g. the enantiopathic [palliative] at the effect; the allopathic at provoking a second distracting energy operation). Despite that, these other systems also have, *nolens volens*, an effect at the level of operation of causal energy, inchoate though this may be. Consequently, the homoeopath takes into anamnestic consideration all other therapeutic approaches, even those that seem innocuous. (See

'Aetiology', 'Aetiotropism' and 'Disease and Drug Action in Homoeopathic Congruity', section 2.)

Causes of Disease

● **The reason for becoming ill is to be found in the body's vulnerability as well as in some other influence, that may interfere mechanically, chemically or, most often, dynamically.**

The Greek homoeopath George Vithoulkas, who speaks of three planes (mental, emotional, physical) which are affected by disease, has summarized the definition of wellness of the whole human being as follows: [1]

> 'Health is freedom from pain in the physical body, having attained a state of well-being; freedom from passion on the emotional level, having as a result a dynamic state of serenity and calm; and freedom from selfishness in the mental sphere, having as a result total unification with Truth.'

He goes on to define the measurement for an individual's comparative degree of illness (or wellness):

> 'What is the parameter that defines, for instance, whether an individual with rheumatoid arthritis is in better health than another one suffering from depression? The parameter which enables such measurement of health is creativity. By creativity, I mean all those acts and functions which promote for the individual himself and for others their main goal in life: continuous and unconditional happiness. To the extent that an individual is limited in the exercise of his creativity, to that degree he is ill. If the rheumatoid arthritis patient is crippled to the extent that his ailment prevents him from being creative more than the patient with depression, then the rheumatoid arthritis patient is more seriously ill than the depressed one . . .'

He adds clarity and coherence to creativity against which mental illness or wellness, the most crucial in an individual's existence, can be measured:

> 'A healthy mind should be characterized in its functions from the following three qualities: clarity, coherence and creativity. To the extent that any or all of these qualities are reduced or missing, the person is ill . . .'

Here Vithoulkas deals with the observable manifestations of disease and/or state of health, but the question that arises is: How does disease take hold? At least two elements constitute disease:

1 The predisposing quality of the organism.
    This is the bias and character of its particular reactive force as evidenced in the particular constitution. It imparts an individuality to each disease state. Moreover, this quality predetermines whether or not, and if at all, in what way, and to which degree, the individual might succumb to the

[1]Vithoulkas, George. *The Science of Homoeopathy,* Wellingborough: Thorsons Publishing Group, 1986, p 41.

secondary determinants of disease. This is the individualizing element of disease.

2 The secondary determinants, the external provocations of disease.

These obey a fixed law of constancy, which allows for the customary grouping of disease patterns in terms of a recognizable aetiology, an identifiable group of common signs, and/or consistent anatomical alterations. This is the generalizing element of disease.

Looking at the question quite differently and applying yet another criterion of classification, as Stuart Close has done,[1] the organism may be said to be acted upon in a disease process in one of three ways:

(i) mechanically, (ii) chemically, or (iii) dynamically. The causes of disease can also be grouped under these three categories.

Mechanical causes of disease include injuries, foreign bodies, extraneous substances, many congenital defects, osteopathic lesions, amputations, or growths. Such conditions would primarily require treatment by osteopathy, chiropractic, physiotherapy, surgery or hygiene, assisted by homoeopathic treatment. Hahnemann repeatedly instructed homoeopaths first to remove the exciting cause or foreign agent that may be present in any diseased condition. For example, parasites and entozoa, when their presence gives rise to disease, must be expelled, either by mechanical means or by such medicines as would be capable of weakening or destroying them, without in any way endangering or adversely affecting the patient ('prima non nocerum' is the Hippocratic precept for all physicians held absolutely inviolate by homoeopathy). As an example Cucurbita pepo (pumpkin seed), which is one of the most efficient and yet harmless taeniafuges, might be used by a homoeopath. [Preparation: Scald the seeds; peel off outer skins when softened; the green inner pulp is the part used. Dose: 50g of seed yield 25g of pulp. May be mixed with cream and taken like porridge, followed in two hours by 15ml Bofareira Θ (castor-oil).]

Chemical causes of disease are acids, alkalis, esters, salts, saponins, alkaloids, a large number of poisons, and the like. Yet such destructive agents also always have secondary dynamical effects, which fall within the ambit of homoeopathy. In such cases the use of chemical or physiological antidotes is required, combined, in some cases, with the means for the physical expulsion of the injurious substance (e.g. stomach-pump). Thereafter, homoeopathic treatment is necessary for the correction of the functional derangements which remain or follow.

Dynamical causes of disease, which influence the reactive functions of the total patient are very numerous: they may be emotional, climatic, electro-magnetic, radiation-induced, atmospheric, telluric or thermic; they may be found in diet, contagion, lack of hygiene, infection, allergic predisposition, pharmacophilia (use and abuse of all hard drugs and medications), or result from pervious constitutional resistance to the pathogenetic effects of specific

[1]Close, Stuart. *The Genius of Homoeopathy*, New York: Boericke and Tafel, 1924, pp 42-44.

toxins exuded by certain micro-organisms. With regard to the last-named, homoeopathy is on record as consistently being highly successful in treating 'serious' disease associated with failing resistance to bacteria, protozoa, rickettsiae and viruses whenever large epidemics permitted statistically significant comparisons with comparable non-homoeopathic approaches, such as in:

Asiatic Cholera, Diphtheria, Typhoid Fever (bacterial)
Malaria (protozoan)
Typhus (rickettsial)
Yellow Fever or Viral Pneumonia (viral).

In all instances this was achieved solely by internal homoeopathic medicines, without resorting to bactericides, chemobiotics, antivirals or antibiotics that might produce allopathic after-effects. (See also 'Disease', 'Epidemiology', 'Homoeopathic Laws, Postulates and Precepts' and 'Miasma'.)

Celsus, Aulus Cornelius (25 BC-50 AD)

See 'Philosophical Premise of Homoeopathy'.

Centesimal Potency

See 'Potentizing Methods'.

Cerate

Unctuous preparation, more solid than an ointment, containing enough wax to preclude it from melting when applied to the skin. Its use has become rare in homoeopathy. (See 'Cetaceum', 'Ointment' and 'Vehicle'.)

Cetaceum

Spermaceti; a waxy substance obtained from the head of the sperm whale, which is chiefly used (now less frequently) to add firmness to the bases of homoeopathic ointments. (See 'Cerate', 'Ointment' and 'Vehicle'.)

Characteristic

Any well-marked, typical feature, attribute or trait which will serve as a distinguishing peculiarity or quality. (See 'Key-Note'.)

Chemical Causes of Disease

See 'Causes of Disease'.

Children's Remedies

See 'Paediatric Remedies'.

Children's Types

See 'Constitutional Type'.

Chilliness

Frissons; sensation of cold, usually with pallor, shivering and cutis anserina (gooseflesh), accompanied by a compensating elevation of temperature in the interior of the body; this symptom signals the organism's reactive engagement and is, therefore, often prodromal of a full disease state. As a symptom component, it features prominently in many homoeopathic drug pictures. As an example of a 'guiding symptom' for prescription some syndetic pointers to two homoeopathic medicines involving 'chilliness' are:

Chilliness commencing generally between shoulder-blades with shuddering after every drink with burning affections of the mucous membranes, or with pain in distant parts on coughing (e.g. in knees, bladder, legs, etc.) – Capsicum annuum

In the debilitated, despondent patient with great weakness in the chest, chilliness and chattering of teeth often with cold hands and numbness of fingertips – Stannum metallicum

Chiropractic

Method of diagnosis, prevention and treatment which deals primarily with mechanical causes of disturbances of the nervous system and their correction by manipulative means. It, consequently, deals with functional disorders (mainly, though not exclusively, musculo-skeletal), caring for the human frame in health and disease, with specific manual spinal adjustments or other forms of manipulation as well as various other forms of supportive treatment. This therapeutic approach is widely considered to be complementary to homoeopathy.

Cholera Epidemics

In 1831 an epidemic of Asiatic Cholera swept with tremendous speed and virulence from Asia through Russia into the Austrian province of Galicia and from there into Prussia and the Electorate of Saxony. Soon it had moved into most other parts of the huge Dual Monarchy (Austro-Hungary), only to proceed westward from there into the rest of Europe. In the absence of adequate sanitary and hygienic conditions anywhere in Europe at that time, the authorities were helpless, while the orthodox physicians had neither an effective treatment nor knew any preventive measures. Hahnemann resolutely published four dissertations on Cholera from June to October of that year, refusing any fee from the publishers. These tracts, of course, aroused bitter antagonism in certain quarters and in a number of districts (including his home county of Coethen) the medical councils had medical censors legally installed by the political authorities who suppressed these dissertations with the words of the Protomedicus: 'Pro typis non est qualificatum' (not suitable for printing). Hahnemann's assessment of the Asiatic Cholera in general, and of that epidemic in particular, is summarized hereunder. It is as well to bear in mind that Louis Pasteur was not nine years old and Robert Koch was yet to be born twelve years hence, when Hahnemann wrote the words quoted here, that are a measure of his intuitively unerring grasp of the nature of things.

1 Cholera Asiatica is an acute miasma (see 'Miasma'), which means it always arises from the same contagion;

2 This contagion he referred to as a 'brood of excessively minute, invisible, living creatures' and as 'the most minute animals of a low order' and he says further 'the Cholera miasma . . . probably consists of a murderous organism, undetected by our senses, which attaches itself to a man's skin, hair, etc. or to his clothing and is thus transferred invisibly from man to man'.

3 The remedy best suited to the character of that epidemic was Camphora, in the initial stage of the disease, to be given in a tablespoonful of water every five minutes (or with some sugar); in the advanced (second or third) stages of the disease he recommended the homoeopathic use of Cuprum metallicum, Veratrum album, Bryonia alba and Rhus toxicodendron (the last two in alternation with one another). (See 'Epidemiology'.)

4 For the removal of the offending cause and as a protective measure against its further propagation his instructions are this: 'In order to make the infection and spreading of Cholera impossible, the garments, the linen, etc., of all strangers arriving there have to be kept in quarantine (whilst their bodies are cleansed by speedy baths and provided with clean clothes of linen or fustian suitable for the house) and retained there for two hours in a stove heat of 80 degrees' [Réaumur =100 degrees Celsius] '(at which a vessel of water would boil). – This represents a heat at which all known infectious matters, and consequently the living miasma, are annihilated.' He continued by laying special emphasis on the greatest cleanliness, ventilation, and disinfection of living and sleeping rooms.

Hahnemann and all those who practised homoeopathy then had astonishingly good results with this approach. For instance in Raab, in Austro-Hungary (now Györ, Hungary) the homoeopath Dr Bakody treated 154 Cholera patients from 28th July to 8th September of that year. Of these six died, making the proportion of deaths to recoveries 2:49. In the non-homoeopathic hospitals of that town there were 122 deaths out of 284 cases treated and in private homes, out of 1271 Cholera patients treated by allopaths, 699 died, making the proportion of deaths to recoveries, over the same period, 6:5. A bigoted attack on Dr Bakody was only averted when 112 of his recovered patients produced officially accredited testimonies. Among the signatories were a Canon (in the name of the recovered Bishop), three other Priests, an Evangelical and a

Reformed Church Preacher, a Councillor of the Consistory, a High Court Advocate, and other dignitaries. Similarly good comparative results are recorded for homoeopathy in other parts of the Dual Monarchy: 1:20 in Bruenn, province of Moravia (now Brno, CSFR); 1:26 in Lemberg, capital of Galicia (now Lvov, Ukraine SR); 1:20 in Daka, Hungary; and 1:42 in Vienna. The least favourable, though still very much better than the non-homoeopathic results, were in Vishnii-Volochok, Russia with a ratio of 1:5 and Berlin, Germany with 1:6. One of the victims cured of Cholera homoeopathically in Tischnowitz, Moravia was Dr Frederick Foster Harvey Quin (1799-1878) who introduced homoeopathy to the United Kingdom. He wrote in July 1832 of his cure, 'I owe my life to the Spirit of Camphor . . .'

All other Asiatic Cholera epidemics that have passed through areas where homoeopathy was established produced equally convincing results. An example is the severe cholera outbreak in Liverpool of 1849. The Edinburgh graduate in medicine, John Drysdale, founded the Liverpool Dispensary in 1837, as with all similar records elsewhere, the results with the exclusively homoeopathic treatment given there were outstanding. They were significantly below Orthodoxy's comparable figures, with only a 25% mortality rate. As a result of these statistics Drysdale was invited to the post of physician to the city's Children's Hospital. Despite the fact that he was a close friend of the famous Scottish obstetrician, Sir James Young Simpson (1811-1870), after whom the 'Simpson forceps' are named and who was first to use chloroform as an anaesthetic both in surgery and in labour, the opposition from the orthodox medical establishment to the appointment of a homoeopath was so considerable that Drysdale was eventually forced to withdraw the official application.

The 1854 Asiatic Cholera epidemic of London is discussed under 'Epidemiology'.

Chopping Board and Knife

See 'Utensils of Homoeopathic Pharmacy'.

Chromotherapy

Uses specific colour rays therapeutically on the patient's body. It is an approach that may be complementary to homoeopathy. (See 'Naturopath'.)

Chronic Disease

One of long duration, marked usually by no very violent symptoms; if left untreated, occasionally ending in recovery with the aid of an intercurrent attack of a similar acute disease, failing which, it may eventually end in death through cachexia (wasting away).

In 1828 Hahnemann published *The Chronic Diseases, Their Peculiar Nature and*

Their Homoeopathic Cure, generally referred to simply as *Chronic Diseases*. This, which ranks with *The Organon* and *Materia Medica Pura* as one of his fundamental works, was translated into French by Dr A J L Jourdan and published in Paris 1832 by Editions Baillière. Hahnemann's enlarged second German edition was published in 1835. This version was first somewhat inexactly translated into English by Charles Julius Hempel (1811-1879) and published in New York by William Radde in the years 1845-6. It was only re-translated (all 1600 pages of it) as late as 1896 by Prof Louis H Tafel, with annotations in the materia medica section by Richard Hughes, edited by Pemberton Dudley, and published in Philadelphia, USA by Boericke and Tafel in 1904. The significance of this monumental work lies in the fact that it represents a profound modification by Hahnemann of his hitherto universally prescribed method of application of the law of similars in therapeutic practice. Hahnemann, the tireless researcher and scrupulous observer, had totally revised his stand in the eighteen years since the first edition of *The Organon* (1810), in the light of his clinical experience with chronic diseases. No longer was the homoeopath to apply the law of similars individually to every particular case at all times, regardless of anything else. Instead, when confronted by the debilitation wrought by chronic disease, the homoeopath would henceforward have to identify the class of chronic disease (chronic miasma) and then prescribe a specific remedy for the miasmatic disease in question. This was such an about-face in scientific therapeutics that many supporters defected for a time from the new Hahnemannian position, including, poignantly enough, Ernst Georg Baron von Brunnow, who had translated *The Organon* into French (in gratitude for having had his sight restored by Hahnemann, after other physicians had failed) and to whom *Chronic Diseases* had, ironically, been publicly dedicated by Hahnemann. (See 'Miasma'.)

Chronic Miasma

See 'Miasma' (and entry under 'Chronic Disease').

Chronology of Symptom Variations in Provings and/or Disease

See 'Therapeutic Science'.

Clarke, John Henry (1853-1931)

Eminent UK homoeopath who trained in Edinburgh. He was consultant at the Royal London Homoeopathic Hospital and the editor of *Homoeopathic World*. He presided over the 1906 International Homoeopathic Congress and attended the 66th Annual Session of the American Institute of Homoeopathy in Los Angeles, California, USA from 11th to 16th July 1910, where he was received as an honoured guest. He fell out with his former friend and influential colleague Richard Hughes, whose bitter opponent he became, accusing him, not without reason, of pandering to the allopaths and of being a prescriber of low potencies only. Hughes, he said, was ready to undermine the whole approach to homoeopathy for the sake of trying to make homoeopathy palatable to allopathy. Clarke himself was not a high-potency prescriber but made full use of the entire range of dynamizations. He revelled in controversy and often seemed deliberately to express the opposite view to Richard Hughes. This became an open rift, which damaged – at least in part – the cause of homoeopathy, as did similar strife in the USA also.

Clarke was a prolific writer who made very major contributions to the homoeopathic literature, undoubtedly the foremost among which is *A Dictionary of Practical Materia Medica*. This, together with *A Clinical Repertory of the Dictionary of Materia Medica*, covers a monumental 1981 pages and has remained the standard reference work for over ninety years. Clarke spent sixteen years collecting all available knowledge on homoeopathic drugs. The homoeopath Robert Cooper organized a Dining Club at the end of the nineteenth century, which consisted of himself, John Henry Clarke, James Compton-Burnett and Thomas Skinner. Cooper possessed a prodigious knowledge of many unusual homoeopathic medicines and was of outstanding assistance to Clarke in his compilation of the Dictionary. The later homoeopath Le Hunte Cooper, who was first to examine the possible poisonous effects of aluminium cooking utensils and the effects of Alumina as a remedy, was this Robert Cooper's son. Clarke's major writings include:

The Prescriber 1885
Dictionary of Domestic Medicine 1890
Rheumatism and Sciatica 1892
Therapeutics of Serpent Venoms 1893
Diseases of Glands and Bones 1894
Diseases of Heart and Arteries 1894
Heart Repertory 1896
A Dictionary of Practical Materia Medica 1900
Clinical Repertory 1904
Life and Work of J Compton-Burnett 1904
Homoeopathy Explained 1905
Whooping Cough, cleared with Pertussis 1906
Thomas Skinner, MD 1907
Radium as an Internal Remedy 1908
Vital Economy 1909
Gun powder as a war remedy 1915
Hahnemann and Paracelsus 1923
Constitutional Medicine 1925
Colds, Hay-fever and Influenza 1928
Indigestion – its causes and cure 1928

This industrious author and busy practitioner was utterly devoted to his wife, Helen, to whom he dedicated *The Sword* (see below) with the words penned on the manuscript: 'To his First and Dearest Auditor this Copy of ''The Sword'' is inscribed by The Author'.

In the late 1890s Clarke had read the Aldine edition of William Blake's poems during a very long train journey. 'From that moment,' he said, 'Blake gripped me with a hold which time has only strengthened.' He became an authority on this poet, painter and mystic, and was often asked to read papers to the Blake Society. His non-homoeopathic writings include:

The Sword printed and bound privately for: London: The Financial News, 1917

William Blake on The Lord's Prayer London: The Hermes Press, 1927

From Copernicus to William Blake London: The Hermes Press, 1928

The God of Shelley and Blake London: John M Watkins, 1930

Classical Homoeopathy

Phrase used to describe homoeopathy very strictly interpreted and applied. Classical homoeopathy insists on the use of single, simple, pure drugs that have been deprived of injurious properties and had their curative (reactive) power refined by the Hahnemannian pharmaceutical process of mechanical comminution to scale. Any such remedy will have been selected and employed on the basis of a correspondence between either the symptom-syndrome, or the constitutional type, or the miasmatic predisposition of the patient, or even a combination of any two or three of these factors, compared to a matching set of symptoms recorded in the materia medica, with a strong emphasis generally placed on the 'mentals'. A drug producing such a matching symptom-similarity is said to be homoeopathic to the patient's condition, constitution or chronic miasma, as the case may be. Classical homoeopathy's maxim is:

'Simplex, Simile et Minimum'.

(See also 'Combinations of Homoeopathic Drugs'.)

Clathrate

Cancellate; reticular; resembling a honeycomb. In botany: meshy, or like lattice-work. In chemistry: a form of compound with such a structural attribute, in which one component is linked to (combined with) another by the enclosure of one kind of molecule within the cage-like lattice structure of another, a macromolecule, as, for instance, the inclusion of an inert gas in 1,4-dihydroxybenzene. Clathrate compounds can be used as so-called 'molecular sieves' (e.g. the synthetic zeolites) that can absorb or separate molecules, which are trapped in 'cages' formed by the shape of the crystal lattice. The sizes of these can be selected to suit the given molecule to be captured. In 1977 this structural attribute led the Austrian homoeopath Gerhard Resch to develop and provide evidence for the analogous hypothesis of 'solvation structures' in liquids, specifically in water and in hydro-ethanol mixtures as employed in the process of dynamization (potentization). (See 'Physiological Response in Homoeotherapeutics, Mechanism of' and 'Solvation Structures'.)

Cleansing of Utensils and Sterilization

All utensils should be washed immediately after use. Glass items and bottles should first be kept in a big basin of filtered or unpolluted rain-water for several hours. Then, by means of a hard brush, or a bottle brush, all the inner or work surfaces are to be scrubbed under water in that basin. They should then be washed again individually in cold water, and rubbed with a soft clean linen cloth. Then each item is to be washed again in distilled water and dried in the hot air oven at maximum temperature. Into any phials that have been washed a small quantity of dilute alcohol is then poured.

Porcelain vessels should be washed first with very hot, or boiling, water and then with distilled water and dried like the glassware. The press should be taken apart and washed first with cold water, then with very hot water, and thoroughly dried. Mortars and pestles should first be washed in cold rain-water, then with very hot water and wiped until they are absolutely dry. Then a quantity of alcohol is burned in the mortar with the pestle inside it. If a mortar and pestle set has once been used for preparing one homoeopathic drug (trituration) it should not be used thereafter for the preparation of another, unless the contact surfaces have first been re-ground (rubbed with glass paper) or reglazed, and then washed as described. After mercurial preparations the mortar and pestle is cleaned with nitric acid first.

In the case of reusable therapeutic instruments, sterilization is essential in almost all instances. Prior to sterilization all such equipment is to be cleaned manually to remove traces of any gross impurities, like blood. Autoclaving thereafter is satisfactory. Minimally, such equipment ought to be boiled under a constant pressure of 2kg per cm^2 for 30 minutes. A common form of sterilizer sold for general medical practitioners' surgeries is not adequate for the purpose of sterilization of, say, reusable (gold and silver) acupuncture needles, or hypodermic needles, whereas the previously described procedure is. Following sterilization, the equipment may either be stored under absolute alcohol, or stored dry, after drying in the hot air oven. (See also 'Utensils of Homoeopathic Pharmacy'.)

Clinical Proving

See 'Sources of Homoeopathic Drug Semiology'.

Clinical Trials

To study the safety, efficacy and quality, and/or more specifically special precautions, possible drug interactions and so-called adverse drug reactions, orthodox medicine conducts trials to establish the effects of its drugs on people. Prior to this, however, mathematical formulae are arrived at to determine a quantitative assessment of the likelihood of the drug's producing toxic effects. They are almost invariably derived from animal experiments and are not necessarily useful in humans. Clinical trials are not to be confounded with 'clinical usage' (refer to this entry).

Definitions

Minimum Lethal Dose: Average between smallest dose that kills and the largest dose that does not kill.

Median Lethal Dose (or LD 50): Dose which kills half of a population, normally expressed as mg of drug/kg animal.

(Note: The homoeopaths were the first to point out, and it has recently been generally accepted, that species differences make these indices useless as guides to the lethal dose in a different species.)

Therapeutic Index: Attempts to measure the therapeutic value of an orthodox drug by relating the useful dose to the toxic dose. Paul Ehrlich (1854-1915), the Nobel laureate for his work on immunity, proposed the ratio – maximum tolerated dose to minimum curative dose. This, however, did not take into account the variability of a normally distributed population. It was replaced by the formula LD 50 : ED 50 (ED = effective dose). Yet this ignored the margins between the safe and the effective doses. So it was replaced by the formula LD 0.1 : ED 99.9 which is the ratio between the dose killing 1 in a 1000 and the dose which would cure all but 1 in a 1000.

Standard Safety Margin: Expressed as the percentage increase above the therapeutic dose which is lethal to a given proportion of subjects. (Example: The standard safety margin of phenobarbitone in mice is 8%: the dose producing sleep in 99.9% has to be increased by only 8% to become lethal to 1% of the mouse population).

There are other tests on animals: e.g. behavioral changes may be assessed (spontaneous motor activity depressed or stimulated?); there may be monitoring of alteration in body temperature and body weight; evaluation of potentiation of the coercive pharmacological effect of substances such as hexobarbital, apomorphine, amphetamine, etc.; gauging reactivity in the hot-plate and writhing syndrome tests; appraisal of any protective effect against electro-shock and pentylenetetrazol-induced seizures; measuring any changes in the concentration of serum oestradiol or the level of serum prolactin; and much more like it.

When these preliminary animal experiments have yielded their formulae and statistics the drug is first tested on human volunteers to begin to establish possible dosage levels for this species. Then the drug will be investigated in patients with the disease that it is hoped to cure, in a therapeutic trial that is usually carefully designed, with the aims set down in great detail, spelling out the type of case to be included and the exact questions it is hoped the trial will answer. Of particular interest are comparisons with existing drugs and pre-existing conditions affecting the patient. Often a double-blind technique is employed and statistical tests of significance are applied to assess the probability of observed clinical effects. (Note: The use of clinical trials denies completely the value of individual cases, which are viewed by orthodoxy as too subjective to allow of generalizations.)

Homoeopathy has never had any truck with the sort of animal experimentation described above (see 'Animal Experiments'). Traditionally, homoeopathy has confirmed, through clinical usage (not to be confused with clinical trials), what the law of similars indicates (see 'Usage, Clinical'). At odd times, however, it has conducted its own double-blind clinical trials (refer to the Mustard Gas 30CH experiment under 'Nitrum cum Sulphuri Praecipitati et Carboni'; the confinements experiments under 'Combinations of Homoeopathic Drugs'; the two hayfever experiments under 'Allergy'; and the Oscillococcinum experiment under 'Isopathy', section 1 Nosode (ii) of animal origin). Three other recent double-blind clinical trials are:

1 Patients with rheumatoid arthritis were individually prescribed a homoeopathic medicine, but only half received it, while the other half received a placebo. Result: 82% of those given the homoeopathic medicine experienced some relief of their symptoms, whereas only 21% of those given the placebo experienced a comparable degree of improvement. [1]

2 Patients with influenza were given either a homoeopathic combination remedy (of ten component drugs) or a placebo. They were two coded unknowns. This was under the direction of Professor Paul Casanova and other medical practitioners who did not practise homoeopathy, at the Department of Infectious Illnesses of the Felix Houphouet-Boigny Hospital, Marseilles, France. Statistically highly significant results in favour of the combination remedy were achieved in improvement in all the following: [2]

   bronchial congestion
   nocturnal coughing
   rhinorrhoea
   day-time coughing
   recourse to antibiotics after treatment
   speed of recovery patients' subjective assessments

3 Female patients between the ages of 20 and 60 with nervous depression were given either a homoeopathic combination remedy (of ten component drugs) or the benzodiazepine diazepam. Result: After 30 days of treatment, the homoeopathic combination remedy was found to be as effective as diazepam on thymo-effective parameters, on hot flushes, tachycardia, shortness of breath, intestinal problems, micturition frequency, dyspareunia and dizzy

[1] Gibson, R G, S L M Gibson, A D MacNeil, *et al.* 'Homoeopathic Therapy in Rheumatoid Arthritis: Evaluation by Double-Blind Controlled Trial', *British Journal of Clinical Pharmacology,* vol IX, 1980, pp 453-459.

[2] Casanova, Paul, *et al.* 'L.52 – A Flu Treatment', published by Dr Ph. Lecocq, Metz: Lehning Laboratories Publications, 1988

spells; there were no weight changes; there was a lowering of the pulse rate, a marked increase in the number of hours of sleep; there were no cases of addiction and no potentiation of the effects of alcohol, although 10% of the large sample was, as it happened, alcohol-dependent.[1]

One of the many problems with clinical trials in homoeopathy is that either (in the single remedy approach) there is a very large number of remedies used (in rheumatoid arthritis, perhaps 200 different ones) which may be continually changed according to the individual and his changing symptoms, or combinations of remedies are used, which many homoeopaths decry as intolerable 'unhomoeopathic' polypharmacy. In an attempt to come to terms with these problems, a double-blind experiment was conducted on patients suffering from a rheumatological disease, fibrositis. The ingenious research design allowed the homoeopaths only a choice of three remedies from which to prescribe (Arnica montana, Bryonia alba, Rhus toxicodendron). There was no statistical difference between the group given a placebo and that given the homoeopathic medicine. However, part of the intricate research design was to evaluate the accuracy in homoeopathic prescription itself. A panel of homoeopaths, who did not know in advance which patients had experienced improvement, were asked to evaluate the accuracy of the prescriptions. Result: This subsequent evaluation showed a statistically significant difference between those given a placebo and those subjects who, in terms of the panel's consensus, had actually received the correct homoeopathic drug.[2] Clearly individualization is essential in single-remedy homoeopathy.

Another problem is by what homoeopathic criterion is medicinal effectiveness to be evaluated? For example, it happens often enough that the physical symptoms of disease may have disappeared but that the patient has developed severe anxiety instead. This could be called a change in the centre of gravity of a disease process. Is Hering's rule of direction of cure to be applied? This states that a homoeopathically well-indicated medicine causes symptoms to disappear in the reverse order of their original appearance (see 'Homoeopathic Laws, Postulates and Precepts' section 14). Perhaps George Vithoulkas' rule of a shift in the 'centre of gravity' as an evaluation of improvement/deterioration is to be applied? This states that any downward shift of signs and symptoms in the listings immediately below clearly signifies improvement is occurring in the individual's general health, with a concomitant shift away from the adverse 'mentals' into the 'emotional' or 'physical' columns:[3]

[1]Drs Depis, Fineltan, Hamzaoui, L'Homme and Magonnier. 'Random Trial of L.72 (a Homoeopathic Speciality) against Diazepam 2 in Cases of Nervous Depression. A Balance Sheet of 60 Random Observations of a Female Population, Age 20 to 60', published by Dr B Heulluy, Paris: Centre for Therapeutic Research and Documentation, 1988.
[2]Fisher, Peter. 'An Experimental Double-Blind Trial Method in Homoeopathy: Use of a Limited Range of Remedies to Treat Fibrositis', British Homoeopathic Journal, LXXVIII, 1986, pp 142-147.
[3]Vithoulkas, George. The Science of Homoeopathy, Wellingborough: Thorsons Publishing Group, 1986, pp 23-44.

Mental	Emotional	Physical
Complete mental confusion	Suicidal depression	Brain ailments
Destructive delirium	Apathy	Heart ailments
Paranoid ideas	Sadness	Endocrine ailments
Delusions	Anguish	Liver ailments
Lethargy	Phobias	Lung ailments
Dullness	Anxiety	Kidney ailments
Lack of concentration	Irritability	Bone ailments
Forgetfulness	Dissatisfaction	Muscle ailments
Absentmindedness		Skin ailments

UK veterinary homoeopath Christopher Day gave Caulophyllum thalictroides 30CH to sows that had an established high rate of stillbirths. Result: Those sows which were given the placebo had a 20.8% rate of stillbirths, whereas those which received the homoeopathic medicine had their rate reduced to 10.3%.[1]

Three UK homoeopathic scientists working at an orthodox school of pharmacy found that rodents given Hypericum perforatum 30CH were able to remain on a hot plate longer than those given water (placebo). During a second test with Hypericum perforatum 30CH, the rodents were also given the narcotic-antagonist naloxone hydrochloride, which is known chemically to inhibit the endorphin (pain-dampening) response of the organism. In fact, the naloxone reduced the protective effects of the homoeopathic Hypericum perforatum 30CH. Since naloxone will reduce the pain-killing effect of morphine, it was inferred that the homoeopathic medicine might work along the same biochemical pathways as morphine.[2] (Note: This last experiment must be considered as an unacceptable infringement of the rights of animals.)

Close, Stuart (1860-1929)

US homoeopath of more than passing relevance during the first quarter of the twentieth century, who was professor of Homoeopathic Philosophy from 1909 to 1913 at the New York Homoeopathic Medical College. These were stirring times at that medical school: for instance, in 1904 Dr V L Getman had begun the original pathogenetic experiments with the sarcode Adrenalinum upon the students, and other similar pioneering work had subsequently been undertaken there. Also the damaging effects of the political manoeuvrings by George Henry Simmons (1852-1937) (see entry under this name) were beginning to have their destructive effect on the homoeopathic medical schools of the USA. Prof Close was consulting physician at the Flower Hospital, NY

[1]Day, Christopher. 'Control of Stillbirths in Pigs Using Homoeopathy', *Veterinary Record*, CXIV, 3rd March, 1984, p 216.
[2]Keysall, G R, K L Williamson, B D Tolman. 'The Testing of Some Homoeopathic Preparations in Rodents', *Proceedings of the XLth Homoeopathic Congress, Lyons, France, 1985*, pp 228-231.

and at the Prospect Heights Hospital, Brooklyn, NY. During that period he was also Assistant Editor of the *Homoeopathic Recorder*. His mentors had been Bernhardt Fincke (1821-1906) and Phineas Parkhurst Wells (1808-1891). His major literary work is:

    The Genius of Homoeopathy: Lectures and Essays on Homoeopathic Philosophy (1924)

Colloid

Submicroscopic aggregate of atoms or molecules of an insoluble substance in a finely dispersed state, either in a solid medium or a liquid, resisting sedimentation, diffusion and filtration, and in this way differing from precipitates. Hahnemann was the first to discover the colloidal solubility of substances insoluble in the crude state. Until as recently as 1915, even homoeopathic pharmacists and their chemical researchers publicly denied the possibility of dissolving insoluble substances in diluted alcohol, as Hahnemann had stated could be done by his method (trituration to the third centesimal potency and then proceeding to further stages of liquid dynamization).[1] A short time later, further chemistry research demonstrated the complete accuracy of Hahnemann's observations about his method of a century earlier. It was proved that all insoluble substances used in homoeopathy, when subjected to Hahnemann's trituration procedures, pass into a colloidal state and remain of a molecular size of 1/1000 micrometre (previously 'micron'). Furthermore, the chemical reactions of such preparations show, even at an 8DH potency, that the effects of a substance dissolved colloidally differ from those of the same solid non-colloidal substance. (See also 'Microscope' and 'Suspension'.)

Colonic Irrigation

Lavage of the lower bowel. This naturopathic treatment consists in the gradual and gentle introduction of water into the colon via the rectum by a gravity-fed machine. It induces peristalsis by massaging the walls of the colon, at the same time cleaning out impacted material that has accumulated on its walls. Up to 50 litres of water are used during the procedure lasting usually about half an hour, but only about one litre is maintained internally at any time. The water is introduced and expelled each time to allow encrusted waste and mucus to be carried away. This therapeutic approach to bowel hygiene is thought by many homoeopaths to be complementary to homoeopathy. (See also 'Naturopath'.)

---

[1] In the *Berlin Homoeopathic Journal* of that year (1915) chemist Hoyer of Dresden, who was interested in homoeopathic drugs and their chemical structure, wrote: 'It is a mistake of Hahnemann when he says that the insoluble substances then dissolve in the diluted alcohol. Modern science has proved that divisibility of insoluble bodies has a limit.'

Colour Therapy

See 'Chromotherapy'.

Combinations of Homoeopathic Drugs

Hahnemann vehemently attacked allopathic and enantiopathic polypharmacy from 1797 onward. For a time, he had seriously considered conducting provings of combinations of homoeopathic drugs, but he abandoned this course. As a result he wrote that no a priori conclusion could be drawn concerning the powers of a compound medicine and, moreover, that nature likes simplicity, effecting much with one remedy, but little with many. He ultimately expressed himself quite unequivocally (section 273 *Organon of Medicine*): 'In no case under treatment is it necessary and therefore not permissible to administer to a patient more than one single, simple medicinal substance at one time.' This has remained the position of all homoeopaths practising in the classical tradition. However, quite recently the thirteen last case-books of Hahnemann's eight final years of practice in Paris have been made public. They are now housed in the 'Institut für Geschichte der Medizin der Robert Bosch Stiftung' in Stuttgart, Germany. From an analysis of these, a rather different picture has emerged. It can be said that Hahnemann, contrary to previously held assumptions:

a) used alternating remedies frequently;

b) employed two remedies simultaneously (he would sometimes use a chronic remedy constantly and not discontinue it when treating an arising acute);

c) would use 'supporting', or 'organ remedies' for particular organs (e.g. unpotentized Digitalis for a heart condition), while using other remedies in potency;

d) was guided by symptoms whenever these appeared and treated them immediately, whether they were the result of aggravation, the reoccurrence of old ones, or the onset of an acute condition, making the most recent symptom the basis for his choice of drug;

e) often administered one remedy to be inhaled and another to be taken orally, practically at the same time (certainly on the same day), and on some occasions the two remedies involved were what are now considered to be incompatible;

f) repeated the remedies frequently (every day, three times daily, up to six times daily);

g) the potencies he used were 3C, 6C, 12C, 18C, 24C and 30C; later he additionally used any potency between 95C and 200C and the quinquagenimillesimal(LM) potencies;

h) diluted the remedies in water and succussed them, thus slightly changing the potency at the time of administration of the medicine;

i) employed placebos whenever he wanted to observe the disease process;

j) had no conception of what later became known as 'constitutional prescribing', but that in all chronic cases he did 'prescribe miasmatically' (e.g. he would prescribe Sulphur to clear any chronic Psora) and then proceeded to treat on other symptoms, as above.[1]

The records also show that he was rather successful with this method of treatment.

In what is cynically seen by many as a politically motivated emulation of orthodox medicine's expedient acceptance of the 'proprietaries' forty-five years previously, the American Institute of Homoeopathy in the USA did a volte-face on the Hahnemannian position on the combination of remedies in homoeopathy. On 17th June, 1948 the American Institute of Homoeopathy, which, in the twentieth century, is often taken to represent the classical tradition, surprisingly approved a resolution, which was, moreover, reaffirmed by this Body on 11th February, 1981, and which has been officially incorporated into the Homoeopathic Pharmacopoeia of the United States (Supplement A – 1982, page 76) stating: 'That combinations of homoeopathic medicines are within the scope and tenets of Homoeopathy provided each component is listed in the Homoeopathic Pharmacopoeia of the United States.' (See 'Simmons, George Henry (1852-1937)' for details of the relevant issues forty-five years prior to 1948.) Combinations of homoeopathic drugs, of which the constituent remedies are nearly always in the Θ to 30CH potency range, are in general use by many homoeopaths (amongst many others, notably naturopaths) internationally now, and through therapeutic observation have come to be accepted by them as an essential part of their 'homoeopathic' armamentarium.

Additionally, many pharmacists provide some of these homoeopathic combinations for simpler cases on an over-the-counter basis, prescribing them pathologically, in preference to non-homoeopathic drugs that may produce injurious reactions. This, in turn, has established widespread confidence in the non-coercive efficacy of the homoeopathic medical system as a whole in the minds of previously sceptical patients. The problem of possible antidotal effects between simultaneously administered homoeopathic drugs of similar action, and other problems, are discussed under the entry for 'Antidote'. On the other hand, the predicament that inevitably arises out of the concomitant non-individualization in such 'homoeopathic shotgun' prescriptions, also resulting, as might be expected, occasionally in total therapeutic ineffectiveness, is highlighted under the entry for 'Headache'. In 1988 the president of the International Institute for Homoeopathic Research, Claude Bergeret, published the *Guide Pratique de Complexisme Homéopathique* [Paris: Maloine, 1988] on this perplexing subject. Yet when all the political, economic and convenience arguments are put to one side, the abiding impression haunting many homoeopaths is that prescribing a combination remedy simply constitutes bad

[1] Handley, Rima. 'Classical Hahnemannian Homoeopathy or What Hahnemann Really Did: Preliminary Observations', based on an address delivered to the Conference of the Society of Homoeopaths in September 1987 at Keele University. *The Wholistic Practitioner*, 1989, vol V(1), pp 25-33.

homoeopathy, at best, because there can never be proper individualization. Homoeopathic medicines are combined in a specific way and then mass produced in order to target them at specific non-homoeopathic disease entities. It means, at the very least, that there is an implicit claim being made for the efficacy of the combination by the manufacturer. In a sense it is a pharmaceutical specific. Legislation worldwide is tending toward requiring the producers of specifics and of such combinations to submit them to clinical trials to substantiate the said claims. This procedure is extremely costly and fraught with numerous difficulties, so that it seems possible that a number of the combination remedies now freely available over the pharmacy counter may disappear in their present form in the near future.

Nonetheless, the question remains pertinent whether it would not be better for some individual to self-medicate with a harmless combination remedy making unsubstantiated claims rather than with, say, phenacetin, paracetamol or aspirin, with the consumption of which, respectively, haemolytic anaemia, necrosis of liver cells, gastro-intestinal bleeding, or even Reye's syndrome, all remain a real risk. The worst that can result from unfounded claims in such instances of self-medication is a self-limiting effect, in that the particular combination remedy may not be bought again.

Experimental Evidence

The legislative requirements imposed by an increasing number of countries in recent times have spurred on a large number of trials of the more popular homoeopathic combination remedies. One such was the following, unusual double blind, placebo-controlled experiment, that was conducted by Drs Pierre Dorfman, Marie-Noel Laserre and Max Tétau in Paris, France during 1987.[1] It showed the effects of a homoeopathic combination remedy, in contrast to a placebo, administered to 93 pregnant women during their ninth month (from their consultation during the eighth month onward), in preparation for their confinement (labour and childbirth). The combination remedy reduced mean delivery time by 3 hours 38 minutes, and the frequency of foetal and maternal dystocia (difficult childbirth) was brought down by 71.75% (incidence: 11.3% with the homoeopathic combination remedy, against 40% with the placebo). The homoeopathic drugs used in combination were:

Arnica Montana
Caulophyllum Thalictroides
Cimicifuga Racemosa (Macrotys, Actea Racemosa)
Gelsemium Sempervirens
Pulsatilla Nigricans.

The main guiding symptoms from the experimental pathogeneses in the materia medica, which prompted the investigators to use these homoeopathic

---

[1]Dorfman, P, M-N Lasserre and M Tétau. 'Préparation à l'Accouchement par Homéopathie: Experimentation en Double Insu versus Placebo'. *Cahiers de Biothérapie*, April 1987, No.94, pp 77-81.

remedies in combination, are reported for each under the entry for 'Antenatal Homoeopathy'.

(See also 'Classical Homoeopathy', 'Eclipse of Homoeopathy (1920-1965)', 'Hempel, Charles Julius (1811-1879)', 'Individualization' and 'Mother Tincture'.)

Comminution

Breaking or grinding of plant material into small fragments.

Commitment to Homoeopathy

The deeply rooted principles of homoeopathy are embedded in a cohesive system of scientific laws, postulates and rules, the practical application of which, in the execution of any technical medical process, permits of no fundamental deviation from these integrated principles. Any elaboration in homoeopathy can only take place within its cohesive scientific system. This, accordingly, demands that homoeopathy be approached universally by its practitioners from an appropriately consistent mental standpoint.

Compatibility of Homoeopathic and Orthodox Drugs

The drugs of orthodox pharmacy are generally suppressive, acting not only on the damaging elements of pathology, but inevitably also on the central healing process itself. Homoeopathic drugs, on the other hand, act by supporting the body's healing efforts. Although the two are, therefore, absolutely incompatible, in that they work in opposition to each other, experience has shown that the power of a well-indicated homoeopathic drug is such that, despite the severely inhibiting consequences of non-homoeopathic medicines, it will override these and act beneficially even where the very pronounced immunosuppressive effects of steroids may be involved, that all but paralyse the vital healing process. In practice, therefore, the homoeopath will not deprive his seriously affected patient of the essential relief (palliation) afforded by orthodox medication until he has managed to set the patient's central healing process in motion in the direction of positive cure. Even then he may prefer to do it gradually, since an abrupt deprivation of habituated allopathica or phytopharmaca can itself produce dynamically adverse effects in the patient, that may sometimes be of a grave nature. Such an adverse rebound effect is likely to be particularly pronounced in the wake of withdrawals of any of the following classes of present-day allopathica:

Class of allopathica	Non-Homoeopathic disease appellations for which commonly used
Anticholinergics	Parkinson's Disease
Anticonvulsants	Epilepsy

Class of allopathica	Non-Homoeopathic disease appellations for which commonly used
Antidepressants	
Antihypertensives	High Blood Pressure
Antispasmodics	Spasticity and Multiple Sclerosis
Beta-Blockers	Angina Pectoris, Myocardial Infarction and Coronary-Artery Disease
Cardiovascular drugs	Cardiovascular problems
Corticosteroids	Allergy, Auto-Immune Disease and diseases thought to be related thereto
Diuretics	Idiopathic Oedema
Hypnotics	Insomnia
Narcotic Anodynes	against intractable pain
Many Psychotropic Drugs	Psychosis, Cyclothymia, Paranoia, Schizophrenia and other psychiatric conditions
Sedatives	
Tranquillizers	

A well-adjusted guide for the homoeopath for effective gradual withdrawal by patients from the 'benzodiazepine' habit is:

Coming Off Tranquillizers and Sleeping Pills by Shirley Trickett (London: Thorsons, 1991, 176 pages).

The fact that all drugs produce multiple reactions in the organism (i.e. a whole range of 'unwanted' effects in addition to its 'desired' action as publicized) means that the homoeopath will want to know exactly what other medication the patient may have been exposed to, before being able to prescribe appropriately. For example, it is not merely the narcotics, hypnotics, barbiturates, anxiolytics, antipsychotics, antidepressants and various other benzodiazepines which can cause pronounced mood modifications in a patient. It has recently been announced by the US Health Research Group[1] that the following commonly prescribed medications, amongst many others, are quite as likely to produce significant mood modifications in patients:

anti-arrhythmics	(disopyramide, procainamide)
anti-arthritics	(diflunisal, fenoprofen, ibuprofen, indomethacin, meclofenamate, naproxen, pentazocine, phenylbutazone, piroxicam)
antibiotics	(cycloserine, ethionamide, isoniazid, metronidazole)
anticonvulsants	(phenobarbital), phenytoin, primidone)
antihypertensives	(clonidine, methyldopa, prazosin)
antiparkinsonians	(bromocriptine, carbidopa, levodopa)
beta-blockers	(metoproplol, nadolol, propranolol, timolol)

[1] Suite 700, 2000 P Street NW, Washington, DC 20036, USA.

corticosteroids	(ACTH [adrenocorticotropin], betamethasone, cortisone, hydrocortisone, prednisone, triamcinolone)
cardiovasculars (each with reserpine)	(chlorothiazide, chlorthalidone, deserpidine, hydrochlorothiazide, methyclothiazide)
H2-blockers (acid secretion suppressors in stomach ulcers)	(cimetidine, ranitidine)

(See also 'Epistemological Assumptions in Homoeopathy' section 7 Holism – Homoeopathic Pharmacology and 'Homoeopathized Allopathica'.)

Complementary Remedies

Those homoeopathic drugs that remove all the remaining symptoms after the action of the simillimum. For example, Lycopodium Clavatum will act with special benefit after Iodium.

Computers and Homoeopathy

See 'Repertorization' and 'Usage, Clinical'.

Concordance of Emotional Symptoms in Disease and Drug Action

See 'Disease and Drug Action in Homoeopathic Congruity'.

Concordance Repertory of the Materia Medica

Comprehensive, convenient remedy-finder in the context of symptom-combinations, inspired by the Biblical concordance compiled in 1737 by the Scotsman Alexander Cruden (1701-1770). The US homoeopath William D Gentry had needed a search lasting several days through the materia medica and repertories available in 1876 to identify a remedy for a particular outstanding symptom-combination. (What had caused the search was: 'Constant dull frontal headache, worse in the temples, with aching in the umbilicus'. The remedy finally found to produce this experimentally was Leptandra virginica). It occurred to Gentry that if only he could have referred in a repertory, under 'Head and Scalp' to the letter U for 'umbilicus' he could have located the homoeopathic medicine without delay. Gentry and his team worked from 1876 to 1890 to produce this homoeopathic classic in six volumes, totalling 5494 pages. Gentry also published two other works:

An Answer to the Question – What is Homoeopathy?
The Rubrical and Regional Text-Book of Homoeopathic Materia Medica.

Condensation

Compression; the change of a gas to a liquid, or of a liquid to a solid. It does not apply to an instance where a gas may go into solution (e.g.: in a liquid like water where carbon dioxide may be in solution, as in 'carbonated water'). (See 'Precipitation'.)

Cones

Hemispherical or conical in shape, these are made from beet and/or cane sugar with Albumen ovi recens (white of chicken egg). Because of the flat base and their shape, as well as their composition, they can absorb more medicinal substance poured over them than any other solid vehicle. The most commonly used size is no. 6, being so designated from the diameter of the base in millimetres. They are not in use as a homoeopathic pharmaceutical vehicle in many parts of the world, largely because Albumen ovi recens is a substance that is simply not sufficiently pharmacologically neutral (see 'Boyd's Drug Classification', Group Eight). (See also 'Dose', 'Granules', 'Pillules', 'Saccharum Lactis' and 'Vehicle'.)

Constitutional Compatibility in Disease and Drug Action

See 'Disease and Drug Action in Homoeopathic Congruity'.

Constitutional Drug

See 'Constitutional Type'.

Constitutional Prescribing

See 'Constitutional Type'.

Constitutional Type

● **Classification according to which a particular medicine suits a specific kind of patient.**

This describes the aggregate of patients' common distinguishing features. The concept was developed, in an attempt to simplify homoeopathic diagnostics, in post-Hahnemannian homoeopathic practice. It is used to identify patients according to their temperament, appearance, certain characteristics of behaviour and their variance from the normal, who each seem to respond to a corresponding polycrest remedy, both

(i) in the earlier, undifferentiated stages of disease and particularly after an acute episode, and

(ii) in chronic disease with pronounced pathological complaints.

If the word constitution describes, as it does, the physical, emotional and mental make-up of a living organism, including the mode of performance of its functions, the activity of its metabolic processes, the manner and degree of its reactions to stimuli and its vital power of resistance to attack, then polychrest remedies are widely applicable but are particularly useful in chronic illnesses where 'constitutional prescribing' is of most value. This is so because polychrests produce a wide range of reactive symptoms in provers, and such a remedy, in potency, through its broad spectrum of action, affects all tissues of the body in some degree. All the polychrest remedies are considered to be 'constitutional drugs' by the majority of homoeopaths, because the proving of these remedies has indicated that certain persons produce a much fuller picture of the total symptomatology than others. This is due to the characteristics and propensity of the individual provers. Identical conclusions have also been reached by clinical experience with these drugs. These characteristics are the common things about people which identify them as being of the type who is hypersensitive to a particular drug. Yet the whole make-up of a patient is still taken into account each time, since homoeopathic prescribing can only be for an individual patient and can never be for a patient group (but see 'Epidemiology' and 'Miasma'). It follows, therefore, that a classification according to 'constitutional type' in homoeopathy is, in reality, a classification more of drugs than of patients, all semantic appearances to the contrary.

'Constitutional prescribing' of an indicated polychrest remedy corresponding to a relevant 'constitutional type' will not alter that patient's basic personality, but clinical experience has shown that it stimulates the total reserve of vital energy of the full person. It increases resistance, improves well-being, prevents relapses and facilitates a wide range of deteriorated physiological and biological functions. It will act the more swiftly, the more appropriate the choice of potency (nearly always a higher one). Discerning the constitutional peculiarities of a patient contributes significantly to the faster prescription of the appropriate homoeopathic drug. Those homoeopaths who prescribe 'constitutionally' for a particular human stereotype frequently prescribe that 'constitutional remedy', compatibility permitting, intercurrently with their main homoeopathic remedy selected, on the totality of the symptoms.

One of the most successful homoeopathic textbooks, originally published in 1853, which in 1981 was in its twentieth edition, lists in its appendix twelve major 'constitutional drugs'.[1] Evident in this list is a pronounced personalization, an anthropomorphism, of the drugs' characteristic general symptomatologies. The drugs are made to appear almost as though they were actual people. This tendency has been adopted by several recent compilers of

---

[1] Müller, Clotar. *Der homöopathische Haus- und Familienarzt: Eine Darstellung der Grundsätze und Lehren der Homöopathie zur Heilung der Krankheiten mit Anhang: Homöopathische Konstitutionstypen*, Heidelberg: Karl F Haug Verlag, 1981, pp 307-320.

descriptive materia medica.[1,2] This, in turn, has reinforced the perpetuation of remedy classifications according to human types, even though this has been deplored by very eminent homoeopaths in this century, e.g.:

1) James Tyler Kent condemns the classification of patients by physical constitutions as useless in prescribing, saying that 'nothing leads the physician to failure so certainly as classification';[3]

2) Herbert A Roberts says that 'many mistakes have been made in prescribing on this so-called type method'; and later: 'prescribing on types, or temperaments, is at best a slack method of using the blessings of homoeopathy. It is really keynote prescribing, and then not on any morbific symptoms, but on a general stature that is present from birth. Keynotes may often give us a clue to the indicated remedy, but this clue must not be allowed to overbalance our judgement in weighing the whole symptom picture'.[4] The upshot is that the phrase 'constitutional type' is interpreted in two different ways by homoeopaths. Some simply mean by it the total symptom-complex presented by the diseased patient, fully as he is found to be at the time. Others, however, also include in its meaning certain unchangeable aspects, such as the patient's build, hair colour, ingrained behaviour patterns and the like, which identify the patient-type with a propensity to be constitutionally sensitive to the particular remedy. The former group, which denies that unaltering morphology can have any meaningful role here, during the process of homoeopathic remedy selection, simply ignores the references to build, hair colour, etc. that have crept into the more descriptive 'constitutional drug' pictures.

A selection of 21 constitutional drug types (there are many more), with the outstanding characteristic features of each drug, follows:

Aluminium metallicum: has greyish tinge in complexion; is on top form only late in the day; has gastro-intestinal discomfort.

Arsenicum album: propelled by nervous restlessness, yet worn and exhausted physically; is intelligent but fussy; has fine skin, is delicate looking with dark shaded rings around eyes.

Baryta carbonica: appears to be a little backward; looks younger than patient actually is; keeps mouth a little open; has large tonsils, a tendency to swollen glands and offensive foot-smells.

Bryonia alba: may be a brunette of bilious tendency and choleric temper with firm flesh; cannot bear a disturbance of any kind, either mental or physical; has dry mucous membranes and rheumatic pains and swellings, relieved from pressure.

[1]Blackie, Dame Margery Grace. *Classical Homoeopathy,* Beaconsfield: Beaconsfield Publishers Ltd, 1986.
[2]Coulter, Catherine R. *Portraits of Homoeopathic Medicines: Psychophysical Analyses of Selected Constitutional Types,* Washington, DC: Wehawken Book Company, 1986.
[3]Kent, James Tyler. *New Remedies, Clinical Cases, Lesser Writings, Aphorisms and Precepts,* Calcutta: Sett Dey and Co, 1958, pp 212-213.
[4]Roberts, Herbert A. *The Principles and Art of Cure by Homoeopathy: a Modern Textbook,* Bradford: Health Science Press, 1942, pp 170 and 173.

Calcarea carbonica: is pasty-faced, soft, fat, flabby and usually fair-complexioned with a rather large head, of pleasant disposition, but mentally and physically slow, which worries the patient; has clammy hands.

Calcarea phosphorica: often has dark hair, long lashes and dark blue eyes, with a rather sallow complexion; may be long-legged (with a short back, though) and tends to have a clammy face; has a weak memory, is fretful and peevish, cannot concentrate and is disinclined to work.

Calcarea silicica: is weak, pale and anaemic-looking; always feels worse after breakfast; is very sensitive to alcohol; cannot stand pain well; has a marked tendency to spraining an ankle.

Carbo vegetabilis: has a heavy, sallow complexion with bluish fingers, toes, nose and face; has not been able to recover from the effects of a previous illness or injury; flatulent stomach and abdomen, pressing upward causing a full feeling in chest.

Cuprum metallicum: is distressed-looking with bluish-pale complexion; makes jerky, twitching or very angular movements; easily bored by idleness yet disinclined to work; complains of metallic taste in mouth; commonly has respiratory symptoms.

Ferrum metallicum: is clear-skinned and fair, and can become pale one moment, then flush up on a little excitement, food, drink or exertion; has pale mucous membranes but colour around the cheek-bone area; is very easily tired and often feels faint; has very cold hands and feet; gets cramps in feet; noise irritates; weeps easily; is definitely anaemic; gets constipated.

Graphites: is stout and flabby, with a slightly mauvish tint in the skin colour; is timid and despondent, intensified by music; cannot make decisions; fingers tend to crack on exposure to cold and in cold water; has droopy eyelids and a large head; easily tired out; commonly has some skin complaint.

Ignatia amara: is highly strung, bright, sensitive and paradoxical; headaches are relieved by heat; is very sensitive to noise; can easily be offended but also smiles readily; gets distressed in a confined place; has changeable moods.

(Trigonocephalus) Lachesis: has venous engorgement visible in the skin; is very restless; can be conceited and narrowly religious; all conditions get worse from sleep or warmth; alcohol produces an unpleasant flushing of the face; disposed to haemorrhages.

Lycopodium clavatum: has pale complexion and looks older than the patient really is; has leathery skin and is given to frowning; is intelligent, imbued with unshakeable viability, nonetheless gets keyed up in anticipation: e.g. is first concerned about making a speech, yet pleased while making it; desires solitude but fears to be alone (will put someone next door); is loquacious but at the same time slow of speech; is strongly intellectual but may be dyslexic or have a faulty memory; is cross on waking up and generally peevish.

Nux vomica: is the bad-natured office drudge with a furrow on the forehead; in Caucasians there is a very red face, in others a deeper colour; has a broad mouth with extruding lips; is a debauchee with sensuous inclination; can be spiteful; predisposed to gastro-enteric complications; awakens tired; is addicted to stimulants, nostrums, patent and psychotropic medications, as well as spices, narcotics, bitters and culinary herbs; can become very officious and overbearing in manner.

Phosphorus: frequently tall, slender and narrow-chested with soft hair and long eyelashes; in Caucasians probably either reddish hair and freckles, or brown hair and eyes; is a waxy person; craves cold things to eat and would be liable to flush with hot food; perspires when anxious; is sensitive to atmospheric changes.

Plumbum metallicum: has a pale, ashen hue on shiny, greasy face and sunken cheeks, with the whites of the eyes a yellowish tinge; has inclination to cheat; suspects someone intends to poison him; is troubled by severe constipation: stools are hard, round, black balls; has impaired memory; sleeps restlessly.

Pulsatilla nigricans: is generally fair-skinned, soft, warm-hearted, with a yielding disposition; is easily moved to tears, being touchy too; has soft muscles; loathes fat in food; is fidgety and changeable; suffers from constant dry mouth but is seldom thirsty; is suspicious of human company of the opposite sex; liable to flush from emotion and then go pale; any pain gets better on movement in open air.

Sepia officinalis: has tendency to perspire with sallow, oily skin; displays negative attitude to everything; is depressed with dull indifference; has chloasma and hot flushes; is apathetic to sex; gets diarrhoea from milk; always complains of a downward-bearing pressure in the lower part of the body.

Silica: is thin (male) or petite (female) or rachitic (child); has clammy hands and poor nails; is faint-hearted; develops spinal headaches ascending from nape of neck to head, which gets worse from looking upward; hands go dead, but improve when placed in hot water; susceptible to septic cuts, boils or eczema, all ending in suppuration or refusing to heal; dislikes speaking; dreads failure; is resentful, but can be witty and good fun if encouraged.

Sulphur: is a self-assured swaggerer with a rough, blemished skin and, in Caucasians, often with a reddish head; is full of plans, ideas and inventions, but chronically untidy; has tendency to blepharitis, styes or red eyelids; is quarrelsome and impatient, but actually lazy; every kind of skin eruption is possible, with burning sensations, giving pleasurable sensation on scratching; has a smelly perspiration; can be bright, interesting, friendly and clever, when stimulated; has noticeable ear discharges, and daily, early-morning diarrhoetic stools.

There is also a drug classification system that has broken completely with the tradition of the majority's emphasis on human types, relying, instead, on the electro-physical properties of each drug. See 'Boyd's Drug Classification'.

Then there is Douglas M Borland's child classification. He did something rather different in his useful and sensitive study on 'Children's Types', in which he divides them into five types, not according to any sterile system, but very simply into:

1 Fat, fair, chilly, lethargic
2 Backward, delayed development
3 With skin indications
4 Warm-blooded, and
5 The nervy type.

He ranges against each child-type about six remedies with all the drug pictures as they apply to children. Each drug picture leads easily on to the next – so to say, naturally blending into, or anticipating, the next drug picture. This way he focuses the prescriber's choice on a short selection of appropriate homoeopathic medicines among which the indicated remedy is likely to be found.[1]

In the German-speaking area Dorcsi has added an extra dimension to the concept 'constitutional type' by adding humoral pathology as an integral component. (See 'Humoral Pathology in Prescribing', where this concept is discussed.)

Veterinary homoeopathy has its 'constitutional types' too. In April 1989, during a lecture at a seminar by the British Homoeopathic Association in Norwich, UK, the veterinary homoeopath George MacLeod said:[2]

> 'Types:
>   It so happens that with experience you find that certain breeds of dog react to certain remedies. It is not a truism exactly, but we find that German Shepherds will react to the remedy Lycopodium in nine cases out of ten, even in a condition where you might think another remedy could be applicable. The Irish Setter is a dog which responds well to Phosphorus. If you study the remedy Phosphorus in the materia medica you will find all the symptoms there a typical Irish Setter will present: he is red-haired, excitable, etc. Spaniels very often fit the Sulphur picture; Great Danes, Whippets and Borzois fit the Silica picture, and so on.'

Quite a distinct system of classification for 'constitutional types' evolved in the entire francophone area. It began with a homoeopath in the Gastein Valley (near Salzburg), Austria, a contemporary and early supporter of Hahnemann, Eduard von Grauvogl, who had observed that patients of a certain type (morphology) were more prone to certain diseases. He classified them into what he called their 'biochemical states' (eight years before Schüssler's biochemical nutritional theories were published, it must be emphasized). These 'constitutional dispositions', published by him in Nuremberg, Bavaria in 1865, are:

the hydrogenoid,
the oxygenoid, and
the carbo-nitrogenoid states.

Lengthy violent disputes were fought in medical circles about this homoeopath's biochemical theories, just when Rudolf Ludwig Karl Virchow's

[1] Borland, Douglas M. 'Children's Types', Monograph, London: The British Homoeopathic Association.
[2] MacLeod, George. 'Veterinary Homoeopathy', *Homoeopathy*, April 1990, vol XL(2), p 35.

Cellular Pathology (first published in 1858) was also creating a turbulence in these same circles. These continued to flare up for a long time and it is more than probable that von Grauvogl's biochemic theories influenced Wilhelm Heinrich Schüssler (1821-1898) to some degree. Hahnemann's chronic miasmata were soon linked to these three 'biochemic constitutions' postulated by von Grauvogl:

the sycotic miasma to the hydrogenoid,

the luetic (syphilitic) miasma to the oxygenoid, and

the psoric miasma to the carbo-nitrogenoid types.

The person primarily responsible for this development was the homoeopath Emil Schlegel (1852-1934) of Tübingen, Württemberg, Germany. To quote Richard Haehl:[1]

'. . . the homoeopathic physician Emil Schlegel . . . gives full recognition to the psora theory. From his clever arguments in the "Reform of the Healing Art by Hahnemann's Homoeopathy" we gather that in his opinion the essential conception of "psora" is superfluous, "for in the healing science it is not merely a question of assuming a mysterious miasma, but rather of recognizing those natural phenomena which have led to this assumption . . . If we can find a simpler and better hypothesis for the explanation of the phenomena present, then it is to be preferred." '

Haehl immediately continues:

'In Schlegel's opinion, Hahnemann's idea of psora coincides to a large extent with that of inherited predisposition to disease, weakened conditions of individual organs or systems, with which our cell centres are burdened.'

According to Francis Treuherz, Emil Schlegel is reputed to have had a long-standing friendship with his near contemporary, the Austrian philosopher Rudolf Steiner (1861-1925), originator of Anthroposophy, whom he may have imbued with the homoeopathic elements evident in Anthroposophic medicine. Moreover, Treuherz reports that both the New York homoeopath Elizabeth Wright-Hubbard and the Franco-Swiss homoeopath Antoine Nebel were pupils of Schlegel.[2] Both accepted the latter's ideas about constitutional types. Each developed these differently. For instance Nebel conducted a full pathogenetic experiment (proving) with Robert Koch's tuberculin preparation in 1901 and was the first to identify the fourth, the tuberculinic, miasma and describe the taint of tuberculinism, that was then further explored by Henry C Allen (of Chicago, Illinois, USA) in some depth.

Earlier, in Lausanne, Switzerland, Antoine Nebel noticed during provings (pathogenetic experimentations) with three drugs, namely with Calcarea

[1] Haehl, Richard. *Samuel Hahnemann: His Life and Work*, two vols, London: Homoeopathic Publishing Company, 1922, vol I, p 151.

[2] Treuherz, Francis. 'Steiner and the Simillimum – Homoeopathic and Anthroposophic Medicine: The Relationship of the Ideas of Hahnemann, Goethe and Steiner', paper read in November 1984 to the Scottish Branch of the British Faculty of Homoeopathy in Glasgow, subsequently published by the *Journal of the American Institute of Homoeopathy*, p 71: He quotes Karl Koenig from the British Homoeopathic Journals, 1951, 1958, 1959 and 1960, and from Denis Demarque's *L'Homéopathie, Médecine de l'Expérience*, Editions Coquemard Angoulême, 1968.

Carbonica, Calcarea Phosphorica and Calcarea Fluorica, that the subjects who produced the largest number of reactive signs were of three discernible morphological types, evidently comparable to von Grauvogl's. Inversely, these types, as patients, seemed often more responsive to treatment in that their pathological complications cleared faster with homoeopathic preparations of substances 'experimentally' corresponding to their type. Nebel's system of dividing people morpho-constitutionally, rather than biochemically, into three types, ultimately superseded von Grauvogl's. The categories under Nebel's influence became:

the carbonic constitution, or carbo-calcic type,

the phosphoric constitution, or phospho-calcic type, and

the fluoric constitution, or fluoro-calcic type.

Here are the morphological characteristics of these 'osseous constitutional types'. The carbonic type was short and fat with hypolax articulations and ligaments; prone to either the psoric or the sycotic miasma. The phosphoric type was tall and thin with normal articulations and ligaments; prone to the luetic (syphilitic) miasma. The fluoric type was of variable height, though tending to small, usually thin, with asymmetry of the face and body; there was dystrophy of the skeleton and hyperlaxity of ligaments resulting in hyper-extension of articular joints; prone to the tubercular taint (pseudo-psoric miasma). The chronic miasmata were the homoeopath's principal guide to 'constitutional prescribing' for each of these 'constitutional types' (See 'Miasma'). These convenient characterisations were popularized by the Centre Homéopathique de France,[1] and for fifty years constituted an integral part of the training of French homoeopaths, even though the three basic morpho-genetic characterizations clearly do not adequately correspond to the plethoric complexity of homoeopathic reality. Therefore, alongside these homoeopathic remedies, others could be chosen on the basis of a so-called typology of temperament (more in line with the rest of the world's version of 'constitutional type'); this meant that medicines like Sepia officinalis, (Trigonocephalus) Lachesis, Iodium, etc. might be supplemented to one of the Calcareas and given in alternation.

In the mid-1930s an embryological basis for the theory of the three 'constitutional types' was proposed, because they were assumed to be hereditary resultants in the light of chronic-miasmatic involvement. This hypothesis, postulated by Henri Bernard, maintains that the constitutional differentiation is brought about by the pre-eminent development of one of the three embryological layers. This was an echo of the concept put forward very much earlier by the homoeopath Philip Rice that idiosyncrasy is a consequence of morphological imbalance (see 'Idiosyncrasy'). Here is a synopsis of these (Bernard's) 'constitutional types':

In the event of a balanced development of the three layers, physiological and

[1] Vannier, Léon. *Homoeopathy: Human Medicine,* translated from French by Mark Clement, London: The Homoeopathic Publishing Co Ltd, ca. 1951, republished Rustington, Sussex: Health Science Press, no date [ISBN 0 85032 101 8], pp 78-110, but particularly p 84.

psychological balance in the individual is said to ensue. In the event of endodermic predominance the appurtenant organs (respiratory and digestive) would preponderate in the constitution's economy and patho-physiology. This is now the 'Calcarea Carbonica', or brevilinear (short-boned), constitutional type. Similarly, in mesodermic preponderance it is taken that the blood, supporting tissue and the immunological system are uppermost. This is now the normalinear (normally-boned) constitution which is seen to react virulently to morbific influences (a pronounced immunological defence) as in the pathogenetic reactions to Sulphur. Hence this is also currently referred to as the 'Sulphur' constitutional type by French-speaking homoeopaths. When the ectodermic layer happens to develop preferentially, from which the skin and nervous system are derived, the constitution that is said to result would seem to be dominated by the nervous system. This is now referred to as the longilinear (long-boned) constitution and because of its affinity to the nervous system and the tall and slender (longilinear) type, it is, at the present time, also called the 'Phosphorus' constitutional type. There is a fourth constitutional type, which is really only a modification of any of these three through the addition of a measure of dystrophy. This is now called the 'Fluor' constitutional type, or the dystrophic type. Combinations of the three principal constitutional types are also recognized.

This embryological hypothesis has, moreover, since been developed further and been placed on a broader patho-physiological basis by Roland Zissu. In its final form[1] it has been widely accepted in the entire francophone area. These four constitutional types each have a very full set of somato-psychical characteristics, sub-divided into:

morphological features,
pathological tendencies, and
neuro-psychic behaviour patterns.

Additionally, the three possible combinations of pairs of 'constitutional types' are variable mixtures of the antecedent components. 'Constitutional prescribing', then, for the resulting seven constitutional types recognized in the francophone area, is along the following lines:

Constitutional Type	**Constitutional Remedy**
[The strong presence of homoeopathic mineral remedies here (see entry) is very striking.]	This is chosen from within the corresponding group (based primarily on chemical affinity with the leading remedy), or from homoeopathically related drugs, as determined by the case.
Calcarea Carbonica (brevilinear type)	Calcarea carbonica (leader) Ammonium carbonicum Ammonium picricum

[1] Jouanny, Jacques. *The Essential of Homoeopathic Therapeutics*, Bordeaux: Imprimeries Delmas for publishers Laboratoires Boiron, 1980, chapter VI 'Typology and Constitutions', pp 55-80.

Constitutional Type	Constitutional Remedy
	Baryta carbonica
	Calcarea acetica
	Calcarea oxalica
	Calcarea picrica
	Carbo vegetabilis
	Carboneum
	Cartoneum hydrogenisatum
	Carboneum oxygenisatum
	Ferrum picricum
	Magnesia carbonica
	Manganum carbonicum
	Natrum carbonicum
Sulphur (normalinear type)	Sulphur (leader)
	Calcarea sulphurica
	Ferrum sulphuricum
	Kali sulphuratum
	Kali sulphuricum
	Magnesia sulphurica
	Manganum sulphuricum
	Natrum hypochlorosum
	Natrum sulphuricum
	Natrum sulphurosum
	Sulphuricum acidum
	Sulphurosum acidum
Phosphorus	Phosphorus (leader)
(longilinear type)	Calcarea phosphorica
	Ferrum phosphoricum
	Ferrum phosphoricum Hydricum
	Ferrum pyrophosphoricum
	Kali phosphoricum
	Magnesia phosphorica
	Natrum phosphoricum
	Phosphoricum acidum
	Phosphorus hydrogenatus
	Phosphorus muriaticus
	Selenium
Fluor	Fluoricum acidum (leader)
(dystrophic type)	Beryllium metallicum
	Cadmium metallicum
	Calcarea fluorata
	Cinnabaris
	Cobaltum nitricum
	Germanium
	Indium metallicum

Lapis albus
Magnesium fluoraticum
Mercurius aceticus
Mercurius biniodatus
Mercurius biniodatus cum. Kali
  iodatum
Mercurius corrosivus
Mercurius cyanatus
Mercurius dulcis
Mercurius nitricus
Mercurius praecipitatus Albus
Mercurius praecipitatus Ruber
Mercurius protoiodatus
Mercurius solubilis
Mercurius sulphocyanatus
Mercurius sulphuricus
Mercurius vivus
Natrum fluoratum
Natrum silicofluoricum
Thallium metallicum
Tellurium

Carbo-Phosphorus Combination — Calcarea hypophosphorosa (leader)
(fat Phosphorus type) — Ammonium bromatum
Ammonium phosphoricum
Carbo animalis

Sulpho-Carbonica Combination — Hepar sulphuris calcareum (leader)
(fat Sulphur type) — Ammonium aceticum
Carboneum sulphuratum
Methylene-blue

Phosphoro-Sulphur Combination — Natrum muriaticum (leader)
(thin Sulphur type) — Ammonium muriaticum
Kali muriaticum
Magnesia muriatica
Sulfonamidum
Sulphur iodatum
Sulphur terebinthinatum
Tuberculinum

Experimental Evidence

There appear to be no published scientific studies specifically concerning either 'constitutional types' or 'constitutional remedies' in the widely accepted meaning of these terms. However, very good work has been done within the French concepts of 'constitutional type', which emphasize the fact that there has to pre-exist a sensitization (idiosyncrasy, susceptibility) which is found only in recognizable 'constitutional types' that are predisposed on the level of their patho-physiology to becoming so sensitized, whether from miasmatic or from inherited determinants, or contingent upon an accelerated growth of one embryonic layer, or merely from induced sensitivity (heightened homoeopathic reactive propensity) brought about by the pathogenetic effects of having participated in a homoeopathic proving, as with Nebel's subjects. Without doubt, it is axiomatic in homoeopathic therapeutics that the patient is hypersensitive to the particular medicine indicated by the law of similars.

A great number of researchers have been sensitizing animals to the very substance to be experimented with, in order, subsequently, to show the activity of the corresponding homoeopathic potencies. Two examples are:

The first large-scale experiment in this area was carried out from 1952 to 1955 at Larriboisière Hospital in Paris by Prof Devraigne, Mr Bagros, a biologist, and Henri Boiron, doctor of pharmacology. After having produced hyper-oestrogenic conditions in female rats, they showed the action of Folliculinum 7CH, 15CH and 30CH. This is natural folliculin (oestrone) in deconcentrations of 10^{-14}, 10^{-30} and 10^{-60}. The extent of this experiment was considerable. It involved more than 2000 animals and was the object of several scientific papers, including a thesis for a doctorate in medicine. This experiment demonstrates the reproducible action of ultramolecular potencies of Folliculinum on the previously sensitized rats.[1]

A second experiment was carried out in 1955 in Strasbourg by Prof Lapp and Miss L Wurmser. They showed the activity of Arsenicum album 7CH (10^{-14}) and Bismuthum 7CH (10^{-14}) upon the subsequent elimination of these two poisons previously fixed in the animals' organisms through subintoxication.[2]

Many variations of this experimental model, as well as reruns confirming previous results, have been successfully undertaken under controlled conditions. They have yielded statistically significant and repeatable results that have been published in the scientific literature.[3,4]

Contagious Principle and Contagion

See 'Miasma'.

[1]Devraigne, Prof, Bagros and H Boiron. 'Etude Expérimentale de l'Activité Biologique de Dilutions Homéopathiques de Folliculine', paper originally read to Societé Rhodanienne d'Homéopathie in 1955.

[2]Lapp, Prof C, and Miss Lise P Wurmser. 'Demonstration that Arsenic or Bismuth, Previously Fixed in the Organism, can be Mobilized and Re-excreted under the Effect of Infinitesimal Doses of those Same Elements', Sainte-Foy-Les-Lyon: Editions Boiron, 1976, p 8.

[3]Sankaran, P. *Some Recent Research and Advances in Homoeopathy*. Bombay: The Homoeopathic Medical Publishers, 1978, pp 70-82 (the bibliography).

[4]Research Committee of the Liga Medicorum Homoeopathica Internationalis, General Secretary to the. *Aspects of Research in Homoeopathy*, Volume I. English translation. Sainte-Foy-Les-Lyon: Editions Boiron, 1984, pp 70-79 (the bibliography).

Contra-indication Against Administering Simillimum

In a patient whose disease is terminal and which may be in its final stages, namely where the life force is hopelessly overwhelmed by the forces of disease, or in many emergencies, it is absolutely contra-indicated to prescribe the simillimum, which would, in the circumstance, only be able to produce an aggravation hastening death. In such an instance functiotropic, organotropic or pathotropic remedies ought to be the homoeopathic drugs of choice, with the intention of inducing a measure of improvement for the limited period remaining to the patient. The attending homoeopath will be mindful of the fact that a terminal case will reach a point where the symptoms call for material doses or very low dynamizations because the susceptibility has diminished to a low level that is unable to react to any other. In such cases the textbook 'maximum dose' may, in fact, be the ideal 'minimum dose' necessary to bring about the desired reaction. (See also 'Pain Relief Methods in Homoeopathy'.)

Convulsion

Paroxysm; violent spasm. (See 'Emergencies – Homoeopathic Treatment', under Convulsions (of infants) and under Epilepsy.)

Coulter, Harris Livermore

This distinguished historian of Western medicine in general (from Hippocrates to the twentieth century) and of homoeopathy in particular, was born in Baltimore, Maryland, USA. He graduated from Yale in 1954, and subsequently wrote a dissertation on homoeopathy's relations with the American Medical Association for which he received his Ph.D. from Columbia University in 1969.

His lasting merit has been to specify accurately the place of homoeopathy's philosophy within the Empirical Tradition of medicine and to identify its irreconcilable antithesis, the ever-changing Rationalist Tradition of medicine. Coulter's is a scholarly approach to the study of homoeopathy's history and philosophy, and to the influences of dominant socio-economic trends in shaping the forces antagonistic to homoeopathy with which it has to interact. His *Divided Legacy* is a monumental and detailed history of Western medical ideologies. Ivan Illich describes this work as 'a vast and well-documented recent attempt to paint the history of empirical medicine in constant tension with the rationalist tradition'.[1] Coulter has lectured at medical schools and universities, has published several articles on homoeopathy, has served on editorial boards for professional journals, and is co-founder of a citizens' medical lobby in Washington, DC where he lives with his wife, Catherine R Coulter, a homoeopath. They have four grown children.

[1] Illich, Ivan. *Limits to Medicine – Medical Nemesis: The Expropriation of Health,* London: Marion Boyars, 1976, p 253, footnote 86.

He has been involved in legal action against the US Food and Drug Administration to lift the secrecy surrounding the testing of orthodox medicines.

His major literary works to date include:

Homoeopathic Medicine, St Louis, Missouri: Formur Inc, 1972 (73 pages)

Homoeopathic Influences in Nineteenth Century Allopathic Therapeutics, Washington, DC: American Institute of Homoeopathy, 1973 (83 pages)

Divided Legacy: A History of the Schism in Medical Thought, (3 vols), Washington DC: Wehawken Book Co, 1973 (vol III), 1975 (vol I), 1977 (vol II) (1947 pages)

Homoeopathic Science and Modern Medicine: The Physics of Healing with Microdoses, Berkeley, California: North Atlantic Books, 1981 (174 pages)

DPT: A Shot in the Dark, New York: Warner Books Inc, 1986 (480 pages; co-authored with Barbara Loe Fisher)

AIDS and Syphilis – The Hidden Link, Berkeley, California: North Atlantic Books, and Washington DC: Wehawken Book Company, 1987 (138 pages)

His English-born wife, who holds a master's degree in European literature from Columbia University, was introduced to homoeopathy in France in 1960. She has published the following gracefully written, original and fascinating works in her own right:

Portraits of Homoeopathic Medicines: Psychophysical Analyses of Selected Constitutional Types, Berkeley, California: North Atlantic Books, and Washington DC: Wehawken Book Company, 1986 (443 pages)

Portrait of Indifference: Supplement to Portraits of Homoeopathic Medicines (Volume Two), Berkeley, California: North Atlantic Books, and Washington DC: Wehawken Book Company, 1989 (49 pages)

Cowperthwaite, Allen C (1848-1915)

US author and minor poet as well as homoeopath who was born in New Jersey and graduated as MD in 1869 from the Hahnemann Medical College in Philadelphia. He studied further, obtaining a Ph.D. and then the doctorate in law, LL D. From 1889 to 1891 he was editor of the *North-Western Journal of Homoeopathy.* For eleven years he was professor of Materia Medica and Gynaecology in the Homoeopathic Medical Department of the State University of Iowa and of Therapeutics at the University of Michigan. Later he became Emeritus Professor of Materia Medica in the Hahnemann Medical College and Hospital of Chicago, Illinois. For some time he was president of the American Institute of Homoeopathy. He made a significant contribution to homoeopathy's position in fundamental medico-legal issues in his writings, particularly:

Insanity in its Medico-Legal Relations.

He also wrote a number of text-books, some of which have become classics:

Science in Therapeutics (1877)

Elementary Text-Book of Materia Medica (1880)

Text-Book of Materia Medica (1882)

Disorders of Menstruation (1888)
Text-Book of Gynaecology (1888)
Text-Book of Materia Medica and Therapeutics (1891)

Cravings

See 'Aversions and Desires' and 'Disease and Drug Action in Homoeopathic Congruity' sections 3 and 9(iii).

Cryotherapy

See 'Actinotherapy'.

Cupping

See 'Acupuncture' and 'Naturopath'.

Cure

A restoration to health or a recovery; to make well or to heal. By properly applying the law of similars as well as correcting any adverse nutritionally and environmentally modifying factor, a cure is brought about with the disappearance of all reversible, sense-perceptible symptoms of disease along with pathological concomitants, where the recovered patient also remains healthy and free from later related (chronic) disorder(s).

Whenever, in any disease processes that were left unchecked or were treated inappropriately, the reversible mode of cellular dysfunction has given way to permanent anatomical changes, as in the bony deformations of osteoarthritis, the likelihood of complete reversion to earlier anatomical morphology is improbable, but not entirely impossible, in the homoeopathic cure.

The progress in the direction of cure needs to be assessed too, if the homoeopath is to gauge therapeutic advance. By which homoeopathic criterion is medicinal effectiveness to be evaluated? For example, it happens often enough that the physical symptoms of disease may have disappeared but that the patient has developed severe anxiety instead. Or that asthma is 'cured', but a new condition, eczema, has appeared instead. This is said to be a change in the centre of gravity of the disease process. Or there may simply be a homoeopathic aggravation.

Hering's rule of direction of cure will be the applicable criterion. This states that a homoeopathically well-indicated medicine causes symptoms to disappear in the reverse order of their original appearance, which may mean that perhaps an old forgotten skin complaint may suddenly reappear for a time (see 'Homoeopathic Laws, Postulates and Precepts' section 14 and 'Therapeutic Science'). Perhaps George Vithoulkas' rule of a shift in the 'centre of gravity' as an evaluation of either improvement or deterioration ought to be applied? This states that any downward shift of signs and symptoms in the listings provided immediately below clearly signifies improvement is occurring in the individual's general health, with a concomitant shift tending away from the adverse 'mentals' toward the 'emotional' or 'physical' columns:[1]

Mental	Emotional	Physical
Complete mental confusion	Suicidal depression	Brain ailments
Destructive delirium	Apathy	Heart ailments
Paranoid ideas	Sadness	Endocrine ailments
Delusions	Anguish	Liver ailments
Lethargy	Phobias	Lung ailments
Dullness	Anxiety	Kidney ailments
Lack of concentration	Irritability	Bone ailments
Forgetfulness	Dissatisfaction	Muscle ailments
Absentmindedness		Skin ailments

(See also 'Clinical Trials', 'Disease' and 'Homoeopathic Laws, Postulates and Precepts'.)

Cuts

See 'Emergencies – Homoeopathic Treatment', section on Wounds.

Cyclopaedia of Drug Pathogenesy

A scrupulously accurate record of homoeopathic drug pathogeneses on the healthy with an emphasis on pathological changes issued under the auspices of The British Homoeopathic Society and The American Institute of Homoeopathy in accordance with identical mandates from the respective memberships which, inter alia, require the publication of

a) the chronology of symptom occurrence;
b) the drug's toxicology, in full;
c) the results of experiments on animals;
d) only the symptoms from attenuations up to 6CH/12DH.

It was published in four volumes (3066 pages) from June 1886 to November 1891 (London: Leath & Ross), edited by:

United Kingdom – Richard Hughes; United States of America – Jabez P Dake; each assisted by the following consultative committee:

UK – John Drysdale, R E Dudgeon, A C Pope; USA – Conrad Wesselhoeft, H R Arndt, A C Cowperthwaite.

[1]Vithoulkas, George. *The Science of Homoeopathy,* Wellingborough: Thorsons Publishing Group, 1986, pp 23-44.

D

Dake's Exclusion Synopsis

A five-point summary of medical and paramedical methods of treatment, that can never be related to the homocopathic law of similars, originally compiled in 1873 and later consolidated by Jabez P Dake of Tennessee, USA. (The summary is listed under both 'Epistemological Assumptions in Homoeopathy', section 1 and 'Homoeopathic Laws, Postulates and Precepts', section 16.)

Dao Yin Jiao Cheng

A form of physiotherapy within Oriental Medicine which, approximately translated, means 'ancient method for health protection and treatment', offering exercise and breathing therapy, the correction of subluxations by manipulation, adjusting the patient's energy, attempting to restore musculo-skeletal structure to the functional optimum by removing tension, tonifying muscles and strengthening the elasticity of ligaments. All this is undertaken by manual techniques alone, and includes some acupressure. It is claimed that the therapy may enhance resistance to disease. This adjunctive modality may be considered complementary to homoeopathy.

David, Pierre Jean (also David d'Angers) (1788-1856)

Renowned French sculptor, born at Angers, who won the Prix de Rome in 1811. The pediment of the Panthéon, Paris, France is his most outstanding work, reflecting his academic, neo-classical training. Of great significance were his evocative sculptures commemorating brilliant persons, their actions and the period and events these influenced. His well-known monuments include 'Gutenberg' in Strasbourg and 'Jefferson' in Washington, DC. The busts he did of many famous men, because of their remarkable quality, have subsequently been replicated many times in a vast corpus of portrait medallions and textual illustrations. He produced portrait busts, among many others, of:

Johann Wolfgang von Goethe (1749-1832) – greatest poet and most versatile genius of German literature;

Johann Heinrich von Dannecker (1758-1841) – classical sculptor of renown from Würtemberg [Weimar library bust of Friedrich von Schiller and Ariadne on the Panther are best-known works];

Johann Ludwig Tieck (1773-1853) – Prussian storyteller, poet and critic, whose works, from 1820 to 1840 had considerable influence on English and US literature;

Christian Daniel Rauch (1777-1857) – after J G Schadow [triumphal chariot on Brandenburg Gate, Berlin] the most influential master of classical Prussian sculpture [sepulchre of Queen Luise and the equestrian statue of Friedrich II, Berlin].

This celebrated sculptor, David d'Angers, also chiselled a bust of Hahnemann soon after the famous man's arrival in France (15th July 1836). Hahnemann himself donated a replica of this bust to the Homoeopathic Academy of Allentown near Philadelphia, Pennsylvania, USA, which Constantin Hering and Heinrich Detwiller had founded in that same year (1836) and to which homoeopathy's founder was very well disposed. Unfortunately the donated bust went down in a shipwreck. (See also 'Goethe, Johann Wolfgang von (1749-1832)', 'van Gogh, Vincent (1853-1890)' and 'Well-Wishers and Supporters of Homoeopathy'.)

Decantation

Pouring off the clear upper portion of a mixed fluid.

Decimal Potency

See 'Potentizing Methods'.

Decoction

An aqueous herbal preparation obtained by allowing a botanical drug to simmer in water for about seven or eight hours. This method is used for woody substances whose constituents are water-soluble but non-volatile. A decoction is made in the ratio of 25g of the cut or crushed plant material simmered in 500ml of water in a slow cooker, below boiling point, until the volume is reduced by one quarter. It is then cooled, strained and, if necessary, pressed. This liquid will only keep for two or three days and ought to be refrigerated.

Dental Surgery and Homoeopathy

Under 'Surgery' homoeopathy's relationship to, and role in, that form of treatment is discussed in detail. *Mutatis mutandis,* all the issues canvassed in that entry likewise apply to the relationship between dental surgery and homoeopathy. Yet there also is a sizeable non-surgical component in dentistry, that involves the administration of medication, which is the preserve of homoeopathy.

Homoeopathy has always had serious misgivings about the use of amalgam as occlusal compact material in dental fillings, because of the leaking of mercury, tin, silver and copper into the host body that is known to occur.

A number of dental surgeons use only homoeopathic internal drugs and external solutions for the medicinal side of dentistry, notably in France, with resounding success. In all the better-known repertories, references to materia medica entries for homoeopathic drugs are to be found for the undermentioned (and other) dental, oral, peri-oral and related maxillo-facial conditions:

alveolar abscesses
aphthous ulcers
bleeding gums
cancrum oris
caries
cracks on the tongue
decayed teeth:
    lower jaw
    molars
    roots
    upper jaw
dental cyst
dental polyp
deterioration of enamel
difficult dentition
epulis
fissures on edges of tongue
fistula dentalis
gingivitis
glossitis
gum boils
halitosis
inflammations (e.g. of the pulpa dentis)
leukoplakia
loose teeth
neuralgic conditions
pain and swelling from wearing dentures
pain produced by filling or preparing tooth/teeth
periodontitis
periostitis dentalis
plumbism
profuse bleeding after extraction of tooth/teeth
pyorrhoea alveolaris
putrid mouth odour and bitter taste
rachitic deficiency
retarded dentition
salivation excessive or acidic
scorbutic gums
septic wisdom tooth
spongey gums

slow suppurative processes
stomatitis:
   aphthous
   catarrhal
   gangrenous
   herpetic
   induced by drugs or chemicals
   induced by electrical action due to dissimilar metals
   mercurial
swellings of jaw, including chondroma, fibroma, osteoma and solid odontomes
swelling of sub-maxillary lymph nodes
tartar
teeth sensitive to hot and/or cold
teeth turn black and crumble as soon as they appear
thrush
tongue cracked, dry, bloodlike fluids exude from cracks
toothache
toothache with earache
trigeminal neuralgia
trismus
unerupted ulcerated tooth
unnatural looseness of roots in sockets
varicose veins on tongue
Vincent's infection

It should be mentioned here that ultra-sound (dental drill) destroys homoeopathic potency.

The pain following extractions can be reduced and healing promoted by Arnica montana perlingually. (See also 'Douche'.)

Experimental Evidence

In *Homéopathie*, no I-1984, pp. 47-49, professors H Albertini and W Goldberg, together with Drs Sanguy and Toulza published the results of sixty randomized placebo-controlled trials demonstrating the highly significant effectiveness of Hypericum perforatum and Arnica montana in patients (age < 65 years) suffering from dental neuralgia. This facial ague is of sudden onset and involves the maxillary and mandibular branches of the trigeminal nerve, with violent paroxysmal episodes of pain, often difficult to localize, which may be provoked by apical root treatment and is often brought on by the act of chewing. It is distinguished from postoperative pain in that dental neuralgia is fulgurating and occasionally accompanied by trismus and/or crepitant temporo-mandibular articulation. The regimen over two days was four pilules of Hypericum perfoliatum or placebo followed four hours later by four pilules of Arnica montana or placebo, once or twice per day. The intensity of pain was evaluated by patients themselves in accordance with a visual scale. There was little difference beween the verum and the placebo pain on day one, but a statistically highly significant mean difference in favour of the Hypericam-Arnica treatment appeared on day two (e = 3.09 p<0.0001) and on day three (e = 4.3 p = 0.00001). The aggregate judgement by the sixty participants (33 women and 27 men) subsequent to the trial was:

Treatment effectiveness	successful	failed
verum (Hypericum-Arnica)	23	7
placebo	12	18

(See also 'Pain Relief Methods in Homoeopathy'.)

Depletion

See 'Exhaustion'.

Derivatives of Homoeopathy

In its vigour, homoeopathy spawns offshoots at regular intervals, the majority of which it eventually reabsorbs. Such tendrils are: Bach's Flower Remedies, Gemmotherapy, Lithotherapy, Organotherapy, Homoeosiniatry, Isopathy and Schüssler's Biochemic Medicine. The only one to have retained its distinct identity is Anthroposophic Medicine. (See entries under these and under 'Acupuncture' for Homoeosiniatry.) (Curiously, the first four of these have each produced a range of remedies numbering in the thirties. Perhaps this is the figure that is small enough so that the emerging therapy will not be regarded as an apostatical threat, though still being large enough to make the desired impact?)

With regard to Anthroposophic Medicine, Francis Treuherz has analysed the relationship of the ideas of Hahnemann, Steiner and Goethe. He pointed out that though Goethe was influenced by Hahnemann, and though Goethean science was the major inspiration for Steiner's Anthroposophy, there is a clear divergence between some aspects of the medicine of Hahnemann and that of Steiner. Treuherz also identifies a more direct link between Steiner and Hahnemann, in the person of the influential homoeopath Emil Schlegel (1852-1934) who is reported to have maintained a long-standing friendship with Steiner.[1] (Schlegel also played his part in the historical development of the homoeopathic concept 'Constitutional Type', qv.)

Desiccation

Removing water content from a substance at a low or moderate temperature.

[1]Treuherz, Francis. 'Steiner and the Simillimum – Homoeopathic and Anthroposophic Medicine: the Relationship of the Ideas of Hahnemann, Goethe and Steiner', paper read at a meeting of the Faculty of Homoeopathy, Scottish Branch, Glasgow, November, 1984 and subsequently published in the *Journal of the American Institute of Homoeopathy* [copies from author: Flat 2, 18 The Avenue, Brondesbury Park, London NW6 7YD, UK].

Desiccator

See 'Utensils of Homoeopathic Pharmacy'.

Desires

See 'Aversions and Desires'.

Destruction of Potency

● **Dynamized homoeopathic medicines are liable to become ineffective if not handled or stored correctly.**

Dehydration, prolonged exposure to sunlight, ultrasound (e.g. from dental drill or electrotherapy apparatus), heating to beyond 120 degrees Celsius, the influence of aromatic substances, and exposure to the types of radiation that destroy long-chain polymers, are all known to destroy potency. In a well-stoppered bottle, and stored in a cool place, to obviate dehydration, potencies will keep for decades.

Determinism

Has three meanings:

1 The religious and psychological proposition that human action is not free but inevitably determined by motives.
2 The doctrine of mechanistic biology which holds that all behaviour is dependent upon genetic and environmental determinants only.
3 The philosophical principle that any phenomenon is always the result of a necessary chain of causation.

Generally in the third sense determinism has been the guiding principle of the Rationalist tradition in medicine, expressed semi-jocularly in the once much used phrase 'ex nihilo nihil fit' (from nothing, nothing comes). The concept of causality contained here was subjected to the most searching criticism by the sceptical Empirical philosopher and historian David Hume (1711-1776). This, however, did not deter Orthodox Medicine from unceasingly looking to many sciences outside itself on which to base its ephemeral diagnostic assessments. The counterpoised philosophical principle guiding the Empirical Tradition in medicine, with homoeopathy in its vanguard, is probabiliorism (in the entry under this word a short differential summation of the contrasting influences and conceptual consequences flowing from both probabiliorism and determinism can be found).

Detoxication

Detoxification; the process of eliminating toxins, accumulated waste products and metabolites from the body through gut, kidneys, bile, mucous membrane, lungs, ceruminous and sweat glands, after the liver has diminished the poisonous quality of these substances in its function as controller of both the carbohydrate and protein metabolism. In homoeopathy certain chronic disease states are frequently seen as being a failure of this function due to one of the following causes:

1 exposure to pollutants;
2 intoxation;
3 overburdening by inordinate indulgence in food;
4 cumulative allopathic drug effect; or
5 allergy.

Some homoeopaths employ sarcodes, nosodes, isotherapeutic agents or even auto-isopathics in such cases to initiate, or stimulate further, this process, but the majority would follow the procedure described under 'Drainage'.

(See also 'Allergy', 'Isopathy' and 'Miasma'.)

Dewey, Willis A (1858-1938)

This eminent US homoeopath was Professor Emeritus of Materia Medica and Therapeutics at the Homoeopathic Medical College of the University of Michigan subsequent to having been Professor of Materia Medica at the Hahnemann Hospital College in San Francisco. In 1888 he was co-author, with William Boericke, of:

The Twelve Tissue Remedies of Schüssler.

His other writings of note were:

Practical Homoeopathic Therapeutics
Essentials of Homoeopathic Materia Medica

and its companion volume:

Essentials of Homoeopathic Therapeutics.

The two last-mentioned works are each a quiz compendium. The former book is a quiz on the principles of homoeopathy, homoeopathic pharmacy and homoeopathic materia medica, while the latter is a quiz on the application of homoeopathic remedies to diseased states. Both books are in like manner systematized, condensed and simplified especially for the use of students of homoeopathy and remain thoroughly practical for the quick selection of medicines in bedside diagnoses.

D'Hervilly-Gohier, Marie Melanie (1800-1878)

Maiden name of Hahnemann's second wife. (See 'Hahnemann, Christian Friedrich Samuel (1755-1843)'.)

Diagnosis

● **The homoeopath's case-making concerning a sick patient to decide on the most suitable treatment.**

Identification of the nature of a particular patient's illness or disability made from the careful study of the presenting sense-perceptible signs and symptoms of that case of disease. Whenever possible, such a study is accompanied by questioning and attentive observation of the patient and pertinent body discharges, further augmented by means of physical measures such as auscultation, palpation, percussion, and local inspection. Moreover, if appropriate, it may include the topographic determination of a disease focus.

The law of similars is the universal precept that establishes the diagnostic frame of reference which endows the homoeopath with remarkably adaptable omniformity of pharmacological application in all conceivable disease conditions, provided these have remained within reversible limits. The scientific link between diagnosis and therapy is permanently established via common homoeopathicity. This means that the sole feature of pharmacological knowledge that is therapeutically relevant is whether or not that knowledge can be applied clinically in accordance with the law of similars. As a consequence, the homoeopathic concept of 'drug diagnosis' denotes the homoeopathicity of the drug's proven action in artificially induced disease to the presenting disease picture; thus references such as to 'a Nitric acid case' or to 'a Colocynthis condition' represent such drug diagnoses. On the other hand, a concept such as 'diagnosis by exclusion' (made in some non-homoeopathic medical disciplines by excluding affections to which some of the symptoms belong, leaving only one to which all the symptoms point) are based on a disease classification system that is foreign to homoeopathy.

Two diagnostic methods, that are occasionally employed and considered legitimately adjunctive in diagnosis by the majority of homoeopaths, include:

1 laboratory techniques for the purpose of:
    obtaining biochemical values
    biopsy examinations
    microscopic studies
    culturing micro-organisms
    and similar technological investigations of secretions, blood, tissue and discharges.

2 pathological investigations involving either:
    forensic procedures and/or post-mortem examinations or:
    the study of lesions present and comparison of symptoms
  to permit:
    assessment of whether or not a disease process is within reversible limits in relation to drug treatment;
    identification of an eventual epidemic disease process;
    distinction of symptoms that are merely secondary to gross structural alteration from those truly part of the patient's altered dynamis, furthering exact homoeopathic disease/drug evaluation; and
    facilitating accurate prognoses in certain types of miasma.

However, there are those homoeopaths who postulate that the simile principle holds beyond the sense-perceptible signs and symptoms as established, into the area of pathology and laboratory investigations. Those are the homoeopaths who follow Hughes' method of prescribing according to organic pathology. They 'prefer to work the rule 'similia similibus' with pathological similarities where these are attainable; though in their default, and to fill in the outline they present, they thankfully use the comparison of symptoms'.[1] Richard Hughes (1836-1902) emphasized what had been derided by his opponents, the Hahnemannian homoeopaths, as 'the luxury of patho-pathogenesis' (where the pathological changes induced by homoeopathic drugs on the healthy are recorded in the materia medica as indications for matching pathological changes in a patient's disease). He said, 'We hold that the true way of learning the physiological action of drugs is the study of a series of cases illustrating the disorder they cause.' He goes on to exhort, 'for the student of drug-action . . . [to study] records of pathogenesy'.[2] This is regarded as superfluous and even misdirected by Hahnemannian homoeopaths, who point to section 14 of the *Organon:*

> 'There is, in the interior of man, nothing morbid that is curable and no visible morbid alteration that is curable which does not make itself known to the accurately observing physician by means of morbid signs and symptoms'.

(See also 'Disease', 'Disease and Drug Action in Homoeopathic Congruity', 'Epistemological Assumptions in Homoeopathy' section 1: Similarity – as a Concept in Science: the Integrating Principle of Homoeopathy, 'Foci', 'History of Homoeopathy before 1900' section United Kingdom, 'Observation', 'Pathology', 'Prognosis', 'Questionnaire', 'Therapeutic Science' and 'Vitalism'.)

Diathesis

A morbid disposition arising from the constitution that may be inherited or acquired. (See 'Constitutional Type' and 'Miasma'.)

Dietary Support

See 'Homoeopathic Practice'.

Dietary Therapy

A therapeutic approach treating disease through the manipulation of the patient's food and drink. While Hahnemann condemned any 'artificial and often mischievous system of diet' and suggested that a patient might do better following his instinctive capacity to eat what agrees with him, he also imposed

[1] Hughes, Richard. *A Manual of Pharmacodynamics,* Sixth edition, London: Leath & Ross, 1893, p 84.
[2] Hughes, Richard, and Jabez P Dake. Introduction to *A Cyclopaedia of Drug Pathogenesy,* Four vols, London: Leath & Ross, 1886, vol I p xv.

stringent supportive diets on patients who were receiving homoeopathic treatment. In the case of treatment for allergy sufferers, the elimination from the diet of offending food allergens is an essential part of homoeopathic treatment. (See 'Allergy', 'Bran', 'Bulimia', 'Foods as Health Problems', 'Homoeopathic Practice', 'Nutritional Equipoise' and 'Obesity'.)

Dietetics

See 'Dietary Therapy'.

Dilute Alcohol

See 'Alcohol'.

Dilution

Rarefaction; the act of reducing the concentration of a solution or a non-fluid mixture, or the resultant solution or non-fluid mixture, proper. Occasionally used erroneously as a synonym for (liquid) potency or dynamization, but correctly used to describe (liquid) non-homoeopathic medicines that have, in the course of their preparation, undergone dynamization procedures resembling those characteristic of homoeopharmaceutics, as in Organotherapeutic or Anthroposophic remedies, for example.

Dioskorides Pedanios (in first century AD)

See 'Philosophical Premise of Homoeopathy' and 'Isopathy'.

Discharges from the Body

Whenever these occur, homoeopathy insists upon the drainage and free flow of all discharges from the body, totally without obstruction. This is as true for the discharge from a fistula, which will heal and close up when the correct treatment is applied, as it is for the periodic passage of menstrual flow. Any interference would bring on a deeper disease process or create a much more serious condition. Such discharges are sometimes potentized and used in treatment of that patient (see 'Isopathy', section on Auto-Isopathics).

Examples of syndetic pointers to two homoeopathic medicines:

Surly patient with bloody discharge (inflamed surfaces tend to bleed; haemoptysis; haemorrhages of eye, nose, cavities; bloody urine; sanguineous semen; buccal bleeding; bloodboils; faeces mixed with mucus and blood) – Ledum palustre
If patient, usually with remarkable perspicacity and heightened mental activity, has discharges (from both ears; profuse sputum, clear, jelly-like and

ropy; due to eczema capitis which cracks, exudes and wets the hair; of strong urine like a cat's) and a possible tendency to choroidopathy – Viola odorata

Disease

● **The body's defensive and corrective dynamic effort in its battle against injurious influences.**

In Elizabeth Wright Hubbard's memorable phrase, homoeopathy's 'concept of disease [is] a protective explosion'[1] manifesting in an individual as a particular set of symptoms. This is any one individual organism's innate, undeveloped healing effort, which homoeopathy supports and stimulates by the administering of that medicine which has been shown to produce, artificially, a matching pattern of symptoms in healthy human beings. Except in cases involving epidemics or miasmata, homoeopathic disease classification, consequently, describes a diseased state by the name of the medicine that acts curatively. For instance, a homoeopath will say he has treated a 'Sulphur case', or that some patient is a 'Phosphorus type': this is known as drug diagnosis.

Standard disease entities, based on a recognised aetiology, an identifiable group of common signs and consistent anatomical alterations, are also used by homoeopaths, as in acute miasmata or epidemics, but otherwise largely for convenience's sake, as in a reference to a 'Phos. Ac. case of typhoid'. This is so, despite the fact that in homoeopathy the unitary concept of disease prevails, which holds that there is really only one collective disease concept, and what are disparately known as 'diseases' are no more than varying manifestations of the damage endured. The use of standard disease nomenclature, as used in many other medical disciplines, facilitates the understanding of how a disease might progress without treatment, and therefore helps the homoeopath assess the response to his treatment. It also allows for the ready identification of symptoms that are truly characteristic to the individual's dynamic reaction in his disease, rather than stereotypical of it.

The Sydenham Society Lexicon of Medicine and Allied Sciences (1879-1899) defines dynamism (in the context of disease) as:

'The theory of the origin of disease from change or alteration of vital force.'
Hahnemann says of disease (*Organon,* section 6):

'The unprejudiced observer – well aware of the futility of transcendental speculations . . . notices only the deviations from the former healthy state of the now diseased individual, which are felt by the patient himself, remarked by those around him and observed by the physician. All these perceptible signs represent the disease in its whole extent, that is, together they form the true and only conceivable portrait of the disease.'

[1] Hubbard, Elizabeth Wright. *Homoeopathy as Art and Science,* edited by Maesimund B Panos and Della DesRosiers, Beaconsfield: Beaconsfield Publishers Ltd, 1990, p 1.

and further – (*Organon*, section 11):

> 'When a person falls ill, it is only this spiritual, self-acting (automatic) vital force, everywhere present in his organism, that is primarily deranged by the dynamic[1] influence upon it of a morbific agent inimical to life; it is only the vital principle, deranged to such an abnormal state, that can furnish the organism with its disagreeable sensations, and incline it to the irregular processes which we call disease; for as a power invisible in itself, and only cognizable by its effects on the organism, its morbid derangement only makes itself known by the manifestation of disease in the sensations and functions of those parts of the organism exposed to the senses of the observer and physician, that is, by morbid symptoms, and in no other way can it make itself known.'

and still more – (*Organon*, section 12):

> 'It is the morbidly affected vital energy alone that produces disease,[2] so that the morbid phenomena perceptible to our senses express at the same time all the internal change, that is to say, the whole morbid derangement of the internal dynamis; in a word, they reveal the whole disease; also, the disappearance under treatment of all the morbid phenomena and of all the morbid alterations that differ from the healthy vital operations, certainly affects and necessarily implies the restoration of the integrity of the vital force and, therefore, the recovered health of the whole organism.'

(See also 'Causes of Disease', 'Cure', 'Detoxication', 'Diagnosis', 'Dynamis', 'Epidemiology', 'Health', 'Homoeopathic Laws, Postulates and Precepts', 'Miasma', 'Observation', 'Pathology', 'Prognosis', 'Therapeutic Science' and 'Vitalism'.)

Disease and Drug Action in Homoeopathic Congruity

● **The sum of the symptoms of an ill patient must agree with or greatly resemble the sum of the symptoms that the curing drug has been found to produce in a healthy person.**

Applied therapeutic science requires a coincident parallelism between the symptom complexes of both the disease and the drug of choice on as many of the first seven undermentioned points of comparison as possible, in other words, the ideal striven for is: they are to be as similar as possible as often as possible. Obvious incongruity in any comparative aspect (negative symptom) frequently amounts to symptom-dissimilarity in the case allowing for the elimination of many otherwise eligible remedies, facilitating the process of repertorization.

[1] Materia peccans! [*footnote from* Organon]
[2] How the vital force causes the organism to display morbid phenomena, that is, how it produces disease, would be of no practical utility to the physician [. . .]; only what is necessary for him to know of the disease and what is fully sufficient for enabling him to cure it, [will have been] revealed to his senses. [*footnote from* Organon]

1 Generic Similarity

Homoeopathicity of type of affliction; describes the identity in the class of affections induced by both the natural disease of the patient and the experimental disease of the drug to be used: for example, (i) if the illness is febrile, the remedy must be pyreto-genetic; (ii) if the disease is an inflammation, the drug of choice will be an irritant, etc.

2 Causal Similarity

Homoeopathicity of formative affectors; means that the antecedent concomitants present when the disease arises will substantially narrow the field of contenders among drugs to be used: for example, (i) neuralgia induced by injury to a nerve is different from one brought on by shingles and that again is also distinct from one that comes with gout; (ii) jaundice from severe emotional shock is different from that arising from tropical heat or a similar disorder due to faulty diet.

3 Parallels in Symptom Modalities

Homoeopathicity of modalities. Meteorological and thermic influences, cosmic rhythms, mental factors, physical conditions (including movements and rest), relation to food and drink, location, laterality and time are circumstances that can contribute to making symptoms (i) better or (ii) worse, (iii) appear and (iv) change. An example is the drug (Solanum) Dulcamara, under the influence of which healthy individuals develop twitching of the eyelids, lips and hands on exposure to cold damp weather, which readily subsides under the application of dry warmth. Other things being similar, Dulcamara should be suitable as a medicine in such affections as are modifiable in this way.

4 Symptom Character Resemblance

Homoeopathicity in the quality of abnormal sensations. All sensations have a distinct character: for instance, a gnawing pain, a burning pain, a tearing pain, or a stabbing pain are distinctly different from one another; and so are a sour taste, a metallic taste, a foul taste, in a patient's mouth. The character of such sensations are to be alike in both the disease and the drug action, for example, the shooting-tearing neuralgia of Arsenicum Album would be homoeopathic to a patient's shooting-tearing pain in the hip, thigh or groin.

5 Constitutional Compatibility

This is discussed in detail under 'Constitutional Type'.

6 Synchronicity of Symptom Evolution

Homoeopathicity of pharmacodynamic devolution; is discussed in detail under 'Therapeutic Science'.

7 Concordance of Emotional Symptoms

Homoeopathicity of disposition; 'matching mentals'. Emotional and/or intellectual symptoms are simply referred to as 'mentals' in homoeopathy (and often erroneously as 'mental symptoms', with the misleading connotation that they represent some 'psychiatric pathology'). Since 'mentals' are in evidence well ahead of functional and morphological changes when disease develops, they frequently provide very early indications for homoeopathic treatment. Patients might be insufferable, aggressive or depressed a long time before the physical manifestation of a disease. A few examples of a vast amount of such symptoms ('mentals') are:

the vindictiveness – of Acidum nitricum;
intense anxiety with fear of death – of Aconitum napellus;
religious mania alternating with suicidal mood – of Aurum metallicum;
morose irritability, peaking in passionate obstinacy – of Bryonia alba;
transient, emotion-induced dyslexia & anger with serious upsets – of
 (Matricaria) Chamomilla;
jealousy – of Hyoscyamus niger;
the distress – of Ignatia amara;
the taciturnity, fault-finding, haughtiness and cruelty – of Platina;
the androphobia, which paradoxically dreams of men, the disgust at
 everything, yet the mild, good-natured disposition – of Pulsatilla nigricans.

8 Matching of Three or More Guiding Symptoms

Multiples of semiological homoeopathicity. Reliance on the coincidence of three, but preferably more, striking symptoms, evident in both the artificial illness of a drug as well as in the phenomena of a disease, rests on the mathematical law of permutations. This says, simply put, that the number of possible rearrangements of the figures of a series increases with near-exponential progression in proportion to their number, so that for five figures it is 120, but for seven it is already 5040. In that same ratio increases the probability against any one combination occurring by chance. Therefore, if three distinctive symptoms of a case can be found to have been experimentally produced by a medicine, there is already considerable likelihood of its acting on the same parts and in the same manner. Certainly the odds in its favour increase rapidly as the points of symptom-similarity are multiplied. Nonetheless, even by a matching of symptom-similarity in only three or four of the above seven points of comparison the likelihood of achieving a good clinical effect is high.

9 Ranking

Many homoeopaths are guided by Robert Gibson Miller, who in 1910 proposed ranking the above points of comparison in the following order of priority:

(i) matching the 'mentals';
(ii) correspondence between the modalities of times, seasons, thermic and
  meteorological factors, motion, locality, position, pressure and touch;
(iii) similarity of pronounced cravings and aversions;

(iv) menstrual, or hormone-related, changes in state in both the natural and the artificial diseases;

(v) resemblance between the particulars as well as the generals of both diseases, where only the peculiar, unexpected, striking or unaccountable symptoms are of significance; and, least of all,

(vi) common symptoms, as featured in standard non-homoeopathic disease classifications.

(See 'Diagnosis', 'Observation', 'Pathology', 'Pathotropism', 'Repertorization', 'Syndetic Pointers' and 'Therapeutic Science'.)

Dispensary

Pharmacy, with three distinct narrow meanings:

1 Office of a practitioner who dispenses his own medicines to patients.
2 Office of a pharmacist, usually part of the out-patient section, from where medicines are given to patients against prescriptions.
3 Public institution where the poor sick obtain subsidized or gratuitous medicinal supplies.

Homoeopathy successfully maintained a sizeable number of dispensaries, of meanings 2) and 3) (see 'History of Homoeopathy before 1900').

Dissension-Causing Issues in Homoeopathy

Four such issues in homoeopathy have at times created major factional splits with strongly held divergent views by both sides in the debate, thereby having an extremely damaging effect on homoeopathy's development:

1 The question of very high potencies, beyond the 30CH level set as the highest by Hahnemann in 1829, that were being introduced by General von Korsakoff and Equerry Jenichen, and have been employed by some homoeopaths ever since (see 'Potentizing Methods', section entitled International Distribution of Scales and Methods).

2 The Isopathy debate which began with veterinarian homoeopath J J W Lux in 1833 and was largely subdued by P W L Griesselich in decisive rebuttals in his journal *Hygea: Periodical for Therapy* about fifteen years later. It has since been revived in the twentieth century but the debate no longer inflames such extreme passions as it originally did (see 'Isopathy').

3 The fundamental 'symptomatology versus pathology' controversy that raged from about 1860 to 1920, when most of the pro-pathology faction opted for integration into orthodoxy's medical associations and disappeared through simple assimilation (see 'Eclipse of Homoeopathy (1920-1965)', 'Hempel, Charles Julius (1811-1879)', 'History of Homoeopathy before 1900' section on United Kingdom, 'Pathology', 'Simmons, George H (1852-1924)' and 'Tessier, Jean-Paul (1811-1862)').

4 The simplex prescription as opposed to the combination remedy in homoeopathy, which since about 1960 has gained in prominence as a contentious issue, although it has been around since Hahnemann's day (see 'Classical Homoeopathy' and 'Combinations of Homoeopathic Drugs').

Distillation

● **First vaporizing then rendering liquid again in order to purify.**

The process of converting a liquid into vapour by heat and then, by cooling, of condensing the vapour back into the same liquid, separating by this process, the volatile from the non-volatile, or the more volatile from the less volatile, part of a liquid mixture.

Distilled Water

Aqua destillata, one of the most important vehicles in homoeopathic pharmacy. (See 'Alcohol' and 'Vehicle'.)

Doctrine of Signatures

See 'Anthroposophical Medicines'.

Do-In

See 'Acupuncture'.

Dosage

The administration of medicine in doses. Also the determination of the proper dose of a remedy. It is not a synonym for the word 'dose'.

Dose

A definite quantity of medicine to be taken, or applied, all at one time, or in apportioned amounts within a given period. As a guideline:

For the following pharmaceutical form	The stated approximate quantity constitutes one standard dose
granules (internationally) or pilules (in English area)[1]	1 salt-spoonful (adult or child) 1 granule (infant) area)
tablets, tabloids or cones	one (adult or child) a quarter, crushed and, perhaps, diluted (infant)

[1] For an explanation of the seeming confusion in the use of the terms 'granule', 'pilule' and 'globule', refer to 'Nomenclature, Discrepancies in'.

solution	10 drops (adult or child)
	1 drop (infant)
globules (internationally)	3 globules (adult or child)
or granules (in English	1 globule, crushed (infant)
area)[1]	
mother tinctures	e.g. Arnica monatana or Calendula to be applied locally as solution 10 drops to 300ml aqua destillata
	e.g. Iberis amara. Convallaria majalis or Crataegus oxyacantha unpotentized, orally, as drops, for heart conditions: orally 5 drops three times daily
low potency solutions	e.g. Hydrastis canadensis or Kali bichromicum or Pulsatilla nigricans, 2DH, or 3DH for nasal and upper respiratory catarrhs: orally 5 drops four-hourly
creams, ointments, eyedrops, lotions, mouthwashes, liniments	are used on an 'as required' basis normally; usefully to be combined with systemic medicine
injectables, pessaries, suppositories, inhalation capsules, powders	the unit dose is self-evident in such pharmaceutical forms

Except with unpotentized homoeopathic medicines, or with very low potencies, the exact quantity of a homoeopathic dose is of minor importance, in contradistinction to the intervals of repetition of dose, which are crucial (see also 'Dose Repetition'). Some authors in the USA of the nineteenth century used the word dose interchangeably with the word potency. A remnant of this usage is to be found in the commonly used phrase 'ultramolecular dose', which really refers to potency (meaning above Avogadro's number, at 23DH) rather than to dose (which might, in theory, even be quite 'substantial').

Dose Repetition

There are no inflexible rules here, only the following ten general principles:

1 Once an administered remedy has elicited a reaction, the progress of this reaction is observed closely by the homoeopath; only when the curative stimulus has become exhausted (i.e. the reaction has stopped, or the condition is regressing) is the homoeopathic drug repeated, or, perhaps, changed (Hering's rule provides a sure guide here, when the homoeopath makes this choice).

[1]For an explanation of the seeming confusion in the use of the terms 'granule', 'pilule' and 'globule', refer to 'Nomenclature, Discrepancies in'.

2   Low potencies (e.g. of the tissue salts) are generally repeated frequently.
3   High potencies (e.g. of constitutional remedies) will act for weeks or sometimes for much longer periods, and are, therefore, not repeated frequently by most homoeopaths, except in acute situations when they are universally repeated at rapid intervals.
4   The 50-millesimal (LM or quinquagenimillesimal) and the medium potencies (used in some chronic conditions) are adaptable: they can be given daily, or just occasionally, or only once.
5   Rising potencies of the same (frequently the constitutional) drug are sometimes given at increasing intervals over a prolonged period.
6   Bowel nosodes are generally administered as a single dose and not repeated for several months, while related remedies are employed in the interval. The exception, here, is that low potencies (usually 6CH) are given in a daily dose over a period determined by clinical observation in disease conditions with advanced pathology.
7   In the case of a collapsed patient dose repetition may be every two minutes, up to the point of recovery.
8   In the case of a lingering acute miasma, where the patient's organism experiences repeated noxious assaults (e.g. in a viral infection) repetition of the dose two or three times daily is often indicated.
9   Where a single noxious impulse, though it has itself ceased to operate, had set off a persisting disease effect (e.g. post-traumatic neurosis), a single dose of the well-indicated homoeopathic drug is usually sufficient.
10 Whenever two or more remedies are prescribed in alternation, there is a distinct time interval between the administration of each medicine, from 15 minutes to 12 hours (or more).

(See also 'Exhaustion' and 'Homoeopathic Practice'.)

Douche

A treatment technique in homoeopathy, being the irrigation of a skin, or other surface, or an orifice, by a water-based solution carrying an active ingredient. Examples are:

Ear – equal parts Plantago major Θ & warmed water;

Eyelids – granular ophthalmia: Calendula officinalis Θ 5gtt to 30ml warmed water irrigating against closed swollen granular lids;

Eyes – purulent inflammation: Eye-bath with a Borax veneta wash;

Mouth – aphthous sores: Hydrastinum muriaticum 200mg in 90ml aqua destillata;

Nose – in ozaena or for ulcerated nasal passages: Hydrastinum Muriaticum 200mg in 90ml aqua destillata;

Teeth & Gums – toothache and painful gums: Plantago major Θ rinse hollow tooth and painful gum area;

Vagina – leucorrhoea and pruritus vulvae: either Vulva Hydrastis canadensis Θ or Calendula officinalis Θ.

(For 'Antiseptic Douche' see entry under that.)

Drainage

The homoeopathic promotion of detoxication. A pathological process is made up of two complementary elements: destruction and healing. Both of these would be opposed by an allopathic drug effect, whilst only healing is impeded by other maladjustments of the detoxication mechanism. In order to promote drainage, a dual homoeopathic drug strategy is generally employed: the coupling of a pathological remedy to the patient's constitutional remedy. Homoeopathy's aim is to attack the fundamental disease, whilst promoting the reactive healing forces of the patient. If the healing potential is obstructed, the central fundamental disease process would be free to seek additional, different focal points of manifestation and modes of expression. A more serious disease may have developed, now also affecting the periphery. Constitutional remedies treat fundamental disease at the core, whereas pathological remedies exert their action on certain types of pathology, that is peripherally. There is, therefore, a bipolar, complementary relationship between the two types of remedy being exploited by this method. The direct peripheral effect of the pathological remedy, which exerts very little action on fundamental disease, boosts the weaker, secondary, peripheral effect of the well-indicated constitutional drug, thereby promoting detoxication. The application of the principle of homoeopathic drainage, first developed in France, is fully explained by E A Maury[1] whose mentor was Leon Vannier. They both followed Antoine Nebel of Switzerland, who, as far back as 1912, began to teach the doctrine of 'organic cleansing' as being indispensable to any well-conceived homoeopathic treatment. The original French term applied to the therapeutic effect aimed at in this approach is 'canalisation', meaning 'channelling' in the sense of 'guiding', which makes 'drainage' appear to be rather an infelicitous translation. (See 'Detoxication', 'Low Potency Prescribing', 'Miasma' and 'Pathotropism'.)

Drug

Substance used in the composition of a medicine, or from which potencies (dynamizations) are run up, or synonym for a medicine.

Drug Diagnosis

In non-homoeopathic pharmacology this is synonymous with pharmacodiagnosis, which is the use of drugs as diagnostic tools. In

---

[1] Maury, E A. *Drainage in Homoeopathy (Detoxication)*. Translated from the French. Rustington, Sussex: Health Science Press, 1965.

homoeopathy it refers to the identification of a diseased state by the name of the medicine that acts curatively in the particular case. (See 'Disease'.)

Drug Picture

This descriptive term is a post-Hahnemannian linguistic embellishment of the concept originally embodied in section 153 of the *Organon of Medicine:*

> 'The whole of the elements of disease a medicine is capable of producing can only be brought to anything like completeness by numerous observations on suitable persons of both sexes and of various constitutions.'

In the phrase 'the whole of the elements of disease', meaning the sum and essence of it, Hahnemann captures the encompassing, holistic feature inherent in the concept of the drug picture, that sets it apart from a mere collection of individual items of otherwise unrelated information. Homoeopathy observes and treats the individual as a whole and the corresponding individual remedy must be known in exactly that way. That drug picture, with the whole of the elements that make up its distinctive image, must be promptly recognizable in its counterpart, the diseased patient. For this to spring to the homoeopath's mind readily, requires continuing study of the materia medica and the assiduous observation of many patients over a long period of time. That way s/he will learn to recognize the characteristics that are quintessential to the type of illness through its resemblance to a particular drug picture. (See also 'Constitutional Type', 'Disease and Drug Action in Homoeopathic Congruity' and 'Sources of Homoeopathic Drug Semiology'.)

Drug Preparation

The three processes of homoeopathic drug preparation are:
(i) serial dilution; (ii) succussion; and (iii) trituration. Refer to Figure 1.

Dilution reduces the toxicity of the original crude drug by serialized deconcentrations (see 'Aggravation', the section on Chemical Aggravation). Serial dilution simply means that each is prepared from the dilution that immediately came before it. For soluble remedies (mother tinctures) the solvent is a water-ethanol mixture, but for insoluble medicinal material, such as Aurum metallicum (gold) the diluent is Saccharum lactis (sugar of milk, lactose). Succussion, for soluble drugs, and trituration, for insoluble medicines, are the mechanical methods that impart the pharmacological message of the original substance (active principle), as all evidence seems to indicate, to the water molecules of the solvent or diluent respectively. (It is worth noting that there is a good deal of water in the Saccharum lactis, and that dehydration destroys the potency of any remedy.) As is clinically and experimentally demonstrable, this message, or perhaps the template thereof, is serially passed on by these means from one dilution to the next, even beyond Avogadro's limit (reached around 23DH or 12CH) where no molecules of the

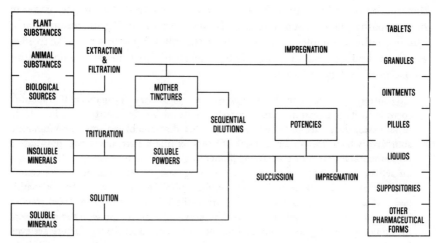

Adapted from: Homoeopathy: Effective Modern Medicine, Durban: SA Homoeopathic Assoc, 1990, p 3.

Schematic Representation: Stages in Preparation of Homoeopathic Medicines

original substance are expected to be present any longer. (See 'Dynamization', 'Pharmacological Message', 'Physiological Response in Homoeotherapeutics, Mechanism of', 'Potency', 'Potentizing Methods', 'Solvation Structures', 'Succussion' and 'Trituration'.)

Drug Strength

Indicates the proportion of the drug's active principle contained in the medicinal preparation. Below Avogadro's number, which is reached at the 23DH potency, there is, at each successive stage of potentization, an ever-decreasing vestige of the original medicinal substance to be found in remedies. Above that number, drug strength is entirely a matter of energies. No verifiable and practical means of measuring drug strength exists, to evaluate accurately the proportion of active principle of either medicinal energy or the residual drug intaglio that a remedy may be endowed with. Experience has shown, though, that the drug strength of well-indicated remedies can be nothing less than abundantly adequate, if, as they do, very small, unrepeated doses of such homoeopathic drugs display such evident effectiveness. (See 'Dose', 'Drug Preparation' and 'Potency'.)

Dunham, Carroll (1828-1877)

Distinguished US homoeopath originally from New York, who graduated in 1850. Like von Boenninghausen he became a homoeopath following a dramatic personal cure after all Orthodox methods had failed. He became a friend of Constantin Hering in Philadelphia and also spent some months working alongside von Boenninghausen in Münster. He was an early advocate of the single remedy approach and strongly favoured the single dose in homoeopathy. His strong convictions about maintaining uncontaminated homoeopathic principles are evident from the following words he spoke in 1870 at the annual general meeting of the American Institute of Homoeopathy, whose president he became:

> 'In contradistinction to any body of physicians, we profess a principle of therapeutics so wide in its application as to express the natural law, in accordance with which, in all cases, drugs are to be selected to restore diseased organisms . . . We have a standard which the other School [Orthodox medicine] does not possess – a fundamental therapeutic law. [In the pioneering days of homoeopathy,] when to avow oneself a homoeopathist required moral courage such as only a profound conviction of truth could give, there was in all members absolute belief in the homoeopathic law and a general acceptance of corollaries [thereto] . . . But as the new practice became popular, men took the name of homoeopathic physician who did not accept the homoeopathic law as of universal application in therapeutics . . . [There are even some] whose massive doses would sometimes astonish the Old School itself.'[1]

This, in retrospect turned out to be the first salvo against the homoeopaths whose leader was to be the British homoeopath Richard Hughes (see 'History of Homoeopathy before 1900', section United Kingdom).

He defined scientific medicine as that possessing the 'capability of infinite progress in each of its elements without detriment to its integrity as a whole.'[2] Homoeopathy conformed to that scientific criterion because its fund of knowledge is stable and cumulative, as opposed to Orthodox medicine which is historically unstable and revisionist. He was an influential contributor to the American Homoeopathic Review. His major literary works are *Homoeopathy, the Science of Therapeutics* and *Lectures on Materia Medica*.

Dynamic

See 'Dynamis'.

Dynamic Causes of Disease

See 'Causes of Disease'.

Dynamic Exhaustion

See 'Exhaustion'.

Dynamical Energy

See 'Dynamis' and 'Energy'.

[1]*Transactions of the American Institute of Homoeopathy*, XXIII, 1870, p 570.
[2]Dunham, Carroll. *Homoeopathy, the Science of Therapeutics*. Philadelphia: F E Boericke, 1885, p 13.

Dynamis

The autarkic life force in each organic being, which Aristotle referred to as entelecheia (entelechy); by this he meant the necessary condition that has enabled a potentiality to have been realized as an actuality. In concrete terms: a conglomerate of chemical components normally found to make up a human being (a potentiality) was enabled, for instance, to be the author of this dictionary (i.e. a human being has been realized as an actuality) through the writer's dynamis (the necessary condition for this development to have been possible at all). Synonymous or related terms for this life force are vital factor, organismic field, immanent organizing principle, and nisus formativus (the formative impulse), inferring, as they all do, that self-determined holistic purposiveness is an unmistakable feature of living organisms. Regeneration, regulation and the curative process are clear expressions of just such a purposiveness.

Philosophical and Scientific Context

The Dutch philosopher Benedict de Spinoza (a.k.a. Baruch Spinoza) (1632-1677) conceived God as the dynamic principle of order within nature as a whole; and he considered the human mind as a 'spiritual automaton' subject to necessary laws of its own. Just as the body was subject to the laws of motion, so the law of inertia applied to ethics and psychology, and he postulated that by its very nature, the dynamis of every form of life endeavours to preserve itself indefinitely unless it is hindered from doing so by some superior force (e.g. an overpowering disease). He recognized that the individual dynamis is universally endowed with the overriding drive for self-preservation, in an epoch when Scholastic philosophy taught that all forms of nature were directed to final causes (immutable ends) and that human nature only existed for the sake of a supernatural celestial end. That newly-discovered nisus, 'the primacy of the endeavour for self-preservation', he termed this faculty 'conatus' (meaning 'directive effort'). A faculty of all living organisms, it became the (usually unacknowledged) pivotal concept for most of biological science's developments since, not the least of these are the evolutionary and biological hypotheses of Charles Darwin. Spinoza also constructed a psychology of the emotions which he viewed as dynamic forces, subject to laws derived from three primary affects: pain, pleasure and desire. He said that human nature must first be understood and obeyed before it may be commanded and controlled. For dispensing with supernatural sanctions, and for other reasons, Baruch Spinoza of the Orthodox Jewish religion, was excommunicated by the Jewish community in 1656 for his heretical views.

Gottfried Wilhelm Baron von Leibniz (1646-1716), born in Leipzig, a Saxon like Hahnemann, a mathematician and philosopher of immense genius, who has many achievements to his credit, propounded dynamism as a philosophical theory in which all the phenomena of the universe are explained by an immanent force or energy – specifically that all substance involves force. A few

Dynamis

pertinent details about his many activities deserve to be recorded here. He developed the theory of differential calculus simultaneously with Sir Isaac Newton, and invented a calculating machine that could extract roots, multiply and divide, as well as subtract and add. Leibniz established the famous logical principle, the identity of indiscernibles. He described space and time as relational, and substance as essentially energy-bearing. He was the first to describe kinetic energy in mechanics, and understood that inertia is itself a force. First nudged by the Catholic archbishop of Mainz, he became greatly concerned with the preservation of peace in Europe after the devastation of the Thirty Years' War and was motivated to seek a rational foundation for Christian philosophy which could be acceptable to Catholics and Protestants alike and thereby to promote tolerance and pacifism. This was the beginning of Leibniz' complete and rational system of metaphysics. He also saw that France's ambitious and powerful Louis XIV constituted the most serious threat to European peace. Leibniz prepared a superbly conceived plan for the conquest of Egypt, saying how much more glory, in keeping with the standing of a Christian monarch, such a conquest would earn the victor in comparison with the rape of insignificant, tiny Christian principalities in Europe. Although he was summoned to Paris to expound his plan, and he spent four years there, he did not persuade Louis XIV; however, his plan was seen in the archives much later by Napoleon, who studied it and was evidently so impressed by it that he seems to have implemented it as his own expedition to and campaign in Egypt (1798-1799, in the hope of destabilizing British rule in India).

The Sydenham Society Lexicon of Medicine and Allied Sciences (1879-1899) defines dynamism (in a medical context) as:

'The theory of the origin of disease from change or alteration of vital force.'

Hahnemann's position on dynamis is, *inter alia*, set out in *Organon*, section 10:

'The material organism, without the vital force, is capable of no sensation, no function, no self-preservation;[1] it derives all sensation and performs all the functions of life solely by means of the immaterial being (the vital principle) which animates the material organism in health and in disease.'

and in *Organon*, section 11, footnote no. 7:

'What is dynamic influence – dynamic power?'

Referring to the forces of orderly planetary interplay, to magnetism, and to the power that produces ebb and flow, as 'dynamic', in a way almost reminiscent of Leibniz, Hahnemann asserts:

'such effects [are] dynamic, virtual, that is, such as result from absolute, specific, pure energy and action of the one substance upon the other substance. For instance, the dynamic effect of the sick-making influences upon healthy man, as well as the dynamic energy of the medicines upon the principle of life in the restoration of health is nothing else than communication and so not in any way material, not in any way

---

[1] It is dead, and now only subject to the power of the external physical world; it decays, and is again resolved into its chemical constituents. [*footnote from* Organon]

mechanical. . . . Substances, which are used as medicines, are medicines only in so far as they possess each its own specific energy to alter the well-being of man through dynamic, conceptualist influence, by means of the living sensory fibre, upon the conceptualist, controlling principle of life. . . . Only upon this conceptualist principle of life depends their medicinal health-altering, conceptualist (dynamic) influence. . . .Far more healing energy is expressed in a case in point by the smallest dose of the best dynamized medicines, . . . than by large doses of the same medicine in substance. That smallest dose can therefore contain almost entirely only the pure, freely developed, conceptualist medicinal energy, and bring about only dynamically such great effects as can never be reached by the crude medicinal substance itself taken in large doses.'

At this point the resemblance to Leibniz' Theory of Monadologie is quite apparent (that theory states that the substantial universe consists of entities without parts or extension, that are really [arithmetical units, or geometrical] points of local intensity or force, possessing, in infinitely varied degrees, the power of perception). Hahnemann refers to a 'conceptualist' faculty, invests medicines with an immaterial force or power by dynamizing them, and subdivides that medicinal power infinitesimally: all in Leibnizian fashion. He continues:

'It is not in the corporeal atoms of these highly dynamized medicines, nor their physical or mathematical surfaces (with which the higher energies of the dynamized medicines are being interpreted but vainly as still sufficiently material) that the medicinal energy is found. More likely, there lies invisible in the moistened globule or in its solution, an unveiled, liberated, specific, medicinal force contained in the medicinal substance which acts dynamically by contact with the living animal fibre upon the whole organism (without communicating to it anything material however highly attenuated) and acts more strongly the more free and more immaterial the energy has become through the dynamization. Is it then so utterly impossible for our age celebrated for its wealth in clear thinkers to think of dynamic energy as something non-corporeal, since we see daily phenomena which cannot be explained in any other manner?'

Dynamis is to be distinguished from the Greek word 'nous' first used by the pre-Socratic philosopher Anaxagoras (ca. 500-430 BC) to denote an all-pervading, all-knowing force, but which later came to mean simply reason, mind or intellect, and has quite recently become part of colloquial English, meaning gumption or common sense. (See 'Disease' and 'Vitalism'.)

Dynamism

See 'Dynamis'.

Dynamization

Potentization; imparting and passing along through serial dilutions the pharmacological message of the original substance (i.e. creating a template of the active principle) by means of trituration or succussion. It describes the process of modification of medicines as invented by Hahnemann. It is characterized by the following four distinguishing features:

a) It is a purely mechanical and mathematico-physical process.
b) The procedure involves neither uncertain, unreliable nor immeasurable factors.
c) The resultant product is stable and can readily be maintained that way.
d) The process is theoretically illimitable, though it becomes laboriously time-consuming in the higher range of potencies.

(See 'Drug Preparation', 'Dynamis', 'Energy', 'Potency', 'Potentization', 'Potentizing Methods', 'Succussion', 'Trituration' and 'Vitalism'.)

Dynamize

Potentize; endow with medicinal power by succussion or trituration. (See 'Drug Preparation', 'Dynamis', 'Dynamization', 'Energy', 'Potency', 'Potentization', 'Potentizing Methods', 'Succussion' and 'Trituration'.)

E

Eclectics

See 'Phytotherapy'.

Eclipse of Homoeopathy (1920-1965)

● Homoeopathy was pushed into the political and scientific background for nearly half a century, at a time when science favoured the lop-sided approach of looking only for mechanical explanations to everything.

From the position of prominence that homoeopathy had attained by 1900 (see 'History of Homoeopathy up to 1900'), its influence went into partial eclipse for nearly half a century, beginning in the 1920s. During this time it is estimated that its sympathizers, institutions, practitioners, pharmacists, colleges, researchers, hospitals and publications were uniformly reduced throughout the world by approximately a factor of fifty. This period coincides exactly with the complete philosophical ascendancy in scientific thought of the materialistic paradigm, which postulates exclusively mechanistic (non-vitalistic) explanations for all the problems raised by biology.

Until then, Aristotelian (non-mechanistic) concepts were freely applied to living organisms by biological scientists.[1] For example, an 'unconscious organic memory'[2] or 'a potential recollection of all that had happened to each one of its ancestors',[3] phrases that are both consonant with homoeopathic miasmatics, represented concepts that were generally considered as appropriate scientific propositions. Suddenly though, soon after World War I, it seemed that life in all organisms, and with it the healing impulse in them, could be explained simply in terms of complex interactions between inanimate molecules, with precise three-dimensional shapes, and nothing more. Atomisms, and variations on it, had conquered all. Life and healing were, it therefore appeared, really just produced mechanistically. This unproven metaphysical assumption, fuelled by the continuing heady successes of technology, was so widely held and soon so profoundly integrated into the then current pool of scientific information that it attained the status of a self-evident truth, which one only questioned at the risk of being permanently scientifically ostracized. Homoeopathy, in that hostile climate, was soon in full retreat. Many of the very few remaining true apologists for homoeopathy during that period took up rear-guard positions that were intellectually and scientifically

[1] Russell, E S. *Form and Function*. London: Murray, 1916, pp 335-344.
[2] Hyatt, A. 'Phylogeny of an Acquired Characteristic.' *Proceedings of the American Philosophical Society*. Vol XXXII, 349-647, 1893, p 4.
[3] Butler, S. *Life and Habit*. London: Cape, 1878, p 297.

inconsequential, and generally dismissed as such. Many practising homoeopaths took refuge in the realms of very high potencies, some even denying that low potencies were part of homoeopathy, believing thereby to have moved to the safety of the high ground of ultramolecular energies and away from the uncomfortable proximity of molecular biochemistry, where, they feared, homoeopathy should never have been able to hold its ground.

This inherent weakness was thoroughly exploited, both commercially and through political manoeuvres, by orthodox medicine and pharmacy, that had themselves, so recently, been retreating on a broad front. That, the retreat of orthodoxy, had happened during the second half of the nineteenth century when the prevailing influences of liberalism permitted a laissez-faire approach in science, leading to signal, consistent successes by homoeopathy in open competition with the mainstream of medical thought. In stunned disbelief established medicine and pharmacy had been helplessly observing homoeopathy's broad acceptance by the general public, while confidence in orthodox methods had declined sharply. When the philosophical tide had begun to turn the orthodox medical establishment engaged in some delicate ethical adjustments followed by a series of astute political manoeuvres.

By around 1910 orthodox medicine had universally managed by an extraordinary volte-face to reconcile its own interests fully with those of the patent and proprietary medicine manufacturers, which is the more remarkable since the latter had been openly castigated at every opportunity as purveyors of dangerous nostrums for the preceding sixty-odd years. This meant that these manufacturers were suddenly permitted: (1) to advertise in the orthodox medical journals and publications; (2) to fund research at orthodox medical schools where their products were investigated along with much other research work for which there had been no funds previously. This provided a steady and very ample flow of much needed money for orthodoxy. The fact that orthodox medical practitioners were then themselves also permitted to prescribe these medicines had an enormous reciprocal benefit for the manufacturers, having significantly boosted sales of the proprietary medicines. The partnership between proprietary medicine manufacturers and the orthodox medical establishment soon became an enduring international cartel of gigantic proportions, wielding an impelling political influence everywhere, which was consistently employed for self-serving ends, though mostly well within the bounds of pragmatic defensibility.

It is a matter of historical record that about forty homoeopathically proven medicines, most of which had been in common use by homoeopaths for decades, were seen as successful remedies and simply taken over by orthodoxy, almost invariably without acknowledging the homoeopathic source.[1] Since ponderal doses are normally used in orthodoxy a certain degree of chemical aggravation unavoidably accompanied the frequent curative effects then

---

[1] Coulter, Harris Livermore. *Homoeopathic Influences in Nineteenth-Century Allopathic Therapeutics.* Washington DC: American Institute of Homoeopathy, 1973, pp 23–72.

achieved with these 'new medicines'. At the same time many of the older, injurious orthodox medicines, and treatment methods like calomel and blood-letting, to which public resistance had become so great, were quietly abandoned.

The radical change within scientific thought during the 1960s – for example, the espousal by the majority of particle physicists of evolutionary conceptions of matter, fields and energy, or the fact that in biology organicism seemed to be displacing the entrenched mechanistic theory – signalled an end to the scientific eclipse of homoeopathy (see 'Epistemological Assumptions in Homoeopathy', section 2. The first concrete political evidence of this, the real turning point, may turn out to have been homoeopathy's official re-appraisal in 1965 in the French Pharmacopoeia. It is, perhaps, also no accident that it was in France that homoeopaths widely adopted the use of combinations of homoeopathic drugs (see entry), which, outside continental Europe, had generally been spurned as unacceptable until then. A proportion of the funds generated thereby for these manufacturing pharmacists was duly invested in scientific homoeopathic research, which, in turn, proved in most studies to be successful while being immensely beneficial for the homoeopathic profession as a whole. (The fundamental, as opposed to the historico-political, reason underlying homoeopathy's identity-loss is analysed under 'Hempel, Charles Julius (1811-1879)'.)

Electrotherapy

● **Electricity is used in different ways to help healing.**

Makes use of negative ion exposure, galvanism, statics, high frequency, (short-wave) diathermy, sinusoidal current and faradism to obtain biological and electrophysiological effects. Magnetic induction therapy belongs here too. In the hands of an experienced practitioner this therapeutic approach can produce very favourable results complementary to the homoeopathic treatment, provided the attending homoeopath is aware of the concurrent electrotherapy. Hahnemann, in sections 286 and 287 of the *Organon of Medicine* said magnets and electricity could be used curatively, especially in disease states involving 'abnormal sensations and involuntary muscular movements'. (See 'Naturopath'.)

Elimination Diet

● **Used to pick out those foods that could upset a patient's health.**

Trial by dietary exclusion, designed to detect what food component causes allergic manifestations in the patient, by successively withdrawing each singly from the diet. This was popularized by Dr A H Rowe about half a century ago, and has been adopted by a sizeable number of homoeopaths to assist in allergen exclusion and the possible selection of an isopathic agent. (See also 'Allergy', 'Aversions and Desires', 'Foods as Health Problems' and 'Isopathy'.)

Emanometer

See 'Bio-electronic Regulatory Medicine', 'Bio-resonance Therapy' and 'Boyd, William Ernest (1891-1955)'.

Embrocation

Liquid applied by rubbing to the distressed part of the patient; a liniment.

Embryological Basis for Constitutional Typing

See 'Constitutional Type'.

Emergencies – Homoeopathic Treatment

All practising homoeopaths will eventually be confronted by one or several emergency situations, whether in their consulting rooms or elsewhere. On these occasions, where pronounced risk (a) of injury or (b) to life is involved, the prudent homoeopath ought to call for emergency support at the first opportunity. There remains, at the very least, the intervening period prior to the emergency team's arrival during which the homoeopath's immediate treatment may be critical to the survival and well-being, or to the mere survival, of the patient. This may be a difficult time for the homoeopath who is normally used to a non-emergency treatment routine in his/her daily practice. Moreover, s/he may not stock the homoeopathic medicine(s) most commonly indicated in such emergencies.

It is expressly emphasized that both the remedies listed below and the potencies given alongside them are no more than offered for consideration to the homoeopath whom it behoves to exercise his professional discretionary judgement in every case. These suggested emergency uses for the remedies stated may be found (at least in a semblant form) in many well-established homoeopathic works of reference that are in current use, particularly in:

Pocket Manual of Homoeopathic Materia Medica Comprising the Characteristic and Guiding Symptoms of All Remedies [Clinical and Pathogenetic] by William Boericke (Philadelphia, Pa: Boericke and Runyon [Boericke & Tafel, Inc]);

The Prescriber: A Dictionary of the New Therapeutics by John Henry Clarke (Rustington: Health Science Press [The C W Daniel Company Ltd Publishers]);

Homoeopathic Vade Mecum by Edwin Harris Ruddock (New Delhi: Ashoka Press [Taj Offset Press]).

Whereas constitutional remedies treat fundamental disease at the core, involving time, both for the correct selection first and for the total curative action thereafter, pathological homoeopathic remedies will exert direct action, peripherally, on specific types of pathology. This immediacy of action where desired makes them fast-acting. It is in the nature of emergencies that speed of action is essential. However, since the reciprocal of the law of quantity and potency requires that the less the similarity to the total disease picture, the lower the potency applicable, all such pathological remedies are generally given in the very lowest potencies, or unpotentized, provided only that they are homoeopathic (though not isopathic) to the immediately apparent pathology or malfunction. Some homoeopaths maintain that the administration of homoeopathic drugs in such ponderal doses in emergencies ceases to be true homoeopathy. Yet Hahnemann went further, when he said in note 67 to section 67 of the *Organon of Medicine:*

'. . . in the most urgent cases, where danger . . . allows no time for the action of a homoeopathic remedy . . . it is admissible and judicious, at all events as a preliminary measure, to stimulate the irritability and sensibility (the physical life) with a palliative . . . When this stimulation is effected, the play of the vital organs again goes on in its former . . . manner. It does not follow that a homoeopathic medicine has been ill selected for a case of disease because some of the medicinal symptoms are only antipathic to some of the less important and minor symptoms of disease . . . ; the few opposite symptoms also disappear of themselves after the expiry of the term of action of the medicament, without retarding the cure in the least.'

He goes on to warn that his statement should not be interpreted as a licence for mixers who wish to

'justify their convenient employment . . . of other injurious allopathic trash besides, solely for the sake of sparing themselves . . . trouble . . . and . . . conveniently appearing as homoeopathic physicians, without being such.'

It is quite clear from Hahnemann's words that the inducing of any serious symptomatic crisis in a patient through the negligent or excessive use of unpotentized, or low-potency, remedies, though they may well be homoeopathic, is absolutely contrary to the fundamentals of homoeopathy (the elimination of adverse drug action, while bringing to the fore the drug's reactive potential) and such a crisis may only be risked when the patient's life is in imminent potential danger. (Cf. 'Contra-Indication against Administering Simillimum'.)

For the sake of emphasis it is clearly stated that, since grave chemical aggravations (see entry) are always possible with pathological homoeopathic remedies that are unpotentized, or of very low potencies, **any such use of homoeopathic drugs must be under experienced professional attention and undertaken with due judicious caution for the minimum time, only as may be considered absolutely necessary in true emergency situations.** (See 'Aggravation' and 'Homoeopathic Laws, Postulates and Precepts'.)

In a number of countries, recently introduced legislation has made access difficult or even illicit to some of the following medicines (or low dynamizations thereof), but exemptions may be applicable in true emergency situations. In all events, the following should not be construed as encouragement to unlawful action.

A recently published reference work which comprehensively covers homoeopathic treatment in many non-emergency ailments and some simpler first-aid situations is *The Family Guide to Homoeopathy* by Andrew Lockie (London: Penguin Group's Elm Tree Books, 1989, 402 pages).

A comprehensive guide for rendering essential physiological assistance concurrent with the homoeopathic treatment to casualties of all ages in any emergency involving injury or sudden illness is indispensable. A relatively complete, easy to use, reference book on the subject is

First Aid Manual – Emergency Procedures for Everyone at Home, at Work or at Leisure being the authorized manual of St John Ambulance, St Andrew's Ambulance Association, and The British Red Cross Society (London: Dorling Kindersley Ltd, Feb 1990 fourth impression). Refer also to details of a manual given in this entry under Toxic Spills and Leaks (of chemical and radioactive materials) for chemical emergencies.

Anaphylactic Shock (Anaphylaxis)

(extremely severe allergic reaction to insect stings, sulphites, penicillin, aspirin, egg, fish, nuts, shellfish, legumes, milk, potato, rice, blood transfusion or serum-based injectables).

a) If provoked by an injectable, place tourniquet above injection site (remove temporarily every 10 to 15 minutes);
b) Patient to be in recumbent position with lower extremities elevated;
c) Adrenalinum 3CH administered with a nebulizer hand-pump and inhaled repeatedly, as often as necessary, to control acute laryngeal oedema; if this comes too late, insert endotracheal tube or perform tracheotomy;
d) Administer potentized Antitoxinum, preferably in suppository form, or as an injectable;
e) Give oxygen at 4 to 6 litres per minute;
f) Monitor vital signs frequently;
g) If blood-pressure cannot be obtained, give normal saline intravenously;
h) If potentized Antitoxinum is unavailable, give Calcarea lactica natronata 1CH (lactate of calcium and sodium) in water to patient to drink.

To prevent a recurrence, identification of allergen is essential, and patient will need to avoid the specific foodstuff, or wear certain colour combinations when outdoors to decrease the chance of being stung, or carry an Adrenalinum nebulizer hand-pump to be used when unavoidable exposure to the hazardous agent has occurred. (See also 'Allergy'.)

Angina Pectoris (stenocardia due to ischaemia of the heart muscle in coronary disease)

Amylium nitrosum, which in its provings produces pain and constriction around heart, palpitations and praecordial anxiety, is homoeopathic to this condition. A small quantity of mother tincture, of not more than 0.2ml, dropped on to a handkerchief and inhaled, will give immediate relief. This remedy's action is only of a short duration. (N.B: The inhalation of large doses is harmful.) This is thereafter to be followed immediately by Glonoinum 3CH at quarter-hourly intervals to normalize palpitations, residual pain and dyspnoea. [Historical note: The name of this remedy is an acronym, derived from **GL**ycerin, **O**xygen and **N**itr**O**gen, because the base substance is nitroglycer**INUM**, which is an explosive discovered by Ascanio Sobrero in Italy in 1846. In the following year Constantin Hering, working with Morris Davis, a Philadelphia chemist, had begun extensive homoeopathic provings of this substance on himself and others stretching over four years. The homoeopathic uses of Glonoinum were published in the *British Journal of Homoeopathy*, vol.VII (1849), pp 412-421; and ibid. vol.XI (1853), pp 268-292. Glonoinum is one of the many monuments to Hering's therapeutic genius, thanks to which this notable remedy was introduced into homoeopathy's materia medica. From there it passed into orthodox medical practice. The first allopath to use it (about thirty years later) similarly for angina pectoris, was Dr William Murrell, who published *Nitroglycerine as a Remedy for Angina Pectoris* in 1882 (Detroit: Davis).]

Angioneurotic Oedema (giant urticaria)
Either Antipyrinum 2DH or Copaiva 1CH in half-hourly alternation with Calcarea lactica natronata 1CH will bring speedy relief. If these remedies are not to hand, the first centesimal Hahnemannian trituration of Chloralum, given once only, will also provide relief. If one of the large oedematous swellings affects the glottis it may endanger life by suffocation. In such a case Adrenalinum 3CH, sprayed from a hand-pump nebulizer, should be inhaled immediately by the patient. (See also 'Allergy'.)

Animal or Human Bites (e.g. one child by another)
To be treated as wounds (see below); bleeding must be stopped (no tourniquet to be used) and the wound cleaned thoroughly (see Bleeding and Haemorrhage below). Aconitum napellus 6CH is to be taken immediately. In an attack by an animal, be alert to the possibility of rabies. Bites are infectious up to five days before rabies symptoms become evident in an infected animal. In any event (Trigonocephalus) Lachesis 30CH or Hydrophobinum (Lyssin) 30CH should be administered in all such cases. As with all dirty wounds (see Septic Conditions and Blood-Poisoning below), complications associated with infection by Clostridium Tetani bacterium, must be borne in mind, and one of the following five remedies should be administered straight away: Curare (Chondodendron tomentosum) 6CH; Passiflora incarnata Θ sixty drops, repeated several times; Physostigma venenosum 3CH; Strychninum 3CH; or Upas tiente 3CH. Sutures may be required. If a snake-bite is involved, do not use a tourniquet, do not cut the wound, and do not allow the victim to walk if the bite is on the leg. Reassure the victim and treat as for oligaemic shock (see below). The antidoting of particular ophiotoxins requires the identification of the snake that bit, but the very great predominance of nervous symptoms

in (Simaba) Cedron gives it the power to antidote, or at least to attenuate considerably, the effects of quick-acting neurotoxic snake-venom (of front-fanged species), that may often cause early death from respiratory failure (asphyxia). The pure tincture of this bean is to be scraped on the wound. If unavailable, (Mikania) Guaco 3CH is to be administered. For the slower-acting snake-venoms, the following remedies may be considered: Euphorbia polycarpa (Golondrina) – tincture locally and internally every 15 minutes; Salaginella – macerate in cow's milk, locally and internally; Sisyrinchium – doses of 15 drops of tincture half-hourly; or Gymnema sylvestra – powdered root locally and internally.

The table [1] below sets out the correlation of snake families with venom-types and symptom group, to assist in deciding which homoeopathic remedy may be more pathotropic:

Family	Venom type	Symptom Group
Adders	Cytotoxic	Intense pain; massive swelling and extravasations. Death due to oligaemic shock.
Front-fanged	Neurotoxic	Little or transient local pain; little swelling; restlessness; difficult swallowing; increased sweating; dizziness; respiratory failure (asphyxia).
Seasnake	Myotoxic	General muscular paralysis. Death due to respiratory failure, hypercalcaemic cardiac arrest, or generalized metabolic toxaemia.
Back-fanged	Haemotoxic	Moderate local pain; haemorrhage at site of bite; dizziness; headache; nauseated feeling; peripheral and internal haemorrhage; haemoglubinuria. Death due to loss of blood.

Appendicism

Acute appendicitis is, almost always, a surgical condition. For appendicism, however, which is a symptomatic discomfort in the region of the vermiform appendix, the routine pathotropic emergency prescription is Iris tenax 2DH two-hourly.

Arterial Hypertension (high blood pressure)

To lower both the systolic and the diastolic pressures Spartium scoparium 1CH is administered three times daily.

Auricular Fibrillation and Arrhythmias

Chinidinum sulphuricum Θ restores normal rhythm in auricular fibrillation,

[1]Visser, John, MSc and Prof David S Chapman, MD, MS, FRCS. *Snakes and Snakebite.* Johannesburg, London and Cape Town: Macdonald Purnell, 1981, p 7.

supplementing the action of Digitalinum 3CH trit (dose: 0.5g two-hourly). Two doses of 100mg each, three hours apart – if patient responds, to be followed by four doses of 200mg each daily. This corrects paroxysmal tachycardia and establishes normal heart rhythm, at least temporarily, though less so in valvular lesions. (See also Tachycardia, below in this entry.)

Bleeding (capillary)

An Adrenalinum 4DH solution sprayed, or applied with cotton wool, where local, direct application is feasible (e.g. bladder, ear, larynx, mouth, nose, rectum, stomach, throat or uterus), provided the capillary haemorrhage is not due to defective coagulation of the blood. If complete ischaemia (bloodlessness) is induced, it is of no serious consequence, because it will not last for long.

Boils and Styes

(also ulcerations on edge of eyelid and catarrhal or purulent conjunctivitis)
    Arctium lappa 1DH three times daily. Locally, a 1% solution of Cuprum sulphuricum Θ.

Bronchial Asthma and Severe Allergic Rhinitis (hayfever) Affecting Chest

Acidum hydrocyanicum 3DH quarter-hourly, if recent and uncomplicated; or Adrenalinum 3CH inhaled with hand-pump nebulizer; or 0.2g of Iodoformum (base powder Θ) placed on to back of tongue will relieve an attack (note: very occasionally an idiosyncrasy exists; this should be eliminated by questioning the patient.) (See also 'Allergy'.)

Burns and Scalds (first degree)

Twelve drops of Urtica urens Θ to 50ml of aqua destillata, or a lotion of Hamamelis macrophylla Θ (20 drops : 50ml aqua destillata) are used to saturate a sterile gauze or dressing that covers the burn; to be moistened again and again when becoming dry, without removing the lint. In the absence of this tincture some boiling water poured on to freshly picked stinging nettles will do as well. Blebs should not be opened or drained. Or, Echinacea angustifolia Θ applied locally as a cleansing wash and then as a moist dressing.

Cold Injuries and Frost-bite

Rest in a recumbent position. Initially, very gentle rubbing of the affected area with snow (forceful massage or compression is harmful) then the application of some cold (i.e. room-temperature: not icy) water. This homoeopathically prevents too sudden a reaction involving the mechanism of vascular changes and sludging of the blood. Then rapid rewarming by moist heat is indicated, keeping temperature of solution between 31 and 37 degrees Celsius. After rewarming, the affected part should be painted with (Lindera) Benzoin Θ. If it is in the feet and hosiery adheres Oleum olivae is to be rubbed over the Benzoin tincture. Thereafter exposure to air at room temperature (21 to 24 degrees Celsius) is the most satisfactory, while use of the affected part is discouraged until the extent of damage can be determined.

Collapse

(with sub-normal temperature and low blood pressure)

Camphora 1DH, three doses to be given in 15-minute intervals.

Congestive Heart Failure

Supportive treatment consists of rest, decrease in cardiac work demand until compensated, and oxygen under positive pressure (6 litres per minute) by nasal catheter. Strophanthus hispidus (a.k.a. Uabaina or G-Strophanthin) Θ should be employed as it is homoeopathic to all the left cardiac and ventricular insufficiency syndromes. It is perhaps twice as efficient as Digitalis, for which the latitude between therapeutic and toxic doses is dangerously small. Strophanthus hispidus is non-cumulative and is only contra-indicated in hypertension with marked arteriosclerosis, in coronary artery disease, in hypercalcaemia, in cases of pronounced electrolyte imbalance and in acute or chronic nephritis. In acute cases, the dosage is 5-10 drops of the tincture three times daily, after an initial emergency dose of not more than 5ml in acute heart failure. Less dramatic, but with an action on the heart very similar to Strophanthus is Convallaria majalis Θ. It, too, has no cumulative action, and it has no contra-indications. Dosage: in symptoms of acute heart failure 15 drops of the tincture. The concomitant use of Chloralum hydratis, that is occasionally recommended in some homoeopathic text-books, is advised against. Digitalis pulverata (powdered leaves) is recommended by Professor William Boericke, E Harris Ruddock and was even used by C F S Hahnemann on such occasions. It is, however, not recommended here since the latitude between the therapeutic and toxic doses is uncomfortably narrow. Moreover, its effects are cumulative, and it is contra-indicated in many conditions that may not be readily identifiable in emergency situations, such as: low serum potassium level, ventricular tachycardia, sinus tachycardia, rheumatic carditis, angina pectoris, pneumonia, following an acute coronary thrombosis, in diphtheritic heart, in thyrotoxocosis, in partial heart-block, and in patients receiving Parathyroidinum or large doses of either Vitamin D or Niacin. Chloralum hydratis that is occasionally recommended in some textbooks is also advised against.

Contusions

(bruising of the soft parts):

Arnica montana Θ or Arnica oil should be applied to the part if the skin is unbroken. If the skin is broken, a lotion of Hamamelis macrophylla Θ (20 drops to 50ml). Arnica montana 3CH internally.

(bruising of the bones):

Lotion of Ruta graveolens Θ (20 drops to 50ml) and Ruta graveolens 3CH internally.

(bruising of the female breast):
Bellis perennis 3DH internally.

(bruising of parts with abundant innervation, such as fingers, toes or spine):
Liniment of equal parts of Hypericum perforatum Θ, alcohol fortis and aqua destillata to be rubbed on to the injured part (if the spine) three times daily, or to be kept applied on lint (if it is in the extremities).

Convulsions (of infants)
Warm bath (34-36 degrees Celsius) and a single dose Oenanthe crocata 6CH. Prevention of self-injury (e.g. dislocation), assurance of adequate airway by positioning and removal of mucus and secretion by suction and support of the jaw are indicated. The causative factor should be determined as soon as possible. (See also under 'Toxic Spills and Leaks' below in this entry.)

Cyanosis Neonatorum (of the newborn infant)
(Cerasus) Laurocerasus Θ to be given in two or three drop doses, as necessary. Patient is best supported in knee-chest position. If heart massage is necessary, for a baby's heart it is sufficient to press with two fingers only, at about one hundred beats a minute.

Delirium Tremens
Restraint may be necessary but should be avoided, if possible. Ranunculus bulbosus Θ in 30 drop doses, or Scutellaria laterifolia Θ in 10 drop doses half-hourly until relieved. Patient may have strong soup or beef infusion.

Dysentery (with high fever)
Along with rest in bed, warmth, and ample fluids by mouth in the form of water or fennel tea, five to ten drops of Cuphea viscosissima Θ is to be administered to the patient in acute cases; in long-standing cases Vaccinum myrtillus Θ ten drops eight-hourly.

Electric Shock (including lightning-stroke)
Current must be switched off. If this is impossible, the person is to be freed with some insulating material intervening, such as heavy duty insulating gloves, or with the aid of something made of wood or rubber, or even with folded newspaper. Without touching the victim's skin, the surrounding clothing, if it is absolutely dry, may be used to free the person from the current. If breathing is failing, or has ceased, resuscitation must be instituted immediately. Morphinum 3CH is the homoeopathic drug of choice for the effects of lightning and electric shock. Phosphorus 6CH is an effective alternative.

Epilepsy
In epilepsy without halo Zincum valerianicum 2DH is the pathotropic remedy

of choice, on the supposition that the patient's convulsions are the only, or at any rate the only serious, departure from health. In other epilepsy, Scutellaria laterifolia Θ will reduce the severity of the attack and diminish the frequency of the convulsive symptoms. During a seizure, self-injury is to be guarded against by gentle restraint and removal of dangerous objects nearby. Some insist on insertion of a rolled handkerchief or washcloth into mouth across the bit (with edges well protruding) to prevent tongue biting and tooth damage. Others advise not to put anything in patient's mouth or to try opening it.

Haemorrhage

With rest, reassurance, avoidance of excitement and all stimulants, and, if the haemorrhage is external, the application of pressure (20 minutes) and sterile cellulose alginate (made from seaweed and absorbed without setting up local irritation) Acalypha indica 6CH (or Achillea millefolium 3CH) is administered, with the possible addition of Menadione (vitamin K3).

Hiccough (persistent, severe and rapid singultus)

The pathological homoeopathic remedy for this debilitating condition consists of 60 drops of Scutellaria lateriflora 3DH repeated every two hours, or a single dose of Moschus moschiferus 1CH. (Datura) Stramonium 6CH is another pathotropic remedy for this condition. The homoeopathic ('like') household cure for it is rebreathing using a paper bag or face mask.

Insect Stings

(non-allergenic, including bluebottle- and scorpion-stings, spider- and horsefly-bites)

Ledum palustre Θ is immediately applied locally. In its absence, equally quick results can be expected from Arnica montana Θ, or Calendula officinalis Θ, or Urtica urens Θ. Internally, two 15 drop doses of Grindelia robusta Θ to be taken ten minutes apart, or, for very red inflammation with burning hyperaesthetic sensation relieved by gentle massage, a single dose of Cantharis vesicator 30CH. For a sting on the tongue or in the mouth one tablespoonful (15ml) Calendula officinalis Θ is to be poured into mouth and kept there for as long as possible. Pyrethrum parthenium is, as its name suggests, homoeopathic to the hot sensations produced by insect stings or bites, and its mother tincture applied to the skin has the added advantage that it repels insects.

(allergenic)

Adrenalinum 3CH, sprayed from a hand-pump nebulizer, should be inhaled immediately and repeated quarter-hourly at first, then less frequently, to control the reaction. Hypericum perforatum 6CH is to be taken perlingually.

Jelly-fish Sting

See 'Externally Applied Homoeopathic Drugs', under Acidum aceticum.

Nausea and Vomiting (from motion or pregnancy)

Where no form of food is tolerated, the remedy of choice is 10 drops Amygdalus persica Θ; also Cucurbita pepo Θ or 1DH as an alternative.

Miscarriage Threatened

The threatened foetus can be secured with the administration of five drops of Viburnum opulus Θ three times daily.

Oligaemic Shock (due to haemorrhage, or plasma-, or electrolyte-loss)

Blood flow is increased to vital centres (e.g. medulla oblongata) by raising the foot of the bed or couch where patient is allowed to lie undisturbed, with warmth in moderation, being given fluids by mouth, when possible. Stimulants are contra-indicated. The remedy to be given is Hypericum perforatum 1DH four-hourly.

Paediatric Emergencies

Infants and children represent a relatively large proportion of emergency cases. Under certain circumstances in these age groups, some conditions require suitable modification in emergency therapy as given here for adults. In all cases ponderal drug dosages must be modified by weight, age or skin surface area, where no specific infant or child doses are given.

Poisonings

Refer to section 'Ingested Poisons' in this entry under 'Toxic Spills and Leaks' (of chemicals or radioactive material).

Subcutaneously Injected Overdose of Drug: Patient is to remain recumbent. A tourniquet (1 x 50cm) is applied proximal to the site of the injection. The pulse beyond the tourniquet should not disappear and it is to be loosened for one minute in every ten. First trituration of Zincum valerianicum to control the excitement may be indicated, as it is homoeopathic to hysteria, epilepsy without aura, violent neuralgias and uncontrollable sleeplessness. For patients with great nervous agitation, restlessness and extreme sensitiveness the first trituration of Codeinum might be employed. In cases of coma, Opium 30CH is usually the drug of choice, whereas in catalepsy it would be Curare (Chondodendron tomentosum) 6CH. Apomorphinum 6CH may be considered where alcoholism plays a part. (Erythroxylon) Coca 6CH may be suitable when diplopia and/or local sensory numbness and formication feature along with talkativeness and cerebral activity. Where there is hallucinatory psychosis or a suicidal tendency Anhalonium lewinii 4DH might be the most homoeopathic functiotropic drug, whilst (Datura) Stramonium 6CH might be appropriate if erotomania, delirium and/or tremors are present.

Pulmonary Venous Congestion and Uraemic Dyspnoea

Aspidosperma quebracho Θ, a 10 drop dose every hour, with patient in

Fowler's position or the position for maximum comfort; oxygen by mask or nasal catheter at 6 to 8 litres per minute to be supplied.

Septic Conditions and Blood-poisoning
Echinacea angustifolia Θ, 20 drops, every two hours, and larger doses. To be used locally at the same time, as a cleansing and antiseptic wash. Pyrogenium (Pyrexin) 6CH intercurrently every four hours may be considered.

Snakebites
See entry for Animal or Human Bites above.

Sun-stroke or Heat-stroke
Glonoinum 6CH is repeated two-hourly till relief of the bursting, pulsating headache, which cannot bear motion, is achieved. At the same time, where there is sun-burnt skin, a solution of Calcarea chlorinata, one part to ten aqua destillata, may be applied locally. In its absence, Citrus limonum Θ in a solution of like proportion applied twice a day will minimize the ill effects. The patient must be kept in a cool shady room. In severe cases the rectal temperature must be reduced to 39 degrees Celsius by whatever means are available, such as constant vigorous massage of the extremities to promote circulation of the blood cooled there to all parts of the body.

Stricture of Tear Duct (in an infant)
Thiosinaminum 3DH is administered twice daily.

Stricture of Urethra
Clematis erecta Θ two-hourly is given first. Once the resolution is established, treatment is continued with Thiosinaminum 2DH four-hourly. Patient is encouraged to drink freely.

Surgical Erisipelas (haemolytic infection of the wound following a surgical operation, accompanied by severe constitutional symptoms)
Cinchona officinalis Θ ten drops two-hourly, while applying Veratrum viride 1DH hourly, when the tissues under the affected area of skin are involved and suppuration threatens. This will often cut short an attack if done right at the outset. When suppuration has occurred, Hepar sulphuris calcareum 6CH is indicated. It is important to pay attention to such foci as chronic fissures, which may be the fount of recidivation. Therefore, Balsamum peruvianum 1DH may be painted on to the part concerned.

Tachycardia (rapid beating of heart, more than 100 bpm)
Crataegus Θ five drops two-hourly should help to control this straight away; Iberis amara Θ would do as weli Patient to rest in recumbent position. In the case of supraventricular tachycardia application of Weber's manoeuvre is

advised: patient to sit up in bed with head bent forward between flexed knees, expelling a deep breath against a closed glottis or blowing into sphygmomanometer tubing to maintain a pressure of 40 mmHg for 15 to 30 seconds; to be repeated several times, with short intervening rest periods. Muscular contractions in chest, abdomen and diaphragm in forced expiration raises the air pressure within the lungs and thereby impedes the flow of blood through the pulmonary capillary bed. In such cases and in auricular fibrillation and arrhythmia 100mg powder of Chinidinum sulphuricum base substance to be administered (dose not to be exceeded to avoid precipitating a symptomatic crisis – see under Auricular Fibrillation and Arrhythmias in this entry above).

Toxic Spills and Leaks (of chemicals or radioactive materials)

Over the past decade chemical substances and other hazardous materials have increased in number, usage and complexity. With the existing diversity both the risk of exposure by individuals (at home or the work place) and the potential for a chemical emergency on a wider scale (on a public thoroughfare or along the railway track) have increased substantially. A very comprehensive 'Chemical Emergency Action Manual' has been published by the C V Mosby Company of London/St Louis/Toronto (second edition, 1983). This is an all-encompassing quick-reference volume that makes the following essential information instantly accessible in a way that is concise, yet easily understood:

Identification of the chemical or noxious agent;
Hazardous attributes associated with it;
Measures to contain the extent of damage caused by it;
Immediate signs and symptoms observable in its victims;
Name and instructions for use of any chemical antidote;
Essential first aid procedures under four headings – skin, eyes, ingestion and
   inhalation.

The signs and symptoms will direct the homoeopath to the indicated pathotropic (lesional) remedy that can be the only one applicable in such an emergency. General guidelines, concerning such accidents are outlined here:

Chemical in the Eye:

Clean, cool water is to be used at once to flush the eye (with lids held open) continuously for at least 15 minutes. Attempt to use chemical antidote should be avoided. Later a lotion (20 drops to 50ml of aqua destillata) of either Hydrophyllum virginiacum 1CH or Euphrasia officinalis Θ or occasionally even the succus (not the spirit tincture) of Cineraria maritima Θ, whichever may be homoeopathically appropriate, may be instilled into the eyes several times daily.

Chemical Burns:

Once contaminated clothing not sticking to the skin has been removed all affected parts are to be flushed with plenty of clean, cool water. (N.B. The clothing ought to be handled in a manner to preclude further contamination.) If hosiery adheres Oleum olivae may gently be applied. A sterilized dressing, with a 1% aqueous solution of the possibly homoeopathic Acidum picricum, may be applied to the exposed damaged skin (not over very large surfaces, however); if indicated the 1% Acidum picricum solution may be continued until granulations begin to form. When chemical burns turn into poisoned wounds (septicaemia) the internal remedy of choice is Echinacea angustifolia Θ, twenty drops every two hours.

Burns and Scalds:

Small burns and scalds (first degree) should be treated by flushing the affected area with plenty of clean cool water and then treating as stated above in this entry under section 'Burns and Scalds (first degree)'. When the burn is large or deep it should be covered with lint soaked in lotio Calcii hydroxidi oleosum (Carron oil, which is equal parts of linseed oil and the homoeopathically proven Aqua calcis [lime water]), while Cantharis vesicator 3CH, or Kali bichromicum 3DH, is given perlingually every hour. Later Causticum 30CH may be substituted.

Gassing and Inhaled Poisons:

Victim is moved to fresh air by someone equipped with respiratory protection. Tight clothing ought to be loosened, and blankets wrapped around the victim, if necessary, so as to conserve body warmth. If breathing is depressed artificial respiration (possibly resuscitation also) should be started, with objects and vomitus removed from the casualty's mouth. Phosphorus is homoeopathic to accidental injuries caused by the inhalation of gases and may be administered in a 12CH potency to the casualty.

Unconsciousness:

Immediate attention is to be given to the victim's air passages, which must be kept open: the mouth must be cleared (of dentures, vomit, etc.); the tongue may not block the back of the throat. Unless there are suspected fractures that cannot be secured with support, the unconscious person would best be placed in the 'recovery position'. Opium is homoeopathic to unconsciousness and may be given in a 30CH potency to the casualty.

Ingested poison:

It is emphasized at the outset that when the victim has ingested a convulsant, a corrosive (alkali or acid) or a petroleum product (benzinum [lighter fuel], thinners, petrol [gasoline], acetone, kerosene [paraffin], solvent naphtha, petroleum ether, toluene, xylene, etc.) the administration of syrup of (Cephaelis) Ipecacuanha is strictly contra-indicated. (The incompatibility arises from the fact that petroleum products pass readily into the trachea where they reactively reduce the cough reflex, and during vomiting the patient may aspirate gastric contents. Whereas with alkalis or acids, emesis presents the possibility of gastric perforation. In the third instance, with convulsants, vomiting may bring on such convulsions.) Nevertheless, Ipecacuanha's chief homoeopathic action is on the ramifications of the pneumo-gastric nerve, producing spasmodic irritation in chest and stomach, with its principal guiding feature being persistent nausea and vomiting. It is frequently indicated for other ingested poisons that produce such symptoms. In such an emergency

15ml of syrup of Ipecacuanha are administered, followed by half a glass of water, for no other purpose than to induce vomiting so as to remove the poison from the stomach. If it has moved further along the intestinal tract, two tablespoonfuls of Natrum phosphoricum monobasicum (phospho-soda) are administered as a cathartic. Succus of Citrus limonum (or, simply, expressed lemon juice) may be administered as an antidote in alkali poisoning; John Henry Clarke in the 'Dictionary of Practical Materia Medica' states that it will allay convulsive fits, while antidoting a variety of poisons. To delay absorption and to ameliorate poisoning with corrosives, undiluted Lac vaccinum (cow's milk) may be administered in small quantities. The first trituration of Carbo vegetabilis, thoroughly mixed with sufficient aqua destillata to make a consistency of thick cream, will make the most effective adsorbent, the prompt use of which prevents the effects of otherwise lethal amounts of poison. For each kilogram of the patient's body weight 5ml of the Carbo vegetabilis may be administered in toto orally (or by gastric lavage) and then removed by suction or emesis. This may be repeated up to twenty times with doses of 15 or 20ml each time. Each gram of Carbo vegetabilis will absorb from 100 to 750mg of poison. The only exceptions here are mineral acids or alkalis against which it is ineffective. Body warmth may be conserved through blankets, but the application of external heat is not appropriate.

Uraemic Dyspnoea

See above, under 'Pulmonary venous congestion and uraemic dyspnoea'.

Wounds

(lacerated):

Lotion of Calendula officinalis Θ (20 drops to 50ml) locally and Calendula 3CH to be taken internally every two hours.

(incised):

Lotion of Hypericum perforatum Θ (20 drops to 50ml) locally and Hypericum perforatum 3CH internally every hour.

(punctured):

Lotion of Ledum palustre Θ (20 drops to 50ml) locally and Ledum palustre 6CH internally every hour.

(poisoned):

Lotion of (Trigonocephalus) Lachesis 6CH (10 drops to 50ml) locally and Lachesis 6CH internally every hour.

Empedocles of Agrigentum (ca. 490-430 BC)

See 'Humoral Pathology in Prescribing'.

Empirical Medicine

More correctly the Empirical tradition in medicine relies on practical experience as a guide to practice or to the therapeutic use of any skill or remedy; avoids all extraneous speculation and abstract reasoning. Historically it has always occupied the probabilioristic minority counter-position *vis-à-vis* the Rationalist tradition in medicine. By its adherents it is seen as scientific medicine. Homoeopathy views itself as the ultimate scientific development within this stream of medical thought. (See 'Determinism', 'Hahnemann, Christian Friedrich Samuel (1755-1843)', 'Philosophical Premise of Homoeopathy', 'Probabiliorism' and 'Rationalist Medicine'.)

Emulsion

A combination of two immiscible liquids in which one is dispersed throughout the other, suspended in the form of very small globules. (See 'Lotion'.)

Emulsoid

Emulsion colloid.

Enantiopathic Method

See 'Allopathy' and 'Phytotherapy'.

Encyclopaedia of Pure Materia Medica

See 'Allen, Timothy Field, AM MD (1887-1902)'.

Enema

Administration of a homoeopathic medicine in a liquid, applied at varying volumes via the rectum, either to treat a local bowel condition or to provide the body with internal medication, to be absorbed via a route different from the standard perlingual. Homoeopathy deplores the use of physiological doses of medicinal components in enemas, because these often alter the bacterial flora of the bowel and are readily absorbed into the body fluids exerting a coercive drug effect.

Energy

The capacity or power to produce an effect. Energy can be potential or kinetic, and comes in a variety of forms: chemical, dynamical, electrical, mechanical, nuclear, radiant and thermal. Dynamical energy is *sui generis* the capacity or power inherent in the life principle. In both its latent and active forms, dynamical energy charges the dynamic field of an organism, that is it exerts a physical influence by interrelating and firmly linking matter and all manifestations of energy in a living entity. Comparable to the dynamic fields of organisms are other fundamental fields within which matter is bound as energy: the electro-magnetic and the gravitational fields and the matter fields in quantum physics. (See 'Dynamis', 'Homoeopathic Laws, Postulates and Precepts', 'Pharmacological Message', 'Radiant State of Matter, Theory of' and 'Vitalism'.)

Entelechy

Entelecheia (see 'Dynamis').

Environment

Occasionally, this is a factor precipitating, or contributory to, the onset of disease (e.g. the occupational diseases or the effects of bad hygiene). If the environment's adverse effects are either long, or profound, enough, they may set off a chronic disease process (chronic miasma) which continues even after the offending environmental influence has been removed (e.g. the grave prognosis in the Morgagni-Laennec syndrome [alcoholic cirrhosis] despite teetotalism; and in a large number of the so-called diseases of occupations). At other times, however, this is a positive modifying factor (e.g. the ideal environment sought to be created in a convalescent home or spa, designed to allow the process of cure to proceed to best advantage). (See 'Miasma'.)

Enzyme Potentiated Desensitization

Technique employed at the Royal London Homoeopathic Hospital for allergy hyposensitization. It was originated in 1966 by Len McEwan originally of St Mary's Hospital Medical School, London, UK and subsequently of the London Medical Centre. The method uses a potentized mixture of a wide variety of highly purified inhalants and foods in conjunction with the enzyme beta-glucuronidase as an adjuvant. Beta-glucuronidase is an enzyme that is present throughout the human body, and the dosage employed is within the range present within the patient's tissues at the time of administration. Two modes of administration exist:

1 The Cup Method – in which a small area of the thigh or forearm is scarified and the hyposensitizing fluid is held in place over the scarification for twenty-four hours by means of a plastic cup;
2 Intradermal Injection – through a fine needle the fluid is introduced into the forearm's skin (not below it), to raise a bleb in the skin from where it is absorbed into the system slowly, via the same route as in the cup method.

This multiple-remedy homoeo/isotherapeutic combination is reported to be very successful in seasonal, pollen-induced hayfever and general house-dust mite allergies, but less reliable in controlling allergies from ingestants or contactants. The most pessimistic assessment on the success rate is: 'Enzyme

Potentiated Desensitization will fail in about 20% of suitable patients with known allergies. The rest will experience varying degrees of improvement.' It is reported that this treatment's effect can be almost immediate, notably in house-dust mite allergies. Seasonal hayfever is said to be treated successfully with one dose per year given not more than four months before the allergenic season; the full benefit, however, will set in only after about three weeks of administering the combination remedy. A moderately severe dietary adjustment, covering only the 48-hour period immediately subsequent to inoculation, is part of the regimen imposed on the patient.

Epidemiology

The study of epidemics and epidemic diseases. When disease, introduced from outside, attacks many people (animals, plants) in a community contemporaneously, it is said to be epidemic, as distinct from endemic, which refers to disease that is continuously present. A temporary increase in the number of cases of an endemic disease is also called an epidemic. Homoeopathy regards epidemics as a class of specific disease (just as it also regards the acute miasmata), quite distinct from the general mass of morbid phenomena evident in each afflicted individual. Each epidemic has features of its own and is distinguishable from other, perhaps superficially similar, epidemics. Homoeopathy regards each epidemic as a product of a single cause, being, therefore, in all instances amenable to one and the same specific remedy, which is to be reached by the study of the phenomena of several cases, carried on until the symptom-totality of the particular genus epidemicus is captured and its simillimum found.

In an outbreak of epidemic stomatitis aphthosa (highly infectious foot-and-mouth disease) among cattle in Switzerland in 1960, Dr Pierre Schmidt of Geneva and a veterinary student of his undertook a trial of homoeopathic prophylactic treatment amongst the cattle not yet infected. They administered RNA picornavirus and another appropriate nosode in rising potencies (30CK, 200CK and 1M), two doses of each potency per drug for three days running, followed by Acidum nitricum 6CH added to the drinking water as a pathological remedy. Not a single animal treated in this way developed the disease although they were fed and dosed by the same cowherd who tended the rest of the herd that was or later became infected.

One of many other instances of the efficacy of homoeopathy in epidemics revolves around the severe outbreak of Cholera Asiatica in London during 1854. The London Homoeopathic Hospital was adapted during the epidemic to treat only cholera victims. When the epidemic was over the Government instructed a medical inspector, Dr Maclouchlin, to gather the results of treatment in the various hospitals. The results of the London Homoeopathic Hospital were so outstanding that they were suppressed by the Medical Council in its Blue Book, containing the report put to Parliament. Fortunately, a homoeopathic patient was there as a Member of Parliament. He questioned why the results of the Homoeopathic Hospital were not included and insisted that they be procured for Parliament. So as not to appear next to the figures for the non-homoeopathic hospitals, a separate Blue Book was produced and put before Parliament together with a letter from Dr Maclouchlin, the inspector, himself an orthodox medical man. It was revealed that the death rate at the Homoeopathic Hospital was 16.4% contrasted with 51.8% at the other hospitals. (The records of the British Museum confirm these figures.) The second Blue Book confirmed that they were all true cases of Cholera Asiatica. In his official report the medical inspector said he had seen cases recover who would have died in other hospitals, while at the conclusion of his letter he wrote: 'If it should please the Lord to visit me with Cholera I would wish to fall into the hands of a homoeopathic physician'. (See 'Causes of Disease', 'Miasma', 'Nosode', 'Verdi, Tullio Suzzara, (1829-1902)' and 'Veterinary Homoeopathy'.)

Epistemological Assumptions in Homoeopathy

● **The nature and validity of homoeopathic science is looked at closely covering the following aspects: similarity, health, disease, disease names, constitution, environment, infinitesimal deconcentrations, placebo, wanted and unwanted drug reactions, as well as objective and subjective symptoms.**

Homoeopathy makes at least ten fundamental assertions, of a scientific and philosophical nature, that have acquired an axiomatic character in homoeopathic therapeutic science, as it is practised. These concern:

1 The universal similarity principle making the curative impulse coextensive with the disease process;
2 The indivisibility of physiology and pathology;
3 The synonymity of disease and drug categories;
4 The primacy of constitutional propensity over environmental influence;
5 The medicinal efficacy carried into the dynamized ultramolecular drug deconcentrations;
6 The untraceability of any substance that is homoeopathically totally inert at all times, consequently reducing the rating of 'placebo' from a status of an absolute to no more than a relative co-ordinate in therapeutics and experimental work; the same can be said, *mutatis mutandis*, for 'vehicle' (in homoeopathic pharmacy);
7 The link between homoeopathy's holistic approach and scientific pharmacology to be in the recognition and in the skilful exploitation of the full multiplicity of drug effects;
8 The parity of scientific validity between subjective experiences and objective phenomena in both diagnostics and therapeutics;
9 The postulating of vitalism as the firm conceptual thesis both for therapeutics in disease and for drug pathogenesis in health; and
10 The biphasic action of medicines, also known as hormesis, where the first

coercive action gradually changes into the second reactive effect, that is more or less opposite to the first.

1 Similarity
● **as a Concept in Science: the Integrating Principle of Homoeopathy.**

Many kinds of symmetry are encountered in nature on all levels: on the atomic level, and beyond, amongst the baryons, hadrons and mesons, and still further amongst the quarks (where each is organized into characteristic repetitive combinations); the same is true for the molecules; it happens in polymerization and in crystallization; it is evident in plants and in animals; based, in all cases, on the similarity principle. For instance, the quality possessed by crystalline substances, by virtue of which they exhibit a repetitive arrangement of similar faces, is the result of their peculiar internal atomic structure. That repetitive arrangement follows a similarity principle. In fact, all repetition, as in reproduction, genetics, cellular regeneration (healing), and much besides, can only take place within the confines of the similarity principle. Likewise, everything that is imitative, such as mimicry, camouflage, and convergent evolution (nature's plagiarism of its own previous handiwork), employs the similarity principle. All adaptations, and, as the word suggests, assimilative processes demonstrate this bias in the direction of similarity. The most pervasive feature of the cosmos is the controlling omnipresence of similarity in a myriad forms. Without that the cosmos would appear as utterly, unimaginably alien. It is, clearly, a mosaic of individuation where nothing is truly identical to anything else, but with similarity in some form ever present as the one unifying bond. It is thanks to the similarity principle that ideas, feelings, judgements and movements are integrated in the minds of individuals and proper associative connections can intelligently, intuitively and instinctively be made there. The process of inductive reasoning (inference from the particular to the general) rests on the phenomenon of recurring similarity. It is through similarity that an individual feels, or rather knows within himself, that he shares a common kinship with everything in the universe. The phenomena of resonance, periodic movements, harmonics, actinomorphisms, cyclic occurrences, and such like more in abundance, are evidence of an imitative affinity expressed as repetition patterned through the similarity principle. Memory could not function without this principle being evident all around. Classification of any sort is only possible through it. Recognition, sorting and other selective actions are only feasible through elements with traces of similarity. Problems are solved through comparisons and contrasts made against the backdrop of similarity. The immune system could not function except through this one constant. The unique sequence along the helical strands of deoxyribonucleic acid, or the templates of messenger-ribonucleic acid, can only fulfil their autoreproductive function by employing the correspondence principle. Cells distinguish between the similar and the dissimilar, accepting the former and rejecting the latter. Most astonishingly, it has been found that chaos, the highly irregular behaviour of bodies in motion, possesses a *de facto* element of 'feedback', becoming evident as a dynamic phenomenon, unfolding as the state of a chaotic system changes into patterned regularity with time. The jargon of the geometry of chaos is clearly rooted in the idiom of similarity and its associations in physics: e.g. topological dynamics, phase space, saddles, mappings, bifurcations, orbits, flows, joined tori, closed loop, endless cycle, periodic behaviour, resonant motion, period-doubling cascades, all speak of coherence through ultimate recurrence. There is, indeed, nothing where the similarity principle does not in some way play a primary role.

The universe consistently conforms to a teleonomic requirement to keep producing patterns of mimesis (close resemblance), seemingly because of the manifest continuity and survival value these have. This generalization describes specified natural phenomena within the limits of empirical and experimental observation; it is also not in conflict with recognized laws of nature comprehending relevant phenomena; moreover, this generalization can be meaningfully related to such other laws. This means that the statement at the beginning of this paragraph meets all the requirements of a scientific law waiting to have its validity tested for inconsistencies. Any exception to this scientific law would be just such an inadmissible inconsistency; it could invalidate it. (See 'Laws of Nature'.)

Given its universality, one would, therefore, expect the similarity law also to apply in matters relating to the mechanism of drug effects. A closer look at a condition called Dermatitis Medicamentosa should provide a conclusive prima facie answer. Cutaneous lesions arising from reactions to drugs taken internally, or administered topically, are collectively referred to as Dermatitis Medicamentosa. Drugs, used non-homoeopathically in ponderal doses, may produce, under favouring conditions, nearly all the diverse primary lesions which occur in the very many skin ailments. Obviously the drugs are given with the intention for them to act in a specified way on the patient, instead, or in addition thereto, these drugs have induced an unwanted reaction in the patient.

First observation: Drugs are capable of producing a primary action coercively, as well as eliciting a secondary reaction.

While the effects of drugs used in ponderal doses upon the skin are not constant, or the same in different individuals, or even the same in the same person at different times, this is also true as regards other external provocations of 'natural disease', where the predisposing quality of the individual organism (constitution), modified by temporal variations, co-determines the variations in symptom-pictures.

Second observation: Diseases can best be known through their symptoms as presenting in individual patients, and are not usefully classifiable with respect to common external provocations, but rather in terms of individual symptom-pictures.

Third observation: Each drug's reactive quality becomes evident only

in the course of pathogenetic experimentation (provings), and/or clinical, veterinary and toxicological evidence, the sum of which provides that drug's symptom-picture.

Occasionally, in Dermatitis Medicamentosa, the drug action on the skin is nearly constant and specific as also may be the action of a specific cause of disease (in a miasma) (see both 'Epidemiology' and 'Miasma'). This occurs frequently and consistently enough to permit a clear generalization to be made in which specific drugs can be said uniformly to have a reactive affinity to specific dermatological disease conditions.

Fourth observation: A demonstrable analogous relation, based on similarity, exists between the symptom-complex of disease and that produced by specific drugs (the homoeopathic agents).

Similarity is the integrating concept of homoeopathy. It links the organism's own curative mechanisms (reaction) to drug effects. It is always the operative principle. Even when it may be obscured by plethoric individuation, flowing from subjective symptoms. Underneath it all, this overt similarity remains the absolute basis for connecting drugs to disease, and can never be absent. In Dermatitis Medicamentosa subjective sensations, such as itching, burning or tingling may precede, attend or follow the outbreak of the eruption. Systemic symptoms may be absent, or fever, headache and malaise may appear. If long continued, some drugs, in non-homoeopathic applications, lead to grave constitutional symptoms or even death. Drug eruptions may appear rapidly such as the congestive and exudative forms or more slowly, such as the eruptions from iodine and bromine salts. Erythemas are more often produced than any other lesions. Next in order are vesicles, papules, wheals, blebs, pustules and tubercles, while pigmentation, gangrene, purpura and desquamation are rarer effects. Some drugs may produce all varieties of lesions while others give rise to only one or two.

The following collation obviously does not include all the drugs which may, here and there, also cause skin eruptions nor does it mention the more subtle drug effects. But quite apart from the illustrative purpose in producing this list, it is important that the attending homoeopath should be familiar with non-homoeopathic drug effects for purposes of differential diagnosis, and the elimination of a pathogenetic agent, if such there be; for this the compilation may serve as a handy reference. It must be pointed out that in some instances (e.g. Acetanilidum) the dermatological effects, though they occur, are uncommon and the drug concerned may tend to be applied homoeopathically as a pathological remedy in areas that feature more prominently in the drug's symptom-complex; in other instances (e.g. Tuberculinum and Antitoxinum) the remedies are never used pathologically for their undoubted dermatological effects, but only systemically (in miasmata) or constitutionally. This list demonstrates homoeopathy's drug-in-phase-with-disease concept with close consistency. This fundamental concept is summed up here in the –

Fifth observation: The symptom-complex, which a remedy can cause in a susceptible organism, is invariably that which the remedy is ideally

adpated to cure in another susceptible organism, on the basis of drug-to-disease symptom-similarity, provided obstacles to cure have been removed.

The broad juxtaposition of the mass of recorded[1] 'incidence of dermatitis medicamentosa & symptoms' (IDM) and 'other prominent pathogenetic effects (OPE) on the one hand, alongside all causative drugs' 'pathotropic application in homoeopathy' (PAH) on the other, is unfortunately not possible here. Yet a representative number, given in some detail, clearly demonstrates, in the randomly chosen sample (the first dozen, taken alphabetically), the incontestable parallelism between the symptom-complex which a drug can cause and another, semblant symptom-complex, due to miscellaneous other causes, which the same drug can cure homoeopathically. Although any other segment of disease phenomena might have been chosen with like results (e.g. occupational diseases),[2] the reasons why dermatological effects were selected as a basis for demonstrating the similarity principle were:

a) their high degree of conspicuousness;

b) the practical usefulness of such a compilation for reference purposes; and

---

[1] The information, given under the first three rubrics (NHU, IDM and OPE) below, is compiled from the following eight sources:

i) The Pharmaceutical Society of Great Britain. *The Extra Pharmacopoeia*, William Martindale. Volume I, 24th Edition. London: The Pharmaceutical Press, 1958.

ii) Bellanti, Joseph A. (Professor of Paediatrics and Microbiology, Georgetown University School of Medicine) *Immunology*. Philadelphia, London & Toronto: W B Saunders & Co, 1971.

iii) Cohen, E Lipman and J S Pegum. (Consultant Dermatologists, England) *Dermatology*. 2nd Edition. London: Bailliere, Tindall & Cassell, 1970.

iv) Coulter, Harris Livermore and Barbara Loe Fisher (the former is a medical historian), referred to for their source documents, particularly for the Pertussis Vaccine in *DPT: A Shot in the Dark*, 1st edition, New York: Warner Books, Inc, 1986.

v) Criep, Leo H. (Associate Professor of Clinical Medicine [Emeritus], School of Medicine, University of Pittsburgh) *Clinical Immunology and Allergy*. 2nd Edition. New York & London: Grune and Stratton, 1969

vi) Dearborn, Frederick M. (Professor of Dermatology, New York Homoeopathic Medical College) *Diseases of the Skin, Including the Exanthemata*. This homoeopathic textbook, of the pre-steroid age, contains 230 photographic plates, providing a large number of visible examples of cured or greatly improved cases of serious dermatological complaints of diverse aetiology, stating for each which of the homoeopathic remedies, and in which potency, achieved the curative effect; also which other methods had been attempted. Originally published New York, 1913; republished New Delhi: B Jain Publishers, 1979.

vii) Lockey, Richard F. (Associate Professor of Medicine, University of South Florida College of Medicine) *Allergy and Clinical Immunology*. New York: Medical Examination Publishing Co, Inc, 1979.

viii) Solomons, Bethel (Consultant Dermatologist in England) *Lecture Notes on Dermatology*. 3rd Edition. Oxford, London, Edinburgh and Melbourne: Blackwell Scientific Publications, 1975.

[2] Hunter, Donald. *The Diseases of Occupations*. Well over one thousand metals, alloys, metallic compounds, salts, alkalis, acids, aromatic and aliphatic carbon compounds, as well as a miscellany of chemical and volatile irritants, toxicants and asphyxiants are given with a detailed description of the disease effects they produce. The great majority of these have also undergone homoeopathic pathogenetic experimentation (provings) and their pathotropic application in homoeopathy demonstrates, exactly as it does in drug-induced dermatitis: 'The like of what it can cause, it can cure.' Sixth Edition. London, Sydney, Auckland and Toronto: Hodder & Stoughton, 1980, pp 248-686.

c) the additional advantage of simultaneously providing consistent and clear evidence of the first part of Hering's rule regarding direction of disease metastasis. (See 'Homoeopathic Laws, Postulates and Precepts, section 14.)

Sixth observation: Though the pathogenetic drug effects begin on the surface as skin lesions, if the exposure to the drug is for a lengthier period, it may lead to grave constitutional symptoms or even death, which confirms part one of Hering's rule, that states: 'With intensification of any disease, symptoms move from the surface to the interior.'

Viewed from the practical, therapeutic angle, Dermatitis Medicamentosa becomes the organism's 'early warning system' of worse to come, if ignored.

Seventh observation: The homoeopathic drug-to-disease similarity principle applies to the use of medicinal agents only (and to nothing else), to be administered in a manner designed to elicit a dynamic curative reaction homoeopathic to the existing disease symptom-complex.

That definitely means the similarity law does not relate to agents simply intended to affect the organism in any of the following five ways:

1 Coercively, by direct chemical or toxic action;
2 By mechanical effects;
3 Through supportive, supplementary or nutritional additives;
4 By methods to incapacitate, remove or destroy infesting parasites directly; and
5 By direct physiological effects.

This is known as Dake's exclusion synopsis; the exclusion succinctly delimits the sphere of the law of similars to scientifically predictable homoeopathic drug effects. This summary is not intended to shut out, a priori, any other medical or paramedical method as such, for each of these may sometimes well be complementary to the homoeopathic effect.

It is colloquially said, that certain procedures are 'homoeopathic' (e.g. the physiological effects intended in 'sweating out a fever in a wet-pack' or by 'gently rubbing snow on to frostbitten parts'). Whereas this is quite proper common usage, it cannot be regarded as strictly accurate.

A final point must be made. The collation that follows is not to be misconstrued. **Under no circumstances are the dermatitogenic drugs that are known to have caused a dermatitis medicamentosa to be prescribed pathologically (pathotropically) for that same dermatitis medicamentosa, in the acute phase.** This would constitute the type of senseless Isopathic treatment against which Hahnemann spoke out in note 63, section 56 of the *Organon of Medicine*: 'Isopathy, as it is called – . . . is . . . a method of curing a given disease by the same . . . principle that produces it. . . . [The noxious principle] is given to the patient highly potentized, and, consequently in an altered condition . . .' Hahnemann then distinguishes between 'simillimum' (the most similar) and 'idem' (the same) in higher dynamizations, and continues, 'To attempt to cure by means of the very same morbific potency (per Idem) contradicts all normal human understanding and hence all experience. Those who first brought Isopathy to notice, probably thought of the benefit which mankind received from cowpox vaccination by which the vaccinated individual is protected against future smallpox infection and, as it were, cured in advance. But both cowpox and smallpox are only similar and in no way the same disease. They differ in many respects . . .' Therefore, the drugs, in and around the very low potency levels, given next to PAH below, might well be prescribed pathologically for similar dermatitis medicamentosa symptom pictures that have other than identical causes. There are, of course, instances where isopathic treatment has its rightful place in homoeopathy (see 'Allergy' and 'Isopathy'), for example, in isopathic hyposensitization procedures in allergies and hypersensitivities, but in such instances, again, the very low potencies used in pathological prescribing would not be applicable. Hahnemann conceded, that the 'idem' could be regarded as a 'simillimum' once it had been potentized beyond the 'lower' stages, because it would take on a different character then, making Isopathic procedures effectively homoeopathic.[1] (See 'Isopathy'.)

Collation on Dermatitis Medicamentosa
Legend:
NHU   = principal non-homoeopathic use(s)
IDM   = incidence of dermatitis medicamentosa and symptoms
OPE   = other prominent pathogenetic effects
HMM = listed in homoeopathic materia medica
PAH   = pathotropic application in homoeopathy, through not necessarily primarily so

Acetanilidum (N-Phenylacetamide):
NHU   — antipyretic, analgesic;
IDM   — not common; erythema, erythematous papules;
OPE   — cyanosis, secondary anaemia, collapse;
HMM — W Boericke, J H Clarke;
PAH   — 3CH perlingually to relieve cyanosis and collapse, also in pallor of the skin;

Acidum benzoicum:
NHU   — preservative in pharmaceuticals, expectorant, used to acidify the urine, antimycotic agent;
IDM   — rare; erythema, papules, wheals;
OPE   — asthmatogenic cough, irritation of gastric mucosa;
HMM — Homoeopathic Pharmacopoeia of US, W Boericke, J H Clarke, C Hering, T F Allen (Encyclopedia), R Hughes and J P Dake (Cyclopedia of Drug Pathogenesy), F. Donner (Provings);

[1] Hahnemann, Christian Friedrich Samuel. *The Chronic Diseases, their Peculiar Nature and their Homoeopathic Cure*, translated in 1896 from the second enlarged German edition of 1835 by Prof Louis H Tafel, Philadelphia: Boericke and Tafel, 1904, p 152.

PAH — 3CH perlingually to relieve gouty syndromes with swellings and red itchy blotches; Acidum Benzoicum is the peculiar principle of all true balsams, used topically for many dermatological conditions;

Aqua amygdalae amarae:
NHU — base for skin lotions;
IDM — rare; erythema, urticaria;
OPE — none;
HMM — Homoeopathic Pharmacopoeia of US, W Boericke, J H Clarke, C Hering, T F Allen (Encyclopedia), F Donner (Provings), T L Bradford (Provings);
PAH — 3DH perlingually for urticarial wheals;

Antimonium crudum and tartaricum:
NHU — against schistosomiasis, leishmaniasis;
IDM — rare; vesicles, pustules, urticaria;
OPE — pains in joints and muscles, bradycardia, colic;
HMM — Homoeopathic Pharmacopoeia of US, E Boericke, J H Clarke, C Hering, T F Allen (Encyclopedia), F Hughes and J P Dake (Cyclopaedia of Drug Pathogenesy), F Donner (Provings), T L Bradford (Provings);
PAH — 3CH-5CH (atten. or trit.) perlingually for eczema with colic; pimples, vesicles and pustules; urticaria; scaly, pustular eruptions; rheumatic pains;

Antipyrinum (2:3-Dimethyl-5-phenylpyrazol-5-one):
NHU — analgesic, antipyretic;
IDM — common: usually morbilliform, occasionally erythematous macules, and less often papules, wheals, blebs, pustules, purpuric spots, desquamation and pigmentation;
OPE — excessive perspiration, nausea, fainting, collapse, occasionally agranulocytosis, seldom methaemoglobinaemia and cyanosis;
HMM — W Boericke, J H Clarke, T L Bradford (Provings);
PAH — 2DH perlingually for erythema, eczema, pemphigus, pruritus, urticaria, angioneurotic-oedema, dark blotches on skin and desquamation, scarlet macular eruptions, nausea, Cheyne-Stokes respiration, fainting spells and, in higher potencies, for leukocytosis and erythema multiforme;

Antitoxins, Tuberculins, Vaccines (Tuberculinum Hominis/Bovis; Diphthericum; Tetanicum; Bordetella Pertussis vaccine):
NHU — to confer passive, or produce active, immunity; in diagnosis;
IDM — occasional: Tuberculin rash may be scarlatiniform, morbilliform, or in irregular patches; Diphtheria Antitoxin causes erythematous, scarlatiniform, morbilliform, purpuric or urticarial lesions;

Tetanus Antitoxin may cause wheals;

Pertussis Vaccine occasionally produces eczema, angioneurotic-oedema, subcutaneous extravasation of blood (ecchymosis) and formation of egg-sized lump at injection-site, and a variety of skin rashes;

OPE — fever, respiratory distress, central nervous system depression, somnolence, spasms, brain damage, pain with high-pitched screaming, systemic shock, irritability, cretinoid retardation, hypsarrhythmia in electroencephalogram patterns (exceedingly irregular), epilepsy;

HMM — Addendum to Homoeopathic Pharmacopoeia of US, T L Bradford (Provings);

PAH — the symptoms given under IDM above, all appear under the Antitoxin and the Tuberculina, but these are not normally used as pathological remedies in the light of the much more serious nature of the systemic symptoms listed under OPE;

Apium virus (Bee-venom):

NHU — employed therapeutically in rheumatic affections, in the form of injection, as ointment and as a solution for external use;

IDM — common: generalized eruption of wheals, erythema and oedema;

OPE — acute anaphylaxis;

HMM — Homoeopathic Pharmacopoeia of US, J H Clarke, W Boericke, T L Bradford (Provings);

PAH — 3DH perlingually for erythema nodosum, venenous, allergic, gouty and dropsical swellings, erythema without vesiculation, nettle-rash, inflammation of labia, phlebitis, oedema glottidis, swollen hands, burning of feet, varicosities, urethritis;

Arsenicum album:

NHU — as a tonic, in the treatment of malaria, in syphilitic skin conditions, against psoriasis, in lupus erythematosus and in secondary anaemia;

IDM — common: nearly every variety of skin lesion, erythema, papules, vesicles, wheals, pustules, purpuric and psoriatic spots, pigmentation, keratosis, gangrene, ulcers, loss of hair and nails, pruritus, inflammation of the conjunctive and nasal mucous memoranes, disposition to oedema (especially in face and around eyelids), varioloid eruptions;

OPE — severe gastric pain, vomiting, diarrhoea, numbness and tingling in the feet, muscular cramps, ischuria, peripheral neuritis, renal or liver disease;

HMM — Homoeopathic Pharmacopoeia of US, W Boericke, J H Clarke, C Hering, T F Allen (Encyclopedia), R Hughes and J P Dake

(Cyclopaedia of Drug Pathogenesy), F Donner (Provings), T L Bradford (Provings);

PAH — the symptoms given under IDM above, all appear under Arsenicum Album, but it has been rarely used as a pathological remedy, because it is one of homoeopathy's constitutional remedies. When, however, it had been so used by homoeopaths (at College of Homoeopathic Medicine of the State University of Iowa, in the Yonkers Homoeopathic Hospital, in the Flower Hospital, and in the Metropolitan Hospital, all of New York) in anthrax, epithelioma, erysipelas, acute glossitis, smallpox, and ulcerative endocarditis a significant rate of success was recorded. The related remedies of Antimonium Arsenicosum, Arsenicum Bromatum, Arsenicum Chloratum, Arsenicum Creosotum, Arsenicum Hydrogenisatum, Arsenicum Iodatum, Arsenicum Metallicum, Arsenicum Stibiatum, Arsenicum Sulphuratum Flavum, Arsenicum Sulphuratum Rubrum, Arsynal (Disodium Methylarsenate), Kalium Arsenicosum and Natrum Arsenicum all present much the same reactions under the IDM and OPE rubrics in non-homoeopathic applications; this group is more frequently used pathotropically in homoeopathy, with a high success rate;

Aurum metallicum:
NHU — in rheumatoid arthritis, in non-disseminated (non-systemic) lupus erythematosus;
IDM — toxic reactions are reported in up to 50 per cent of patients undergoing gold therapy; in some 5 per cent of patients these reactions are severe and, occasionally, even fatal; pruritus, exfoliative dermatitis, wheals and nodules (these like erythema induratum or syphilitic formations), purpura;
OPE — nephrosis, agranulocytosis, anaphylactoid reaction including flushing of the face, oedema of the tongue and eyelids, dyspnoea, cyanosis, precordial distress, severe depression, unconsciousness and intensification of secondary skin rash;
HMM — Homoeopathic Pharmacopoeia of US, W Boericke, J H Clarke, C Hering, T F Allen (Encyclopedia), R Hughes and J P Dake (Cyclopaedia of Drug Pathogenesy), F Donner (Provings), T L Bradford (Provings);
PAH — for this medicine and its related remedies, Aurum Arsenicicum, Aurum Bromatum, Aurum Fulminans, Aurum Foliatum, Aurum Iodatum, Aurum Muriaticum, Aurum Muriaticum Kalinum, Aurum Muriaticum Natronatum and Aurum Sulphuratum, the homoeopathically proven and curative dermatological component of the symptom-complex comprises collectively: discoid lupus erythemetosus, erethism, scrofula,

eczema, indurations, pruritus vulvae, alopecia areta, bubos,
fistulae and nodules on tongue; but, since the Aurum
component in each of these drugs is very deep-acting,
profoundly affecting the patient's entire organism, none of them
are normally prescribed pathologically in homoeopathy.

(Atropa) Belladonna:

NHU — to first stimulate and then depress the central nervous system;
to antagonize the peripheral activity of parasympathetic and
certain sympathetic nerves, especially those innervating smooth
muscle, glands and the heart; for its depressant action on the
vagus nerve, while increasing heart rate; in ophthalmology as a
mydriatic and cycloplegic; as a liniment for muscular
rheumatism, sciatica and neuralgia; to reduce secretions, except
bile, milk and urine; as a spasmolytic; as an analgesic in
dysmenorrhoea; in enuresis;

IDM — common: scarlatiniform erythema, vesicles, pustules, gangrene;

OPE — glaucoma, pyrexia, suppression of sudoresis, photophobia,
excessive dryness of mouth, burning and constriction of throat,
severe thirst, difficulty in swallowing and speaking, stupor;

HMM — Homoeopathic Pharmacopoeia of US, W Boericke, J H Clarke,
C Hering, T F Allen (Encyclopedia), R Hughes and J P Dake
(Cyclopaedia of Drug Pathogenesy), F Donner (Provings), T L
Bradford (Provings);

PAH — for this medicine and its related remedies, Atropinum and
Atropinum Sulphuricum, the homoeopathically proven and
curative symptom-complex includes those under IDM above,
but it is generally prescribed, say, in a 3CH potency for such
dermatological conditions only if they appear together with
symptoms given under OPE, e.g. for Roseola with fever,
scarlatina, or Vincent's tonsillitis with erythema;

Borax veneta (Natrum boricum):

NHU — bacteriostatic, fungistatic, antiseptic in eye and skin lotions,
mildly astringent mouth-wash;

IDM — rare: morbilliform erythematous rash, papules, vesicles,
pustules, scales;

OPE — depression of circulation, subnormal temperature, meningeal
irritation and convulsions, aphthous sores in mouth, vomiting,
diarrhoea, coma;

HMM — Homoeopathic Pharmacopoeia of US, W Boericke, J H Clarke,
C Hering, T F Allen (Encyclopedia), R Hughes and J P Dake
(Cyclopaedia of Drug Pathogenesy), F Donner (Provings), T L
Bradford (Provings);

PAH — 1CH perlingually or as irrigation in aphthous stomatitis or
buccal thrush, as well as in cystitis, in pruritus pudendi and

eczema in vulva, similarly in exfoliative dermatitis and erythema multiforme; Acidum boricum is a related remedy with a comparable sphere of homoeopathic action.

Bromium:

NHU — antiseptic and deodorant lotion for chronic ulcers;

IDM — common: acneiform papulopustules, affecting parts abundantly supplied with sebaceous glands (face, back, shoulders), varicelloid vesicles, pustules and furuncular formations; more rarely: erythematous, urticarial, nodular, bullous, papillary or fungoid lesions; in children: lesions are usually condylomaform;

OPE — severe gastro-enteritis and violent irritation of respiratory tract and mucous membranes, caustic burns on skin;

HMM — Homoeopathic Pharmacopoeia of US, W Boericke, J H Clarke, C Hering, T F Allen (Encyclopedia), F Hughes and J P Dake (Cyclopaedia of Drug Pathogenesy); [Bromium Iodatum only] F Donner (Provings), T L Bradford (Provings);

PAH — [must be prepared fresh – liable to rapid deterioration] 1CH–3CH perlingually of this medicine, and related remedies Bromium iodatum and Acidum hydrobromicum, and primarily used pathotropically in asthma and other respiratory tract complaints, but scrofula, indurations, fistulas and skin ulcers are homoeopathically indicating symptoms.

The remainder of this collation on Dermatitis Medicamentosa only indicates (due to lack of space) the rate of incidence and briefly describes the known inflammatory or other conditions of the skin, brought on by the ingestion or absorption of the medicinal substances in orthodox pharmaceutical application. As in the twelve examples given above, the law of similars applies consistently. It is uniformly established through the corresponding curative homoeopathic effects. Each of the sixty undermentioned medications appears in all three of the following: (a) Martindale's [footnote 1 above, section i]; (b) Prof F M Dearborn's dermatology textbook [footnote 1 above , section vi]; and (c) the Addendum to the Homoeopathic Pharmacopoeia of the US, 1974, making such a comparison possible.

Bryonia alba (Bryony): Rare: erythema, papules, vesicles;

Calcarea carbonica (Carbonate of Lime): Rare: wheals, sometimes linear, wart-like lesions;

Cantharis vesicator (Spanish Fly): Rare: erythema, papules;

Capsicum annuum: Rare: papulovesicles;

Carbolicum acidum (Phenol): Rare: vesicles, pustules, erythema;

Chloralum (Hydrate of chloral): Common: scarlatiniform or morbilliform erythema; more rarely: vesicles, papules, wheals or furuncular, carbuncular and pruric lesions;

Chloroformum: Common: erythema; occasionally: pruric spots;

Chrysophanicum acidum (Goa powder): Common: coppery-red erythema, like erysipelas; marked desquamation;

Cicuta virosa: Rare: erythema, large papules, tubercles;

Cinchona (Quinine): Common: scarlatiniform erythema, desquamation, exfoliation; itching and pricking sensation with fever; less commonly: wheals, vesicles, blebs and purpuric spots;

Conium maculatum: Rare: papules, pustules, erysipelatous erythema;

Copaiva and (Piper) Cubeba: Common: most eruptions observed from the combined use of these drugs (as urinary antiseptics and expectorants) are due to Copaiva; vesicles, bullae, wheals, scarlatiniform and morbilliform erythema;

(Gonolobus) Cundurango: Rare: furuncular, acneiform lesions;

Digitalis purpurea, Digitalinum and Digitoxinum: Rare: erythema, vesicles, bullae and wheals;

(Solanum) Dulcamara: Rare: erythema, wheals, scales;

Euphorbium officinarum: Infrequent: oedema, erythema, vesicles with pain and fever; occasionally: pustules, ulcers and gangrene;

Graphites (Ferrous carbon): Occasional: erythema, papules, vesicles, dryness, induration, fissures, itching and exudation;

Guaiacum: Rare: miliary erythema;

Hydrastis canadensis: Rare: erythema with severe burning;

Hyoscyamus niger and Hyoscyaminum: Occasional: oedema, erythema, wheals; exceptionally: pustular and purpuric lesions;

Iodium: Common: papules, and papulopustules (so-called 'iodide acne') generally on the face, neck and shoulders; the lesions may become confluent and give rise to papillomatous, condylomaform, carbuncular or crusted lesions; occasionally: a multiforme or polymorphous eruption;

Iodoformum: Uncommon: erythema, papules, bullae, vesicles;

(Cephaelis) Ipecacuanha: Very rare: fiery red erythema with elevated borders; occasionally: wheals and vesicles;

Iris versicolor: Rare: vesicles, pustules, crusts, with neuralgic pain;

Jaborandi (Pilocarpus pinnatifolius): Rare: erythema, miliary papules, vesicles and wheals;

Kali chloricum (Potassium chlorate): Rare: erythema, papules, cyanosis;

Liquidum argenti nitratis (Silver Nitrate eye-drops): Rare: grayish-black pigmentation, erythematous papules;

Lycopodium clavatum: Very rare: erythema, pustules, vesicles, with itching, burning and bleeding;

Malonal (5:5 Diethylbarbituric Acid) & long-acting Barbiturates: Rare: scarlatiniform or morbilliform erythema;

Mercurius (Hydrargyrum) and its salts: Common: erythema, papules, pustules, vesicles, bullae or purpuric, furuncular and ulcerated lesions;

(Daphne) Mezereum: Rare: vesicles, pustules, abundant exudation, yellowish crusts;

Nitricum acidum: Rare: erythema, vesicles, pustules;

(Strychnos) Nux vomica and Strychninum: Rare: scaralatiniform erythema, vesicles, acneiform papules and pustules with pruritus;

Oleum jecoris aselli or Oleum morrhuae (Cod-liver Oil): Rare: acneiform papules, or erythematous vesicles;

Oleum ricini (Castor oil): Rare: pruritic erythema;

Oleum santali (Oil of sandalwood): Rare: simple erythema, petechial purpura;

Oleum terebinthinae (Oil of turpentine): Occasional: scarlatiniform or morbilliform erythema; in Terebene (as expectorant): papules with pruritus;

Opium, Morphinum and derivatives: Common: all forms of erythema, the exudative being the most common; wheals, vesicles, pustules, oedema with itching;

Phenacetinum (Acetylphenetidin, Paracetophenetidin): Rare: erythema;

Phosphorus and acidum Phosphoricum: Rare: grouped vesicles, wheals, bullae and haemorrhages;

Piper methysticum (fermented juice of Kava-kava): Common: erythematosquamous exfoliation and desquamation;

Pix liquida (Tar): Rare: morbilliform erythema, wheals;

Plumbum (Lead) and its salts: Rare: erythema, vesicles, pustules and purpuric lesions;

Pulsatilla nigricans and Pulsatilla nuttaliana: Rare: rubeoloid and urticarial eruptions;

Rheum officinale and Rhaponticinum (Rhubarb root extract): Rare: scarlatiniform desquamative erythema;

Salicylicum acidum and Salicylate derivatives (Aspirin): Rare: erythema, wheals, or, rarely, vesicles, bullae, purpura and gangrene;

Salol (Salicylate of phenol): Rare: wheals;

Santoninum and Natrum santonatum (Sodium santonate): Rare: wheals with desquamation and oedema, vesicles;

Sarsaparilla (syrup vehicle): Uncommon: erythema, vesicles; rarely: papillary or wart-like elevations;

Secale cornutum (Ergot): Rare: vesicles, pustules or furuncular, gangrenous, purpuric eruptions;

(Delphinium) Staphisagria: Rare: miliary papules and vesicles;

(Datura) Stramonium: Rare: scarlatiniform erythema; petechial, vesicular or pustular lesions;

Sulphonal (2:2-Di(ethylsulphonyl)propane): Occasional: desquamative erythema, with intense itching;

Tanacetum (Oil of tansy): Very rare: varioliform eruptions;

Tanninum acidum (Tannin): Rare: erythema, wheals;

Thallium metallicum and Thallium acetatum (Thallous acetate): Occasional: alopecia, more or less complete;

Valeriana officinalis (Valerian): Very rare: urticarial papules;

Veratrum viride (Alkavervir): Rare: erythema, pustules;

Viburnum prunifolium: Rare: scarlatiniform, desquamative erythema.

Treatment of Dermatitis Medicamentosa

In the majority of cases, the discontinuance of the drug or medicine is sufficient. Occasionally an antidotal drug (in homoeopathic application) will hasten recovery or correct any residual damage. Externally, protective measures are required when open lesions exist to prevent possible infective complications, or, it may be, that soothing applications are needed to relieve irritations or subjective sensations. Drug antidotes (refer to this entry) can be found in most works on Materia Medica; the correct antidotes will often be found to be the best in relieving any discomfort from which the patient may be suffering.

2 Physiology – Pathology

● **the Spectrum from Illness to Wellness as a Continuum.**

Consistent clinical experience and the cumulative experimental evidence of homoeopathy demonstrate that the terms 'health' and 'illness' represent mutually supplementary and very relative concepts, that are inclusive of one another. They are nothing if they are not the mutable expressions of one single entity: a particular individual's constitutional state. One man's health may be another's illness. Homoeopathy interprets both the propensity to heal and the tendency to illness – inherent aspects of every constitution – as essential constituents among those elements that drive life inexorably toward the mosaic of individuation and ever-abundant uniqueness. This is in conflict with, and, in fact, challenges, the older but more widely held Cartesian paradigm of the organism viewed as a stereotypical physiochemical machine, monotonously alike to any other of its species. More recently, in the biological sciences, post-mechanistic concepts, have attained prominence, such as:

the semi-empirical quantum models of electronic structure in biochemistry
(where the mechanistically conceived shape of molecules no longer has any
significance);
the chreodes of developmental biology;
the theory of cerebral morphogenetic radiation in psychophysiology;
the isomorphic phenomena of Gestalt psychology;
the archetypal form patterns of Jungian psychology;
formative causation in genetics;
teleonomic mutation (specifically to enhance survival) in evolutionary theory;
deterministic chaos;
morphic resonance in the theories of diffuse cognitive transference; and the
like.

These are in full accord with the epistemological assertions that have been made for about two hundred years by homoeopathic science.

3 Disease – Drugs

● **the Dynamic Patterns of Constituent Symptoms as Namesakes of their Curative Remedies.**

Homoeopathy rejects attempts at superficial symptomatic cures as ultimately worthless and as occasionally dangerous. No single symptom, nor even a few symptoms, outside their individual constitutional context, can have significance standing alone. The homoeopathic method consists of describing the whole reactive symptom syndrome of one individual's disease condition, within which each constituent symptom has a contributory meaning, as modified only by the constitutional inherency. Only with the aid of this dynamic pattern, as applied to any individual patient's case, can both the disease and its namesake remedy be accurately identified. The underpinning axiom for systematic homoeopathic disease classification is that all disease names are synonymous with the names of the medicines that act curatively by virtue of their being able to call forth the cognate illness patterns in the healthy.

4 Constitution – Environment

● **Constitutional Structuring Predetermines the Environmental Influence Eventually Manifest in any Living Being.**

Homoeopathy asserts that the well-indicated medicine (or an appropriate external psychological stimulus) can only heal within the possibilities, and into the limits of, a set individual constitutional pattern, and never beyond it. It also states that environmental factors, whether these impinge adversely or supportively, can only have an effect to the extent that either the corresponding vulnerability or receptivity pre-exists in the individual organic whole. Moreover, in the issue of how much any environmental formative influence (parental, educational, social) might itself contribute toward the structuring of somatopsychic features in an individual constitution (nurture versus nature), homoeopathy's understanding is

(i) that the almost unalterable potential endowment is there from conception; and

(ii) that the realization of previously dormant somatopsychic features in an individual is only brought about by his or her responding selectively (almost like a harmonic vibration of a string in a musical instrument to a particular note played elsewhere), by responding reactively only to the antidotal (the 'like') stimulus produced in such a person by parental, criminal, educational, social or other environmental influences.

It follows that, according to homoeopathic tenets, neither the predispositions nor the limitations would be capable of any fundamental transformations. This is of profound and far-reaching significance not only in daily homoeopathic clinical practice, but also in its interaction with psychotherapy, education, criminal rehabilitation, etc., because here homoeopathy is on the cusp of the Cartesian body-mind dichotomy. It can and does, for instance, profitably alert parents, penologists, educationists, social scientists, etc. to concealed limitations, tendencies or potentials in an individual. Although homoeopathy sees these constitutional features as being relatively fixed, allowance is made during assessment for the individual's degree of susceptibility. This is capable of being modified, though not removed, by factors such as age, noxious habits, long-term occupational insalubrity, accidental impairment, pathological conditions, or any similar radical somatic alterative. (See also 'Foods as Health Problems'.)

5 Base Drug – Ultramolecular Dose

● **Reactive Propensity: from Coarseness to Indefectible Correspondence. Quantity alone (in Chemical Terms) does not Constitute an Effective Pathogenetic Dose (Antidote): Homoeopathicity of a Drug Relative to a Disease Remains Intact from the Medicine's Crude Stage to any of its Finely Honed Infinitesimal Potencies.**

Quality, proportionality, dosage and patient susceptibility are the four factors homoeopathy says must be taken into account to achieve the desired curative stimulus. Quality represents the best attainable symptom-similarity between drug and disease action. Proportionality and dosage refer to the law of quantity and dose, which states that 'quantity (i.e. potency and dose repetition) of the drug required is in inverse ratio to the similarity' (see 'Homoeopathic Laws, Postulates and Precepts' section 4. Patient susceptibility to a drug is assessed in terms of the rule that the clearer and the more positively the finer, more peculiar and more characteristic symptoms of a remedy are evident in a patient, the higher the degree of susceptibility to the medicine to be anticipated, and hence the higher the likely choice of potency. It is the aspect of drug susceptibility that may induce a homoeopath to change the potency of a drug administered, or to employ 'rising potencies' (see 'Dose Repetition', particularly section 5). The underlying assumption made here by homoeopathy is that while there is no change in a drug's homoeopathicity as it is taken from base substance or mother tincture, through the low potencies, beyond Avogadro's number, to the high potencies, there is a subtle change along the way. It is not in the drug's strength or weakness, nor, except in the first few potency stages close to the crude state, does this change have anything to do with 'chemical aggravation' (see 'Aggravation' and [the introduction to] 'Emergencies – Homoeopathic Treatment'). This subtle change is in the development of the peculiarities of the remedy, as it rises in the scale of potencies. Provings of the crude drug and its lowest potencies produce only the more common and general symptoms, whereas the special and peculiar character of a medicine, revealed by its finer and most characteristic symptoms, becomes evident higher up the scale of dynamization. Yet both clinical experience and consistent experimental evidence, stretching over nearly seventy years, show that there is not a straight linear progression of refinement of symptoms, just as there is not such a progression in the patient's receptivity to the curative stimulus. Particular potencies will produce results while others below or above will not, but may once again further up or down the scale of dynamization (potentization). There are those homoeopaths who largely prescribe on the basis of the more common and general symptoms.

They tend to employ the lower potencies in most instances, and to shun the higher dynamizations by and large. There are also those homoeopaths who generally prefer the high potencies in drugs where the special and peculiar character is evident that exactly matches the patient's presenting disease picture. They will employ the low dynamizations only in a few very specific circumstances, but would actually prefer to avoid using them. There is no scientific reason why the whole potency range should not be available to benefit all patients.

Experimental Evidence

In 1927 K König bred Rana fusca larvae (from fertilized egg to embryo to young tadpole) in homoeopathic potencies, from 10^{-1} to 10^{-30}, of lead and silver nitrate. After Avogadro's number, from 10^{-24} to 10^{-29} there was a significantly higher death rate than in the controls, and strangely enough the results were ranged along a sinusoidal curve through the potencies.

During the 1930s W Persson of Leningrad tested the effect of various potencies of mercuric chloride on the rate of fermentation of starch by ptyalin (salivary amylase) and of the effect of a number of other potentized substances on the lysis of fibrin by pepsin and trypsin. In the starch experiment, which was well-controlled, he obtained a sinusoidal curve showing reactions to all potencies up to 10^{-120}, whereas none of the controls were affected abnormally. The results in the fibrin series of experiments were comparable.[1]

In 1988 Jacques Benveniste and his colleagues at the South Paris University found that human white blood cells (basophils), which are part of the immune system, responded to a solution of antibodies potentized serially all the way through to 10^{-120}. Basophils carry certain antibodies of the immunoglobulin E type on their surface and when these cells encounter antibodies directed against the immunoglobulin E molecules, they release histamine which they store in granules in the cell. Once they have become degranulated in this fashion, they respond differently to certain chemical stains. As was the case previously, Benveniste found a periodic fluctuation all the way up the scale of dynamization. The degranulation response of the basophils falls off at one potency, only to return at a higher one.[2]

---

[1]Stephensen, James. 'A Review of Investigations into the Action of Substances in Dilutions Greater than 1 x 10^{-24} (Microdilutions)' *Journal of the American Institute of Homoeopathy*, XLVIII (1955), 327 – 335. These two experiments, amongst many others, are described with full bibliographical references.

[2]Benveniste, Jacques, F Beauvais, E Davenas, P Belon, J Sainte-Laudy and B Poitevin, Université Paris-Sud, France. 'Human Basophil Degranulation Triggered by very Dilute Antiserum against IgE.' *Nature*, vol 333, pp 816-818, 30th June 1988. The editor of this scientific journal, the British journalist John Maddox, who publicly announced his strong antipathy to homoeopathy in a BBC Television interview in October, 1988, and two other men from the USA, the professional conjurer, James 'The Amazing' Randi and Walter Stewart, a scientific-fraud detective of the National Institutes of Health in the USA, set out to debunk this experiment two weeks after its publication. They created a momentary tumult around Prof Benveniste, a respected immunologist, but have nowhere claimed to have detected fraud; in fact, they only managed to point out that his group

6 Placebo – Nocebo

● **Appraisal of Such Co-ordinates in Homoeopathic Therapy aand Experiment**

Homoeopathy has established that no substance is absolutely medicinally inert, and that, consequently, there can be no absolute placebo. It follows that only a relative value can be assigned to placebo assessments both in therapeutic and experimental investigations, this is so whether the placebo is known or unknown, active or wrongly said to be inactive. The corollary concept of a 'nocebo effect' – any changes that occur as a result of placebo therapy that are perceived as negative or counter-productive to the path of cure – is regarded as homoeopathically tautological, for obvious reasons. (See 'Foods as Health Problems', 'Isopathy', section 2 – Sarcode: entry under Saccharum Lactis, and 'Placebo'.)

7 Holism – Homoeopathic Pharmacology

● **Multiplicity of Drug Effects Inevitably Leads to Holism in Homoeopathic Practice and to Permanence in its Pharmacology.**

Homoeopathy regards the concept of the selective action of drugs as canvassed by orthodoxy, and now sometimes emulated by phytotherapy, as misleading to some extent, since such a selectivity can be no more than relative. It is quite evident that any drug has more, many more, than one action, even leaving aside other related effects of great importance such as individual variations, drug reactions, dependence, hypersensitivities, teratogenicity, addictions, and the like. Homoeopathy maintains that any given action of a drug is either wanted or not wanted, in its orthodox application. Disingenuousness lies in the fact that what is therapeutically desired is simply labelled as the main action pharmacologically and is then given undue

---

had omitted some detail in the protocol set down for the experimental design (note: when there is inadequate succussion at one stage of dynamization, or for several other reasons [see 'Destruction of Potency'], the original message ceases to be carried forward into subsequent ultramolecular (sub-physiological) deconcentrations: the 'potency' becomes effectively non-potentizable from there onward; Benveniste *et al* discarded these inert potencies, but negligently omitted to say so in the preamble to their published work).

Parts of this experiment were, however, successfully duplicated in Canada, Israel and Italy by the following:

P Fortner and B Pomeranz, Departments of Zoology and Physiology, Ramsay Wright Zoological Laboratories, University of Toronto, 25 Harbord Street, Toronto, M5S 1AI Ontario, Canada;

J Amara and M Oberbaum, Ruth Ben Ari Institute of Clinical Immunology, Kaplan Hospital, 76100 Rehovot, Israel;

B Robinzon, Department of Animal Sciences, Faculty of Agriculture, P O Box 12, The Hebrew University of Jerusalem, 76100 Rehovot, Israel;

A Miadonna and A Tedeschi, Department of Internal Medicine, Infectious Diseases and Immunopathology, University of Milan, Ospedale Maggiore Policlinico, Milan, Italy.

prominence. At the same time the range of unwanted effects, on the spectrum from the trivial to the fatal, are relegated in the literature to the minor position of adverse, toxic or side effects, remaining more or less unpublicized. The fact that drugs produce multiple reactions in the organism, though publicly passed over in silence this may often be, is tacitly acknowledged by orthodoxy in that the same neglected side effect of one application may, often, on another occasion become the one wanted effect (e.g. the sedation caused by the competitive antihistamines). The strong tendency to a unitary-effect-per-drug approach in orthodox medicine takes its origins in orthodoxy's constant search for medicines that are specific for certain standardized disease categories. Yet as each drug's many effects, other than the one that was targeted as the main effect in the publicity effort surrounding the drug, become more and more difficult to conceal from its users, so these drugs are abandoned as therapeutic agents, only to be replaced by others chosen on the same faulty premise, destined to end the same way, and so on: orthodoxy's familiar march-past of short-lived remedies.

By contrast, homoeopathy's insistence 1) that the entire spectrum of a drug's reactive potential be skilfully utilized inevitably places its approach solidly in a holistic position; and 2) that homoeopathy will never need to jettison any of its drugs makes for the durable basis underpinning its scientific approach to pharmacology.

(See also 'Compatibility of Homoeopathic and Orthodox Drugs'.)

8 Subjective Experiences – Objective Phenomena

● **The Scientific Necessity for the Inclusion of the Patient's (or Prover's) Subjective Symptoms along with Objective Ones is Asserted by Homoeopathy, Believing These to be Inseparable.**

The arbitrary positing by Orthodox Medicine of an exclusively external medical world that is totally independent of both the individual patient and the attendant homoeopath is seen as scientifically unsound and misleading for two reasons:

1   the homoeopath could not help but use a subjectively contaminated mental model to assess the patient, quite like any non-homoeopathic practitioner cannot ever avoid doing; and
2   the patient, or prover, would be reduced to a human caricature devoid of consciousness, leading to the problems experienced by some non-homoeopathic disciplines, but particularly acutely by Orthodox psychiatry and neurophysiology, or Behaviourist psychology, that allow no place in the patient's brain for consciousness or mind. (This is discussed in some detail under 'Philosophical Premise of Homoeopathy', in the section entitled Contribution by Christian Friedrich Samuel Hahnemann.)

9 Vitalism – Physicalism

● **The Thesis for Postulating Vitalism as a Firm Conceptual Base both for Therapeutics in Disease and for Drug Pathogenesis in Health.**

This is discussed under 'Vitalism'.

10 Biphasic Drug Action

● **The Observed Action of Medicines, where the First Direct, Coercive Action Gradually Changes into the Second Reactive Effect, Which is More or Less Opposite to the First.**

The uniform pattern, first described by Hahnemann, manifests palpable similarity between the patient's disease symptoms and the primary symptoms of the drug. The homoeopathic effect amounts to the exploitation of the fact that the disease irritation would always be reliably extinguished by the later secondary symptoms of the medicine, which are, in reality, the patient's appropriate reaction, now reinforced, that will overwhelm and annihilate the disease – provided the organism's dynamic reactive capacity is adequate. (See 'Homoeopathic Laws, Postulates and Precepts', section 5.)

Equivalents Established Between 'K' and 'H' Potencies

The technical differences between the Korsakovian ('K') and the Hahnemannian ('H') dynamizations are set out in detail under 'Potentizing Methods' section The Specifications Relating to Potentization Methods. However, the average correspondences of experimentally measured ('tagged') molecular deconcentrations permit the establishment of the following table of comparative approximations.[1]

Korsakovian 1M (1000K)	9CH
200K	8CH
30K	7CH
12K	6CH
9K	5CH
6K	4CH
4K	3CH

This is the generally accepted formula for comparison between medicines dynamized by the two potentization methods. It is evident that this 'equivalence' is only based on the mean residual quantity of molecules remaining behind from previous (lower) dynamizations, since due to normal adhesion to the phial's glass sides there is comparatively much more such residue left behind after any Korsakovian attenuative step, than there would

---

[1] Boiron, Jean. 'Scientific Proofs of the Action of Homoeopathic Medications', sub-item 'The Making of Homoeopathic Medicines', medical seminar – public lecture, Johannesburg, RSA on Saturday 21st February 1981.

be using the Hahnemannian method. This assessment, however, simply ignores every other pertinent aspect, particularly the fact that a 30K would have been succussed twenty-three times more than the 'equivalent' 7CH.

Older versions of such tables[1] gave different equivalents, due to mensuration inaccuracies, for the two highest clearly measurable potencies: 8CH was taken to be 60K or 70K, and 9CH was taken as 100K. A contributory factor to this error probably was the preconceived conception that there would have to be a straight-line progression of approximately 30K steps for each 1CH increment from 7CH to 8CH to 9CH. In reality, this progression on the Korsakovian scale of dynamizations has turned out to be an asymptotic curve, as shown on Figure 6 under 'Potentizing Methods'.

Ethanol

See 'Alcohol'.

Euthenic (Nosode) Treatment

A homoeopathic prophylactic therapy during the first three months of pregnancy to benefit the growing foetus, by tending to better both its prenatal environmental influences as well as its own developing innate qualities, although the drug choice, apart from the nosodes in the 1st, 3rd and 4th weeks, is guided by the constitution of the mother-to-be.

- 1st week – Psorinum or a constitutionally indicated psoric drug (see 'Miasma');
- 2nd week – Tuberculinum residuum hominum (Koch's) or Tuberculinum aviarum or Tuberculinum bovinum or Tuberculinum hominum (Marmorek's) [formerly in favour in francophone area] or Bacillinum (Compton-Burnett's) or one of the two tuberculinic drugs Phosphorus and Stannum;
- 3rd week – Medorrhinum or one of the three sycotic drugs Acidum nitricum, Natrum sulphuricum and Thuja occidentalis;
- 4th week – Lueticum (Syphilinum) only.

(See also 'Antenatal Homoeopathy', 'Euthenics', 'Foubister, Donald (1902-1988)', 'Gynaecology', 'Obstetrics and Homoeopathy' and 'Pregnancy'.)

Euthenics

Deals with determining optimum living conditions for plants, animals or humans, especially through care for proper environment and provisioning. (See 'Drainage', 'Environment', 'Nutrition' and 'Miasma'.)

[1] Chavanon, Paul. For example, this laureate of the Faculty of Medicine of Paris and of the Societé d'Homéotherapie de France, published such a table with his preface to *Memento Homéopathique d'Urgence*, Paris: Editions Dangles, 1973, p 35.

Evaporator

See 'Utensils of Homoeopathic Pharmacy'.

Exclusion Diet

See 'Elimination Diet'.

Exercise

This, like Remedial Dance Therapy, is corrective therapy that is complementary to homoeopathic treatment. (See 'Naturopath'.)

Exhaustion

Utter fatigue; depletion; in homoeopathy, dynamic exhaustion is a state characterized by an inability to respond to stimuli; a using up, or removal, of contents from any material supply of, or stored power in, anything. Nervous exhaustion is neurasthenia. Mental exhaustion constitutes an inability by the brain to respond adequately. Heat exhaustion describes a reactive state of the organism in response to exposure to heat, which is marked by dehydration, prostration or collapse. Exhaustion of a drug's action, as a phrase, describes the stage of completion reached after the stimulatory effects exerted by a homoeopathic medicinal agent (see 'Dose Repetition').

Experimental Research in Homoeopathy

The field of research in homoeopathy may be divided into seven broad categories:

1 Experiments designed to substantiate the law of similars in the drug-to-disease relationship, by showing that a like-disease substance provokes a defensive reaction in the body;
2 Work concerned with establishing up to what potency there is a discernible presence of the original drug substance;
3 Experimental demonstrations of the biological activity of dynamizations, whether physiological or ultra-molecular, upon animals and plants, aimed at obviating the ubiquitous placebo-effect inference;
4 Investigations into the nature and physical structure of homoeopathic potencies, exploring the hypotheses concerning their mode of action;
5 Experimental laboratory studies (in vitro) to establish the minutiae of a great variety of homoeopathic effects and phenomena, such as, for instance: preventive and inhibiting effects by 73 mother tinctures on the pathogenic action by 20 strains of microbial organisms (including Staphylococcus aureus [MRSA], resistant to virtually all known orthodox 'antibiotics', and a strain of Pseudomonas aeruginosa regarded

by orthodox medicine as multi-drug resistant);

mercuric chloride potencies on lymphoblasts;

various dynamizations on macrophages;

changing effects using different degrees of succussion;

changing effects due to different rest periods between succussion of one potency and employing it to prepare the next higher dynamization (it is postulated that the minimum of three minutes required between succussion and dilution is the length of time for the long-chain polymers to stabilize after the destabilizing succussion process);

anti-viral activity in developing chick embryos;

protective effects from potencies of Mercurius Corrosivus on mercury-poisoned human skin fibroblasts;

prevention of degranulation of allergen-sensitized basophils (occurring in allergic reactions) in response to dynamized Apis Mellifica, as also to Histaminum 7CH; and

a miscellany of biochemical effects.

6   Clinical trials on human disease conditions; and

7   Clinical trials on animal disease conditions.

A representative selection of some experimental work is given in the appropriate place throughout this text: see, for example, 'Allergy', 'Antibiotic', 'Boyd, William Ernest (1891-1955)', 'Clinical Trials', 'Combination of Homoeopathic Drugs', 'Constitutional Type', 'Dental Surgery and Homoeopathy', 'Epistemological Assumptions in Homoeopathy', section 5 on Ultramolecular Potencies, 'Isopathy', 'Lithotherapy', 'Miasma', 'Mother Tincture', 'Nitrum cum Sulphuri Praecipitati et Carboni', 'Opsonic Index', 'Physiological Response in Homoeotherapeutics, Mechanism of', 'Potency', 'Potentizing Methods', 'Solvation Structures', 'Veterinary Homoeopathy' and 'Yeast'. This accumulating evidence, at the very least, constitutes a case to be answered.

A fascinating compendium of a representative selection of comparable experimental work in homoeopathy, done largely in north America, the bulk of which is not featured in this Dictionary will be found in *Homoeopathic Science and Modern Medicine: The Physics of Healing with* by Harris Livermore Coulter, Ph.D., Berkeley: North Atlantic Books, 1981 [170 pages, fully referenced]. This book is an exposé of the fundamental basis of homoeopathy as seen by the author, an outstanding medical historian who is able to marshal homoeopathy's historical resource and contemporary theoretical speculation together with experimental evidence in a cogent presentation that defines homoeopathy's position in the world today. Coulter deals with the momentous issues of homoeopathy with masterly ease, covering

its doctrinal basis

symptoms as adaptive phenomena in the context of an organism's curative-assertive effort

the biphasal action of medicines (hormesis)

pathogenetic experimentation
the organism's ultrasensitivity to the similar medicine
evidence for the infinitesimal homoeopathic dose from
    biochemical investigations
    botanical investigations
    bacteriological investigations
    zoological investigations
    investigations within the field of physics
    homoeopathy's rejection of the monotonicity rule
    orthodox medicine's non-conscious use of homoeopathy's law of similars
homoeopathy's scientific method
clinical evidence
clinical trials in homoeopathy and in orthodoxy.

A second well researched summary of relevant homoeopathic advances within the natural sciences, in the context of historical influences both prevailing upon it and exerted by it, as well as the therapeutic potential of these challenging advances, is to be found in *Homoeopathy: Medicine for the 21st Century* by Dana Ullman, MPH, Wellingborough: Thorsons, 1989 [295 pages, completely referenced].

Thirdly, the 'Berlin Documentation Project on Research in Homoeopathy' (Universitätsklinikum Steglitz, D-1000 Berlin 45, Germany) has begun to publish, from September 1990, a journal each alternate month under the name *The Berlin Journal on Research in Homoeopathy*. In this publication original laboratory and clinical research are both to be brought together and hypotheses to be invited on the broad topic of homoeopathy. The intention is to encourage an unhindered exchange of ideas among homoeopaths and homocopathic researchers themselves. As it is interdisciplinary, other sciences, like biophysics and biochemistry, are also encouraged to contribute ideas and experimental studies to address the problem of how homoeopathic dynamizations (potencies) work. The overall aim of the journal is said to be to construct a well-grounded view of what homoeopathic medicines actually are and how they interact with biological systems – and ultimately with the dynamis. (See also 'Clinical Trials'.)

Expression

Changeable features of a face, a saying, a gesture, a look, or a message emitted through body mobility or posture. Another meaning is expulsion through pressure. In homoeopathic pharmacy, a process employed in the preparation of a succus, where the plant juices are forced out of fresh plant material by pressure (see 'Utensils of Homoeopathic Pharmacy', section on Presses). By immediately adding the succus, in pharmacopoeial proportions, to a water-ethanol mixture, the resultant is the homoeopathic mother tincture (see 'Mother Tincture').

External Events and Scientific Development in Homoeopathy

See 'Nitrum Cum Sulphuri Praecipitati Et Carboni'.

Externally Applied Homoeopathic Drugs

The following are the more common external applications of remedies as found in the undermentioned four reference works:

Prof William Boericke's *Pocket Manual of Homoeopathic Materia Medica Comprising the Characteristics and Guiding Symptoms of All Remedies* [Clinical and Pathogenetic], ninth edition, Philadelphia: Boericke and Runyon, 1927;

Edwin Harris Ruddock's *Homoeopathic Vade Mecum* revised by J C Nixon, MRCS, LRCP, re-print, New Delhi: Ashoka Publishing, 1978;

John Henry Clarke's *The Prescriber: A Dictionary of the New Therapeutics* ninth edition, Rustington, Sussex: Health Science Press, 1972;

John Henry Clarke's *Dictionary of Practical Materia Medica* in three volumes, third edition, Bradford, Holsworthy, Devon: Health Science Press, 1977.

N.B. Care must be taken not to provoke a symptomatic crisis through extended use of unpotentized remedies, or drugs of very low potencies. As a general rule, any of these homoeopathic medicines should be discontinued as soon as the curative effect has set in, or if it is clear that the remedy is not working:

Name	Base & Usual Potency		Indicated Uses
Acidum aceticum	Dilution	1DH	Jelly-fish and insect stings: rubbed in well at point of sting
Acidum boracicum	Lotion of (1g : 50ml aqua destillata)	Θ	Conjuctivitis
Adrenalinum	Dilution	4DH	Epistaxis: nose to be plugged with soaked cotton wool
Aesculus hippocastanum	Cream/Ointment	Θ	Haemorrhoids
Aristolochia clematis	Ointment	1DH	Skin ulcers
Arnica montana	Cream/Liniment/ Ointment/Tincture	Θ	Contusions (on unbroken skin)
Balsamum peruvianum	Cerate/Lotion	2DH	Cracked nipples, indolent ulcers, is scabicidal
Bellis perennis	Tincture	Θ	Blows, muscular injuries in falls, naevi

Name	Base & Usual Potency	Indicated Uses
Bofareira (a.k.a. Ricinus communis)	Oleum Θ (as daily oil massage of breasts, and internally 5 drops every 4 hours)	As galactagogue
Calendula officinalis	Cream/Ointment Θ Pessary/Soap/Tincture	Fissures, sores, burns, wounds, leukorrhoea, suppurations, skin ulcers, erysipelas
Camphora	Oleous Solution Θ (dilution: one part tincture to four parts oleum olivae)	Erysipelatous skin eruptions, itching chicken- or smallpox vesicles [applied to the pocks by camelhair brush]
Cantharis vesicator	Lotion 3DH	Herpes zoster (shingles): to be kept applied on linen
Carboneum sulphuratum	Lotion 1CH	Facial neuralgia and sciatica
Ceanothus americanus	Aqueous Solution 1DH	Hair tonic
Cedron-simaruba ferroginea	Tincture Θ	Snake-bites and insect-stings: applied locally
Chrysarobinum	Ointment 1DH (paraffinum mollis flavum)	Psoriasis, ringworm, crusty eczema behind ears
Cineraria maritima	Succus Θ (not for spirit tincture)	Corneal opacity, senile cataract
Cochlearia armoracia	Tincture Θ and Aqueous Solution	Dandruff: as a gargle and mouthwash in scorbutic gums and sore throat
(Gonolobus) Cundurango	Tincture Θ	For pain in cancer of tongue
Cuprum sulphuricum	Tincture Θ (in 1-3% solution)	For inoperable sarcoma; for other uses see 'Emergencies – Homoeopathic

Name	Base & Usual Potency	Indicated Uses
Cuprum sulphuricum (cont.)		Treatment', under Boils and Styes
Echinacea angustifolia	Ointment/ ⊖ Tincture	Burns
Eupatorium aromaticum	Tincture ⊖	Infant's sore mouth, sore nipple
Euphrasia officinalis	Tincture ⊖ (15 drops:50ml in aqua destillata)	Soft cataract, capsular opacity and conjunctivitis
Gaultheria procumbens	Liniment 1DH (in oleum olivae)	Rheumatoid arthritis, pruritus, epididymitis
Golondrina (Euphorbia polycarpa)	Tincture ⊖	Poisonous insect and snake bites
Graphites	Cream/Ointment 6DH	Dermatitis
Hamamelis angustifolia	Cream/Ointment ⊖ Tincture	Haemorrhoids, Varicosities
Hydrastis canadensis	Tincture/Lotion ⊖ (dilution: in glycerinum one part to nine parts) Pessary	Varioloid eruptions, impetigo; leukorrhoea
Hypericum perforatum	Cream/Ointment ⊖ Tincture	Puncture-wounds, antitetanic, relieves post-operative pain for animal bites and street injuries
Ichthyolum	Ointment/ 1DH Aqueous Solution	Rheumatic joint, chronic eczema and psoriasis, acne rosacea, scabies and chilblains
Ilex aquifolium	Lotion 1DH (5 drops q.i.d.)	Staphyloma, burning pains in orbits at night
Iodoformum	Base Powder ⊖ (0.2g on to back of tongue) Ointment	Asthma

Tubercular meningitis |
| Lavandula angustifolia | Oleum ⊖ (affected parts to be painted over) | Parasitic itch |

Name	Base & Usual Potency		Indicated Uses
Ledum palustre	Tincture	Θ	Insect bites, stings, carbuncles, puncture wounds
Lemna minor	Dilution	3DH	Nasal polypi, swollen turbinates
Mentha piperita	Tincture	Θ	Pruritus vaginae
Naphthalenum	Ointment	1DH	Dermatitis
Paeonia officinalis	Cream/Ointment Tincture	Θ	Haemorrhoids
Passiflora incarnata	Tincture	Θ	Erysipelas
Phytolacca decandra	Tincture	Θ	Mastitis, follicular pharyngitis
Plantago major	Tincture	Θ	Toothache, earache, otorrhoea
Platanus occidentalis	Tincture (must be used for some time)	Θ	Tarsal tumors, ichtyosis
Ratanhia	Tincture	Θ	Anal fissures, haemorrhoids, pruritus ani, pin worms
Rhus glabra	Tincture	Θ	Aphthous stomatitis, soft and spongy gums
Rhus toxicodendron	Cream/Lotion	Θ	Rheumatic pain, where indicated
Ruta graveolens	Ointment	Θ	Strains, Ganglia
	Lotion (15 drops:50ml aqua destillata) (not the alcoholic dilution)	1CH	Eyes
Sabadilla officinarum	Lotion (1:20 parts aqua destillata) (to be bathed in lotion, after daily hair-wash)	Θ	Head lice
(Juniperus) Sabina	Tincture	Θ	Warts
Sempervivum tectorum	Succus	Θ	Indurations of tongue
Skookum chuck	Ointment	Θ	Eczema
(Delphinium) Staphysagria	Lotion (30ml:200ml aqua destillata)	Θ	Pediculosis – capitis; – corporis; – bubis

Name	Base & Usual Potency		Indicated Uses
Sulphur	Ointment	Θ	Scabies itch: inunction every night, hot bath with thorough soaping followed by change of all bed and body linen every second night
Sulphur iodatum	Ointment (400mg:100g paraffinum mollis flavum)	Θ	Barber's Itch
Symphytum officinale	Tincture, warm Lotion (1:1 aqua destillata) or Poultices	Θ	Dressing for ulcers, sores, pruritus, animal wounds penetrating to perineum and bones, irritable stump after amputation, in non-union of fractures
Taraxacum dens leonis	Tincture	Θ	Skin of tongue peeling off, mapped tongue
Tamus communis	Ointment	6DH	Chilblains
Terebinthina	Stupes	3DH	Tympanites in fevers and inflammations
Teucrium marum	Base Powder (as snuff)	Θ	Nasal polypi, swollen turbinates
Thuja occidentalis	Tincture	Θ	Warts: to be painted on each morning and night nasal polypi;
	Lotion (10 drops:50ml aqua destillata)		Granular Ophthalmia
Urtica urens	Cream	Θ	Blisters in burns and sunburn, bee stings
Verbascum thapsus	Oleum (a.k.a. Mullein oil)	Θ	Otalgia, dry scaliness of meatus, partial

Name	Base & Usual Potency	Indicated Uses
Verbascum thapsus cont.		deafness with sense of obstruction
Vinca minor	Glycerole $\ominus$ (6g:50g glycerinum)	Eczema capitis
Zincum sulphuricum	Dilution/Lotion 1CH (5ml:20ml aqua destillata) (not the alcoholic dilution)	Corneal opacity (to be warmed a little before irrigating)

Externalization of Disease

● **Common development in the end phase of the dynamic healing effort, involving a reaction in the patient's skin.**

An ephemeral skin rash is often the end stage of the process of cure, in accordance with the first part of the reciprocal of the rule of the direction of disease metastasis (Hering's rule): ' . . . symptoms move from the interior to the surface . . .' in the curative process. (See also 'Clinical Trials', 'Epistemological Assumptions in Homoeopathy', section 1 (Dermatitis Medicamentosa) and 'Homoeopathic Laws, Postulates and Precepts' section 14.)

Extractive

An extract; a preparation containing the active principle of a substance in a concentrated form, obtained by treating any matter with solvents followed by evaporation, leaving viscid material. This residue can then be adjusted to the pharmacopoeial standard for the preparation of a mother tincture or base substance.

F

Farrington, Ernest Albert (1847-1885)

US homoeopath of some consequence. He was professor of Materia Medica at the Hahnemann Medical College of Philadelphia and, for a while, editor of the Hahnemannian Monthly. His major writings are:

Clinical Materia Medica

and published posthumously by his son, the homoeopath Harvey Farrington:

Therapeutic Pointers and Lesser Writings with Some Clinical Cases.

Fever

Elevated body core-temperature usually part of the reactive state evoked in a disease condition, particularly when infection by certain pathogenic micro-organisms has occurred, but also at other times, as in many acute miasmata. This term is also used in non-homoeopathic disease classifications to describe a distinct category of illness where a high body temperature is present. Common examples of acute miasmata are: cholera, diphtheria, glandular fever, influenza, malaria, measles, meningitis, mumps, pertussis (whooping cough), pneumonia, poliomyelitis, puerperal fever, q-fever, rheumatic fever, scarlet fever, typhoid fever and yellow fever. Fever, as a leading homoeopathic symptom component, features particularly prominently in:

Achyranthes-calea
Aconitum napellus
Agrostis vulgaris
Arsenicum album
Baptisis tinctoria
(Atropa) Belladonna
Ferrum phosphoricum
Histaminum hydrochloricum
Hoitzia-coccinea
Paronichia illecebrum
Phytolacca decandra
Rajania subsamarata
Spiranthes autumnalis
Terebinthina chios (not to be confused with either Oleum terebinthinum or
    Terebinthina)
Triosteum perfoliatum

Fevers swiftly respond to well-indicated remedies, but bed-rest and fluids-only regimens (preferably fruit juices) are indicated, with sponging down with warm water until the temperature has subsided. With profuse perspiration, the 'like' method is the so-called wickel (wet body pack) for which the procedure is as follows. A wrung-out linen sheet that has been soaked in cold (tap) water, is wrapped two or three times around the entire trunk of the patient; then covered with flannel cloth and secured in place tightly. The patient is then covered with a blanket or several blankets. In this manner the body heat is trapped inside and 'the fever is sweated out' as the saying has it. Hot bricks, wrapped in flannel, may be packed to the sides of the body to increase the reaction to the full body pack.

Examples of syndetic pointers to four homoeopathic medicines:

Violent intermittent heartbeat, body temperature above 38 degrees Celsius, with muscular and mental power significantly diminished – Gelsemium sempervirens

In a fever, flushes of heat that come in waves of heat upwards; occasionally patient may also have pulsating headache – Glonoinum

In scarlet fever with pains alternating from one side to patient's other side and back again, or pains constantly flying from one part to another – Lac caninum

Patient has a violent cough from the very beginning with a pronounced heartbeat with hyperpyrexia, or a rapidly oscillating temperature, or cerebro-spinal fever – Veratrum viride

(See also 'Miasma' and 'Pack'.)

Fifty Millesimal Potency

LM potency; quinquagenimillesimal dynamization; 50-milles potency; the only high potency devised by Hahnemann. (See 'Potentizing Methods'.)

Filtration

Process for purifying a liquid of solid insoluble matter by pressing it through some porous medium that arrests suspended solid particles.

Fincke, Bernhardt (1821-1906)

See 'Philosophical Premise of Homoeopathy' and 'Homoeosis'.

Fleury, Rudolph (born 1916)

Distinguished contemporary Swiss homoeopath, resident in Berne, a graduate of Zurich, who also studied in Paris and Vienna. President of the Swiss Homoeopathic Society from 1950 and member of the Liga Medicorum Homoeopathica Internationalis from before World War II. He introduced some innovations into the method for homoeopathic case-taking. He was editor of the *World Directory of Homoeopathic Physicians* from 1967.

Fluid

Generally refers to liquid, more rarely to gas. It is a condition in which the particles can move about (flow) from one part of the substance to another with freedom, yet still cohesively, in the case of a liquid. (See 'Solvation Structures'.)

Fluoric Constitution

See 'Constitutional Type'.

Foci (plural of Focus)

Focus, in disease, is the term for primary lesion, the centre, or the starting point from which the disease process radiates. The simillimum will often produce a complete cure, including the clearing up of foci that may have been present. During the reactive healing process foci generally attract attention to themselves. This notwithstanding, the matching medicine will lead to a cure and the focus will be cleared. If, for example, a dental focus is going to be cleared by dental surgery, prior treatment with Arnica montana 12DH (or 6CH) ten drops once daily for five days may be prescribed, or some other appropriate functiotropic remedy. (See also 'Diagnosis'.)

Foods as Health Problems

Many homoeopaths maintain that the very frugal diet, to the influence of which the human species was exposed during the major part of its existence (i.e. for more than 3 million years of its pre-history), enduringly forged the species' constitutional intaglio. During that time humans seem to have existed on a diet the modern approximation of which is the recently promoted, so-called 'stone-age diet'. This long habituating exposure brought with it a process of assimilation that is known as homoeosis. In one of its aspects homoeosis produces a beneficial miasma-like constitutional impress by which the organisms so leavened are in resonance with the foods of their staple diet. These foods have by then ceased to produce any pathogenetic effects on the consumer; i.e. the items to which they have thus grown constitutionally attuned have become bland. On the other hand, exposure since then to items different from these results in many individuals experiencing pronounced health problems. This has been demonstrated with foods only introduced within the last 30 000 years (like barley, chicken eggs, rye, cow's milk and meat, oats, salt and wheat), and in the case of others introduced a mere few hundred years ago (e.g. beet sugar, cane sugar, potatoes, coffee, maize, cocoa, common tea, many spices and aromatic herbs), or still more in the case of those paraaliments introduced very recently, in the twentieth century (preservatives, colourants, flavourings, taste enhancers, anti-caking-, curing-, gelling-, thickening-, raising-agents, stabilizers, emulsifiers, antioxidants and sequestrants). [It should be noted that even a period of 30 000 years represents less than one percent of man's total exposure to his conditioning to 'stone-age' type foods.] An excellent scientific summation of evidence in this field is *The Retardation of Aging and Disease by Dietary Restriction* by Richard Weindruch and Roy L Walford [Springfield, Illinois: Charles C Thomas Publisher, 1988, 453 pp].

One might say that in the Western diet and the diverse deleterious effects it can be seen to have on the health of individuals the world is witness to the largest uncontrolled homoeopathic 'proving' ever carried out. (See also 'Aversions and Desires', 'Bran', 'Epistemological Assumptions in Homoeopathy', sections 4: Constitution – Environment, and 6: Placebo – Nocebo, 'Genetic Assimilation', 'Gutman, William', 'Homoeopathic Practice', section Supportive Diet, 'Homoeosis', 'Miasma', 'Nutritional Equipoise' and 'Vitamin'.)

Foubister, Donald MacDonald (1902-1988)

This homoeopath came from the treeless, windswept, folklorish main island of the Orkney Isles, to the north of Scotland. He was born in Kirkwall, the capital, where he attended the Grammar School. His family usually went south to the Scottish Highlands for their holidays, where the magic of trees cast a spell over the young boy. He resolved to make forestry his life and with this goal he went to Aberdeen University where he obtained a degree in geology, botany and zoology. He then left for Canada.

He worked there for five years, mostly for a seed company in Nova Scotia. A sporting injury in Canada produced a prolonged back problem, which did not respond to orthodox medical treatment. This was finally cured by an osteopath, which aroused his deep interest in osteopathy. He resolved to make this his life's new focus. He returned to Scotland and paid his way through medical school at Edinburgh University. In the practical tutorials he was paired with a fellow student who had an intense interest in homoeopathy. It occurred to him that this may be the one complete medical system, even more so than either orthodoxy or osteopathy. After graduation he went to London to pursue this avenue.

At the age of 35 (in 1937) he was appointed house physician at the London Homoeopathic Hospital. There he received tuition from Douglas Borland, Margaret Tyler, Sir John Weir and Dame Margery Blackie, all top ranking homoeopaths. During World War II he served as a medical officer both in the UK and abroad. He always used homoeopathy in his treatments, despite some official disapproval. In 1946 he became assistant paediatrician in the Children's Department of the Royal London Homoeopathic Hospital and in 1956 he became consultant homoeopath there. He held the Diploma in Child

Health of Great Ormond Street Children's Hospital. He was admitted as Fellow of the Faculty of Homoeopathy in 1955 and was appointed Dean of the Faculty in 1960. He was elected President of the Faculty from 1970 to 1972.

His study of the important but infrequently prescribed Lac caninum is scholarly (*British Homoeopathic Journal,* vol XXXIX, April 1949, no 2, pp 114-120), but his paediatric wisdom is captured by him in his book

Tutorials on Homoeopathy (Beaconsfield: Beaconsfield Publishers Ltd, 1989, 216 pages).

Functiotropism

See 'Organotropism'.

Funnel

See 'Utensils of Homoeopathic Pharmacy'.

G

Gemmotherapy

● **A form of near-homoeopathic treatment that resembles phytotherapy.**

Described by its supporters as a 'tissue potentialization therapy'. It uses a low homoeopathic potency (1DH) of glycerin macerates prepared from fresh embryonic plant tissue, harvested at a time when this is in the process of incipient growth. It is aimed at promoting drainage and is always prescribed pathologically (see 'Drainage'). Customarily 50 to 100 drops per 24-hour period (say 12 to 25 drops three times daily) is the prescribed dosage. In the materia medica of gemmotherapy the principal clinical indications (for which no homoeopathic provings have been conducted and for which only clinical observations, extending over nearly two decades, serve as pointers to their possible benefits) are the following:

1 Abies pectinata (fir buds) – decalcification, rickets, dental caries
2 Acer campestris (maple buds) – sequellae of paralysis, poliomyelitis, herpes zoster
3 Aesculus hippocastanum (horse chestnut buds) – haemorrhoids, varicosities
4 Alnus glutinosa (alder buds) – sequellae of cerebral haemorrhage, chronic rhinitis
5 Ampelopsis weitchii (virginia creeper young shoots) – rheumatoid arthritis, chronic rheumatism
6 Betula pubescens (birch buds, catkins & root-bark) – psychasthenia
7 Betula verrucosa (birch seeds) – intellectual overwork
8 Birch-sap – tonic restorative for nerves
9 Carpinus betulus (hornbeam buds) – rhinopharingitis, spasmodic cough
10 Cedrus libani (cedar young shoots) – dry eczema, ichthyosis, pruritus
11 Citrus limonum (lemon tree stem bark) – sore throat, excessive menstruation, sub-clinical scurvy, haemorrhages, chronic rheumatism, pain from tongue cancer, oedema, hydrops, anasarca, ascites
12 Coryllus avellana (hazelnut shrub buds) – pulmonary fibrosis, emphysema
13 Crataegus oxyacantha (hawthorn buds) – cardiac insufficiency, tachycardia, precordial pain, sequellae of myocardial infarction
14 Fagus sylvatica (beech buds) – renal lithiasis and/or insufficiency
15 Ficus carica (fig tree buds) – obsessional and anxiety neuroses, gastric or peptic ulcers
16 Fraxinus excelsior (ash buds) – acute or chronic gout
17 Juglans regia (walnut tree buds) – varicose ulcers, skin infections (e.g. impetigo, infected eczema)

18 Juniperus communis (juniper young shoots) – major hepatic insufficiency and cirrhotic syndromes

19 Olea europaea (olive tree young shoots) – elevation of triglyceride level, hypertension, atherosclerosis, hypercholesteraemia

20 Pinus montana (pine buds) – vertebral osteoarthrosis, chronic rheumatism, osteoarthrosis of hips and knees

21 Populus nigra (poplar buds) – obliterative arterial disease of the lower limbs and associated trophic disturbances

22 Prunus amygdalus (almond tree buds) – arteriosclerosis, hypertension

23 Quercus pedonculata (oak buds, young acorns, rootlets and root bark) – spleen dropsy, vertigo, tinnitus, aureus, alcohol addiction, recurrent malaria, nervous headache

24 Ribes nigrum (blackcurrant buds) – hayfever, migraine, chronic coryza, allergic problems

25 Rosa canina (dog rose young shoots) – migraine and headache

26 Rosmarinus officinalis (rosemary young shoots) – biliary colic and dyskinesia, hepatic insufficiency

27 Rubus idaeus (raspberry bush young shoots) – for easing and improving labour, pelvic pain, metritis, vaginitis, mouth and throat infections, conjunctivitis

28 Sequoia gigantea (sequoia redwood young shoots) – prostatic hypertrophy and adenoma, uterine fibroids

29 Sorbus domestica (sorb buds) – venous problems, sequellae of phlebitis, haemogliasis

30 Tamaris gallica (tamarisk shrub young shoots) – hypercholesteraemia, various types of anaemia

31 Tillia tomentosa (lime tree buds) – nerve sedative, neuralgia, insomnia

32 Ulmus campestris (elm buds) – weeping eczema, acne, impetigo

33 Vaccinum vitis idaea (mount ida vine young shoots) – chronic Escherichia coli infections, dysbiosis, various intestinal syndromes

34 Viburnum lantana (guelder rose buds) – asthma, simple, and with complications

35 Viscum album (mistletoe young shoots) – epilepsy, low blood pressure, metrorrhagia, retained placenta, ovaralgia, sciatica, muscles in fibrillary contraction

36 Vitis vinifera (grape-vine buds) – benign bone tumours, painful osteochondritis deformans, Scheuermann's disease, painful rheumatism, arthritis in small joints

37 Zea mais (maize rootlets) – produces fall in blood transaminase level and favours healing of post-infarction cardiac tissue.

There appears to be a fair number of homoeopaths, particularly in the francophone area, and increasingly elsewhere, who have incorporated this range of remedies into their armamentarium and most of these speak highly of the supportive role they play in drainage. It remains to be seen whether gemmotherapy ever becomes fully integrated into homoeopathy the way Bach's Flower Remedies or Schüssler's Biochemic Medicine both were.

'Generals' and 'Particulars' (Symptom Types)

These terms denote two sorts of homoeopathic symptoms.

General symptoms (the 'generals') are the subjective symptoms of the patient as a whole, whenever the patient uses the personal pronoun in the first person singular as either the subject or object of the sentence, e.g.:

I dare not move at all during a thunderstorm or I shall get dizzy.

I will always feel there isn't enough sugar in my coffee.

I just cannot stand damp heat.

Cold weather always disagrees with me.

Blustery weather knocks me all to pieces; it gives me a twitch in my right eye.

A terrible thirst comes over me in the mornings.

All these are 'generals', the I-symptoms, that describe the whole patient. Many homoeopaths, following the example of James Tyler Kent, rank these symptoms as equivalent to mentals, because the whole being is involved here.

Particular symptoms (the 'particulars') are the attributive personal symptoms, whenever the patient uses the possessive form of the personal pronoun in the first person singular, e.g.:

The numbness in my foot never goes away.

My ringing ears are a real nuisance.

That stomach of mine is so sore.

My knees are better now: all the swelling has gone down.

After supper my headache gets really awful.

All these are 'particulars', the my-symptoms, which deal only with particular parts of the patient. These are the symptoms that indicate the second, the pathologically-prescribed, remedy in, say, a drainage procedure. (See 'Kent, James Tyler (1849-1916)' and 'Pathotropism'.)

Generic Similarity in Disease and Drug Action

See 'Disease and Drug Action in Homoeopathic Congruity'.

Genetic Assimilation

Lamarckian hereditability of acquired miasmatic effects that were merely phenotypical to the originally affected individual, but have since become genetically transmissible. (See 'Foods as Health Problems', 'Lamarckism' and 'Miasma', particularly under Experimental Evidence.)

Genius of the Remedy

See 'Key-Note'.

Genus Epidemicus

See 'Epidemiology'.

Georgenthal Mental Hospital

See 'Asylums for the Insane'.

Gibson Miller, Robert

A homoeopath from Glasgow, Scotland, who, on 1st December 1910, in a paper read to the Medicine and Pathology Section of the British Homoeopathic Society, proposed a set of comparative values to grade symptoms in the selection of any remedy (detailed under section 9 of 'Disease and Drug Action in Homoeopathic Congruity'). His views on 'Hot and Cold Remedies' inspired Dr William Ernest Boyd (as told more fully under that entry). His method of repertorization and details of the hot and cold remedies are described at length by Drs Margaret L Tyler and Sir John Weir on pages 1432-1443 of the *Repertory of the Homoeopathic Materia Medica* by James Tyler Kent. He also compiled a 44-page reference manual entitled *Relationship of Remedies with Approximate Duration of Action* covering the following rubrics after each remedy: Complements; Remedies that follow well; Inimicals; Antidotes; and Duration of Action (see 'Antidotes').

Glauber, Johann Rudolf (1604-1668)

See 'Spagyric'.

Globules

See 'Granules'.

Glycerinum

Glycerin; a clear colourless, odourless, hygroscopic, syrupy liquid with a sweet taste but practically no nutrient value, that contains not less than 97% of $C_3H_8O_3$ and weighs 1.255 to 1.26 g per ml, in terms of the Pharmacopoeia Internationalis. A solution of it in water is neutral to litmus. It is miscible with both water and alcohol, but insoluble in chloroform, ether and fixed oils and is sterilized by heating to 150 degrees Celsius for one hour. Crystallization may occur if kept at a temperature below 17 degrees Celsius and if other glycerinum has been allowed to crystallize in the general vicinity. The crystals will not melt until the temperature is raised to about 20 degrees Celsius. It is used as a solvent in pharmacy in concentrations of 30% and over for its antiseptic properties, particularly in aqueous and non-alcoholic extracts and because of its hygroscopic action it is used in non-greasy applications to prevent drying out. It is a vehicle for several homoeopathic preparations:

1   For the preservation of certain animal products, e.g. Crotalus horridus, Elaps corallinus, etc.
2   For preparing mother tinctures and the lower dilutions of certain remedies, e.g. Apis mellifica, Buthus australis, Naja tripudians, Tarentula cubensis, Vespa crabro, etc.
3   As an essential component of the drug Glonoinum.
4   As a homoeopathic suppositorial base (glycerinated gelatin).
5   For preparing external applications, such as eye-drops, ear-drops, vaginal douches, enemas, lotions and ointments; in some of these one part mother tincture is mixed with nine parts Glycerinum.

(See 'Vehicle'.)

Goethe, Johann Wolfgang von (1749-1832)

This contemporary of Hahnemann, the greatest poet and most versatile universal genius of German literature, shared some of the contempt for orthodox medicine with the founder of homoeopathy, if the views he expresses in *Faust* are taken as representative. One of several expressions of this can be found in the words that Goethe has Faust address to his assistant Wagner during their walk on the outskirts of the city:

'That was the physic! True, their patients died,
But no-one ever asked them who was cured.
So, with a nostrum of this hellish sort,
We made these hills and valleys our resort,
And ravaged there more deadly than the pest.
These hands have ministered the deadly bane
To thousands who have perished; I remain
To hear cool murderers extolled and bless'd.'[1]

In the second part of *Faust* he explicitly supports homoeopathy by having Mephistopheles say:

'To like things like, whatever one may ail;
There's certain help.'[2]

Goethe expressed his strong inclination towards homoeopathy in five of his published letters written in 1820 from Karlsbad and Jena.[3] In 1829 he acknowledged the value of Hahnemann's dietary restrictions, as he also did

[1] Goethe, Johann Wolfgang von. *Faust – Part One,* translated by Philip Wayne. Harmondsworth: Penguin Books Ltd, 1956, p 65.
[2] Haehl, Richard. *Samuel Hahnemann: His Life and Work,* 2 vols. London: Homoeopathic Publishing Co, 1922, vol I, p 170, quoting the English rendering of Sir T Martin.
[3] Ibid., pp 113-114.

in a letter to Grand Duke Karl August.[1] In December 1830, however, orthodox medicine had its revenge on this great man, then in his eighty-second year: after having had a severe haemorrhage (a very large wash-basin was used to collect the blood – and it was half filled by the haemorrhoeia), this octogenarian was bled of a further litre of blood by the attending physician.[2]

In *Zerstreute Blätter,* vol II, Goethe has the following to say of Hahnemann and his system:

'Hahnemann, that rare combination of philosophy and learning, whose system must eventually bring about the ruin of the ordinary prescription-crammed heads, is but still little accepted by practitioners, and rather shunned than investigated'.[3]

It is perhaps appropriate to quote one of Goethe's passages from *Faust,* with the perennial two-pronged dilemma of orthodox medicine – the wilful shunning of homoeopathy on the one hand and the impasse of iatrogenic effects on the other – in mind:

'What one does not know is just what one might need,
And what one knows one cannot use'.[4]

Francis Treuherz has succinctly analysed the relationship of the ideas of Hahnemann, Steiner and Goethe. He pointed out that though Goethe was influenced by Hahnemann, and though Goethean science was the major inspiration for Steiner there is a clear divergence between some aspects of the medicines of Hahnemann and of Steiner.[5] (See also 'Anthroposophical Medicine', 'David, Pierre Jean (also David d'Angers) (1788-1856)', 'Steiner, Rudolf (1861-1925)', 'van Gogh, Vincent (1853-1890)' and 'Well-Wishers and Supporters of Homoeopathy'.)

Gonorrhoea

The chronic miasma of sycosis. It is a contagious catarrhal inflammation of the genital mucous membrane involving Neisseria Gonorrhoeae. Beginning usually from the lower or upper genital tract, and the uterine tubes in women, it may spread to the peritoneum and occasionally to the heart, joints and other structures of the body primarily by way of the bloodstream. The term sycosis (condylomatous disease) is used because condylomata acuminata (venereal verrocose excrescences, moist fig- or cauliflower-like) are a secondary symptom

[1] Ibid., p 271.
[2] Ibid., pp 303-304.
[3] Danciger, Elizabeth. *The Emergence of Homoeopathy: Alchemy into Medicine,* quoted on p 83.
[4] Goethe, op. cit., p 66.
[5] Treuherz, Francis. 'Steiner and the Simillimum – Homoeopathic and Anthroposophic Medicine: the Relationship of the Ideas of Hahnemann, Goethe and Steiner', paper read at a meeting of the Faculty of Homoeopathy, Scottish Branch, Glasgow, November, 1984 and subsequently published in the *Journal of the American Institute of Homoeopathy* [copies from author: Flat 2, 18 The Avenue, Brondesbury Park, London NW6 7YD, UK].

associated with gonorrhoea, as are the chronic miasmatic complications of gonococcal arthritis, serosynovitis, etc. (See 'Miasma'.)

Granules

Globules, spherical in shape and made of pure beet and/or cane sugar ($C_{12}H_{22}O_{11}$). These are hard and approximate the size of a poppy seed. The sizes commonly used are generally numbers 15 or 20, this being the number of millimetres taken up by ten granules lined up in a straight row. Homoeopathic use: vehicle for administering the medicine with which they may have been impregnated. (See 'Dose', 'Nomenclature, Discrepancies in', 'Vehicle' and also 'Pilules'.)

Grauvogl, Eduard von (1811-1887)

German homoeopath who practised in Nuremberg, Bavaria and later in Gastein, Austria, where he discovered a species of gneiss in the mineral springs of that town. It is Calcarea silico-fluorata to which he gave the name Lapis albus by which it is still known in homoeopathy. It is used in cretinism and goitre resulting from suboptimal iodine uptake (clinical authorities: ten such successfully treated cases were reported in the *American Homoeopathic Observer,* 1867, vol 411; and Von Grauvogl's own reports appeared in English in the *Hahnemannian Monthly,* 1874, vol 10, p 182). He had a very keen intellect. He formulated the law of quantity and dose ('Homoeopathic Laws, Postulates and Precepts', section 4) and in 1865 he provoked a minor storm – which he clearly enjoyed – when he announced that he had observed that certain homoeomorphic types of individual were prone to certain disease syndromes; and proceeded to classify them into what he called their 'biochemical states' as these were held to pertain to 'three constitutional dispositions', namely the hydrogenoid, the oxygenoid and the carbo-nitrogenoid. He assigned homoeopathic drugs to each of these states. For example, the polychrest Causticum is one of Von Grauvogl's hydrogenoid remedies, and hence 'a chilly medicine'. Violent disputations were fought out in both homoeopathic and non-homoeopathic circles, for a long time, certainly well beyond his demise. His other major writings are:

Textbook of Homoeopathy (1870)
The Homoeopathic Law of Similarities (1879).

Grauvogl's Biochemical States

See 'Constitutional Type'.

Grimmer, Arthur Hill (1874-1967)

US homoeopath who was a graduate of the Hahnemann Medical College, Chicago, Illinois. He was a pupil of James Tyler Kent (1849-1916) and later became his secretary, working closely with him on his repertory. He practised in Chicago for a long time, then he moved to Florida. He was a lecturer for many years at the American Foundation of Homoeopathy.

Groups of Remedies (According to Natural Orders)

See 'Aversions and Desires'.

Guernsey, Henry Newell (1817-1885)

US homoeopath, born in Vermont, who graduated from the New York University in 1842. He was one of the very early members of the American Institute of Homoeopathy, practised in Philadelphia, and should not be confused with William Jefferson Guernsey. In 1857 he was appointed Professor of Obstetrics, Gynaecology and Paediatrics in the Homoeopathic Medical College of Pennsylvania. Later he became Professor of Materia Medica and Institutes in the Hahnemann Medical College of Philadelphia and Dean of the Faculty. He was also consulting physician to the West Philadelphia Homoeopathic Hospital for Children. He strongly advocated both the single remedy and the general use of high potencies in homoeopathy. He is the originator of the 'key-note' system in drug diagnosis (see 'Key-Note'). His major literary works include:

Introductory Lectures on Obstetrics and Diseases of Women and Children (1867)
The Key-Note System (1868)
Uterine Haemorrhage (1870)
Homoeopathic Treatment of Disordered Dentition (1870)
The Homoeopathic Materia Medica (1870)
Key-Notes to the Materia Medica (1872)
Ovarian Tumours (1877)
Plain Talks on Avoided Subjects (1882)

Guernsey, William Jefferson (1854-1935)

US homoeopathic author, not to be confused with his namesake Henry Newell Guernsey, whose son was the homoeopath Joseph C Guernsey. The major writings published by William Jefferson Guernsey include:

The Travellers' Medical Repertory and Family Adviser for the Homoeopathic Treatment of Acute Disease (1879)
Haemorrhoids (1882)
Desires and Aversions (1883)
Menstruation (1884)
The Card Repertory (1885)
Guernsey's Boenninghausen (1889)

Guiding Symptoms of the Materia Medica

● Leading 'pathogenetic' characteristics of drugs, as these were shown to affect the healthy, which together point the homoeopath to the disease pictures these are capable of curing with certainty.

So named, a colossal, comprehensive, practical homoeopathic reference work compiled by Constantin Hering, which was completed posthumously by his son Walter E Hering, and carefully edited by Dr Calvin B Knerr, with Professor Carl Gottlieb Raue and Dr Karl ('Chas') Mohr. Its ten volumes appeared, staggered from 1879 to 1891, totalling 5708 pages. It is a complete record of characteristics of verified homoeopathic medicines, which presents only such symptoms, as they have been shown, experimentally, both to have produced and, in consistent clinical application, to have cured. Hering made a very judicious selection of symptoms, including only that pathogenetic semiology which had stood the test of time and thorough clinical experience. There are, therefore, symptoms in Hahnemann's *Materia Medica Pura* and in Allen's *Encyclopaedia of Pure Materia Medica* which are omitted by him here, whereas others of comparatively low gradation in such pathogenetic records are emphasized in his Guiding Symptoms, because they had subsequently been verified and frequently reconfirmed in actual practice.

Hering was motivated by Orthodox Medicine's concerted philosophical attack at that time on homoeopathy summarized by the then current phrase 'post hoc, ergo propter hoc' (subsequent to this, therefore because of this), expressing the fallacy which alleges that a thing which follows another is, therefore, caused by it. The thrust of the anti-homoeopathic argument ran as follows: If, indeed, there were the same or similar symptoms in provings (pathogenetic experiments) of the same drug as it cured in sick patients on various occasions, these symptoms could at best be construed as no more than **probably** produced by the medicine. Physiological and pathological corroborations did no more than magnify that probability, but could not, in any way, provide certainty, nor much less prove that these medicines could subsequently, therefore, cure such symptoms in the sick. If they did sometimes appear to do that, it could just as easily be spontaneous remission or be due to some other impalpable factor(s). Hering, who to his dying day remained at the centre of North American homoeopathy, assiduously collated in his momentous *chef-d'oeuvre* symptoms confirmed through cures from fifty years' homoeopathic records. As he says in the preface to the *Guiding Symptoms* (p 7), in compiling it he 'never walked on pathological stilts, but always took the symptoms as a reality, on the one side observed by the prover, and on the other side observed on the sick'. The welter of overwhelming evidence provided for him the verification of the law of similars and the rebuttal against the 'post hoc, ergo propter hoc' casuistry.

Gutman, William

US homoeopath, who is a graduate of the Medical Faculty of the University of Vienna, Austria. He was Professor for Homoeopathy at the otherwise non-homoeopathic New York Medical College for a long time. From 1965 to 1966 he was President of the American Institute of Homoeopathy. He supported research in homoeopathy with enthusiasm before this became the general norm. For a time he was President of the Foundation for Homoeopathic Research, Inc., as well as later becoming first Secretary-General, and then Chairman for many years, of the International Homoeopathic Research Council, an agency of the Liga Medicorum Homoeopathica Internationalis. A significant literary work by him appeared in 1986 (Bombay: The Homoeopathic Medical Publishers), entitled:

Homoeopathy – the Fundamentals of its Philosophy, the Essence of its Remedies.

Yet, probably, his most interesting work is the much earlier:

The Prolongation of Life: A Study in Longevity (Rustington, Sussex: Health Science Press, 1961, 196 pp), which is a profound and exhaustive study of practically all the relevant factors in longevity, covering the great field of the (essentially homoeotic) preservation of individual health. The material of this absorbing book is based upon research covering all the then available literature from antiquity to modern times. Furthermore, questionnaires were sent to a large number of old age homes, to ascertain the life habits of nonagenarians and centenarians, and many persons (all aged over ninety years) were interviewed personally. (See also 'Foods as Health Problems'.)

Gynaecology

Study of disease peculiar to women, principally of the genital tract, but involving also the female endocrine system and reproductive physiology. A C Cowperthwaite, MD, Ph.D., LL D, for eleven years professor of Materia Medica and Diseases of Women at the University of Iowa, Iowa City, USA, published a comprehensive homoeopathic *Text-Book of Gynaecology*, New Delhi: Jain Publishing Co, second reprint 1975 [533 pages, 215 illustrations, wide-ranging bibliography]. Four other works of reference on the subject are:

Homoeopathy in Practice by Douglas Borland, pages 75-90, Beaconsfield: Beaconsfield Publishers Ltd, 1982;

Tutorials on Homoeopathy by Donald Foubister, pages 70, 125, 136 & 137, Beaconsfield: Beaconsfield Publishers Ltd, 1989;

Repertory of Pregnancy, Parturition and Puerperium by Alberto Soler-Medina, Heidelberg: Karl F Haug Verlag, 1989, 79 pages.

Homöopathie in Frauenheilkunde und Geburtshilfe by Erwin Schlüren, Heidelberg: Karl F Haug Verlag, 1980, 211 pages.

(See also 'Antenatal Homoeopathy', 'Euthenic (Nosode) Treatment', 'Obstetrics and Homoeopathy' and 'Pregnancy'.)

H

Habitat

Usual natural surroundings and conditions of animals and plants, sometimes with the wider meaning of ecological niche. In homoeopathic materia medica, when plant remedies are dealt with, reference to habitat identifies the place inhabited by a plant community. From individual constituents of that plant a succus is, generally, prepared. Sometimes plants in symbiotic combination with other plants are taken together to prepare the succus (e.g. Cetraria islandica, Sticta pulmonaria, Usnea barbata and all lichens). The location indicated as the habitat is naturally suitable for abundant growth of the plant(s), or the life and development of an animal, together with all influential external factors, such as the habitat group (set of unrelated plants, or other organisms, which inhabit the same kind of situation) or habitat form (evidence of features, such as luxuriant growth, or dwarfing, or changes in glycosidal or alkaloidal levels, which can be related to the place where it is growing or living).

Haehl, Richard (1873-1923)

Eminent German homoeopath from Stuttgart, who was a senior member of the Homoeopathic Central Society (hom. Zentralverein) in Germany. In addition to his German qualifications he received an honorary doctorate from the Hahnemann Medical College of Philadelphia for his significant two-fold contribution to homoeopathy in the period 1920 to 1922. From the age of about 25 years he collected whatever documents related to Hahnemann he could lay his hands on. He also visited relatives, reconstructing from conversations with them a comprehensive background of this peerless medical innovator. This ultimately culminated in the publication in German and English of the authoritative two volumes (983 pages) entitled:

Samuel Hahnemann: His Life and Work (London: Homoeopathic Publishing Company, 1922).

This represented a considerably more accurate historico-biographical testimony of the discovery of the scientific system of homoeopathy and of its discoverer than had hitherto been available, namely Thomas Lindsley Bradford's *The Life and Letters of Dr Samuel Hahnemann* (Philadelphia: Boericke and Tafel, 1895, 521 pages).

His other outstanding action had been two years earlier, in 1920, when he was finally successful in obtaining Hahnemann's manuscript for the sixth edition of the *Organon* (completed 1842, but totally inaccessible to homoeopathy for fully 78 years, because it would not be released, successively, by Hahnemann's widow, by their adoptive daughter Sophie, then by her widower

Karl Baron von Boenninghausen, or their heirs, until 1920). (Different aspects of the background and some events leading up to Haehl's ultimately successful endeavour to procure this priceless manuscript are described under 'Boenninghausen, Clemens Maria Franz Baron von (1785-1864)', 'Boericke, William (1849-1929)', 'History of Homoeopathy before 1900', section on France, and 'Organon'.)

Hahnemann, Christian Friedrich Samuel (1755-1843)

The founder of homoeopathy. He was born on 10th April, 1755 at Meissen in Saxony (now part of Germany). The entry in the church register at the Frauenkirche of Meissen inaccurately shows the date of birth as Friday, 11th April, 1755 apparently because Hahnemann was born at or just before 24.00 on the night from the 10th to the 11th, which has led to later confusion, resulting, *inter alia,* in the incorrect date being inscribed on the Hahnemann monument in Washington, DC, USA. After studying medicine at the medical schools of the universities of Leipzig and Vienna, he ultimately graduated on the 10th August, 1779 as a Doctor of Medicine from the University of Erlangen, Kingdom of Bavaria (now part of Germany). His thesis had the following title:

'Conspectus adfectuum spasmodicorum aetiologicus et therapeuticus' (Compendium of conditions of cramp with corresponding therapy, listed in accordance with their aetiology).

Hahnemann married twice and had eleven children by his first wife and an adopted daughter with the second. In his lifetime he moved his residence and medical practice frequently, but despite that he managed to generate a prodigious literary output. In his translation of William Cullen's *A Treatise on the Materia Medica* in 1790 he attacked the author's opinion about the pharmacodynamics of the medicinal mechanism of Peruvian Bark (Cinchona) in a footnote (vol II, p 108), and then resolved to test the effect of that medicine upon himself, a healthy person. Other such tests followed which convinced him of the principle of homoeopathy. The first public announcement of the new principle appeared six years later in 1796 in Hufeland's *Journal for Practising Physicians* (vol II, p 434) under the title 'Essay on a New Principle for Ascertaining the Curative Powers of Drugs'.

The year 1796 has, consequently, been officially recognized by followers of homoeopathy as the year of this system's birth.

From then on, as his new scientific medical system evolved, he waged a constant polemical war with all those who disagreed with him. He passed away on 2nd July, 1843 in Paris, France, where he was buried at Montmartre cemetery nine days later, after being embalmed. His body was exhumed on the 24th May, 1898 and transferred to a dignified, fitting tomb in the beautiful Père Lachaise cemetery of Paris, the resting place of many illustrious individuals. There his monument and final resting place is in the company of the graves of such great men as the composers Rossini, Donizetti and Auber, the poet Racine, the fable-writer La Fontaine (a granite fox sits on his grave), the physicist-chemist Gay-Lussac, the anatomist and physician Franz Joseph Gall, and the physicist-astronomer Arago. Nowhere to be read, however, is the inscription Hahnemann, ever the German Romantic, had desired for his own epitaph:

Non Inutilis Vixi (I have not lived in vain).

Constantin Hering wrote in an essay, entitled 'Requisites to a Correct Estimate of Hahnemann', published in the *Hygea* in 1847: 'In order to be able to form an opinion concerning this man who belongs to history, it is necessary to describe in clear and firm outlines the period in which Hahnemann was born . . . The first essential is to represent the moral man . . . Then let us describe him as the physician, teacher, colleague and debater.' Therefore, in an attempt to place in context the enormous contribution Hahnemann made to scientific medicine during his more than eighty-eight year life-span, a condensed perspective of the two streams of philosophical traditions in medicine (as identified by Harris Livermore Coulter in *Divided Legacy*), to both of which he was exposed, is provided. The time-span covered here for the Rationalists begins with the European Middle Ages and ends shortly before 1900; for the Empirics it begins in Antiquity and ends just before Hahnemann.

The Rationalist Medical Tradition

This represents the mainstream of Orthodox Medicine. It has always derived its rationalist models for understanding disease and for determining therapy from systems, disciplines, sciences and paradigms outside of itself, even though, historically, these constantly change with time. Causal assumptions derived from elaborations in other sciences always form the basis of therapeutics. Diagnosis on an 'a priori' basis is always considered extremely important to the choice of therapy, whereas prognosis is not. It attempts to obtain, and occasionally to enforce, practitioner conformism to each successive model that happens to be in vogue at the particular time. The principal emphasis of orthodox medicinal therapy throughout has been 'contraria contrariis curentur' (let the adverse [symptoms] be cured by their contraries) leading, as it does, to symptom-repression. This tendency, though largely subconscious, is still fully evident today in the nomenclature of symptom-negatives used as labels for a plethora of orthodox pharmaceutical categories (for example: antidiarrhoeals, antianginals, antihypertensives, anaesthetics, antipsychotics, antidepressants, anticonvulsives, antigalactics, anti-emetics, antibiotics, antacids, anti-inflammatories, antipyretics, antidiuretics, antitussives, anticatarrhal salts, anti-allergic drugs, antispasmodics, antimitotics, antiperspirants, analgesics or anodynes, m.a.o. inhibitors, c.n.s. depressants, anxiolytics, immunosuppressants, contrastimulants, analeptics, ataractics (also ataraxics), decongestants, muscle relaxants, vasodilators, counter-irritants, desensitizing agents, etc.).

The roots of the Rationalist tradition in medicine lie in antiquity. It found its initial inspiration, outside itself, in Formal Logic, the rules of which were rigidly applied for many centuries in order thereby to attain the ever-elusive medical certainty that was sought. Symptoms were seen as in themselves morbific and the idea that cure comes from the opposition between remedy and disease (the doctrine of contraries) took its origin in Aristotle's Logic, specifically his 'principle of contradiction' (a thing cannot be and not be at the same time).

Historical Overview

Time of greatest influence:	Salient features of the nationalist models, underpinning diagnostics and therapeutics, taken from the dominant external non-medical paradigm of the time:
after the Arab Period, until about 1490	**Mediaeval Period** disease was presented as a punishment; therapy involved charms and amulets, penance, fasting, fanciful concocotions, and prayer, while astrology ruled the prognosis. Scholastic Theology provided the Rationalist model.
ca. 1490–ca. 1590	**Iatrochemical Period** disease was seen only in chemical terms: therapy consisted in neutralization by either alkalis or acids, the opposition between which became the fundamental physiological principle. Chemistry provided the Rationalist model; Galenic contraries were reformulated strictly in chemical terms.
ca. 1590–ca. 1690	**Iatromechanical Period** disease was interpreted as either a problem of hydraulic engineering (blood, lymph, heart) or a defect in mechanics (structure, locomotion): therapy consisted in applying hydraulic and mechanical methods (e.g. blood-letting to alter various perceived pressures), Hydraulics and Mechanics provided the Rationalist model); the discovery by William Harvey (1578–1657) of the circulatory system, which was taken to function autonomously (independent of the heart), lent confirmatory impetus.
ca. 1690–ca. 1750	**Iatromathematical Period** disease and health were taken to be governed by the permanent rules of goemetry and arithmetic; for instance, there were formulae to calculate the exact date of an individual's death, well in advance of the event. Mathematics provided the Rationalist model,

specifically the analytical geometry of Rene Descartes (1595-1650) and the infinitesimal calculus of Sir Isaac Newton (1642-1727).

ca.1750–ca. 1810

Brunonian Period

disease was stated to be due to weakness from deficient stimulation, so that 'heroic' doses of many medicines in one prescription, and similar prodigious means, were needed to stimulate the sick organism back to health; examples of standard therapy: in diphtheria – simultaneous application of leeches, sinapisms, vesicatories, and poultices with hydrochloric acid applied directly to the larynx; in emphysema – simultaneous administration of alkalis, salts, soap pills, and hydrogen sulphide, in order to increase mucous secretions and reduce their viscosity, to promote expectoration so as to clear the airway obstructions; as a treatment against any supervening suffocation, emetics and blood-letting were added.

Physics provided the Rationalist model: Descartes' *Treatise of Man* (published 1662) introduced corpuscular (atomic) particles as the basic constituent of physiology, postulating either blockages or superabundant flow, obeying the laws of Physics; this did away with dynamic spontaneity in an organism; in Newton's *Philosophiae Naturalis Principia Mathematica* (published 1687) the third law of motion (every action is opposed by an equal and opposite reaction) supported the orthodox medical concept of deficient stimulation in disease, if health is seen as an established equilibrium.

ca. 1810–ca. 1870

Period of 'Physiological Medicine'
(also Broussaisism or Contrastimulism

was no more than a Brunonian inversion) disease was now defined as excess energy producing acute or chronic inflammations (sensitizations, or irritations), always beginning in the gastrointestinal tract: the sensitivity (contractility, irritability) thus evoked would be subdued successfully by drug sedation, by withholding food (for days), by the simultaneous introduction of purges and clysters or enemas, and by blood-letting and/or the application of leeches, in addition to medicines in 'heroic' doses (see 'Physiological Dose', and for the more recent period in Rationalist Medicine see 'Eclipse of Homoeopathy (1920–1965)').

Inspired by Physics, as the Brunonian Period had been [Hahnemann comments in some detail on 'Broussaisism' in footnote 66 to section 60 of the *Organon*].

To illustrate the magnitude implied in 'heroic', the following historical statistics are provided: in the ten year period ending in 1836 the orthodox hospitals of the city of Paris alone are recorded to have acquired between 5 and 6 million leeches annually; about five hundred were used daily on every ward, applied mostly to the patient's abdomen (and occasionally to the anus), until the belly looked like a black glistening coat of chain mail; (venesection, with the lancet, was often performed in addition thereto); since a leech draws off 17g of blood and could only be used three times, it was easy to calculate that at least 1 680 000 litres of blood were collectively sucked off each year in these hospitals, quite apart from the amount lost in standard blood-letting. The homoeopaths spoke of 'medical vampirism', that caused more loss of French blood in a few months than had the Napoleonic wars and the French Revolution combined, over years.[1] One reminder of this long blood-thirsty period in Orthodox Medicine is still to be found in the name of a prestigious medical journal (*The Lancet*, published in the UK).

The Empirical Medical Tradition

This has, at all times, represented the minority's contraposition in medicine. The Empirics have always held that each organic constitution, each disease process and each remedy is unique and irreducible. Their two guiding principles have remained, as ever: 1) 'primum non nocere' (first of all not to injure) and 2) 'Natura sanat' (Nature heals). And further, that the appropriateness of medical techniques and the usefulness of remedies in disease can only ever be learned through observation and experience, in other words 'a posteriori', in accordance with the dictum 'nihil in intellectu nisi prius in sensu' (nothing in the intellect was not first in the senses). For this reason it is also referred to as the Medicine of Experience. The Empirics, from antiquity to the present day, view the organism as reacting correctively to morbific stimuli in order to maintain equilibrium with its surroundings (see 'Heterostasis' and 'Homoeostasis'). Therefore, symptoms are seen, not in themselves as morbific, but as the body's own beneficial healing effort, to be

[1]Glasscheib, H S. *The March of Medicine* translated from German, London: Macdonald & Co (Publishers) Ltd, 1963, pp 165-166.

fully supported (hence the doctrine of similars). The Empirics discounted as therapeutically irrelevant the causal assumptions derived from elaborations in other sciences and refused to base their therapeutics on such 'a priori' Rationalist knowledge. Prognosis is generally considered to be an indispensable element in the therapeutic interchange, while diagnosis had no very significant place. To the Aristotelian 'principle of contradiction' (a thing cannot both be and not be at the same time) the Empirical medical retort is that whereas that is undoubtedly true, 'a thing can, however, very well be similar to another thing, without falsely claiming to be the identical thing.' This, moreover, fully accords with the Aristotelian Logic's Laws of Association governing the processes of establishing connexions through contiguity and/or similarity.

Empirical Medicine regards itself as the only true scientific medicine, in the sense of being a scientifically developed method of practice wholly contained within the bounds of the medical endeavour, which in its gradual unfolding has remained tenaciously untouched by the turmoil of politics, deaf to the clamour of false prophets, and undeflected from its path by the mass commercial successes achieved through the hyperbole of persuasion. But, curiously, its scientific arguments have never managed to demolish what are seen by it as the cherished illusions of the day. These, they say, are only eroded by time. Much resentment is often aroused when Empirics point to the recurring historical datum which shows it was the grotesque lot of mainstream medicine to have repeatedly played pimp to human credulity, while they, the Empirics, have advanced steadily along what they see as a scientific path of self-fulfilling trial-and-observation.

Historical Overview

ca. 430 BC	Hippocrates	pointed out the simile principle in medicine.
ca. 240 BC	Serapion of Alexandria	founded the non-dogmatist Empirical School of Medicine.
ca. 60 BC	Lucretius	constructed a sense-perceptible model of the wholeness of an individual's response.
ca. 5 AD	Celsus	established that fever was not evil but, in fact, a beleaguered organism's effort to combat and eliminate morbid material.
1st century AD	Dioskorides	observed that 'where the disease is, there also is the remedy'.
ca. 200 AD	Sextus Empiricus	condemned explanations in terms of 'formal logic' in medicine; and advocated Empirical skepticism.
ca. 1520	Paracelsus	is the father of modern experimental

		Empirical medicine, occupational diseases, and chemistry.
in 1566	Girolamo Cardano	coined the Empirical aphorism: 'Omne Simila Similibus Confirmatur' (everything similar is confirmed by/in the similar).
ca. 1570	Thomas Sydenham	recognized that illness is an attempt by the body to get its vital healing forces back to normal; held that single similar remedies were the best; was the first to distinguish between symptom and illness; and had a direct influence on his friend the Empirical philosopher John Locke.
ca. 1690	Georg Ernst Stahl	set down the distinct role of the dynamis, which he called the 'anima sensitiva'.
ca. 1700	Giorgio Baglivi	urged greater attention to 'peculiar and constant' symptoms and to ignore the 'common' ones; wanted to avoid disturbing the natural course of disease through medicines; accepted the adjunctive role of acupuncture; and searched for Empirical knowledge, disparaging Rationalist opinions.
ca. 1760	John Hunter	emphasized the importance of the patient's constitutional predisposition; held that two or more diseases cannot exist in the same organism at the same time; maintained that medicines act through setting up an artificial irritation (without suggesting there was to be any drug-disease similarity) which might extinguish the existing competing disease irritation, hence proposed the proving of drugs on people; he vigorously cautioned against over-medication; and observed that infection depended only on quality, rather than mere quantity, of the contagion or poison.

(A more detailed overview is to be found under 'Philosophical Premise of

Homoeopathy'; for an example of the profound incompatibility of the Empirical and the Rationalist traditions in medicine, and the reprehensible effects of an attempt at mixing these, refer to 'Hempel, Charles Julius (1811-1879)'.)

Hahnemann's Contribution to Science and his Impact on the Practice of Medicine

He studied medicine first in Leipzig, Saxony, then in Vienna, Austria (for details about the latter, see 'Quarin, Dr Joseph Baron von (1733-1814)' and 'History of Homoeopathy before 1900', section Austria-Hungary). At both universities he had to absorb the Rationalist medical scholasticism of the day in large doses. The Orthodox medical textbooks of the time propounded an obscure, semi-comprehensible jargon which instilled in Hahnemann's highly principled mind an ever growing despair. Phrases that commonly served as 'scientific' diagnostic descriptions at that time were:

'proclivity to the absence of internal stimuli'

'perverseness of the vitality'

'nervous asthenia'

'bilious rheumatism'

and much more in like vein. The student Hahnemann became slowly convinced that the scholarly gibberish the qualified doctors were mouthing served only as a device to impress patients and their relatives, while designed to conceal an abysmal ignorance. With his student's early enthusiasm for medicine eventually shattered, he secretly began to nurse the painful, desolate conviction that he was actually learning nothing from his professors that might enable him to heal the sick. His unimpeachable moral fibre would not permit him to reconcile himself – as distinct from others all around him – to the idea of using the ruses and devices to deceive suffering humanity. It utterly repelled him to have to stoop to what appeared to be blatant quackeries. Furthermore, he was devastated by the evident lack of any genuinely durable scientific method to underpin the practice of medicine.

He had qualified, but in his mind he had again jettisoned most of the therapeutics he had been taught. That made it difficult for him to offer his patients the care he felt they all deserved. Moreover, it made friendship with medical colleagues impossible.

The loner Hahnemann, strongly influenced by the ethos of German Romanticism, began to cast about for a medical system that could guarantee, or would at least approximate, therapeutic certainty. His chosen motto was 'aude sapere' ('dare to know', or a free rendering might be 'be bold and think for yourself'). This gifted, pedantic man and paragon of moral rectitude was transformed into a latter-day Dr Faustus, displaying similar brilliance and energy: every night, by the light of his oil lamp, he would pore over all kinds of medical texts in many languages. By translating some of these he earned extra income as well, which helped to support his growing family. He wrote about his state of mind thus:

'After the discovery of the weakness and misconceptions of my teachers and my books I sank into a state of morbid indignation, which might almost have completely vitiated for me the study of medical knowledge. I was about to believe that the whole science was of no avail and incapable of improvement. I gave myself up to my own individual cogitations and determined to fix no goal for my considerations until I should have arrived at a decisive conclusion.'[1]

It is quite clear that he was soon drawn to the Empirical medical tradition. The most recent exponent of this second stream of medical thought had been John Hunter.

In 1789 Crusius of Leipzig published Hahnemann's *Instructions for Surgeons Respecting Venereal Diseases: together with a New Mercurial Preparation*. In this Hahnemann acknowledges Hunter's 1786 *Treatise on the Venereal Disease* in no less than twenty-three references. In the last-mentioned book Hunter put forward a number of the essential fundamentals that were later incorporated by Hahnemann into homoeopathy. Hence the Empirical line of succession to Hahnemann is clearly established.

One serious defect impeded the evolution of scientific medicine, within the paradigm of medical Empiricism, beyond the point it had reached at the time of John Hunter's death in 1793, and that was that it lacked an exact and serviceable theory of drug action. The problem, as formulated by Hahnemann, was:

'How could you divide up medicines with reference to the pathological states for which they are created?'[2]

He called for the unpredictable element of chance effects to be eliminated from Empirical medicine by demanding

'investigation of the effects of remedies in order to adapt them to disturbances of the body. One should rely as little as possible upon chance and proceed as rationally and conscientiously as possible'[3]

by experiments of drugs on the healthy human body. Only by this means

'can the true nature, the real effect of the medicinal substances be conscientiously discovered; from them [the experiments] alone can be ascertained to what maladies they are safely and successfully adaptable.'[4]

The general principle underlying an effective medicinal method he stated as follows:

'Every effective remedy incites in the human body a kind of illness peculiar to itself, the more particular, the more marked and the more acute, according as the medicine is the more effective.'[5]

[1] Hahnemann, C F S. *Aesculapius in the Balance.* Leipzig: Steinacker, 1805 (70 pp).
[2,3,4,5] Hahnemann, C F S. 'Essay on a New Principle for Ascertaining the Curative Power of Drugs, and Some Examinations of the Previous Principles'. *Hufeland's Journal,* 1796, vol II, parts 3 and 4, pp 391-439 and pp 465-561.

And further, with the sublime certainty of genius, he advises:

'One should apply in the disease to be healed, particularly if chronic, that remedy which is able to stimulate another artificially produced disease, as similar as possible; and the former will be healed – similia similibus – likes with likes.'[1]

Hahnemann then continued by stating the principle of hormesis, the biphasic action of drugs:

'Most medicines have more than one kind of effect – the direct one at the beginning, passing gradually into the second (I call it the indirect after-effect). The latter state is generally exactly opposite to the former.'[2]

In summary, Hahnemann's mandate for a reliably effective medical method became this:

'To obtain a quick, easy and lasting cure, choose for every attack of illness a medicine which can produce a similar malady to the one it is to cure (similia similibus curentur).'[3]

All the while Hahnemann experimented first on himself, later on others also, with remedies that were known to be useful in certain disease conditions – and could demonstrate a clear parallelism for each drug between the natural disease cured by it and the artificial disease it induced experimentally.

On a later occasion Hahnemann set out the premises of the principles of homoeopathy as these pertain to what he called the Medicine of Experience:

'At the bottom of every malady there is a peculiar stimulation contrary to nature and disturbing the harmonious working of our organs.'[4]

He succinctly re-stated John Hunter's earlier position:

'If two general stimuli contrary to nature operate on the body at the same time, and if they are dissimilar, then the action of the one (the weaker) will be lulled and suspended for a time by that of the other (the stronger).'[5]

Hahnemann's own discovery based on empirical observation linked to the experimental evidence he had obtained, however, was:

'If the two stimuli are very similar to one another, then the weaker will be totally annihilated with the whole of its action by the analogous power of the other (the stronger).'[6]

His experimental work had inevitably led him to formulating the following conclusion:

[1,2]Hahnemann, C F S. 'Essay on a New Principle for Ascertaining the Curative Power of Drugs, and Some Examinations of the Previous Principles'. *Hufeland's Journal*, 1796, vol II, parts 3 and 4, pp 391-439 and pp 465-561.
[3]Hahnemann, C F S. *Organon of the Rational System of Medicine*, first edition, Dresden: Arnold, 1810, p v of the Introduction.
[4,5,6]Hahnemann, C F S. 'Medicine of Experience'. *Hufeland's Journal*, 1806, vol XXII, part 3, pp 5-99. Thereafter, separate reprint, Berlin: Wittich.

'To be able to cure, we need only have a suitable medicine for the unnatural stimulus present of the disease. That is, we need only apply another diseased power with action similar to that exerted by the disease itself.'[1]

Homoeopathy had at last burst on the medical scene. Suddenly Hahnemann's reliable technique for establishing and applying 'similarity' in medicine had closed the troublesome lacuna in Empirical Medicine. Hahnemann's brilliant and revolutionary contribution to science explained the interactive drug-in-phase-with-disease phenomenon in verifiable terms which have become axiomatic and this they did totally within the bounds of medicine proper. By taking known medical facts, forming a theory which explained them in pharmacodynamic terms, deducing consequences from the theory, and comparing the results with observed and experimental facts, Hahnemann united, for the first time, the explanation of the physical phenomena (of disease and drug effects) with the means of prediction (prognosis). He converted medical practice from a mere 'science of deductive explanations' into a versatile medical system through the discovery of a powerful technique of universal application. Or as he himself said, in 1819, in the preface to the second edition of the *Organon,* this discovery had elevated medicine to 'a pure science of experience' quite like 'physics and chemistry'.

From here on Hahnemann only needed to work on the extension, refinement, unbroken verifiability and polemical defence of his viable system of medicine. This he did untiringly, and in the process he has additionally earned credit, amongst other things (as evident in this Dictionary), for the following:

a) The discovery of the colloidal solubility of substances insoluble in the crude state (see 'Colloid').
b) The synonymity of disease and drug categories.
c) The indivisibility of physiology and pathology.
d) The parity of scientific validity between a patient's subjective experiences and objective phenomena in both diagnostics and therapeutics.
e) The multiplicity of drug effects on the total person (for b), c), d) and e) see 'Epistemological Assumptions in Homoeopathy', under the first section of which the whole 'similarity principle' is also discussed in some detail).
f) The projection of medicinal efficacy into ultramolecular deconcentrations by means of the process of dynamization (potentization) devised by him, which would, moreover, appear to have made him a pioneer in polymer chemistry (see 'Epistemological Assumptions in Homoeopathy' and 'Potency').
g) Introducing the olfactory pathway for medication (see 'Olfactory Medicines').

[1] Hahnemann, C F S. 'Medicine of Experience'. *Hufeland's Journal,* 1806, vol XXII, part 3, pp 5-99. Thereafter, separate reprint, Berlin: Wittich.

Hahnemann's Literary Output[1]

Hahnemann was a highly gifted linguist. In addition to his native German, he was proficient in English, French, Italian, Greek, Hebrew, Latin and Arabic. His work encompassed:

Sixteen medical, veterinary, chemical, pharmaceutical as well as balneotherapeutic volumes translated from English.

One agricultural volume and one biographical history translated from English.

Albrecht von Haller's *Materia Medica* translated from the Latin.

Six medical and chemistry volumes translated from French.

One volume on manufacturing chemistry translated from Italian.

At least 103 original dissertations, essays, books and scientific articles.

More than 200 scholarly letters concerning homoeopathy are extant (collected and annotated by Richard Haehl in Volume II of *Samuel Hahnemann: His Life and Work*, English translation, London: Homoeopathic Publishing Co, 1922).

Hahnemann's Family

Grandfather: Christoph Hahnemann was a painter, who resided in Bad Lauchstädt, Saxony (now part of Germany). A prominent inhabitant, he had three sons and four daughters.

Father: Christian Gottfried Hahnemann, second son and fifth child, was born on the 24th July, 1720 at Lauchstädt, died 15th November, 1784 at Meissen. Around 1733 the family left Bad Lauchstädt. He became a painter of the world-famous delicate Meissen porcelain and married on the 27th November, 1718 at the Evangelical Lutheran Frauenkirche in Meissen. Nine months later his wife died giving birth to twins, one of which was stillborn, the other surviving its mother for nine months. He published a book on the techniques of water-colour painting.

Mother: Johanna Christina Spiess became the second wife of Christian Gottfried Hahnemann on the 2nd November, 1750. She was the only daughter of the Captain and Quartermaster of Kötzschenbroda, near Dresden, Saxony. After she had the first child, a daughter, her husband bought a house on the corner of Neumarkt Street and Fleisch Walk. Saxony became impoverished by the Seven Years' War (1756-1763) and she and her husband were not particularly well to do.

Siblings: August Hahnemann, his brother, became a Field Apothecary in Austria. Sister Charlotte Hahnemann married twice – first, Pastor A B Trinius of Eisleben, by whom she had one son, Bernhardt; second, General-

---

[1]A bibliography is provided of Hahnemann's writings by Thomas Lindsay Bradford, in *The Life and Letters of Dr Samuel Hahnemann*, Philadelphia: Boericke and Tafel, 1895, pp 515-521. All Hahnemann's extant literary work, letters and other documents are listed, and much material is reproduced, by Richard Haehl, in *Samuel Hahnemann: His Life and Work* translated from German, 2 vols. London: Homoeopathic Publishing Company, 1922, vol II.

Superintendent Müller, also of Eisleben. The other sister, Minna Hahnemann, married M Aubortin of Stuttgart; their daughter married minor nobility by the name of von Landech and settled in Rosswein, near Leipzig, Saxony.

Children: Nine daughters and two sons. One son, Ernst, was killed as a baby by a fall from a wagon. The other son, Friedrich, was born at Dresden on the 30th November, 1786. He graduated as a medical practitioner from Leipzig Medical School in 1812, and married a Dresden widow that year, which estranged him from his father. Friedrich Hahnemann had a daughter, Adelheid, who married Rector Hohlfeld of Dresden; she died in 1829. Friedrich settled in Wolkenstein where he opened a pharmacy. He followed his father's system of medicine faithfully, for which he was relentlessly hounded by the local medical authorities. Finally, something is said to have snapped in him, and he left wife and child to become a wanderer. He spoke Greek, Latin, French, English and Italian, and understood enough Arabic as 'was required by a highly educated physician'. He played both the guitar and the piano exceptionally well. In 1818 he was in the Netherlands, the following year he was in London, UK, in 1823 he was in Dublin, Ireland, in 1828 he was reported to be in Tomkins County, NY, USA, and in 1832 and 1833, during the Cholera epidemic, he was apparently sighted in St Louis, Missouri, in Dubuque, Iowa and in Galena, Illinois, USA. In all these places he practised the homoeopathic method, when the need arose, always with astonishing success, and latterly (in the Cholera epidemic) without charging. Thereafter all traces of him were lost.

One of Samuel Hahnemann's daughters was stillborn, while two further of his daughters, called Karoline and Charlotte, never married. Three others, Louise, Frederika and Eleonore, had childless marriages. Henriette was born at Gommern in 1783; she married Pastor Förster and lived in Dresdorf, near Sangerhausen, in the Hartz Mountains of Thuringia (now part of Germany); she had four children: Louis, a merchant; Robert, a farmer; Adelheid, unmarried; and Angeline, who married Mr Stollberg. Wilhelmine was born at Dresden in 1788; she married music conductor Richter of Gera, Thuringia and died in 1818; she bore one son, Hermann Friedrich Siegmund Richter, who died at Coethen on the 13th May, 1866. Amalie was born in 1789 and married Dr Leopold Suess, by whom she had one son of like name, who, until his death in 1914 at 89 years, practised as a homoeopathic physician in London, UK and had taken on the name Leopold Suess-Hahnemann; her second husband was Mr Liebe with whom she lived in Paris and London; she died in Coethen on the 7th December, 1857.

Wives: First wife – Johanne Henriette Leopoldine Küchler, daughter of Gottfried Heinrich Küchler and later the step-daughter of Master Häseler, the apothecary of of Dessau, was born on the 1st January, 1764; Hahnemann married her at Dessau on the 17th November, 1782; she bore him all eleven children, and died at Coethen on the 31st March, 1830.

Second wife – Marie Melanie d'Hervilly-Gohier, daughter of a painter from Savoy, and an accomplished painter herself, was born in 1800; she was adopted by a senior member of the last Directory Government overthrown by

Napoleon Bonaparte on the 18th Brumaire (9th November), 1799, which allowed her to suffix his name 'Gohier' to her original name; he, Louis Jerome Gohier, died in 1830; Hahnemann married her at Coethen on the 28th January, 1835; she died childless in Paris on the 27th May, 1878, though she and Hahnemann had adopted a Bavarian girl, Sophie Bohrer, who later married Dr Karl Baron von Boenninghausen (see 'History of Homoeopathy before 1900', section on France).

Hahnemann's Itineracy

1755 – 1774 Meissen – childhood and school years in his parents' house;

1775 & 1776 Leipzig – studying at Medical School;

1777 Vienna – studying at Medical School, under the benign influence of Dr von Quarin, who accepted no remuneration from Hahnemann;

1778 Hermannstadt, Transylvania, Dual Monarchy – von Quarin arranged for Hahnemann to be the personal assistant to Samuel von Bruckenthal, Austro-Hungarian Governor of Transylvania; had first-hand experience of ague in that region;

1779 Erlangen – graduated from the University as Doctor of Medicine;

1780 Hettstedt, Saxony – began his medical practice here; from here on he began his private studies and his literary output, that only really stopped with his death 63 years later;

1781 Dessau, Duchy of Anhalt (now eastern Germany) – met Miss Küchler;

1782 – 1784 Gommern, Saxony – became the town's Medical Officer; was married on 17th November, 1782 to Miss Küchler;

1785 – 1789 Dresden – temporarily relinquished the practice of medicine; devoted himself exclusively to the study of chemistry and to writing;

1790 – 1791 Leipzig – his first fight against blood-letting; beginnings of drug provings; the concept of homoeopathy takes shape in his mind; from here on systematic elaboration of the homoeopathic therapeutic method;

1792 Gotha, Thuringia (now eastern Germany) – temporary sojourn, here during the Spring only;

1792 & 1793 Georgenthal (near Gotha) – first homoeopathic asylum for the insane (see this entry);

part 1794 Molschleben – medical practice; auto-provings; writings;

1794 & 1795 Pyrmont – medical practice; auto-provings; writings;

end 1795 Brunswick – medical practice; auto-provings; writings;

1796 – 1798 Königslutter – medical practice; auto-provings; writings;

1799 & 1800 Hamburg – medical practice; auto-provings; writings;

1801 Mölln, Lauenburg – medical practice; auto-provings; writings;

1802 & 1803 Machern – medical practice; auto-provings; writings;

1804 Dessau – literary work only, in his wife's home;

1805 – 1810 Torgau – wrote *The Organon of Medicine;* medical practice; auto-provings;

1811 – 1820 Leipzig University: Hahnemann as lecturer; opposition from professors and some students; collaborator group forms to undertake drug provings on a wider scale; further elaboration of tenets of homoeopathy; involvement with 'The Homoeopathic Hospital and Clinic of Leipzig';

1821 – 1834 Coethen – wrote *Materia Medica Pura* [the painstaking record of years of provings by himself and his collaborators on themselves and *The Chronic Diseases, Their Nature and Their Homoeopathic Cure;* the Theory of the Miasmata; the family had completely settled down here; he had a very prosperous practice; he remained under constant attack;

1835 Coethen – second marriage to Marie Melanie d'Hervilly-Gohier on 18th January, 1835; departure for Paris, arriving there 21st June;

1835 – 1843 Paris, France – medical practice; preparation of sixth edition of the *Organon;* lived and practised at No.7, rue de Madame, at first; from 1837 at No.1, rue de Milan; here he finally passed away apparently from complications following a bronchial catarrh of nine weeks' duration.

Trevor M Cook has produced a biography entitled *Samuel Hahnemann: The Founder of Homoeopathic Medicine* which is appealingly fresh in that its emphasis is not solely on the scientific and medical work of the system's discoverer; instead it gives a fascinating insight into the man himself and the triumphs and tribulations that faced him and his family on a domestic, personal and professional level (Wellingborough: Thorsons Publishers Ltd, 1981, 192 pages).

Hale, Edwin M (1829-1899)

US homoeopath whose study of Amerind and other ethnopharmacy led him to prove (to experiment with, pathogenetically) and thereafter introduce a whole series of new and valuable remedies to homoeopathy, including: Hydrastis canadensis, Iberis amara, Lycopus virginicus, Passiflora incarnata and Phytolacca decandra. As a result he was known as the 'Father of the New Homoeopathic Drugs' and together with others he was also primarily instrumental in introducing some major medicines into the homoeopathic materia medica, such as Gelsemium sempervirens and Plantago major. For a number of years he was Professor of Therapeutics at the Hahnemann Medical College, Chicago, Illinois. His writings, which included the newly introduced homoeopathic drugs, are:

Specific Therapeutics of the New Remedies (1875)
Materia Medica (1881)

Hartmann, Franz (1796-1853)

One of the original medicine-proving group around Hahnemann, that pioneered the development of new remedies and ultimately the Materia Medica Pura. He retained, in all circumstances, a devoted veneration of Hahnemann, and it is from his pen that the most detailed and affectionate descriptions of a great but occasionally querulous Hahnemann have flowed.

When difficulties arose in filling the position of Consultant Director at the homoeopathic hospital in Leipzig, he twice sprang into the breach. From 1828 onward he wrote monographs on Nux vomica, (Matricaria) Chamomilla, (Atropa) Belladonna, Pulsatilla nigricans and Rhus toxicodendron. His greatest work appeared in 1831: *Therapy of Acute Diseases,* which saw three editions and was translated into French and English. This, together with the book he published two years after it, is commonly referred to as Hartmann's *Acute and Chronic Diseases,* which was the earliest attempt at a pathological treatise. (The one that immediately followed this appeared in the USA 36 years later (in 1869) under the title *The Science of Therapeutics According to the Principles of Homoeopathy* by Charles J Hempel, and relied heavily on the work of Bernhard Baehr of Prussia and Jakob Kafka of Austria). Hartmann's four major writings, available in English, are:

Practical Observations of Some Chief Homoeopathic Remedies (1841)
Hartmann's Theory of Acute Disease and Homoeopathic Treatment (1847)
Hartmann's Theory of Chronic Disease and Homoeopathic Treatment (1849)
Diseases of Children and Their Homoeopathic Treatment (1853).

Hawkes, Alfred Edward (1849-1919)

Scottish homoeopathic gynaecologist, a graduate from Edinburgh, who worked most of his life in Liverpool as physician to the Hahnemann Hospital. He was an active contributor to the homoeopathic journals, writing on subjects as diverse as Tuberculinum, Addison's disease, Alcohol, Seborrhoea, and the Heart. His major homoeopathic writings include:

Mucous Colitis Treated with Iso-Tonic Sea-Water (1913)
Gastric Ulcers (1914)
Retroversion of the Gravid Uterus (1916)

Hayfever

See 'Allergy', 'Emergencies – Homoeopathic Treatment', under Bronchial Asthma and Severe Hayfever, and 'Rhinitis'.

Headache

Cerebralgia; cephalea; a diffuse pain in the head, of varying intensity, which may principally, or exclusively, affect any part of the head. It may be one in a collection of symptoms, or constitute the entire disease of which it is the only symptom. In all cases a full investigation should be undertaken to establish whether or not adjunctive osteopathic, chiropractic, surgical, dietetic or hygienic approaches may be advisable, if the headache turns out to have structurally or exopathically determined aspects that may, in part, be beyond the normal reversible limits to the homoeopathic curative impulse. According to the antecedents in which they have their roots, headaches may be classified into eleven broad divisions:

1) Anaemic; 2) Nervous; 3) Reflex; 4) Rheumatic; 5) Dyspeptic; 6)

Hemicrania (Migraine); 7) Hyperaemic; 8) Neurologic; 9) Toxic; 10) Catarrhal and 11) Allergic.

No other common condition rebukes the inattentive homoeopathic prescriber quite so unmistakably, by the total non-alleviation of suffering in every case of negligent, near-hit remedy selection. There is no margin for slackness in the treatment of headaches, for reasons outlined below. In no other disease is careful discrimination and judgment more necessary in choosing the correct homoeopathic drug than in headache, if the best results are to be obtained; it is equally true that with the simillimum being found, no other disease is more amenable to treatment (see 'Disease and Drug Action in Homoeopathic Congruity' for details of the careful discrimination and judgment to be exercised).

Most applicable remedies are listed below. They are effective only because they are homoeopathic to particular headaches, that means when they are selected on the basis of full likeness, as exemplified in the first of the undermentioned drugs:

Belladonna: Suited to nervous, neuralgic or congestive form; with heavy eyelids and blindness or flashes of light before eyes; also sense of burning in eyeballs; it is ineffective in true gastric headaches, although secondary vomiting does not contra-indicate it; hyperaemia & hyperaesthesia are essential characteristics, like flushed face and hot head; dilated pupils; throbbing carotids; predominantly right-sided; aggravated from slight noise, jar, motion, light, lying down and least exertion; ameliorated from pressure, being at rest, standing erect.

Other remedies are to be selected with equally diligent precision from one of the following 130 homoeopathic medicines, which have all produced very distinct drug pictures, each with its own prominent, characteristic headache. This welter of homoeopathic drugs, all producing headaches of diverse types, highlights the homoeopath's time-consuming task of finding the exact remedy:

Acidum carbolicum, Acidum hydrocyanicum, Acidum phosphoricum, Acidum picricum, Aconitum napellus, Aesculus hippocastanum, Aethusa cynapium, Agaricus muscarius, Agnus castus, Aloe socotrina, Aluminium metallicum, Ammonium carbonicum, Anacardium orientale, Antimonium crudum, Antimonium tartaricum, Aranea diadema, Argentum nitricum, Aristolochia clematis, Arnica montana, Arsenicum album, Asarum europaeum, Asclepias syriaca, Aurum metallicum, Baptisia tinctoria, BCG, (Lycoperdon) Bovista, Bryonia alba, Cactus grandiflorus, Calcarea carbonica, Cannabis indica, Cannabis sativa, Capsicum annum, Carbo animalis, Carbo vegetabilis, Caulophyllum thalictroides, Causticum, (Simaba) Cedron, (Matricaria) Chamomilla, Chionanthus virginica, Cimicifuga racemosa, Cinchona officinalis, Cocculus indicus, Coffea cruda, (Citrullus) Colocynthis, Cornus circinata, Crocus sativus, Cyclamen europaeum, Digitalis purpurea, (Solanum) Dulcamara, Epiphegus virginiana, Ergotinum, Eupatorium perfoliatum, Euphrasia officinalis, Ferrum metallicum, Flavus (= Neisseria pharingis flava), Formica rufa, Gelsemium sempervirens, Gingko biloba

(Galisburin adiantinfolia), Glonoinum, Graphites, Helleborus niger, Helonias dioica, Hepar sulphuris calcareum, Histaminum hydrochloricum, Hydrastis canadensis, Hypophysis posterium, Ignatia amara, Indigo, (Cephaelis) Ipecacuanha, Iris versicolor, Juglans cinerea, Kali bichromicum, Kali sulphuricum, Kalmia latifolia, Lac deflorata, (Trigonocephalus) Lachesis, Lachnanthes tinctoria, (Cerasus) Laurocerasus, Leptandra virginica, Lilium tigrinum, Lithium carbonicum, Lobelia inflata, Lycopodium clavatum, Magnesia muriatica, Magnesia phosphorica, Mandragora officinarum, Melilotus alba et officinalis, Mercurius protoiodatus, Mercurius solubilis hahnemanni, Naja tripudians, Natrum carbonicum, Natrum muriaticum, Natrum salicylicum, Niccolum sulphuricum, Nux moschata, Nux vomica, (Nerium) Oleander, Opium, Palladium metallicum, Paris quadrifolia, Penicillinum, Petroleum, Phellandrium aquaticum, Phosphorus, Phytolacca decandra, Platinum metallicum, Plumbum metallicum, Pneumococcus, Psorinum, Pulsatilla nigricans, Pulsatilla nuttaliana, Ranunculus bulbosus, Rauwolfia serpentina, Rhus toxicodendron, Sabadilla officinarum, Sanguinaria canadensis, Selenium, Sepia officinalis, Silica, Spigelia anthelmia, Stannum metallicum, Sticta pulmonaria, Sulphur, (Lycosa) Tarentula, Tellurium, Theridion curassavicum, Thuja occidentalis, Tuberculinum residuum, Usnea barbata, Veratrum album and Zincum metallicum.

Of the 131 remedies mentioned above (including Belladonna) 118 are pertinently discussed in an easy-to-read, concise style in:

B F Underwood, *Headache – and its Materia Medica,* second edition, Calcutta: Roy Publishing House, 1972.

The other 13 remedies are to be found in:

Othon André Julian, *Materia Medica of New Homoeopathic Remedies,* revised (translated) English edition, Beaconsfield: Beaconsfield Publishers Ltd, 1979.

One of the reasons why this entry features so much detail is that the 'common headache' confronts the manufacturers, prescribers and dispensers of ready-to-use homoeopathic medicine combinations with an insuperable dilemma. Such combinations are usually composed of three, four or perhaps five separate headache remedies. These must, therefore, exclude at least 126 remedies, with as many alternatives in each of the following variable categories: (i) type (febrile, neurologic, etc.); (ii) cause (food allergy, herpes, etc.); (iii) modality (heat, strain, change in altitude, barometric pressure, etc.); (iv) character (quality of pain, effect on vision, fatigue or loss of sleep, etc.); (v) constitutional compatibility; (vi) symptom development (chronologically); and (vii) concomitant emotional symptoms. It is clear that such a large number of remedies must represent a large number of individually different headaches, each responding curatively only to the appropriate (matching) homoeopathic remedy. At best the mathematical probability is only around 1:25 to have administered a homoeopathically effective drug whenever a non-individualized drug combination is given to the patient 'for a headache'. In practice, that seems to be the experience with complex homoeopathic drug preparations for cerebralgias.

Examples of syndetic pointers to three homoeopathic medicines, guided principally by time modalities:

Congestive headache starting over the eyes, with a feeling of heat and heaviness in head, worse mornings, evenings and during menses, and after food as well as from warmth or jarring motion, but better from pressure and on lying down, in patients who may have a tendency to haemorrhoids – Kali sulphuricum

Recurring headaches, at their worst between 09.00 and 11.00 and between 16.00 and 20.00; may also be brought on after extreme nervous strain or from exposure to cold; patient often develops a superficial hyperaesthesia whereas the headache is relieved by firm pressure – Magnesia phosphorica

Around the menstrual period, the patient wakes up with a slight headache in the morning which increases as the day wears on, becoming very severe; eyes become hot and tired – Natrum muriaticum, or:

Headache comes on before 11.00 and eases off by 16.00, increasing and decreasing with the heat of the sun; cannot use eyes for close work like sewing or reading – Natrum muriaticum

(See also 'Combinations of Homoeopathic Drugs'.)

Healing Crisis

Denotes the acute symptoms that occur during the homoeopathic treatment of disease when progress is being made in the direction of cure. They indicate that the dynamis has been stimulated into redoubling its efforts at overcoming the morbific influences affecting the organism. The symptoms experienced at these times are those that have been suffered in the past by the patient. (See 'Aggravation', section entitled 'Homoeopathic aggravation', and 'Homoeopathic Practice'.)

Health

● **Dynamic balance.**

The state of an individual organism when it functions optimally, with its cells dynamically in phase and resonance, and without any reactive disease symptoms, disequilibrium or abnormality. (See 'Causes of Disease', 'Disease' and 'Therapeutic Science'.)

Heart Problems

See 'Emergencies – Homoeopathic Treatment'.

Heliotherapy

The therapeutic use of the sun's rays, as a prophylactic against infection, osteoporosis, cancer, tooth decay, and depression, as a stimulant of the immune system, for the promotion of cardio-vascular fitness, to increase the oxygen-carrying capacity of the blood, to reduce blood cholesterol, to normalize both blood pressure and blood sugar levels, to stimulate sexuality, to reduce hyperkinesis in children, to increase the mental performance in sufferers from arteriosclerotic dementia, to alleviate acne, psoriasis and certain forms of eczema (non-lupoid and non-photosensitive eruptions), and many other therapeutic applications. This is a naturopathic treatment that is complementary to homoeopathy, provided the attending homoeopath is made aware of it.

Hempel, Charles Julius (1811-1879)

A Prussian homoeopath, originally Karl J Hempel, who travelled widely and acquired a cosmopolitan education, in Paris and elsewhere. In 1835 he finally settled in the USA, where he graduated in homoeopathy. He was co-editor of the *Homoeopathic Examiner* from 1843 to 1845. During that period he translated Hahnemann's (then in three volumes) *The Chronic Diseases, Their Peculiar Nature and Their Homoeopathic Cure* (New York: William Radde, 1845 and 1846;). Then he was appointed as professor of Materia Medica and Therapeutics at the Hahnemann Medical College of Philadelphia. Hempel had a wide-ranging mind and thoroughly enjoyed intellectual confrontation. He became a prominent figure of that period exerting a very major influence on homoeopathic thought in the USA and indirectly also in the rest of the English-speaking area of the world. His distinctly Rationalist-materialistic philosophical stance was similar to that of Richard Hughes of the UK, from whom he later often took his cues. Hempel's distinct views may be summarized as follows:

1 He regarded as placebos the very high potencies that were beginning to be used by some in homoeopathy (such as are produced by continuous fluxion with the Skinner apparatus; see under 'Potentizing Methods'). He said that a homoeopath 'may use high potencies without being a high-potentialist. With . . . discretion . . . [the homoeopath] may use high potencies or nothing at all, according as the best interests of the patient may seem to require. This has nothing to do with the foolish high-potency dogmatism which bids fair to subvert all scientific correctness in the labours of our physicians and to destroy the very spirit and soul of homoeopathy'.[1] But elsewhere,[2] only two years later, he had become considerably less apodictic, stating: 'We admit that high potencies exert a curative influence. But there is no evidence that they act better than the lower potencies up to the

---

[1] *Proceedings of the Michigan Institute of Homoeopathy*, 1867, p 41.
[2] Hempel, Charles Julius. *The Science of Therapeutics, According to the Principles of Homoeopathy*, two volumes, originally published 1869. New Delhi: World Homoeopathic Links, reprint 1980, vol I, p 46.

thirtieth' [centesimal dynamization, fixed as the upper permissible limit by Hahnemann on 12th September, 1829[1]].

2 Contrary to what has occasionally been imputed to him, he uncompromisingly rejected the idea of compound homoeopathic remedies, saying, 'Every drug must be administered without the admixture of any other medicinal substance. . . . It is undoubtedly this law which has exerted the greatest influence upon [orthodox] Medicine generally. In proof of this it is well known that apothecaries have heaped upon Hahnemann their bitterest curses for introducing this reform. . . . This law is an inevitable consequence of the law of similarity. . . . [But should combination remedies ever be adopted in homoeopathy,] then, definite mixtures that have been proved would be like single remedies, since they would have to be prescribed in every case in the same identical combination'.[2]

3 He pleaded the case for the full integration of the science of pathology into homoeopathy, saying it had become 'indispensable . . . to show in what manner this new system of treatment affects the science of Pathology. In this respect [homoeopathy's] general system of Therapeutics must necessarily differ from that of other therapeutic[s] . . . ; [its] position in the domain of Medicine . . . compels [homoeopaths] to touch certain questions which, though not necessarily included within the range of Therapeutics, yet are of essential importance . . . Of particular value are . . . the material post-mortem changes, which alone render it possible in many cases of a most subtle pathological diagnosis to determine what drug-diagnosis corresponds to it very fully'.[3]

4 He recognized four tolerably workable, albeit unpredictable, non-homoeopathic therapeutic methods:

(i) Disease can be cured by removing the cause that produces it;

(ii) Disease symptoms are removed by exciting an artificial condition directly contrary to the natural malady (enantiopathic method – contraria contrariis curentur);

(iii) Disease is sought to be extirpated by alterations excited in non-affected organs or systems by artificial means (allopathic method, which Hempel called 'the revulsive method');

(iv) Morbid conditions are counteracted by neutralization through either supplementing deficiencies or reducing states of excess.

About the new reliable scientific therapeutic method, he said this: 'In opposition to these vague and defective doctrines, Hahnemann set up a [fifth] maxim alike applicable to the treatment of every kind of disease: Similia similibus curentur, the law of similarity; in other words, a disease is cured most safely, speedily and easily by a drug which, when acting upon

[1] *Neues Archiv für die homöopathische Heilkunst*, 1829, vol III, part 2, p 182.
[2] Hempel, op. cit. p 39.
[3] Ibid., pp 1 and 12.

the healthy organism, produces all the symptoms of the disease in their greatest possible similarity'.[1]

5 He rejected the idea that diet can in any way contribute positively to a homoeopathic cure, but encouraged exercise, hydrotherapy and balneotherapy, while remaining benignly neutral toward surgery.[2]

6 He defended the use of palliative (enantiopathic) remedies in certain circumstances: 'No truly humane homoeopathic practitioner is opposed to the use of palliatives, provided they really do palliate suffering without aggravating the disease after the palliating effect has passed off . . . A true comprehension of the spirit of the homoeopathic method of treatment is utterly opposed to the contracted opinions of the few exclusivists of our school, who would subordinate the victim of the disease to the technical letter of a formula'.[3]

The most far-reaching effects in homoeopathy arose from Hempel's determined canvassing around 1869 of two concepts: (i) that lower dynamizations are probably preferable to very high ones, and more particularly (ii) that the integrating of the science of pathology with the homoeopathic materia medica was, he maintained, indispensable, as this would not only add an extra dimension to homoeopathic drug diagnosis, but would fully establish the then fledgling science of homoeopathic pharmacology. It is here that Hempel crossed the Rubicon. By introducing causal assumptions derived from elaborations of another science (pathology) he moved from the Empirical to the Rationalist medical tradition, or at least opened the floodgate for all manner of other sciences and their elaborations to be seen as equally indispensable. The first effect was that his prompting ultimately bore fruit fifteen years later. In June 1884 the American Institute of Homoeopathy adopted a recommendation, subsequently likewise adopted by the British Homoeopathic Society, that an Anglo-American 'Cyclopaedia of Drug Pathogenesy' be produced with a mandate, inter alia, to record verified data on each single drug's pathogenesis on the healthy comprising: (a) chronology of symptom occurrence; (b) its toxicology, in full; (c) results of experiments on animals; (d) only symptoms from attenuations up to the 6th centesimal or 12th decimal. This enormous undertaking was, in fact, completed and a painstakingly accurate record of homoeopathic pathogenesis within the parameter of the mandate was published in four volumes (3066 pages) from June 1886 to November 1891 in London by Leath and Ross under said title.

The baleful attempt at amalgamation of an extraneous science (pathology) with homoeopathy had a calamitous effect. It produced a whole generation of blighted homoeopaths in the English-speaking world. They were more ready to be guided by pathological assumptions than by the presenting signs and symptoms, which, in turn, led inevitably to non-homoeopathic disease

[1] Ibid., pp 18-20.
[2] Ibid., pp 51-55.
[3] *American Homoeopathic Observer*, 1866, vol III, p 424.

classification being used, rather than homoeopathic drug-diagnoses being made. The fateful consequences of this obliteration of distinctness only became apparent some time after Orthodox Medicine had successfully paralysed homoeopathy in the USA by an insidiously prepared enchantment, containing a high coefficient of allure. This happened during the first decade of the twentieth century when the American Medical Association suddenly offered to recognize homoeopaths as 'regular' practitioners, for which the homoeopaths had secretly yearned for so long. It was further intimated to them that the AMA would not concern itself whether or not such practitioners actually employed the homoeopathic method, provided the tag 'homoeopath' was no longer used in public and no touting for the homoeopathic cause or its system was undertaken by any such 'born-again regular'. With the scientific tide turned implacably against vitalism at that time, and the homoeopaths having been ostracized for a full century before then, this dire lure proved irresistible to most of the blighted homoeopaths (the younger ones). With acceptance of this ingenious package-deal, homoeopathy's own social base, organizational structure and educational foundations were doomed at one fell stroke to a process of irreversible atrophy. Soon thereafter homoeopathy ceased to be the high-profile, well structured alternative to Orthodox Medicine it had been for so long. (See also 'Allopathy', 'Combinations of Homoeopathic Drugs', 'Eclipse of Homoeopathy (1920-1965)', 'Hahnemann, Christian Friedrich Samuel (1755-1843)', both sections – Rationalist Medical Tradition & Empirical Medical Tradition, 'History of Homoeopathy before 1900' section United Kingdom, 'Pain Relief Methods in Homoeopathy', 'Pathology', 'Phytotherapy', 'Potentizing Methods', 'Science of Therapeutics' and 'Simmons, George H (1852-1924)'.)

Henderson, William (1811–1872)

Scottish homoeopath, who had graduated from Edinburgh and later became professor of Pathology at the University of Edinburgh. He achieved prominence by striving to establish a scientific status (within the Rationalist paradigm) for homoeopathy by his outstanding perception in research and attention to physical detail. He placed a strong emphasis on the science of pathology for his interpretation of homoeopathic phenomena. Although he did not go quite as far as Professor Charles J Hempel in the USA (refer to this entry), many contemporary homoeopaths disapproved of his approach because he was thought to be ignoring the centre-piece of homoeotherapeutics, which is the overall sense-perceptible symptom-complex of any given patient. He also strove toward developing specific remedies for acute miasmata, such as pneumonia and other chest illnesses. Richard Hughes (1836-1902) strongly supported his emphasis on the science of pathology. His major writings include:

Homoeopathy Fairly Represented (in reply to Dr Simpson's 'Homoeopathy Misrepresented')

An Enquiry into the Homoeopathic Practice of Medicine.
(See 'Hempel, Charles Julius (1811-1879)'.)

Herakcleides of Tarentum (around 280 BC)

See 'Philosophical Premise of Homoeopathy'.

Herbal Medicine

See 'Phytotherapy'.

Herbalism

See 'Phytotherapy'.

Hereditary Miasma

See 'Miasma'.

Heredity

The transmission of characteristics from ancestor(s) to descendent(s). (See 'Genetic Assimilation', 'Lamarckism' and 'Miasma'.)

Hering, Constantin (1800-1880)

Homoeopathy had the good fortune to have at its disposal the inexhaustible resources of this man of profound and lasting influence. This certainly extended across the entire USA for the largest part of the nineteenth century. It was very largely on account of his imperturbable equanimity and steady dynamism that homoeopathy experienced an extraordinary flourishing period in that country for about seventy years (until about 1910). Yet Hering contributed above all to homoeopathy's permanent foundations in a way that quite transcends national boundaries or linguistic groupings. Hering's motto throughout his life was: 'Die milde Macht ist gross' (loosely: the force of gentleness is magnificent).

Hering was born on 1st January 1800 as the son of the assistant rector at Oschatz in the Electorate of Saxony and went to school at Zittau in the same country (both now in eastern Germany). In 1817 he attended the Surgical Academy of Dresden for three years. From 1820 he studied medicine at Leipzig University. During that time he attended Hahnemann's lectures, without entering into any closer contact with either the discoverer of homoeopathy or the exclusive circle of Hahnemann's other students, who were much older than he was. Hering was the student-assistant to Dr Robbi, a decided antagonist of homoeopathy. Baumgärtner, a Leipzig publisher, proposed to Robbi that he write a book against the 'homoeopathic heresy' in general, and Hahnemann in particular. Hahnemann, by then expelled from Leipzig, was to be expunged scientifically too. Robbi declined, pleading lack of time, but referred Baumgärtner to his assistant, who was thoroughly flattered by the publisher's offer. The young, enthusiastic Hering devoted himself to the study of Hahnemann's entire published work. Hering actually repeated provings of medicines and undertook other practical experiments within the new homoeopathic paradigm, as research for his anti-homoeopathic book. At the end of this, Hering was converted by the evidence of his own investigations at first hand, which result he boldly declared both to his teachers and to Baumgärtner. The latter also changed his allegiance later and helped to propagate the new medical movement by publishing homoeopathic journals and books. Hering went to Würzburg University, in the Kingdom of Bavaria, for the last term since he had aroused his Leipzig teachers' implacable animosity. He graduated there on 23rd March, 1826. In his doctoral thesis he put his previous research to good use. It was entitled 'De Medicina Futura' (On the Medicine of the Future). In it he confessed himself unreservedly to be a homoeopath.

He returned to his own country for a state-examination so as to be permitted to practise medicine in Saxony. During this time he became science instructor and house physician in Dresden at the Blochmann Educational Institute. This Institute with the backing of the Saxon Government sent Hering and the scientific researcher Weinhold to Surinam on a botanical and zoological expedition. He spent more than five years there (1827-1833). As a member of the research association he was prevented from publishing homoeopathic material, but after a while he resigned from the association and became the Physician-in-Attendance of the governor of Surinam's capital, Paramaribo. He then undertook energetic researches in materia medica for homoeopathy, and sent his results both to Hahnemann and the periodical *Archiv für die homöopathische Heilkunst*. In 1833 he returned to Saxony for a short visit and then left for America once more. He decided to go via Philadelphia in the USA, where friends prevailed upon him to stay. In 1835 he and others established the 'Nordamerikanische Akademie der homöopathischen Heilkunst' in Allentown, Pennsylvania. All instruction was in German, which limited the student intake. It eventually closed in 1841. But in 1848 Hering obtained a charter for the English-medium 'Homoeopathic Medical College' of Pennsylvania, in Philadelphia, which was to become the world's greatest homoeopathic teaching institution. From 1835 to 1838 Hering produced the *Domestic Physician* in two volumes, which went through twenty-nine editions. He also devised the so-called 'Homoeopathic Domestic Kit', an important factor in the spread of its domestic practice. On the 10th April, 1844 the American Institute of Homoeopathy was founded and elected Hering as its first president. Hering was the first to use nitroglycerine in medicine, for headaches and for cardiac problems (see 'Emergencies – Homoeopathic Treatment', section Angina Pectoris), more than thirty years earlier than its first use in

Orthodox medicine. In the pathology vs symptomatology dispute within English-speaking homoeopathy, Hering clearly sided with the latter, although he did not take an active part in the parallel dispute between the so-called 'highs' and 'lows'. Hering prescribed low, medium and high potencies. In 1865 Hering published his rule on the correct interpretation of symptoms (see 'Homoeopathic Laws, Postulates and Precepts', section 14), which has since become a key-stone in homoeotherapeutics.

The homoeopath Catherine R Coulter, MA, of Washington, DC, USA reports the following delightful anecdote about the venom of the bushmaster snake, (Trigonocephalus) Lachesis mutus, in her richly textured study of selected homoeopathic medicines: 'Hering, the "Father of American Homoeopathy", discovered the remedy in 1828 . . . . He proved it on himself . . . and in the process of dosing himself with ever higher potencies paralysed his left arm for life. To obtain the invaluable mental picture we now possess, Hering with characteristic Germanic thoroughness also used the unattenuated form (tincture) of the poison, making his wife stay by his bed for several days, notebook in hand, taking down every word that he said in his delirium.' [In a footnote she recounts: The 2.13m snake 'is now preserved in the Philadelphia Academy of Natural Sciences, entered in the ledger as item no.7039 and listed as "Lachesis Mutus, collected in Surinam by Dr Hering" '. Then she continues the story as follows:] 'For several decades thereafter, most of the Lachesis in the entire world was made from Hering's single milking of this one snake until in 1868 the homoeopathic pharmacists in America decided that they could not go on diluting the substance ad infinitum and ordered a second bushmaster to be shipped up from Brazil. When the animal arrived, it caused a sensation in the homoeopathic world: "Lachesis II arrives in America!" was the headline in the homoeopathic journals. Photographs of the snake from different angles were displayed, and its habits and physical dimensions were described as lovingly as if it was a film star!'[1]

In the pathogenetic experiment (proving) that Hering conducted on himself with Lachesis he underwent a series of symptoms resembling a muted version of the symptoms one expects from this snake's bite. It is as well to remember that at that time Hering was looking for an improved substitute for the cowpox inoculation that John Hunter's pupil Jenner was then doing, which was viewed as extremely dangerous and very heavy-handed homoeopathy. His experience with the snake venom led him to surmise that the saliva of a rabid dog, or powdered smallpox scabs, or any other disease products, viruses or venoms might be prepared in the new Hahnemannian way to have a failsafe way to treat disease. In this manner Hering unwittingly became the first in the Isopathic movement (see 'Isopathy'), which was to take on great importance within homoeopathy.

Constantin Hering, the eighty-year-old discoverer of what in orthodoxy

---

[1] Coulter, Catherine R. *Portraits of Homoeopathic Medicines: Psychophysical Analyses of Selected Constitutional Types*, Washington, DC: Wehawken Book Company, 1986, pp 301-302.

became the 'heart remedy' nitro-glycerine, died suddenly one evening of a heart attack after returning from a house call to a patient on the 23rd July, 1880.

The major writings of Constantin Hering include:

A Concise View of the Rise and Progress of Homoeopathic Medicine (1833)

The Homoeopathist, or Domestic Physician [2 vols] (1835)

Wirkungen des Schlangengiftes, zum ärztlichen Gebrauche vergleichend zusammengestellt (1837)

Amerikanische Arzneiprüfungen [7 parts] (1852-1857)

Hahnemann's Three Rules Concerning the Rank of Symptoms (1865)

Analytical Therapeutics (1875)

The Guiding Symptoms of Our Materia Medica (1879-1891)

Hering's Rule of Disease Metastasis

See 'Homoeopathic Laws, Postulates and Precepts', section 14).

Hernia Implantation Graft

See 'Surgery'.

Herophilos of Chalcedon (in 3rd century BC)

See 'Philosophical Premise of Homoeopathy'.

Heterostasis

● **The ability to cure or heal when prompted from outside the body by well indicated treatment.**

Describes the capacity of an organism to potentiate its dynamic curative self-correcting process in response to homoeopathic treatment. (See also 'Altered Receptivity in Disease' and 'Homoeosis'.)

Heuristic Thinking

Probabilioristic reasoning that essentially exploits a kind of teleologically controlled trial-and-error by attempting the most promising avenues of solution to a problem first. Heuristic principles may be used in making decisions, in a learning process, in assessing the effect of a set of steps to be taken in a given operation, etc. For example, a chess player cannot work out all the possible effects of all possible moves and so will use probabilioristic reasoning to guide the choice of moves. Heuristic thinking is normally applied whenever a homoeopath is confronted by a polysymptomatic case. (See 'Probabiliorism'.)

Hildegard, Abbess Saint (ca. 1098-1179)

See 'Phytotherapy'.

Hippocrates (ca.460-ca.377 BC)

See 'Philosophical Premise of Homoeopathy'.

Hippocratic Corpus (School of Kos) (from 430 BC)

See 'Humeral Pathology in Homoeopathic Prescribing'.

History of Homoeopathy Before 1900

The summaries presented here have been compiled from five sources:

1 Transactions of the International Homoeopathic Congresses held quinquennially since 1876;
2 Haehl, Richard. *Samuel Hahnemann: His Life and Work,* English translation, 2 vols, London: Homoeopathic Publishing Company, 1922 (958 pages);
3 Hughes, Richard. *The Principles and Practice of Homoeopathy,* London: Leath & Ross, 1902, pp 164-178;
4 Coulter, Harris Livermore. *Divided Legacy: A History of the Schism in Medical Thought,* 3 vols, Washington, DC: Wehawken Book Company, 1973, *Volume III: Science and Ethics in American Medicine: 1800-1914,* pp 101ff.
5 Bradford, Thomas Lindsley. *The Life and Letters of Dr Samuel Hahnemann,* Philadelphia: Boericke and Tafel, 1895 (521 pages). [This last source was drawn on to a lesser extent than the others.]

Elizabeth Danciger has written an absorbing study of the historical roots of homoeopathy entitled *The Emergence of Homoeopathy: Alchemy into Medicine* (London: Century Hutchinson Ltd, 1987, 117 pages). She places this scientific culmination of medical systematics in the context of its antecedent sources, some of them remote, among which she includes Islamic alchemy, the neo-Platonism of Paracelsus, the Hermetic-Cabalistic tradition, the diverse tides of Renaissance science, Cartesianism, the Enlightenment, and other pre-homoeopathic philosophical currents. (This volume was not consulted in the preparation of this entry.)

Germany

Until 1812 Hahnemann was the sole practitioner (and advocate) of homoeopathy which he had conceived by, and first published in, 1796.

After that, from the time he began to lecture at the University of Leipzig, he attracted a band of followers, who learned from him, assisted him in his pathogenetic experiments (provings), and then each went off to practise the method he had learnt. To this group of early disciples belong the names of

Franz, Gross, Hartmann, Herrman, Lehmann, Moritz Müller, Rückert, Stapf and Wislicenus. Johan Ernst Stapf established the first homoeopathic journal, the *Archiv für die homöopathische Heilkunst*, published in 1822 in Naumburg, and fourteen years later Gustav Wilhelm Gross joined him as co-editor, which continued to appear until 1843. In 1832 another journal, the *Allgemeine homöopathische Zeitung* (AHZ), was founded; this excellent scientific publication has survived more than one and a half centuries to the present day. By 1830 the number of homoeopaths had grown so large that a regular exchange between them was needed and the Central-Verein was constituted. Its first meeting was held in Leipzig, with Müller in the chair. A proposal was adopted for establishing a hospital there, which was accomplished in 1832. Ten years later a dispensary was incorporated and it was upgraded to the status of a polyclinic. It flourished as such under the son of Moritz Müller, Clotar (see footnote 1 to 'Constitutional Type'), for thirty-five years, carrying out its homoeopathic functions on a reasonably large scale, also providing a training centre for the periods of housemanship for the freshly qualified homoeopaths of Germany.

There was one distasteful episode, however, which permanently aroused Hahnemann's profoundest suspicions thereafter of all 'half-homoeopaths', as he called those homoeopaths who also used non-homoeopathic medicines in their practice (as, indeed, some do to this day). It involved Dr Karl Wilhelm Fickel, the fourth Director and Chief Physician of the Leipzig Homoeopathic Hospital (Moritz Müller, Franz Hartmann and G A B Schweikert Snr were the three that had preceded him). He was in office for seven months, from 1st January to 10th August 1836. This young man was a convinced allopath, who (as he afterwards confessed) had used the most elaborate deceit to insinuate himself into that position to expose what he called 'the prevailing charlatanry of our time with the prejudicial influence it is exerting on our science.' He began his fraud by writing homoeopathic books, regurgitating previously established knowledge, under the pseudonyms 'Ludwig Heyne', 'C E Herting', 'Julius Theodor Hofbauer' and 'Union of several Homoeopaths'. Under the last of these he published Part I of *A Cyclopaedia of the Whole of Theoretical and Practical Homoeopathy, for the Use of Physicians, Surgeons, etc.* When this volume, despite its obvious deficiencies, was favourably reviewed in the AHZ he felt it safe to introduce himself personally to the publisher, Ludwig Schumann, as the author of this and other books published through him. Schumann, as one of two Inspectors of the Homoeopathic Hospital, wielded some influence with the Board of Directors, and introduced Fickel to the Leipzig circle of trustful homoeopaths. He also later successfully proposed the appointment of Fickel, when the vacancy arose, to the top position at the Hospital. When this most gigantic deception was uncovered, Schumann's publishing house suffered severely. But it was the patients that paid an exorbitant price undeservedly for Fickel's monstrous fanaticism. In a way his perverse experiment worked, although it never seemed to occur to the swindler that this was a most inappropriate method to arrive at the desired judgement. It did plainly prove that under Fickel's homoeopathically incompetent and untrained tenure the normally statistically much more favourable results declined noticeably: of 59 patients that were under his fraudulent 'care' only 13 were cured, while 17 were discharged as uncured and two died; the remaining 22 were shown as 'recovering'. It is astonishing that this deceiver was not discovered sooner. It was Dr Alphons Noack who exposed Dr Fickel's speciousness in homoeopathy. Fickel was taken before the District Court where on the 10th June 1836 his intent to commit this fraud was proven. He had the consummate effrontery to declare 'mundus vult decipi, ergo decipiatur' (the world wishes to be deceived, therefore let it be deceived). Then followed a long silence, until the year 1840, when Fickel published an uninspired lampoon in which he attempted to defend his dishonourable activity with the plea of 'zeal for science and truth'. Extraordinarily, for the next half century some of this untrustworthy man's words, taken out of their true context from that lampoon, were quoted ad nauseam in attacks on homoeopathy by orthodox medicine.

There were two distinct factions in the homoeopathic camp, almost from the beginning. There were those to whom tradition was dear and who wished to depart as little as possible from the established ways, and there were those who wanted to cut themselves entirely adrift from the past and live solely by the prospects of the future: a classical conservative/progressive polarity. A strong representative of the conservative element was Dr Clotar Müller, who was soon reinforced by Griesselich (see 'Isopathy'), Rau, Schron, Trinks, Arnold and Paul Wolf (of Dresden; arch-opponent of high potencies). They had their views expressed for a fifteen year period (from 1834) in the *Hygea* (a journal named after the goddess of health, daughter of Asklepios), ably edited by Dr P W Ludwig Griesselich up to his fatal riding accident. These views were further expounded for about 25 years thereafter by three journals that followed: two inspired by Clotar Müller (*Vierteljahrschrift* and *Internationale Presse*), the other (*Zeitschrift*) by Hirschel. Eventually these three disappeared when their editors died. With a more progressive approach, only the *Zeitschrift des Berliner Vereins homöopathischer Ärzte*, which always was a credit to homoeopathy both in form and substance, endured into this century, alongside the AHZ already mentioned, appearing monthly from 1882.

In the later part of the nineteenth century the names that added lustre to homoeopathy were Bernhard Bëhr (author: *The Science of Therapeutics*, two volumes, English rendering of which was published in Grand Rapids, USA in March, 1869), Ferdinand Bilfinger (the first homoeopathic hospital physician), Professor Buchner (University of Munich – under him was the homoeopathic lectureship and the conduct of the Munich Homoeopathic Hospital), Elb, Elwert, C A Eschenmayer (of Württemberg; Chief Medical Officer in Sulz-on-the-Neckar, later Professor at Tübingen University, retired as homoeopath at Kirchheim), Dietz (Chief Medical Officer in Freudenstadt, Württemberg), Fielitz (in Lauban), Heinrich Goullon Snr (in Weimar), Eduard von Grauvogl (see entry under his name and 'Constitutional Type'), Carl Haubold (of Leipzig; commanded an extraordinary knowledge of remedies; was elevated, for merit in medicine, to the Court of Dessau in the 1850s), Heinigke, Hirschfeld (in Bremen), Hoppe, Kammerer (in Ulm), Kramer (Privy Councillor of Karlsruhe, Baden and Physician in Ordinary to Grand Duke Karl I of Baden), Kurtz (in Dessau), Lohrbacher, Baron von Lotzbeck von Lahr (Privy Councillor of Bruchsal), Veith Meyer, Quaglio (of Bavaria), Professor Rapp (Tübingen University, later Physician-in-Ordinary to Queen Olga of Württemberg), Röhl (in Halberstadt; in 1831 he publicly challenged any allopath to a fight for 1000 Talers), Johann Joseph Roth (who migrated to Paris; see under 'France' below), G A B Schweikert Snr (of Grimma; Director of the Leipzig Homoeopathic Hospital), Sorge, Stüler (in Berlin), Villers and Weber (Physician-in-Ordinary to the King of Hanover). Interestingly, Prof Hugo Schulz and Dr Arndt, after whom the Arndt-Schulz law is named, supported homoeopathy in a very effective manner, from within the University of Greifswald, although they never openly declared themselves. By the turn of the century, besides the hospital in Leipzig, there were similar ones in Berlin, Munich and Stuttgart, and lectureships, similar to the one existing at the University of Leispic, were held at the University of Munich and at the Berlin Dispensary. These had a lasting effect. In 1900 there were about 550 homoeopaths in active practice in Germany.

Austria-Hungary

It was in the Dual Monarchy's south-eastern areas that Hahnemann, the medical student from Vienna, had seen much swamp-fever at the age of 23 (from autumn 1777 to spring 1779 he was in Hermannstadt in Transylvania [now Sibiu in Rumania]), and had there seen Cinchona used regularly. It was this experience in Austria that induced him to write a translator's footnote on William Cullen's *Materia Medica* contradicting the author about the effects of fever remedies; it was this experience that then led him to experiment with Cinchona upon himself and to conclude that the homoeopathic approach could well be the only true scientific approach in medicine. It was also at the University of Vienna that Hahnemann completed his study of medicine, before graduating at Erlangen.

As seems natural, the Dual Monarchy, speaking the same language, was the first to catch the spark of the homoeopathic fire that had been kindled in the Electorate of Saxony and now burned in other German-speaking states. There were a number of cross-border contacts maintained by the Austrians with their north-western neighbours, the Germans. Eduard von Grauvogl, who was a very influential homoeopath, had moved from the Nuremburg area in the Kingdom of Bavaria to the Gastein Valley in Austria. The contagion spread quickly, so much so that as early as 1819 homoeopathy had made sufficient impact to be forbidden by Austrian Imperial Decree, issued (at the behest of orthodox medical men) by Emperor Ferdinand I. This notwithstanding, homoeopathy continued to assert itself so very successfully there, that in 1837 this ineffective Decree had to be rescinded. Those principally responsible for homoeopathy's dissemination were Drs Marenzeller and von Sax, who were the Regimental Physicians of Prince Schwarzenberg; the priest-physician Father Veith; the Duchess of Lucca's Physician-in-Attendance Anton Schmidt; Drs Fleischmann and Wurmb in Vienna; Johann J Hirsch in Prague; Drs Attomyr and Rosenberg in Pressburg (now Bratislava); Dr Schreter and General Korsakoff in Lemberg (now Lvov); Dr A H Gerstel in Bruenn (now Brno); and Drs Balogh and Bakody in Budapest; Dr Bigel, of Galicia, translated Hahnemann's *Chronic Diseases* into French (he was physician to the wife of the Grand Duke Constantin and settled in Warsaw, Poland). Most of these men maintained an active correspondence with Hahnemann during the Paris period. (The outstanding results they achieved with homoeopathy, when it was still an officially illegal form of medical practice, during the Asiatic Cholera epidemic of 1831, when compared with orthodox therapy, are summarized under 'Cholera Epidemics'.)

After homoeopathy had won its freedom, a further crop of able men flocked to it: Arneth, Huber, Mayerhofer, Wachtel, Watzke and Zlatarowich are the most prominent among them. They founded the Austrian Society of Homoeopaths and published a scientific journal (*Österrreichische Zeitschrift*). They conducted, in a most exemplary fashion, substantial series of pathogenetic experiments of new and important remedies and a large number of re-provings. These feature prominently in the standard reference works of homoeopathy's materia medica (viz. *The Encyclopedia of Pure Materia Medica*, 12 volumes, by Timothy Field Allen [1874/79] and *A Cyclopaedia of Drug Pathogenesy*, 4 volumes, by Richard Hughes and Jabez P Dake [1886/91]). One public hospital and two private hospitals in Vienna were placed in the hands of the homoeopaths. Fleischmann's outstanding results at the Gumpendorffer Krankenhaus and Caspar's and Wurmb's thorough clinical studies conducted at the Leopoldstedter Krankenhaus made these men and the institutions famous. Homoeopathy soon spread over the entire Dual Monarchy. Homoeopathic hospitals were established in Linz and several other places, including Budapest, in the University of which two chairs (homoeopathic doctrine and practice) were founded and given to Drs Haussmann and Bakody, respectively. With the exception of Dr Jakob Kafka of Prague (1809-1893), who, in 1872 became editor of the AHZ, the succeeding homoeopaths did not show quite the same degree of dedication as the earlier ones had. During a period of relative stagnation, they lost one of the chairs at Budapest University, but they did maintain all the homoeopathic hospitals. Homoeopathy had a large following in Austria-Hungary, particularly among the upper classes. By the year 1900 the number of homoeopaths had actually decreased a little, from an earlier peak, to around 450.

Italy

Austria transmitted homoeopathy to Italy. An Austro-Hungarian occupation of the Kingdom of Naples took place in 1821, and the commander of the invading troops, Franz Freiherr von Koller, was a devoted disciple of Hahnemann. Soon he sent for his physician, Dr Georg Necker, who had been one of Hahnemann's pupils, to come and settle in the Italian city. In the ensuing four years this homoeopath made a profound impression with the new method. By the time he had to leave, three of the top physicians of Naples had come to adopt homoeopathy. Unfortunately they were in the 50-60 year age group, which meant that they no longer had many decades of active life ahead of them at the time. These men were de Horatiis, Mauro and Romani.

Later Dr Severin also came from Dresden to lend support to the newly implanted homoeopathic science there, and soon afterwards Wahle moved from Leipzig to Rome which became another centre for proselytizing this method in medicine. The three Italian pioneers translated the *Organon of Medicine* and the *Materia Medica Pura;* they founded a journal in 1832 entitled *Effemeridi di Medicina Omiopatica.* Through their successful work they made converts all over Italy.

But this auspicious beginning did not fulfil its promise later. In 1847 Romani passed away and de Horatiis three years later. Mauro was almost a centenarian when he died in 1857. There was only one prominent man, Rubini, among the converts and successors of the original pioneers. He lived into the twentieth century and has earned profound respect by introducing to homoeopathy the valuable remedy Cactus grandiflora, and demonstrating, as Hahnemann had done before him, what astonishing effects Camphora, freely administered, can work in cholera, so prevalent in Naples. Other important names in the development of homoeopathy in Italy are Bonino, Centamori, Dadea, de Rinaldis, Ladelci, Panelli and Pompili, but they could not match the ardour generated earlier. The position in 1900 was: the monthly journal founded and edited by Dr Pompili (*Rivista Omiopatica*) was in existence; the Instituto Omiopatico Italiano, initiated by Dr Bonino, which met annually, periodically published bundled scientific papers (i.e. fasciculi) entitled *L'Omiopatia in Italia,* and it sustained a hospital in Turin and dispensaries in this and other Italian cities. The number of homoeopathic practitioners in Italy, which was once 110, had diminished drastically, to about 55, by 1900.

France

The homoeopathic medical system preceded Hahnemann to France by about half a decade. In 1829 Hahnemann or his medical discovery was scarcely known in France. It was at this time that the Comte des Guidi, a doctor of medicine and of science, and Inspecteur of the University of Lyons, was in Naples. He and the best medical experts to whom he had access had been unsuccessful in arresting the grave illness of his wife, with a putative fatal prognosis. She was to undergo balneotherapy at the Baths of Pozzuoli and he accompanied her. There he was persuaded to consult Dr Romani. Her remarkable cure by his homoeopathic treatment made a profound impression on des Guidi, and induced him to study Hahnemann's scientific medical method. He also attended the practical clinic which Romani, with de Horatiis, was then running at the Ospedale della Trinita. In 1830 he returned to Lyons. He set about actively promoting homoeopathy while devoting himself to its practice. One of his earliest converts was a man of very high social standing, the eminent physician Antonie Petroz. He, in his turn, won many others over: so that, when Hahnemann, after his second marriage in 1835 (to Mlle Marie Melanie d'Hervilly-Gohier), migrated to Paris, he found a body of disciples there, already organized into the Gallic 'Institut Homéopathique', who gave him a ceremonial welcome. In other quarters, the chagrin at Hahnemann's arrival in France may be gauged by the fact that a sizeable group of members of l'Académie de Médicine immediately wrote to M Guizot, Minister of Education and Public Health, urging him to forbid this intruding Saxon founder of homoeopathy to practise his medical method in France. The Minister gave a balanced reply to l'Académie de Médicine, of which the following is a digest:[1]

> Hahnemann is a scholar of considerable merit. Science must remain accessible to, and free for, all. If homoeopathy is a chimera, or a system with no effective application, it will quickly collapse by itself. If, on the other hand, it is a manifestation of scientific progress, it will persist in spite of anyone's preventive measures, and that, gentlemen, is what l'Académie de Médicine should pre-eminently be seen to desire: for l'Académie has the enshrined mission of furthering science and encouraging her discoveries.

With the Minister holding these views it was a mere thirty days after Hahnemann's arrival in France (13th July, 1835) that he was granted the right to practise medicine, by decree. The French homoeopaths already published two high-quality journals, *Les Archives de* . . . and *Le Journal de la Médicine Homéopathique*. When Hahnemann passed away in 1843, he left his medical system firmly established in France – as, indeed, it is to this day – among its early adherents having been the respected professor of the ancient University of Montpellier, Dr d'Amador. Nor was there ever, as in the case of Austria and more particularly Italy, any subsequent stagnation or decline here. In 1847, Tessier, one of the hospital physicians of Paris, became an enthusiastic convert, and maintaining his appointments, took advantage of his position to show, by abundant clinical evidence, the relative superiority of the homoeopathic treatment. He brought with him into the ranks of homoeopathy a number of pupils and friends, who were subsequently among France's brightest luminaries. The important names are Charge, Claude, Cretin, Croserio (for many years president of the Institut Homéopathique, and, together with Jahr, witnessing signatory on Hahnemann's death certificate), August Paul Curie (published *Le Journal de la Médicine Homéopathique* with Leon Simon, Senior; his one son, Dr Paul F Curie, became a friend of England's pioneer, Dr F F H Quin, and moved to England to set up the Homoeopathic Dispensary that became the base for the London Homoeopathic Hospital, he published *Practice of Homoeopathy*, [London: Bailliere, 1838]; August P Curie was the grandfather of Pierre, one of the famous discoverers of Radium), Dessaix, Devasse, Dion

[1] Haehl, op. cit., vol I, p. 231.

(who had been to Hahnemann in Coethen and had been cured of Asiatic Cholera by homoeopathic remedies), Duplat, Espanet, Fredualt, Foissac, Gabalda, Gonnard, Jourdan (who published *Les Archives de la Médicine Homéopathique*), Jousset (who survived into the twentieth century), Meyhoffer (see 'Homoeopathic Laws, Postulates and Precepts', section 5), Milcent, Molins (father and son), Mure (conducted excellent pathogenetic experiments [provings]), Ozanam (who pointed out that, in homoeopathy, potentization was a method analogous to the infinitesimal calculus of mathematics, upon which the atomic theory of chemistry is based, and that dynamization at once illustrates, and harmonizes with, the theory of the radiant state of matter [see 'Radiant State of Matter, Theory of']), Peschier (through whom it spread into Geneva, Switzerland), Rapou, David Roth (translated Hahnemann's *Chronic Diseases* and Jahr's *Handbook* into French), Leon Simon Snr (delivered a series of lectures on the main features of homoeopathy, and these were subsequently published by Bailliere, Paris, 1835: entitled *Leçons de la Médicine Homéopathique*), Jean-Paul Tessier (1811-1862; the Anatomical Society unanimously expelled this prominent man in 1856 for publishing his scientific work in homoeopathic journals: this was after the Society had adopted ethical rules prohibiting members from consulting with 'a hypnotist, a homoeopath, or any other charlatan of this species'), Alphonse Teste (published, in 1854, *The Homoeopathic Materia Medica, Arranged by Systems* [meaning any complex of structures functionally or anatomically related] and later *A Homoeopathic Treatise of Diseases of Children*), and Timbart.

Dr Imbert Gourbeyre, Professor at the Medical School in Clermont-Ferrand later took over d'Amador's place as homoeopathy's senior academic representative; he enriched homoeopathic literature by a number of valuable monographs. In fact, the literary output of French homoeopathy as a whole was, and has remained, prodigious, both in quantity and in quality, especially in view of the relatively small number of homoeopaths in France. This number never exceeded 300 until the turn of the century. The individuals that have shed special lustre on homoeopathy are:

1) The Simons, grandfather, father and son – after Dr Théodore Simon, born 1873 of that family, the Binet-Simon test, for determining an individual's mental age, is named.

2) The Curies – Dr A P Curie's two grandsons, Pierre and Paul-Jean, the famous physicists, were greatly influenced by their family's involvement with homoeopathy's affinity to the theory of the radiant state of matter, which led to their investigation of both magnetism and piezoelectricity in crystals, and the effects of temperature on the disappearance of ferro-magnetism. After Becquerel's discovery, in 1896, of the radioactivity of certain phosphorescent uranium salts, Pierre, together with his wife Marie, in 1898, discovered the radioactive elements polonium and radium. This family's influence on science can hardly be over-estimated. They gave their name to the unit of radioactivity (curie); to a torsion balance for measuring the magnetic properties of nonferro-magnetic materials (curie-balance); to the temperature points, above which,

and below which, ferro-electric materials lose their polarization (upper, or lower, curie points); to the change of ferro-magnetism into paramagnetism at the curie point (Curie-Weiss effect); and to a law of physics that states, 'For paramagnetic substances, the magnetic susceptibility is inversely proportional to the absolute temperature' (Curies' law). Dr Paul F Curie moved to London where he, the close friend of Quin, opened a dispensary, which was to become the base for the (later Royal) London Homoeopathic Hospital.

3) Georg Heinrich Gottlieb Jahr (1800-1875) was born in Thuringia (now part of Germany) to an Austrian (Moravian) family and qualified in Bonn, but spent most of his very productive life in France (see entry under his name). He is second only to Hahnemann himself in promoting the spread and development of homoeopathic principles in Europe during the nineteenth century. Amidst his prolific literary output he produced the first standard Homoeopathic Pharmacopoeia, as well as two other classical reference works: a four-volume Manual of Homoeopathic Medicine, and the Symptom Codex. Jahr pointed out that patient susceptibility to a drug conforms to the rule that the clearer and more positively any finer, or peculiar, or even any characteristic symptoms of a remedy are evident in a patient, the higher the degree of receptivity that may be anticipated to that medicine, and, hence, the higher the potency of choice is likely to be. Jahr further observed that while there is no change in a drug's homoeopathicity as it is taken from crude substance, through the low potencies, beyond Avogadro's number, to the high potencies, there is a subtle change along the way. It is not in the drug's strength or weakness: it is in the development of the drug's peculiarities (away from the commoner symptoms) as it rises in the scale of dynamizations. (See 'Epistemological Assumptions in Homoeopathy', section 5, 'Homoeopathic Laws, Postulates and Precepts', section 10, and 'Therapeutic Science', referring to Jahr's description of symptom concentricity.)

4) Dr Karl Baron von Boenninghausen, the son of Clemens M F Baron von Boenninghausen, requires some mention here too. Not long before Hahnemann's death in Paris (2nd July, 1843), Madame Melanie Hahnemann had adopted, at his special wish also, a little Bavarian girl of five, Sophie Bohrer (born in Munich 10th October, 1838). She grew up to become the French Miss Hahnemann and eventually (July, 1857) married Karl von Boenninghausen. The young couple lived with Madame Hahnemann in her house and he practised from there, with his mother-in-law translating for him as she had done in the past for Hahnemann himself. However, in 1870 they all left for the Boenninghausen estate at Darup near Münster in Germany for reasons set out under the entry for 'Organon'.

In France, at various periods (1836/45, 1863/69, 1880/85 and continuously from 1898 onward) homoeopathy was taught systematically and regularly. The Société Francaise d'Homéopathie was formed. The Parisian homoeopaths spawned two journals of a very high calibre: *L'Art Médical* (founded by Tessier and carried on by Jousset, father and son) and *La Revue Homéopathique Francaise*. As in Germany, the French homoeopaths were divided into two camps: the older school of Parisian homoeopaths revered Hahnemann and disparaged the more progressive school that called Tessier its leader, rather than Hahnemann. Fine distinctions were drawn between the practice and theories of the two groups. For a long time the practitioners of Paris remained divided into these two healthily competing camps, each having its hospital, its society and its journal, with the patients as the ultimate beneficiaries. The two homoeopathic hospitals, the Hôpital Hahnemann and the Hôpital St Jacques, disposed over about 100 beds between them in Paris; at Lyons, founded in 1875, and endowed and flourishing at the turn of the century, was (and still is, as, indeed they all are) the Hôpital St Luc. Dispensaries abounded everywhere in France. Although the number of homoeopaths was only around 300 in 1900, they were dedicated and generally of such excellence, that from here homoeopathy gradually spread to the world's vast francophone area, which was, at that time, home to approximately 100 million people.

United Kingdom
Simultaneously with Comte (Dr) des Guidi, Dr Frederick Foster Hervey Quin (1799-1878), a graduate from Edinburgh in 1820, and said to have been the grandson of the famous Earl-Bishop of Bristol, Frederick August Hervey, attended the clinic at the Ospedale della Trinita run by de Horatiis and Romani. They were there demonstrating this astonishing new scientific form of medicine in vivo. Quin, who was a permanent resident in Naples, practised among a fair-sized English-speaking colony there. He had had his attention already drawn to homoeopathy earlier (1825) by Dr Georg Necker, who then regularly supplied him with reading material on the subject. In the course of time, Quin saw the consistently better results achieved by patients who had turned from orthodoxy to homoeopathy. All this persuaded him that the new system deserved serious investigation. After attending the clinic this favourable impression of homoeopathy was strengthened. So he resolved to go to Leipzig to make an in-depth study of it, but before he set out he studied the system privately at a most prodigious rate, putting in nine hours at a stretch every day, in the hope of fully mastering the new theory and the ramifications of its application. In July 1826 he arrived in Leipzig, having stopped in Venice, Trieste and Vienna on the way. Through the Leipzig lecture course, a visit to Dr Stapf in Naumberg and a ten-day stay with Samuel Hahnemann in Coethen, he became more and more satisfied of homoeopathy's scientific value. Yet the event that can be regarded as the precise time of his conversion to the new method was in 1831, when he was touring through Austria, and was struck down in Tischnowitz, Moravia, by the Asiatic Cholera epidemic then raging across Europe, and was there cured homoeopathically (see 'Cholera Epidemics'). That then completely convinced him of the signal value of Hahnemann's medical method. In 1832 he settled in 19 King Street, London determined to advocate and practise homoeopathy, although he found all opinion ranged against him in his espousal of that system. His success was such that he came under personal attack from medical journals, that called his

qualification into question. The animosity and indignation at the popularity that his successes aroused, reached such a pitch, that he was challenged by notice from the Censors of the Royal College of Physicians with the imputation that he was practising illegally in London or within seven miles (11.26km) of the city limits. He decided to ignore this. He responded to the follow-up notice, the tone of which had become more menacing, simply and with dignity, saying that he had not replied to the first one since he did not think the situation applied to himself. Thereupon the matter was dropped. It was Quin's manner always to return vindictive scorn with good humour. He never had to fear any enquiry, as he was always very scrupulous in giving no grounds for complaint in matters of medical etiquette. His good connexions and high social qualities, combined with his ability, abundant energy and extensive knowledge made him the best advocate of the new medical method in the conservative British environment. He gradually gathered colleagues around him and twelve years later (in 1844), with seven others, he founded the British Homoeopathic Society, which continued to meet monthly throughout the nineteenth century from its formation. It issued its transactions first under the title of the *Annals of the BHS*, then of the *Journal of the BHS*. He enjoyed the presidency of this Society, by being honoured with repeated re-elections, until his death in 1878.

Whereas in Germany and France there was philosophical bipolarity, in the United Kingdom the division was tripartite.

Dr T Fletcher, the Edinburgh Professor of Physiology, took great interest in Hahnemann's method, and proposed a physiological explanation of its rationale, based on the primary and secondary action of drugs (i.e. action and reaction) and the essential opposition between them. This greatly influenced John Drysdale and Russell and so they subsequently spent their early post-graduate years in a study of homoeopathy in Austria and Germany. They, in turn, taught Black, who then went to Paris to study and practise under Hahnemann himself. Drysdale moved to Liverpool, while Black returned to Edinburgh where Russell already practised. In 1844, Sir William Henderson, Professor of General Pathology at the University of Edinburgh, fervently and openly espoused homoeopathy, for which he was later expelled by the Edinburgh College of Physicians, which formalized its blind opiniatry by declaring that 'no physician can, without derogation from his honour and that of his profession, consult with a homoeopath or co-operate with him in any medical act'. His conversion was followed by not a few of his students, the most famous of which was Madden (partner of Richard Hughes in Brighton, where they were physicians to the Homoeopathic Dispensary). This was the beginning of the Scottish School of British homoeopathy, which has consistently produced a good number of outstanding men, notable among whom, during the last century, were Ker, Reith, Ruddock and A C Pope (co-editor of the *Cyclopaedia of Drug Pathogenesy* in four volumes [1886-1891]). They loyally embraced the method of Hahnemann without deviation, representing the conservative wing of the body homoeopathic. John Drysdale, in Liverpool, converted R E Dudgeon. They both later also became co-editors of the said

Cyclopaedia. Chapman and Hilbers were two other important men to follow Drysdale into homoeopathy. The Liverpool School of homoeopathy represented its philosophical 'left wing' at that time. Dr R E Dudgeon, probably their most outstanding man, collected and translated *The Lesser Writings of Samuel Hahnemann* (New York: William Radde, 1852); he edited Richard Hughes' *The Principles and Practice of Homoeopathy* (London: Leath & Ross, 1902); he translated the fifth edition of Hahnemann's *Organon of Medicine* (revised again, in 1893, by him); and published his own *Lectures on Homoeopathy*. Yet this man's most remarkable contribution to scientific medicine was the construction of the original sphygmomanometer (blood-pressure gauge) as it has been used ever since in homoeopathy (and soon thereafter also in most other forms of medical practice), namely the instrument with the usual arm sleeve, inflating bulb and mercury manometer. His original prototype can still be viewed today at the Faculty of Homoeopathy, Great Ormond Street, London WC1. Homoeopathy's third growth centre was London, around Quin. This represented the philosophical centre party, at least until Richard Hughes gained the ascendancy. The names of renown here were: Cameron, Forster, Hamilton, Richard Hughes (1836-1902), Kidd, Leaf and Yeldham. There was also a minister, Thom R Everest, who had visited Hahnemann in both Coethen and Paris. One year before Quin had formed the British Homoeopathic Society, the *British Journal of Homoeopathy* had been founded, and it continued to appear until 1884, with Black, Drysdale, Dudgeon, Hughes (from 1862 to 1884) and Russell in its editorial staff at different times. The *Monthly Homoeopathic Review*, with perhaps a marginally wider appeal, joined the first-named in 1856. Its two most outstanding editors were A C Pope and Dyce Brown. In the second half of the century there additionally appeared the *Homoeopathic World*, a semi-popular monthly, edited successively by men most of whom were prolific, first-rate writers themselves, namely Drs Edwin Harris Ruddock (1822–1865), Shuldham, James Compton Burnett (1840-1901) and John Henry Clarke (1853-1931).

Under persistent pressure from Quin, the London Homoeopathic Hospital was eventually founded in 1850 (this is now the Royal London Homoeopathic Hospital). Dispensaries sprang up wherever homoeopaths settled for practice. There were a number of prominent converts to homoeopathy in the 1850s. Among these were: a former President of the British Medical Association, Dr Horner; a lecturer at St Bartholomew's Teaching Hospital, Dr Conquest; and a Fellow of the Royal Society, Dr Sharp of Rugby, whose 'Tracts' persuaded many others to join homoeopathy. The groundswell was such that by 1857 the number of British homoeopaths was already around 200. During the next 43 years the number of homoeopaths grew further to over 300.

During that time, one of the major advancements in homoeopathic theory to emanate from Great Britain was J Compton Burnett's concept of 'vaccinosis' as a new category of chronic miasma (see that entry). This is the term for an immediate disease reaction known as vaccinia, along with that profound and often long-lasting morbid constitutional state engendered by the vaccine virus implant. J Compton Burnett, who studied medicine in Vienna, but returned to Glasgow, to take his MB there in 1872, was persuaded by the case made for homoeopathy by Richard Hughes in his *Manual of Pharmacodynamics* (Third Edition, London: E Gould & Son, 1876), that he began to apply the principles with enthusiasm straight away. An inspired enthusiasm remained with him throughout his life and he made a number of valuable contributions: one is his monograph on Natrum muriaticum; another was his homoeopathic pioneering work, experimenting with: (a) Bacillinum and Bacillinum testium, nosodes of tuberculosis, long before Robert Koch and his work were ever heard of [the Portuguese homoeopath Martinho, in Rio de Janeiro, Brazil, who died in 1854, was first to have developed the homoeopathically prepared sputum of tuberculous patients as a medicine: he called this nosode Tubercina; Swan took this up from him in 1874 and renamed it Tuberculinum; a few years after that Compton Burnett triturated a portion of a tuberculous lung with lactose and called that Bacillinum, because this preparation would necessarily have to include any associated bacillus; whereas it was only in 1882 that Robert Koch discovered and isolated the tuberculosis bacillus]; (b) Ceanothus americanus, the 'spleen remedy'; (c) Urtica urens in low potency as a 'urinary remedy'; and (d) Thuja occidentalis, establishing it as one of the best remedies for vaccinosis. John Drysdale was another innovator for homoeopathy: he must be credited with the introduction of Pyrogenium (Pyrexin, Sepsin), since he published his original work *On Pyrexin, or Pyrogen, as a Therapeutic Agent* (London: Bailliere, Tyndale & Cox, 1880).

During the 1890s the London Homoeopathic Hospital was rebuilt on its foundations, offering a capacity of 100 beds. It published an annual volume of reports, effectively recording the homoeopathic experience gained there. By 1900 there were other homoeopathic hospitals in many parts of the United Kingdom: in Liverpool, Plymouth, Bath, Birmingham, Bromley and St Leonards, all of whom were doing very successful work. During the twelve year period from 1852 there were sporadic courses of lectures at the London Homoeopathic Hospital, given by Quin, Leadham, Russell and others. Then in 1877, under the auspices of the British Homoeopathic Society, but largely at the instance of Dr Bayes, and his sustained effort over a period of three years, the London School of Homoeopathy was established. From inception its Chair of Practice was filled by Dyce Brown, and that of Materia Medica successively by Richard Hughes, A C Pope, J Compton Burnett and J H Clarke. After some eight years of existence it was incorporated into the Hospital that housed it, which since then had always added 'and School of Medicine' to its title (in the twentieth century this became 'The Faculty of Homoeopathy'). These courses of instruction have been continued ever since (in the twentieth century the most influential British homoeopath from the last was honoured annually by the holding of the Richard Hughes Memorial Lectures at the Faculty).

Hughes' philosophical approach to homoeopathy, which can be said to have carried some of the seeds of homoeopathy's decline within it, may be condensed as follows:

1 Homoeopathy, Hughes said, is a working method, framed by scientific processes, reached by inductive generalization, and tested by deductive verification, but it is, itself, not a law of science, it is a methodology. Hughes in all his concise written exposition and brilliant vindications attempted to confine himself to verifiable facts.

2 He reverted to the non-homoeopathic idea that the 'disease' was an objective entity, quasi-real, composed of customary, unastonishing symptoms that a patient had in common with all other cases of the same 'disease', and that these symptoms, in practice, would generally have precedence over any unique symptoms that the patient may manifest.

3 Hughes preferred to prescribe homoeopathic remedies in potencies below 12CH (Avogadro's number).

4 He insisted that the pathology, the site of action of the disease, the organs affected, all causative factors, and the evolution of symptoms during an illness, need always be taken into account on prescribing the most homoeopathically suitable remedy (see 'Diagnosis', where this is discussed in more detail).

5 At a time when a formidable band of prominent British homoeopaths, namely Fletcher, Dudgeon, Drysdale, Bayes, Sharp, Dyce Brown, Reith, Pope, Herbert Nankivell and Percy Wilde (the last two through the *Monthly Homoeopathic Review*), all put about the concept of 'antipraxy' as a fact to be generally accepted, Hughes, on his own, in open debate successfully challenged this as erroneous, and demonstrated it as being quite untenable. (Explanatory note: These men proceeded from the premise that all medicines have two actions in health, according to the dose in which they are given – the effect of a large dose being the direct opposite to that of a small one. The dividing line is a shifting one, according to the drug used, and the individual experimented upon; but in all cases it is there, and constitutes a real point of transition between the two reverse actions. This supposed general fact they denominated 'antipraxy'. They went further by stating that when, in disease, a drug is given in small doses, which in large doses had caused a similar condition to that in evidence, in fact, an agent was being administered whose influence is in direct opposition to the morbid state. Therefore, Hahnemann's method could only depend on the size of the dose and the pharmacodynamic process would, when using the sufficiently small dose, accurately, have to be referred to as 'antipathic', and the name 'homoeopathy' ought, therefore, to be reserved for the principle of selection alone.) The seemingly logical explanation offered by these men in scientific publications appeared to commend homoeopathy to many orthodox medical practitioners who had hitherto been hostile to it. Hughes, being mindful of this politically useful fact, was magnanimous in his victory, stating, 'If the explanation now current commend our method to those who have hitherto refused it, render it in their eyes reasonable and admissible, what is it if to some amongst us, as to myself, it seems to give an inadequate account of the facts? We must say so, but we may be wrong; and in the

meantime the facts are true, the method no less precious though the theory affixed to it be disputable. I only plead that the method be not so bound up with its explanation that the two must stand or fall together; and then I am quite content to allow the latter as plausible enough for provisional acceptance. If our liberty to practise apparent Homoeopathy be acknowledged, we care little about it being considered real Antipathy: and if, because so considering it, our colleagues of the other school will join us in following it, our content will merge into gladness'.[1]

6 Hughes was motivated in all the above by his publicly declared aspiration to achieve acceptance of the homoeopathic principle by orthodox medicine, thus hoping to end the medical ostracism of homoeopaths. In pursuit of his goal, he unfortunately seemed to adopt almost a radical 'either-or' position with regard to the therapeutic employment of either the high or the low potencies by homoeopaths, on a number of occasions scathingly disparaging the former.

From the 1860s to his sudden death in Dublin in 1902 Richard Hughes, MD, LRCP, MRCS ranked head and shoulders above all others in the international arena of medical politics within the English-speaking world, including the USA. He effectively became the leader, in that entire area, of the 'enlightened' (progressive) homoeopaths who wished to de-mystify homoeopathy, to prescribe low potencies, to conduct experimental work along orthodox lines, to use standard disease nomenclature, to cleanse the materia medica of doubtful pathogenetic semiology, to approximate medical education to the orthodox model of the time (by placing greater emphasis on chemistry and pathology), and hoped for some way to procure a position of homoeopathy's acceptance within orthodox medicine. To the pure Hahnemannians, who reacted by retreating into ever higher potency prescribing and spurning the crude 'lows', the homoeopaths led by Hughes appeared as 'hybrids motivated, not by scientific idealism, but by scurrilous indolence'. The upshot was that almost everyone felt obliged to take sides, so that there were soon only 'highs' or 'lows' about. From then on very few homoeopaths (John Henry Clarke was one) had the courage to make use of the whole gamut of potencies. The international standard-bearer and effective polemicist (from the USA) for the Hahnemannian homoeopaths, ranged against Hughes, was Adolph Lippe (more accurately, Adolph Graf zur Lippe-Weissenfeld, a Silesian count who had studied law as well as medicine), but he passed away too soon, in 1888. After Lippe there was no effective international political leader for the conservative wing of homoeopathy. James Tyler Kent (1849-1916), himself a homoeopathic convert from the Eclectic School of Medicine, encouraged high potency prescribing very much in his teaching, and he certainly later exerted a long-term influence, having taught some of the greatest Hahnemannians (Pierre Schmidt, Sir John Weir, Douglas Borland, Margaret Tyler, for

---

[1] Hughes, Richard. *The Principles & Practice of Homoeopathy*. London: Leath & Ross, 1902, p 162.

instance), but he wielded no real cohesive influence yet on the conservatives as an international group, to counter that of Hughes. This doctrinal split caused political and organizational vulnerability, which, after the death of Hughes was fully exploited by the Englishman, Dr George H Simmons (1852-1924), the ex-homoeopath who was to become president from 1899 to 1910 of the American Medical Association (see entry under his name). In fact, it is probable that Hughes himself conditioned his followers into a state of submissiveness to the process of assimilation and identity-loss, exploited by the manoeuvres of Simmons, that overtook the progressive homoeopathic faction (the 'lows'), beginning soon after the demise of Hughes in 1902, and coinciding with the advent of crass materialism in science (see 'Eclipse of Homoeopathy (1920-1965)'; but the ultimate cause for the process of assimilation and identity-loss is analysed under 'Hempel, Charles Julius (1811-1879)').

United States of America

Dr Hans Burch Gram (1786-1840), born of Danish parents in Boston, took his medical degree in Copenhagen, where he practised for a while and was converted to the new method of homoeopathy. He practised only this upon his return to New York in 1825, where, on account of his Masonic activities and his presidency of the Medical and Philosophical Society of New York, he soon persuaded a number of others to adopt homoeopathy. The best known of these are Channing, Curtis, Gray and Hull. A few years later Dr Heinrich Detwiller became a homoeopath, quite independently of Gram, through private study and extensive correspondence with German and Austrian homoeopaths. He was a Swiss immigrant, who had graduated from Freiburg and settled in 1817 in Allentown, Pennsylvania, among the German-American population there. Detwiller was joined, in 1833, by the German homoeopath Constantin Hering (1800-1880), the father of US homoeopathy. Hering was possessed of a vigorous and original mind, a vast store of knowledge, and an indefatigable energy (refer to 'Hering, Constantin (1800-1880)' and 'Isopathy'). Under his powerful influence Philadelphia became the second, but more important, centre for homoeopathy in the USA: together with Wesselhöft, he founded a medical college, the North American Academy for Homoeopathic Healing, to teach the new medical system; provings (pathogenetic experiments) were conducted to supply materials for the practise of homoeopathy; from here, in the 1830s, the new medical method was carried both east and west by German homoeopath-immigrants and German-speaking graduates of the Academy.

Observing the comparative results of orthodox and homoeopathic treatment of the Asiatic Cholera during the 1832 epidemic, swelled the ranks of the homoeopaths by about twenty percent by converts from orthodoxy. In Gram's area of influence, the Homoeopathic Physicians' Society of New York was constituted in 1834. Soon similar organizations sprang up in many other parts of the USA. The increasing number of converts to homoeopathy made it necessary to establish an official body to monitor non-homoeopathic medical qualifications, and ethics in homoeopathic practice, quite apart from the requirement to function as a clearing house for homoeopathic pharmaceutical information. Thus, at the invitation of the Homoeopathic Physicians' Society of NY, a convention was held in the NY Lyceum of Natural History, and on 10th April, 1844 the American Institute of Homoeopathy was founded, to which Constantin Hering was elected as the first president.

Orthodox physicians, who had no such regulatory body, began to be alarmed at the rate of expansion shown by homoeopathy in the liberal climate of the USA. Dr Nathan Smith Davis began to spearhead the agitation for the formation of an equivalent umbrella organization for orthodox practitioners in the US. His efforts culminated in the first National Medical Convention ever to be held, in New York during May, 1846, which then founded the American Medical Association as orthodoxy's defensive response to try to neutralize homoeopathy's advantage gained through having set up the American Institute of Homoeopathy two years earlier. It was the existence of precisely such governing bodies in the European countries, exercising relentless censorship and implementing draconian rules, that impeded the free growth of homoeopathy to some considerable extent there. The late formation of the American Medical Association meant that homoeopathy had had a head start in a liberal, competitive climate. The results speak for themselves. The famous names among the US homoeopaths, about each of whom many chapters could be written, are: Timothy Field Allen (author of the 12-volume *Encyclopedia of Pure Materia Medica*), Jabez P Dake (US leader of the 'lows', and has the 'exclusion synopsis' attributed to himself), Carroll Dunham (a prominent 'high', presided over the World Homoeopathic Convention, 1876 in Philadelphia, during the US Centennial Exposition), Ernest A Farrington, Bernard Fincke (a 'high', introduced the CM potency, originator of the concept of 'homeosis'), Flagg, Gardiner, Gregg, Arthur Hill Grimmer, William Jefferson Guernsey (Professor of Obstetrics, Pennsylvania, and a 'high' proponent), Edwin M Hale (Professor of Materia Medica, Chicago; introduced very important new drugs to homoeopathy, including Gelsemium, Hydrastis, Iberis, Lycopus, Passiflora, Phytolacca and Plantago), Helmuth (Leader of the surgeons in the US who used homoeopathic drugs, and who broke with the tradition of heroic surgery, under which surgeons vied with each other, as it were, as to who was able to remove the most from a patient without killing him or her), Carl Julius Hempel (very prominent among the 'lows', translator of Dr Bernhard Bähr's *The Science of Therapeutics, According to the Principles of Homoeopathy*), William H Holcombe (son of an orthodox practitioner, and an orthodox graduate who converted and later became a president of the American Institute of Homoeopathy), John Jeanes together with Hering and Williamson, founded the Hahnemann Medical College in Philadelphia in 1848), James Tyler Kent (the last leader of the 'Highs' in the nineteenth century), Kitchen, Lord, Ludlam, McClelland, Neidhard, Carl Gottlieb Raue (Professor of Special Pathology and Diagnostics, Hahnemann Medical College of Philadelphia, a protagonist of the 'lows'), Reichel, Small, David Smith, Swann (made prophylactic treatment of rabies first possible through homoeopathy with the nosode Lyssin, described the first proving of Lueticum in 1880, developed Anthracinum), Talbot, Temple, Bruno von Gersdorff (son of Heinrich August von Gersdorff, the lawyer who had come with Blücher in the Austrian Light Horse Regiment to the Battle of Leipzig where he received several severe head wounds, and later became a close friend of Hahnemann and one of the original band of 'provers'), Wesselhöft (together with Hering, co-founder of the North American Academy), and Williamson (together with Hering and John Jeanes, founded the Hahnemann Medical College in Philadelphia in 1848).

By 1900 the Hahnemann College in Philadelphia, with the hospitals attached and its extensive polyclinic, had become the most important homoeopathic educational institution in the world. The German, Richard Haehl, MD reported: [1]

'Its buildings are valued at several million dollars. The College and hospitals are modern in their equipment and abundantly provided with materials of instruction, laboratories, apparatus, etc. The libraries comprise approximately 20 000 volumes and homoeopathic literature in every language is completely represented. For practical training the Hahnemann College offers advantages which are scarcely to be equalled in any European University. More than seventy professors and lecturers are at the disposal of approximately 300 students of medicine. The large number of cases in the hospitals and the polyclinic, where more than 50 000 patients and 6000 accident cases are treated every year, affords the professors abundant material for their clinical instruction. Besides the General Hospital containing about 200 beds, the College possesses a special institution for midwifery, directly attached to it, and allowing the students ample opportunity for observing obstetrical cases. In addition numerous confinements are attended amongst the poor people in the town and these also serve for instruction. . . . In the introduction of four and five years' courses it preceded all others with its good example' [at a time when some orthodox medical colleges in the USA had only just been coerced into introducing a compulsory three years]. 'By the practical training of more than 3500 homoeopathic physicians the Hahnemann College has contributed more to the development and propagation of homoeopathy than any other instructional institution in the world.'

By 1900 the number of homoeopaths was estimated to have been close to 15 000, although only very few of these (1958 then, and 2727 a decade later) were members of the American Institute of Homoeopathy. Most homoeopaths were in thriving general practice, where virtually each one had a large patient following, as opposed to the Orthodox Medical practitioners, who were left with too few patients to support them adequately, largely due to the inroads of the 'proprietary medicine' manufacturers. That meant the Orthodox practitioners felt threatened and they pressed the AMA to find a solution for them, while the homoeopaths were financially secure and therefore cared little what the AIH did or planned to do. The homoeopaths falsely regarded their

[1] Haehl, Richard. *Samuel Hahnemann: His Life and Works*. 2 vol. London: Homoeopathic Publishing Company, 1922, vol I, pp 432-433.

position as impregnable. At that time the homoeopaths of the USA controlled 112 hospitals of various sizes (offering 11 421 beds between them), 34 sanatoria and nursing homes, a large number of maternity homes, 62 orphanages and geriatric homes, 149 dispensaries, and 16 mental hospitals. Some of the country's best endowed special hospitals, such as the New York Ophthalmic Hospital (actually an eye and ear hospital) were in homoeopathic hands. Homoeopathic education of the highest calibre was being taught at 22 medical schools throughout the USA, either on their own account or under the aegis of a University to which they were affiliated (turning out around 500 graduates annually). It seems hard to believe that about thirty-five years later all that in the USA had almost completely disappeared (see 'Eclipse of Homoeopathy' and 'Simmons, George H (1852-1924)').

Brief historical summary up to, and homoeopathy's state as at 1900, in some other countries which are of lesser significance to the development of homoeopathy in the nineteenth century:

India:
- Begun 1867 by Dr Mahedra Lal Sircar;
- number of homoeopaths: 60 qualified and many semi-qualified practitioners;
- three professional journals;
- many homoeopathic pharmacies prescribing over-the-counter.
- This country was yet to become important to homoeopathy in the twentieth century.

Canada:
- Begun 1846 by Dr A Lancaster;
- five homoeopaths had seats on Ontario Medical Council, the licensing and governing body of the profession;
- sections of hospitals in Toronto and London, Ontario under homoeopathic control, and one fully homoeopathic hospital in Montreal (25 beds);
- number of homoeopaths 110.

Australasia:
- Introduced to both Melbourne and Sydney in 1851;
- Melbourne had homoeopathic hospital since 1869 (60 beds), which did outstandingly in Typhoid outbreak;
- hence received large support and Government grants to construct new building;
- sections of hospitals in Bathurst and Adelaide under homoeopathic control;
- and fully homoeopathic clinics in Launceston and Hobart, Tasmania.
- Introduced in 1853 to New Zealand, but had only progressed relatively slowly.

South Africa:
- In the area composed of the Cape Colony, the Natal Colony, the Orange

Free State Republic, the Zuid-Afrikaansche Republiek, the British South Africa Company's land (named Rhodesia by 1895 proclamation), and the British Protectorates of Swaziland, Basutoland and Bechuanaland: In 1900, in that entire area it was the Afrikaans- speaking Boers (at that time the two Republics were at war with Great Britain [1899-1902]) who used and supported homoeopathy almost exclusively, next to simple home remedies;

● amongst the English-speakers there was only one homoeopath, namely Dr Kitchen in Cape Town.

Portugal:
● In 1838 the Professor of Medicine of the Medical School of Lisbon requested permission for practical experiments in the homoeopathic method; this was denied;
● in 1839 he was elected president of Lisbon's Society for Medical Sciences, on whom he prevailed to have Hahnemann elected an honorary member (1st class) [this must have been the only distinction from an orthodox medical source ever bestowed on him], thereby granting the automatic right to have his scientific work examined experimentally there;
● from then on homoeopathy grew;
● Brazilian homoeopaths came to settle in Portugal also adding to the number;
● in the 1850s it acquired a solid footing by support from the Duke of Saldanha, the foremost statesman of Portugal;
● number was 96 in 1900
● homoeopaths ran a ward in Oporto General Hospital, and had a Homoeopathic Children's Hospital.

Switzerland:
● Introduced largely by Dr Charles Caspard Peschier in 1832 who became the secretary of the Homoeopathic Society then formed in Geneva;
● Dufresne and Longchamp, who had travelled extensively in South America, were ardent supporters of homoeopathy;
● by 1900, 33 practitioners with Dr Bruckner at their head, ran one small hospital in Basle.

Scandinavia:
● No proper organization; total number of homoeopaths in Iceland, Denmark, Sweden, Greenland, Finland and Norway was estimated at 30 by 1900;
● the prominent names were Drs Hagemark, Grundal and Liedbeck.

Netherlands:
● In 1827, 3rd edition of the *Organon* was translated by Prof S Bleekrode;
● other prominent homoeopaths were Drs A J Gruber, F W O Kallenbach, J P E Schoenfeld, S J van Rooyen, von dem Borne, and N A J Voorhoeve;
● in fact, merely six men were listed by Dr von dem Borne at the 1896 Congress as having been the only homoeopaths practising at that time in

a country, that before 1914, was very receptive to cultural changes originating in neighbouring Germany, so that the discovery of the homoeopathic method was very widely known to patients;

● he had reported: 'There are regions, as in the province of Zeeland, where the totality of the inhabitants are partisans of our method of treatment, where physicians of the other school cannot earn their livelihood, and where yet it is quite impossible to find a homoeopathic doctor.' Dr von dem Borne was the first and only representative of the Netherlands ever to attend any of the quinquenniel Homoeopathic Congresses. Yet he gave no details, names, dates or events relating to homoeopathy's past in the Netherlands, that might have explained why that country's development of homoeopathy was at variance with that in other countries. Certainly, the records seem to show that the delegates were not made aware of what is known as Thorbeke's Law, which dates from 1865, whereby the Dutch Parliament made it totally illegal for anyone, regardless of qualification, to practise any of the empirical medical methods that were not specifically approved by the orthodox medical authorities of the Netherlands. This was specifically aimed at homoeopathy.

● Noteworthy was only one speech to the Dutch Parliament in the debate on Thorbeke's Law in 1865, by Major Revius, M.P., who is on record as having said: 'The monopoly of medicine is evidently designed to protect the medically entrenched from charlatanism and quackery. . . . Whereas the law grants to each citizen the freedom to exercise his chosen form of religious worship, to decide upon the upbringing and education of his children, to expose himself even to the dangers of employment in a munitions factory or a power plant, he may not entrust his ailing body to the physician of his choice, he may not rely on any curative method not previously approved by the monopolists, without becoming an accessory to an infraction of the law. This state of affairs, this legal anomaly, flies in the face of all reason, right and fairmindedness.'

Russian Empire:

● Here distinguished men promoted the spread of homoeopathy: State Councillor Steegemann, Admiral Mordwinoff, Chamberlain Lwoff, Margrave Skuratoff, General von Korsakoff (after whom one of the potentization methods is named), Drs Trinius [Hahnemann's nephew], Ochs and Adams in St Petersburg (now Leningrad), [the great nephew of Hahnemann] Hermann, Markus and Goldenburg in Moscow, Sahmen in Dorpat (now Tartu in Estonian Rep.), Bojanus, Brasol, Deriker, Villers Snr, Dahl and Dittmann;

● twelve Russian Homoeopathic Societies spread throughout the Empire, most supporting dispensaries and pharmacies;

● a hospital was built in St Petersburg with 50 beds, opened in 1898, which enjoyed enthusiastic public support.

Poland:

● Apart from Dr Bigel (mentioned under Austria-Hungary), Dr Wieniawski attained eminence, but the most important was Dr Drzwiecki, Professor at the Hospital of the Holy Ghost in Warsaw;

● very strong lay support.

Belgium:

● The Titular Surgeon of Alost, De Moor, introduced homoeopathy to the Civil Hospital of that city in 1829, his son Dr Charles De Moor continued to do so;

● in Brussels Carlier and Varlez propagated it and founded an active society and dispensary eventually in 1837;

● in Antwerp the Department of Welfare placed one of its dispensaries under homoeopathic control;

● by 1900 there were about 100 practising homoeopaths, plus some specialists (surgeons, oculists, dentists, etc);

● famous names include Bernmard, Gaillard, Gaudy, Martiny, Mersch, Schepens and Stockman;

● two journals existed: *Revue Homéopathique Belge* (still extant) and *L'Homéopathie Militante*, edited by the intrepid controversialist Gaillard, whose energy and erudition were quite astonishing.

Spain:

● In 1833 Drs Hurtado, Pinciano and Querol began translating homoeopathic publications;

● in 1844 the homoeopath Nunez who had been the founder of the Hahnemannian Society of Madrid and the prime mover behind its periodical *Boletin* (later *El Criterio Medico*) was knighted by Queen Isabella and appointed her personal physician;

● he established the St Joseph's Homoeopathic Teaching Hospital, opened in 1878 containing 50 beds;

● one year later Nunez, who had been to Spain what Quin had been to England, passed away, leaving all his not inconsiderable fortune to that Teaching Hospital;

● metropolitan Spain had around 350 homoeopaths by 1900;

● Barcelona had its own flourishing society which published the *Revista Homoeopatica*.

Jamaica:

● Drs Reinke and Navarro were two prominent homoeopaths tending to a fast growing group of patients.

Brazil:

● Though still strongly linked to Portugal homoeopathy took root there sooner than in the former mother country;

● a student from Leipzig University made the method a subject of his graduation thesis and persuaded Dr Estrado of Brazil to study and practise

homoeopathy, so as to be able to compare the results obtained with the two treatment methods by the same practitioner on the same uninitiated patient community;
- Estrado was delighted with the vast improvement in his patients and homoeopathy made rapid progress from 1837;
- by 1900 there were about 100 practitioners, organized in two societies.

Cuba, Puerto Rico, the Philippine, Balearic and Canary Isles, Ifni, Rio Muni, Rio de Oro, Brunei, Ladrones, Haiti, Santo Domingo, Caroline Island, Oran and Spanish Morocco:
- By 1865 the colonies and (ex-)dependencies of Spain already recorded as many as 359 homoeopaths;
- a rapid growth was evident but relevant information was unobtainable for later than about 1880.

Hispanic (mainland) America:
(The Spanish-American War of 1898 resulted in the loss of the last Spanish colonies and some upheaval in the social order.) Concrete information exists for two of the republics independent of Spain only: Mexico and Uruguay;

- in 1853 Navarette, a homoeopath from Havana, Cuba and Cornellas from Spain settled in Mexico; homoeopathy has rapidly expanded since;
- two societies were founded in the late 1860s, which then still flourished, and as at 1900 three journals had been published, one of which, *La Homoeopatia*, was known to be doing extremely well.
- In Montevideo, Uruguay, it is known that there were seven homoeopaths in 1900.

Hohenheim, Theophrastus Bombastus von (1494-1541)

Paracelsus (see 'Philosophical Premise of Homoeopathy' and 'Spagyric').

Holism

Also Wholism. The doctrine, consonant with homoeopathic science, that wholes are more than the sum of their parts. Contrasted with Atomism.

Home Remedy Kits

Most larger homoeopathic dispensing pharmacies throughout the world are able to supply these, complete with rudimentary instructions – perhaps on printed sheets, on demand at relatively low cost. Homoeopathy is well suited for domestic self-help treatment, although the basis for remedy self-administration rests on the following generalizing assumption: In certain classes of disease condition the human response is relatively stereotyped, or even when this is diverse, a particular sub-type turns out to be rather common, which allows a particular homoeopathic remedy to be most frequently indicated and, therefore, very often astonishingly effective. These kits contain up to forty remedies for various minor acute situations, such as: injuries, fevers, diarrhoea, vomiting, frights, shocks, burns, non-union of fractures, rashes, coughs, sprains, flatulent gastro-enteritis, laryngitis, influenza, stomach troubles, depression, colics, wounds, boils, nose-bleeds, hayfever, cystitis, earache, stings, etc.

One of the most successful homoeopathic textbooks, originally published in 1853, which in 1981 was in its twentieth edition, is a vade-mecum for the domestic practice:

Der homöopathische Haus- und Familienarzt by Clotar Müller (Heidelberg: Karl F Haug Verlag, 1981, 328 pages)

Three useful English-language guides to assist in the choice of remedy and auxiliary treatment are:

Everybody's Guide to Homoeopathic Medicines by Dana Ullman, co-authored with Stephen Cummings; this was awarded the Medical Self-Care Book Award and has been translated into five languages from the original English

The Complete Homoeopathy Handbook: A Guide to Everyday Health Care by Miranda Castro (Basingstoke and London: Macmillan London Limited, 1990, 270 pages)

The Family Guide to Homoeopathy by Andrew Lockie (London: Elm Tree Books of the Penguin Group, 1989, 402 pages)

Two smaller, handy guides to medicines for common ailments are:

Homoeopathic Medicine by Trevor Smith (Wellingborough: Thorsons Publishing Group, 1982, 256 pages); and

Homoeopathic Medicine at Home by Maesimund B Panos and Jane Heimlich (London: 'Corgi Books' of Transworld Publishers Ltd, 1986, 304 pages).

Homoeocyte

Lymphocyte; white blood cell formed in lymphoid tissue throughout the body, i.e. spleen, lymph nodes, Peyer's patches, thymus, diverse tonsils, and occasionally in the bone marrow. Homoeocytes were first described by William Hewson in a series of papers published in the 1770s. They are the major cellular elements involved in an organism's defensive immune response. Homoeocytes contain several enzymes (lipolytic, oxidative, proteolytic and non-specific esterases); they synthesize plasma protein (alpha-, beta-, and gamma-globulins [antibodies]), complement compounds, anti-haemophilic factors; they can release different lymphokines when required, and a host of other substances; the bursa-derived homoeocytes (B-lymphocytes) can transform into plasma cells after encounter with antigens and both synthesize and secrete antibodies; receptor molecules are at the cell surface of both the B-homoeocytes as well as the thymus-dependent homoeocytes (T-lymphocytes). Immunologists, in sympathy with the homoeopathic approach to medical science, have long suspected that it is the homoeocyte itself, or something in its immediate proximity, that acts as receptor for the homoeopathic curative stimulus. Hence some of their experimental work has been concentrated on this area of homoeopathic research. (See 'Experimental Evidence' and 'Opsonic Index'.)

Homoeomorphous

Of like appearance (shape, size and other outward characteristics), but not necessarily of the same composition.

Homoeopathic Ethnopharmacology

Homoeopathy examines medicines that are in use in the various traditional cultures throughout the world. These are of scientific interest both anthropologically and medicinally. Homoeopathy regards all ethnopharmacological studies as valuable sources of primary 'clinical' information that may lead on to standard placebo-controlled Hahnemannian pathogenetic experimentation (provings), followed by incorporation into the materia medica. As an example, the homoeopath Dr Willmar Schwabe studied Pio Carrera's 'Brazilian Phytotherapy' and was struck by Lophophytum leandri (a.k.a. Flor de Piedra) which grows in the tropical forests of Paraguay, Argentina and Brazil, and is used by the natives in rickets, epilepsy, for hepatic and gastric disturbances. He brought it back to the FRG, where in 1964, together with homoeopaths W Herz and E Freiwald, he conducted an extensive symptomatological proving on sixteen provers using 2DH, 3DH, 4DH and 6DH potencies. The English homoeopath Dr J R Raeside undertook another three provings during 1966/7 with potencies 6DH, 6CH and 12CH. During 1967 the French homoeopath Dr Juliette Fourmon undertook yet another thorough proving.

Another example is Ayurvedic medicine (refer to that entry), which has yielded quite a number of its ethnopharmaca to homoeopathy in the normal way.

Two ethnopharmacological compendia that have recently attracted the attention of French homoeopaths and homoeopathic laboratories, for instance, are:

1) Koenen, Eberhard von (homoeopath of Windhoek, Namibia), *Heil- und Giftpflanzen in Suedwestafrika,* Windhoek: Akademischer Verlag, 1977 (272 pages); and

2) Watt, John Mitchell, ED, MB, ChB, FRCPE, and Maria Gerdina Breyer-Brandwijk, DSc, PhilDoct, Apotheker, *The Medicinal and Poisonous Plants of Southern and Eastern Africa: Being an Account of Their Medicinal and Other uses, Chemical Composition, Pharmacological Effects and Toxicology in Man and Animal,* Edinburgh and London: E & S Livingstone Ltd, 1962 (1457 pages).

(See 'Anthropology and Homoeopathy'.)

Homoeopathic Laws, Postulates and Precepts

The test of validity of any law of nature is twofold (see 'Laws of Nature'):

- I) that it is capable of connecting and explaining, without exception, two series of natural phenomena and
- II) that it is in harmony with other known laws, through which relevant phenomena can be comprehended.

Homoeopathy connects the following two series of natural phenomena:

- A) Drugs, when intentionally tested on healthy human subjects, or through accidental exposure by either animals or humans, produce a demonstrable symptom-complex often accompanied by pathological changes; to
- B) Human subjects, as do animals, in a diseased state, produce a demonstrable symptom-complex, often accompanied by pathological changes.

Homoeopathy explains the connexion between these two phenomena through the constant relationship existing between them, evident by virtue of the fact that the best curative effect is induced in a diseased patient by the drug whose artificial disease symptom-similarity is the greatest (see 'Epistemological Assumptions in Homoeopathy', section 1). This biological law, resembling a law of physics, is not in conflict with any known law and is the foundation of all homoeopathic practice (see also 'Laws of Nature' and 'Philosophical Premise of Homoeopathy'). It is known as:

1) The biological law of similars (equivalents), usually expressed by the formula **Similia similibus curentur,** meaning 'Let Similars be treated (cured) by Similars'.

From this all other therapeutic and pharmacodynamic laws, postulates and precepts derive. It was Christian Friedrich Samuel Hahnemann's perceptive genius that discovered the existing parallelism of action between the toxicological and pathogenetic effects of a substance, on the one hand, and its corresponding, replicative therapeutic powers, on the other. Which immediately leads on to homoeopathy's corollary of Newton's third law of motion:

2) The law of bioenergetic drug action, expressed as: **Action and reaction are equal and opposite** (see also 'Antidote' and 'Philosophical Premise of Homoeopathy').

Then there is the aspect of accuracy of prescription relative to the speed of cure, as there is an established direct relationship between homoeopathic congruity, drug to disease, and the speed of cure. This has been summarized under:

3) The law of homoeopathic efficacy, expressed as: **The more accurate the parallelism between the experimental and the actual disease, the greater the therapeutic effectiveness.**

In his *Lehrbuch der Homöopathie* (Nuremberg, 1865) Eduard von Grauvogl, having regard to these three laws, viewed jointly in their combined effects, expressed the opinion, that the curative dose, like the remedy itself, must be similar in quantity and quality to the dose of the morbific agent which caused the disease. But since quantity and quality (i.e. appropriateness of dosage and similarity) are mutually complementary, he concluded, that 'for the purpose of therapeutics, the right dose must and can be nothing else than that amount of the indicated quality (remedy) which is equal to the amount of the force of the cause of disease'. In fact, he mused, a quantity or dose of morbid substance so small as to be imperceptible in any way except by its effects, might set up an action of such violent character in quality as to lead one to suppose that the quantity must have been great. Succinctly put, von Grauvogl found that an optimal matching of any drug symptom-complex to a disease symptom-complex would vouchsafe therapeutic precision, but that the drug action could only effectively counterpoise the force of the disease process if the former were at least of equal force to the latter. Yet given that the two attributes which define any drug dose, the quantitative and the qualitative, are complementary and inseparable, and given further that the quantitative aspect is almost invariably infinitesimally small in homoeopathic dosage, this must mean that, to compensate, the quality must be a stimulus of a correspondingly overwhelming magnitude, if its homoeopathic effect can, as it so often does, subvert and overpower a raging disease. Of course, this is only true when the drug's artificial disease matches the actual disease of the patient superlatively. This leads to the formulation of:

4) The law of quantity and dose, expressed as: **The quantity of the drug required is in inverse ratio to the similarity** (see also 'Antidote', 'Homoeopathic Practice' and 'Therapeutic Science').

During the third quarter of the nineteenth century Professor Hugo Schulz and Dr H R Arndt, both orthodox medical men of the University of Greifswald in Germany, without openly identifying themselves with homoeopathy, were strongly sympathetic to its clear-cut scientific approach to medicine. They were particularly interested in the question of the homoeopathic stimulus, and gave to homoeopathy the so-called Arndt-Schulz law:

5) The law of stimuli, formulated as: **Minute stimuli encourage life activity, medium to strong stimuli tend to impede it, and very strong stimuli to stop or destroy it** (see also 'Biphasic Drug Action', 'Epistemological Assumptions in Homoeopathy', section 10), and 'Potency').

This was amplified by a distinguished French homoeopath, Meyhoffer, as quoted in translation by Prof Boericke: 'From the moment a drug produces pathogenetic symptoms, it exaggerates the function of the tissue, exhausts the already diminished vitality, and thence, instead of stimulating the organic cell in the direction of life, impairs or abolishes its power of contraction.' (William Boericke, in his ever-popular *Pocket Manual of Homoeopathic Materia Medica* Ninth Edition. Philadelphia: Boericke & Tafel, 1927, p 372.)

In 1930 this homoeopathic law underwent a refinement by the German Karl Kötschau, in what he called the 'type effect hypothesis' laying down five stereotypical effects of any medicinal drug, dependent solely on quantity (dose):[1]

i) **stimulating** – with small doses, a stimulant effect is evoked only;

ii) **inhibiting** – with moderate doses, the effect is initially stimulating, but becoming depressant later, eventually settling at the starting position;

iii) **toxic** – with large doses, a fleetingly brief stimulating effect is followed by an unrelenting depressive sequel which is ultimately lethal.

The actual dose quantities are determined by the substance involved. With some specific substances two alternative effects are posited, namely, that the effect given under i) above will be a straight **depressing** effect, and that given under ii) above will be a mirror-image of it, i.e. first depressant, then stimulating, and eventually unchanged.

In 1957 homoeopathy's Arndt-Schulz-Kötschau law was reformulated yet again by taking full account of the varying reactive sensitivity of individual living organisms to any given pharmacological dose (the quantity). It was done by Joseph Wilder in what he called 'the law of initial value'. This time the law more completely corresponded to Hahnemann's original concept of the biphasic drug action on individual patients (hormesis). In passing, Wilder pointed out that virtually no Orthodox pharmacological investigations take the initial state of the organism into account, as they ought to, though they feel compelled to introduce all manner of other rigid controls. Moreover, the omnipresent phenomenon of biphasic drug action had been totally ignored in such investigations, though often mentioned anecdotally. Wilder stated:[2]

> 'Not only the intensity but also the direction of a response of a body function to any agent depend to a large degree on the initial level of that function at the start of the experiment. The higher this "initial level", the smaller is the response to function-raising, the greater is the response to function-depressing agents. At more extreme "initial levels" there is a progressive tendency to "no response" and to "paradoxic reactions", i.e. a reversal of the usual direction of response.'

Obviously the inverse is true too: the lower the 'initial level', the less the response to function-depressing, the greater the response to function-raising agents. The phenomenon first described by Hahnemann, as always the keen observer, the reversal of the usual direction of response, is seen to be ever evident whether as a function of size of dose, or of a varying state of organic sensitivity, or of both these. (See 'Altered Receptivity in Disease'.)

This leads on to Bernard Fincke's pharmaceutical precept, strongly reminiscent of the fundamental principle of mechanics – enunciated one and a half centuries earlier by the French mathematician and physicist Pierre Louis

[1] Kötschau, Karl. 'The Type Effect Hypothesis as a Scientific Basis for the Simile Principle', *Journal of American Institute of Homoeopathy*, 1930, vol XXIII, pp 972-1045.

[2] Wilder, Joseph. 'The Law of Initial Value in Neurology and Psychiatry: Facts and Problems', *Journal for Nervous and Mental Disease*, 1957, vol CXXV, pp 73-86.

Moreau de Maupertuis – known today as the principle of least action, which states: 'The quantity of action necessary to effect any change in nature is the least possible'.

6) In posology the rule of least action, is: **The rule of least action ('maxima minimis') prescribes that the decisive momentum, in the application of the similia principle, is always the minimum, frequently an infinitesimal** (see also 'Philosophical Premise of Homoeopathy').

A corollary of the three preceding epitomes is:

7) The postulate on remedial quality, expressed as: **The quality of the action of a homoeopathic remedy is determined by its quantity, in inverse ratio.**

Then follows:

8) The rule on drug non-repetition during treatment, expressed as: **There is to be no repetition of the remedy administered so long as it continues to be active.**

And logically also:

9) The rule on drug non-repetition in pathogenetic experiments, expressed as: **There is to be no repetition of the dose until symptoms have run their course and completely abated from the dose already administered.**

This leads on to Georg Jahr's propositions, which are based on the essential difference between low and high dynamizations (see 'Potency'), which consists not in their strength or weakness, but in the development of the peculiarities of each remedy, as one rises in the scale of potencies. He developed this a good deal further (see 'Jahr, Georg Heinrich Gottlieb (1800-1875)'). Since this affects pathogenetic experimentation (provings), the following three precepts were laid down:

10) The three rules concerning potencies in provings, expressed as:

a) **Any drug which in its natural state affects bioenergy (dynamis) just a little will develop a proving in a high potency only;**

b) **Any drug which in its natural state disturbs the bioenergy (dynamis) to functional manifestations only may be proven in crude form;**

c) **Any drug which in its natural state disturbs the bioenergy (dynamis) to destructive manifestations should be proven only in a dynamized form.**

In accord with the preceding is:

11) The postulate on posological appropriateness, expressed as: **The dynamization, dose and quantity of a remedy that will thoroughly permeate the organism and make its essential impress upon the bioenergy (dynamis) is that which will affect the functional sphere of the individual.**

This, in turn, is in harmony with homoeopathy's more general tenets concerning natural phenomena, e.g:

12) The postulate on biological evolutionary development, expressed as: **Functional requirement creates and develops an organ.**

From this, again, homoeopathy draws the inverse inference to establish:

13) The dual postulate on disease development, expressed as:

a) **Functional symptoms are produced bioenergetically in exact**

proportion to the profundity of the disturbance;
   b) Functional symptoms precede structural changes.

In *Chronic Diseases* (published 1828) Hahnemann observed that the abuse of medicine in allopathic treatments (see 'Allopathy') produced a metastasis of disease, tending to drive the disease deeper, where it assumed a chronic form (chronic miasma). By 1865, Constantin Hering had developed this concept of disease metastasis, to allow for the correct interpretation of symptoms, into the proposition known as:

14) The rule on the direction of disease metastasis, expressed in these words: **With intensification of any disease, symptoms move from the surface to the interior, from the extremities to the upper parts of the body, and/or from the less vital organs to the more vital** (see 'Therapeutic Science').

A self-evident inference from this proposition, known as the rule of direction of cure, is that a well-indicated remedy causes symptoms to disappear in the reverse order of their original appearance.

A blended version of homoeopathic conceptualizations is poetically captured in:

15) The homoeosis postulate, expressed as: **The simillimum will modulate to nothing but the existing, though perhaps muted, harmonics of the patient's bioenergy (dynamis), which will resonate in response with ever-increasing intensity, though only for the duration, and to the degree, of co-extensive symptom-similarity, up to the full attainment of cure, manifested through the normalization of all symptoms and reversible abnormalities** (see 'Energy', 'Epistemological Assumptions in Homoeopathy' particularly section 4, and 'Vitalism').

Finally, as the homoeopathic drug-to-disease similarity principle applies to the use of medicinal agents only, and to nothing else, and then only if administered in a manner designed to elicit homoeopathically a dynamic curative reaction, the scope of the law of similars, with its scientifically predictable drug effects, must be clearly defined. This was begun by Jabez P Dake in 1873 and later consolidated to what is now known as:

16) Dake's exclusion synopsis, summarized as: **The law of similars does not relate to agents simply intended to affect the organism in any of the following five ways:**

i) **Coercively, by direct chemical or toxic action;**
ii) **By mechanical effects;**
iii) **Through supportive, supplementary or nutritional additives;**
iv) **By methods to incapacitate, remove or destroy infesting parasites directly; and**
v) **By direct physiological effects.**

Homoeopathic Pharmacist

Prepares and dispenses homoeopathic drugs and has knowledge concerning their properties.

Homoeopathic Practice

Homoeopathy's condensed rules of practice are summarized here:

Recognition of Disease
Is on the basis of the total symptom-syndrome, of what is essentially an imbalance in the self-correcting forces within the patient.

Case-Taking (Anamnesis)
Recording a carefully individualized case history,

1 using the patient's own words as far as possible.
2 Local symptoms are to be elicited in a head-to-foot sequence.
3 Mentals, generals and particulars might follow this sequence:
   mind, memory, emotions;
   vertigo, sleep, dreams;
   elimination and water metabolism;
   modalities affecting whole patient;
   skin, humoral pathology, sexuality;
   appetite, aversions, cravings;
   morphology, diathesis, constitution.
4 Previous medical history should cover environmental factors, familial illnesses, predispositions and idiosyncrasies, diathesis, constitution, attitude to others, occupation, past illnesses, inoculations, suppressive therapies, treatments and medications received.

A questionnaire is a useful, time-saving device.

Highlights
To be noted particularly are any peculiar, unusual, outstanding or characteristically (perhaps, uncharacteristically) singular symptoms and signs, or a possible chronic miasma.

Drug Action
Is defined by a set of morbid symptoms in the healthy, the so-called artificial disease, as determined in drug tests, toxicology, clinical and veterinary evidence and listed in works of materia medica.

Cure
The drug-induced disease stimulus brings about a corrective reaction that will, predictably, overcome the natural disease, if the artificial symptom-complex matches the patient's, and provided that the condition is within reversible limits and the patient's reactive forces retain sufficient vital potential.

Drug Preparation
Is by dynamization (potentization), which eliminates any direct drug effect but refines the drug's stimulant effects.

Potency Applicable

The most appropriate to the case is to be administered (see 'Drainage', 'Emergencies – Homoeopathic Treatment' and 'Potency').

Quantity and Dose

Are in inverse ratio to the extent of similarity between the two co-extensive symptom-pictures of disease and matching drug.

Appropriateness

The patient demonstrates the congruity of a particular stimulus as being specifically antagonistic to the disease by the nature and degree of the reaction induced, including, at times, evidence of the reciprocal of Hering's rule of disease metastasis.

Healing Crisis

A well-indicated remedy most often brings about an aggravation which heralds the fact that the patient is being taken in the direction of cure.

Repetition

Progress is assessed first; the choices are:

1 the remedy is left to continue acting,
2 a placebo is administered to allow the changed symptom picture to emerge fully,
3 the same remedy in the same potency is repeated,
4 the potency is altered, or
5 a new remedy is given on the symptom-complex now presenting, if changed from before.

Precautions

Most homoeopathic remedies are taken perlingually, unless specifically directed to be swallowed or employed in some other manner. The mouth should be clean and free of drink, food, tobacco, strong gum or toothpaste when remedies are taken. These should also not be handled needlessly, nor be left in direct sunlight, or be exposed to strong odours, like menthol, naphthalene (mothballs), camphor, eucalyptus, perfumes or potpourris. Nor should ultra-sound (e.g. dental drilling, electrotherapy) be allowed the possibility of degrading the effect of dynamizations. Such things may reduce or completely overwhelm a remedy's action.

Obstacles

Anything that might hinder the cure (e.g. a domestic cat, in the case of an established allergy to its dander) will have to be removed. In slow, or inconsistent, treatment response, aspects such as sequellae of allopathic treatment, miasmatic influences or suppression are to be examined. That any new symptoms may only represent an elimination crisis, in terms of Hering's rule, should not be overlooked. When new remedies are prescribed, the correct sequence of drugs, in terms of the compatibilities given in the materia medica, are to be observed, to achieve the best possible response.

Supportive Diet

This must be individualized, particularly with respect to possible hypersensitivities (see 'Foods as Health Problems'). Regular, light and simple meals (to conserve the patient's reactive forces and to remove anything which could have a medicinal action) are to be prescribed, along these five guidelines:

1 The complete exclusion of: coffee, common tea, cocoa, spices, aromatics, teas made of medicinal herbs (e.g. chamomile), and the concurrent use of household, patent or folk remedies, as well as processed foods (these often contain homoeopathically active substances) and white wheat flour (contains many chemicals and places an excessive load on the patient's insulin-producing cells).
2 The moderate consumption of: sugar, alcohol, fried foods, eggs and fats.
3 The increased consumption of: fresh fruit and vegetables (half the latter preferably raw, the remainder to be steamed or stir-fried or scalded, but not boiled).
4 Drastic reduction in, or preferably the total exclusion of, added salt whether to cooking or at table.
5 Food to be chewed well and is not to be consumed in haste, nor when it is very hot; moderately sized meals are to be consumed at regular intervals.

(See also 'Nutritional Equipoise'.)

Homoeopathicity

Term describing ideal match of symptoms and signs pertaining both to a drug's artificial disease and a patient's natural disease.

Homöopathisches Arzneibuch

Abbreviated as HAB, is the German Homoeopathic Pharmacopoeia. (See 'Potentizing Methods'.)

Homoeopathized Allopathica

Are remedies used tautopathically, i.e. to counter the injurious effects of coercive medication, or may be employed medicinally in their own right. From toxic medicines homoeopathic remedies are produced that may either be administered to stimulate a chronic miasma of iatrogenic origin to manifest all its symptoms, or be employed along standard homoeopathic lines. Many allopathica (under their generic names) have been subjected to placebo-controlled Hahnemannian provings. For unproven allopathica the homoeopath is guided by the observed adverse drug reactions and the known toxic effects associated with each pharmaceutical product; this serves as the toxicological record which then becomes the basis for a fragmentary *ad hoc* drug picture. The remedial administration of such dynamized pharmaceutical products along homoeopathic principles provides a much broader spectrum of indicating symptoms to prescribe on, than its administration purely along isotherapeutic lines. (Refer to 'Isopathy' for a list of recently-proven homoeopathized allopathica; see also 'Miasma' and 'Tautopathy'.)

Homoeopathy

Self-consistent scientific system of medicinal therapy, which was finally developed to its full potential from 1796 onward by Christian Friedrich Samuel Hahnemann (1755-1843), although prodromous beginnings of it had constantly been apparent since antiquity. It is based on the observed biological fact that a diseased deviation from an organism's bioenergetic mean, within reversible limits, can predictably be restored to normal by specially-prepared medicinal stimuli, that need only be administered in small doses, or more often in sub-physiological deconcentrations, owing to an altered receptivity of tissue to such stimuli in disease, provided always (a) that in healthy organisms the medicinal agents chosen would produce symptoms and clinical features like those of the disease, and (b) that obstacles to cure have been removed.

Although homoeopathy was initially applied only in human medicine, Johann Joseph Wilhelm Lux, a veterinary surgeon, and the physician Ernst Ferdinand Rückert, jointly introduced it into veterinary medicine in Leipzig in 1819 with immediate success. Much more recently homoeopathy has tentatively also been applied in phytopathology, again with extraordinary initial success. (See also 'Dental Surgery and Homoeopathy' and 'Surgery'.)

Homoeosiniatry

See 'Acupuncture' and 'Derivatives of Homoeopathy'.

Homoeosis

The beneficial effect of homoeosymptomatic pharmaceutics upon growth, vigour, physical or mental qualities, and the curative capacity of an organism. Bernhardt Fincke (1821-1906), began to develop this concept which others took further. In its final form it describes the homoeopathically induced process, or state of universal assimilation, as Fincke also called it (also the state of quiescent equilibrium between a species and its staples nutrients described under 'Foods as Health Problems'), which is nothing other than the eliciting of any increase in the corresponding bioenergetic reactive force by means of the most similar agent, leading on to the consequent manifestation of physiologic, psychic and pathologic curative normalization. This can be put another way: the organically absorbed similar remedy, in a higher potency, cannot have any direct action of itself, but will modulate only to the existing but muted harmonics of the bioenergetic force-field of the patient, which, in turn, will resonate ever more forcefully, responding to the feedback, until the body-own energy output is amplified to a pitch where other effects are obliterated, either eventually leading on to cure, or conferring immunity against a corresponding actual disease onslaught. To illustrate this: if one holds a tuning fork in one's hand one can absorb the energy of a piano at the other end of the room through resonance.

The Greek suffix -osis denotes a process, condition or state, not necessarily abnormal or diseased, involving increased physiological (pathological) responsiveness secondary to, or in anticipation of, an exopathic influence. Examples are: leukocytosis, tuberculosis, coccidiosis, lymphocytosis. Hahnemann, the perspicacious observer, recognized that some people (in epidemics and at other times) were immune, and, moreover, that a few of these were disease-carriers (he called them 'healthy miasma-bearers' [*Lesser Writings*, p 761.]). This would have to mean that they, who were spared by disease on such occasions, had somehow prophylactically acquired the antidotal homoeopathic component enabling their reactive force (dynamis) to resist the attacks of disease. The process, condition or state involved in such a circumstance is correctly termed homoeosis. (See 'Homoeopathic Laws, Postulates and Precepts', section 16.) In a philosophical mood, Fincke, some time before 1865, writing on the subject of high potencies, said: 'Disease originates in the specific action of noxious matter which is either produced within the organism, or brought in from without, and it is always carried on by a process of assimilation. Assimilation, everywhere, is accompanied by potentiation, by rendering the infinitesimal particles of matter susceptible and active, according to their inherent affinities. . . . The whole organism is the product of assimilation of matter. . . . And so is disease. And so is health. And so is all life. The hypothetical ether is, possibly, infinitesimal comminuted matter, forming, as it were, the reservoir of the high potencies required for the Universal Assimilation or Homoeosis, which is continually going on and mediating all life in the world.' (See 'Radiant State of Matter, Theory of'.)

Developed in biological science from this homoeopathic concept, but in the malefic sense only of an induced inherited miasma, is 'homoeotic mutation' (hence 'homoeotic mutant') meaning a type of genetic variation in which a plant member takes on the characteristics of a member of a different nature of that same plant, as when a petal is changed into a stamen in the plant's offspring due to, say, traces of herbicide or insecticide having entered that plant's food chain. Biology also refers to the malefic process of such an assimilative process as 'homoeosis'. (See 'Foods as Health Problems', 'Heterostasis', 'Immunization and Homoeopathy' and 'Miasma'.)

Homoeostasis

Term coined by the Canadian Professor of Physiology at Harvard University Medical School, USA, Walter B Cannon, in 1932, describing a state of equilibrium in the organism:[1] i.e. a balance between opposing tensions and pressures in the body with respect to various functions, as well as in relation to specific biochemical, dynamical, electrical, mechanical, radiant or thermal antagonisms within the self-containment of the body. One example is the delicate balance of one person's heart rate, temperature, blood pressure, water content, blood sugar, electrolytes, etc. One of the features of homoeopathic treatment is that the well-indicated drug will nudge toward self-correction the organic system (i.e. the holon constituting that individual) which may be in disequilibrium (a bioenergetic reaction; see 'Vitalism') and, when feasible, initiate the processes through which such bodily equilibrium is maintained, provided obstacles to cure are identified and removed.

Homoeotherapy

Similar in meaning to 'homoeopathy'; yet the word is less specific in its semantic connotation than homoeopathy, in that homoeotherapy is generally taken to mean treatment or prevention of disease by means of a medicinal agent similar to, but not identical with, the active causal agent; this meaning would exclude potentized allergens, but include Jennerian vaccination, for instance. Yet neither of these would be understood by the word homoeopathy, were it employed instead. A Division of the American Institute of Homoeopathy is known as the American Academy of Homoeotherapeutics. This last word is new, cumbersome yet found serviceable by those who would have homoeopathy be one of many variants in medical method – amongst the other orthodox medical procedures and methods complementary thereto. Be that as it may, the word has not quite taken on synonymity with the word homoeopathy.

Homoeothermal Organism

See 'Organic Clock'.

Homoeotypical

Of or resembling the given type.

Homoion

Single term for the law of similars; now rarely used. (See 'Homoeopathic Laws, Postulates and Precepts' section 1.)

[1]Cannon, Walter B. *The Wisdom of the Body*. London: Kegan Paul, 1939.

Homotoxicosis

Term coined in 1952 by Hans-Heinrich Reckeweg in his publication entitled *Biotherapie der Homotoxikosen,* which he developed further in *Homotoxine und Homotoxikosen* (1957), *Homotoxikologie – Ganzheitsschau einer Synthese der Medizin* (5th edition 1978), and in two volumes of *Homoeopathica Antihomotoxica* (1981). Homotoxicosis describes a state of subnormal health due to a toxic burden arising from poor elimination of accumulated, potentially poisonous, by-products of both endogenous and exogenous origin. Reckeweg also devised the word 'Homotoxicology' to describe the science of these poisons: their source, composition, action, insidious effects, etc. as well as what he called homoeopathic antihomotoxic therapy.

Hormesis

Biphasic medicinal dose/response action; describes the reversed biological effects in various ranges of concentrations of the same medicinal agent. This is the biphasic dose response first described by Hahnemann when he wrote, 'Most medicines have more than one kind of effect – the direct one at the beginning, passing gradually into the second (I call it the indirect after-effect). The latter state is generally exactly opposite to the former'.[1] (See 'Epistemological Assumptions in Homoeopathy', section 10), 'Hahnemann, Christian Friedrich Samuel [1755-1843]', section entitled 'Hahnemann's Contribution to Science and his Impact on the Practice of Medicine', and 'Homoeopathic Laws, Postulates and Precepts', section 5.)

Hospital, Homoeopathic

Homoeopathic nosocomion (see 'Nosocomial'); an institution with fixed location, or on a ship

a) offering homoeopathic treatment, and care, to cure the sick and wounded and to help prevent illness in those at risk;

b) for the study of each individual patient; and

c) for the training of homoeopaths, surgeons and nurses;

that is equipped to attend to homoeopathic, surgical, or maternity cases, having a resident homoeopathic staff.

The terms nursing home, sanatorium and insane (lunatic) asylum also refer to hospitals, but have special meanings. A nursing home is a convalescent home or a small private hospital. A homoeopathic sanatorium treats chronic diseases (e.g. tuberculosis, neuropsychologic disorders, rheumatoid arthritis), or is an institution for recuperation under homoeopathic supervision. The insane

[1] Hahnemann, Christian Friedrich Samuel. 'Essay on a New Principle for Ascertaining the Curative Power of Drugs, and Some Examinations of the Previous Principles', *Hufeland's Journal,* 1796, vol II, parts 3 & 4, pp 391-439 and 465-561.

(lunatic) asylums run by homoeopathy are, in fact, special hospitals and, therefore, more correctly referred to as homoeopathic mental hospitals (see 'Asylums for the Insane').

For some details concerning homoeopathic hospitals refer to 'History of Homoeopathy before 1900'. (See also 'Cholera Epidemics', 'Emotional and Intellectual Reactive States and Some 'Mentals'', specifically footnote 1 [there are some interesting statistics favourably contrasting homoeopathic mental hospitals with others], 'Epidemiology' and 'Epistemological Assumptions in Homoeopathy', specifically footnote 6 to section 1 [Prof Frederick M Dearborn was homoeopathic consultant for dermatology to a number of homoeopathic hospitals in the New York area, among which are: The Flower Hospital, N.Y.; The Hahnemann Hospital, N.Y.; St Mary's Hospital, N.J.; and The Yonkers Homoeopathic Hospital, NY].)

Hot Air Oven

See 'Utensils of Homoeopathic Pharmacy'.

Hufeland, Christoph Wilhelm (1762-1832)

An enlightened, generous-hearted and unprejudiced orthodox medical contemporary of Hahnemann, who was the celebrated editor of the very influential *Journal für praktische Arzneikunde*. It is a pleasure to observe the distinguished and dignified position Hufeland took in his public attitude to homoeopathy, as opposed to the spiteful attacks on Hahnemann and his theory that were rampant all around. Hufeland had frequent occasion to set down succinctly what he thought were the disadvantages of homoeopathy, though always offering reasoned criticisms. Yet he also felt honour-bound to admit publicly (in 1828, *Journal*, Vol I, page 23) the 'Advantages of Homoeopathy', which he enunciated as follows:

'1) It will attract attention to the all-important question of individualization.

2) It will help to bring dietetics back to its own.

3) It will prohibit large doses of medicines.

4) It will lead to a simplification of prescriptions.

5) It will lead to more accurate testing and determination of the effect of remedies on the living subject, as it has to a certain extent already done.

6) The homoeopathic process will direct attention more to the preparation of medicines and bring about a stricter supervision of the apothecaries.

7) It will never do positive injury.

8) It will give the sick organisms more time for quiet and undisturbed self-help.

9) It will lessen the costs of curing to an extraordinary extent.'

In the concluding paragraph Hufeland wrote, 'Time will judge. Till then we shall continue to test without prejudice, keep more to the facts than to theory and above all found no new sects endowed with intolerance and a desire to persecute.'

Probably Hufeland's most famous aphorism is: 'The great experiment that man began upon himself – Medicine – is not yet ended, nor will it ever be completed.'

Hughes, Richard (1836-1902)

One of the most prominent of UK homoeopaths and a brilliant scholar of the second half of the nineteenth century, whose influence on homoeopathy can hardly be underestimated. He insisted that a prescriber was to take into account the site of action of the disease, the evolution of symptoms, any causative elements, and the organs affected when making his choice of homoeopathic medicine. He always questioned dogmatic attitudes and, like Prof Charles J Hempel in the USA, all but incorporated the science of pathology into the homoeopathic method. He worked at the London Homoeopathic Hospital, though he was based in Brighton where he was in partnership with Dr Madden, and where he was also the physician to the Homoeopathic Dispensary. This man's historico-philosophical impact is discussed in the section on the United Kingdom under 'History of Homoeopathy before 1900'. His major literary contributions to homoeopathy include:

A Manual of Pharmacodynamics
Hahnemann as a Medical Philosopher
Knowledge of the Physician
Principles and Practice of Homoeopathy
and, together with Jabez P Dake of the USA, and others:
A Cyclopaedia of Drug Pathogenesy.

Humoral Pathology in Prescribing

Primarius Mag Dr Mathias Dorcsi, Chief Consultant at Lainz Hospital in Vienna, Austria and head of the Ludwig Boltzmanninstitut für Homöopathie is considered by many to be the most respected living homoeopath of the German-speaking world, whose outstanding efforts to have homoeopathy widely accepted are generally acclaimed. He developed a useful method for quicker guidance to arrive at the correct homoeopathic drug diagnosis by relating particular drugs to the presenting constitutional skin type of the patient. The indicators are six variables (cold, red, dry, pale, moist and warm) which may, additionally, be linked with four other variable indicators relating to general appearance (restless, tranquil, powerful, weak) and/or with the four Ionic temperaments (choleric, sanguine, melancholic, phlegmatic).[1]

[1] Dorcsi, Prim Mag Dr Med Mathias. *Homöopathie – Band sechs: Symptomenverzeichnis.* Vol VI. 2nd Edition. Heidelberg: Karl F Haug Verlag GmbH, 1982, pp 58-67, where the said constitutional attributes and the four temperaments are listed with all the corresponding drugs together with one or two outstanding or peculiar guiding symptoms for each.

For example:

Constitutional		Ionic
appearance of skin	– corresponds to –	temperament
warm, dry, red	(1)	choleric
moist, warm, red	(2)	sanguine
pale, dry, cold	(3)	melancholic
cold, pale, moist	(4)	phlegmatic

The universality of such a diagnostic initiative is remarkable. Homoeopaths who may also be trained in the Four Diagnostic Examinations used in Oriental Medicine find that Dorcsi's parameters translate directly from tongue diagnosis, and the evidence gleaned from facial colour, secretions, appearance and from touch examination of the patient. Likewise, the dermatoscopic approach to constitutional assessment accords with other established Western humoral pathological classifications. In fact, it was Alcmaeon of Croton (around 500 BC), the first Empirical medical philosopher (probably belonged to the school established around 530 BC by Pythagoras at Croton on the south-western coast of the Gulf of Taranto in the Ionian Sea), who taught then, that what today is called homoeostasis depends on the 'equal balance of dynameis', as evidenced by an indefinite number of polarities such as moist and dry, pale and flushed, hot and cold, etc. and that 'the supremacy' of one of these over its opposite is the cause of disease.

Concordance with other Western humoral pathologies:

Numbers as above:	Empedocles (ca. 490–430 BC) and Philistion of Locri (ca. 415–360 BC):	Aristotle (ca. 384–322 BC):	Hippocratic Corpus (school of Kos) (from 430 BC):
(1)	Fire	Warm-blooded	Yellow Bile
(2)	Air	Volatile, fluid	Blood
(3)	Earth	Heavy, viscous	Black Bile
(4)	Water	Cold-blooded	Phlegm

(See also 'Constitutional Type'.)

Hunter, John (1728–1793)

See 'Philosophical Premise of Homoeopathy'.

Hydro-Alcoholic Mixture

Water-ethanol mixture (see 'Alcohol' and 'Vehicle').

Hydrometer

See 'Utensils of Homoeopathic Pharmacy'.

Hydrogenoid Constitution

See 'Constitutional Type'.

Hydrotherapy

Water cure: internal and external, as sauna, baths, enemas, eye baths, steam, wet-packs (wickels), sitz-baths, ice packs, jacuzzis, aerated or ozonated baths, stomach lavages and colonic irrigations. This form of therapy is widely considered to be complementary to homoeopathy. Hahnemann said cold water could be used curatively as a 'physical means of assistance'; it was only the common use of mineral baths with which Hahnemann would have little to do, because the mineral ingredients act medicinally, usually in an indiscriminate non-homoeopathic way. A compendium of simple hydrotherapy treatments, compatible with homoeopathy, for a wide variety of common ailments is *Modern Magic of Natural Healing with Water Therapy* by J V Cerney, AB, DM, DPM (Bombay: D B Taraporevala Sons & Co Pvt Ltd, by arrangement with Parker Publishing Co Inc, reprint 1979 [216 pp]). Two other excellent textbooks are: *Hydrotherapie Elektrotherapie Massage,* J. Christoph Cordes *et al.*, Berlin: V.E.B. Verlag Folk und Gesundheit, 1989 [326 pp] and *Hydrotherapie und Balneotherapie,* Otto Gillert and Walther Rulffs, Munich: Pflaum Verlag, 1988 [265 pp]. (See 'Naturopath'.)

Hygiene

Science devoted to the preservation of health (see 'bad hygiene' under 'Miasma').

Hygroscopic

Capable of readily absorbing and retaining moisture.

Hypnotherapy

See 'Mesmerism'.

I

Iatrogenic Miasma

See 'Allopathy', 'Homoeopathized Allopathica', 'Injurious Treatment' and 'Miasma'.

Idiosyncrasy

● **Bodily or temperamental peculiarity of any person.**

Individual mental, constitutional, physical and/or temperamental characteristic or tendency; mode of expression manifesting an individual bent of mind; susceptibility to the action of drugs, to environmental influences, to emotional affects, to items of diet, and the like, peculiar to an individual patient. A century ago, in the wake of professional disputes (after 1865) over Eduard von Grauvogl's 'three biochemic states' and later over Antoine Nebel's 'three morphological types', Philip Rice stated what has remained the view held by many homoeopaths: 'The fundamental cause of every idiosyncrasy is morphological imbalance; that is an organic state in which, through excess and defect in development there results excess and defect in function, with a corresponding degree of hyper-excitability or non-excitability'.[1] This foreshadowed Henri Bernard's embryological basis for homoeopathic constitutional types postulated in the 1930s. (See 'Allergy', 'Altered State of Receptivity', 'Constitutional Type', 'Epistemological Assumptions in Homoeopathy', 'Homoeosis' and 'Morphology'.)

Immanent Organizing Principle

See 'Dynamis' and 'Laws of Nature'.

Immunity

See 'Homoeosis', 'Immunization and Homoeopathy' and 'Isopathy'.

Immunization and Homoeopathy

It is held by many homoeopaths that the nosodes of the specific diseases (acute miasmata) and/or non-nosodial homoeopathic specifics may be used to properly achieve an inoculative immune resistance in the individual, of an

---

[1] Rice, Philip. Quoted by Stuart Close (1860-1929), Professor of Homoeopathic Philosophy at New York Homoeopathic Medical College (1909-1913), in *The Genius of Homoeopathy*, New York: Boericke and Tafel, 1924, p 113.

order that would safeguard that individual against all but minor attacks of the corresponding acute miasma, or even to provide total prophylactic immunity. Many other homoeopaths view this with deep scepticism.

A) Examples, where efficacy appears to be well established at least on historical grounds, are:
Diphtherinum or Pyrexin (Pyrogenium) against Diphtheria
Influenzinum or Oscillococcinum or Bacillinum against Influenza
Morbillinum or Pulsatilla nigricans against Measles
Parotidinum against Mumps
Pertussinum (Coqueluchinum) or Drosera rotundifolia against Whooping Cough
Rubellinum or Pulsatilla nigricans against German Measles
Rubini's Camphora or Cuprum aceticum against Asiatic Cholera
Scarlatinum or (Atropa) Belladonna against Scarlet Fever
Tuberculinum against Tuberculosis
Typhoidinum against Typhoid Fever
Varicella against chickenpox
Variolinum or Malandrinum against smallpox
(Where the first-mentioned remedy is unavailable, the second – less well-established one – may be employed.)
B) Examples where efficacy is clinically not yet fully established are:
Hydrophobinum (Lyssin) against Rabies (in man)
Hyoscyamus niger or Baptisia tinctoria against Typhus
Lathyrus sativus or Gelsemium sempervirens against Poliomyelitis
Upas (Strychnos tiente) or Strychninum or Physostigma venenosum against Tetanus

Dr A Pulford, in his *Homoeopathic Materia Medica of Graphic Drug Pictures and Clinical Comments* (New Delhi: B Jain Publishers, 1971, p 6 ff) speaks of predisposition to a disease as a prerequisite for contracting it. He goes on to point out that it is precisely the homoeotic absence of such a predisposition to any particular illness, which makes an individual immune to it. Moreover, as historical evidence shows, the homoeopathic form of treatment on its own appears to be capable of reliably removing such predispositions.

The nosodes and remedies mentioned under examples A) above were very widely used to protect children from the corresponding diseases in the days before the existence of Orthodox 'vaccination' and immunization schemes. As is clear from the entry under 'Isopathy', homoeopathy was at least half a century ahead of orthodox medicine in inoculative therapy on a wide front (smallpox vaccination excepted). Additionally there was a great deal of self-medication with homoeopathic remedies in the last century, where parents would obtain the remedy from a pharmacist or a dispensary and simply give it to their children, 'just to be safe'. Homoeopathy cannot test these now because orthodox 'immunization schedules' are so widespread, nor did it carry out any trials of efficacy at that time (from the 1830s). Still, hard historical statistical data strongly suggest that they were effective as protective inoculants, and that this manifest effectiveness, moreover, had also since become heredo-transmissible. In the brief historical discussion that follows, it is important to keep the following two aspects distinctly apart: (1) a medicine's effectiveness in disease prevention, or reduction of its virulence, in specific individual cases on the one hand, which has not been fully established, and (2) its contribution to the total incidence volume of a particular disease, on the other. Homoeopathic medicine has done exceptionally well in the latter, and emphasis is laid on the latter in the discussion below.

The death rate from tuberculosis in New York, for instance, in 1812 was higher than 700 per 10000. Then intervened homoeopathy's frenetic isopathic period, in the 1830s. Only much later, in 1882, followed Koch's first isolating and culturing of the tubercle bacillus. Yet by that year the death rate had already declined to 370 per 10000. By 1910, when the first orthodox sanatorium was opened, the rate was down to 180 per 10000. After World War II, but still before antibiotic treatment had become regular orthodox prescription practice, the death rate had dropped to 48.[1] Likewise, the combined death rate from whooping cough, diphtheria, scarlet fever and measles among children (below 15 years old) analysed over the 105-year period prior to 1965 shows that nearly 90% of the total decline in mortality had occurred well before the introduction of antibiotics and widespread Orthodox immunization.[2] Similarly dysentery, typhoid fever and Asiatic cholera dwindled inside the period when homoeopathy was a strong contender against orthodoxy for the position of medical dominance.[3,4] A comparison of the Vaccine Lymph (used in orthodoxy) and homoeopathy's nosode Variolinum is not possible because the former's use was already very widespread during the isopathic high-water mark in the nineteenth century. All that can be said is that certainly no risk of either infection or post-vaccinal encephalitis, which both surround the former, attend the use of the nosode. Perhaps acting in unison, they jointly eradicated smallpox entirely, as happened in the late 1960s. An area where homoeopathy unfortunately did not do a great deal of prophylactic work during the nineteenth century was in poliomyelitis (infantile paralysis). The apparent dramatic reduction of this much feared illness is said to be due to successful orthodox immunization programmes initiated in 1955. With these the attendant risk seems to be confined only to pregnant women, who should not be immunized during the first four months of gestation, as there is a 20% increase in the risk of incidence of stillbirths associated with this.

[1] Dubos, René and Jean. *The White Plague: Tuberculosis, Man and Society* Boston: Little, Brown, 1953.
[2] Porter, R R. 'The Contribution of the Biological and Medical Sciences to Human Welfare', being the Presidential Address to the British Association for the Advancement of Science, Swansea Meeting, in 1971, published London: the Association, 1972, p 95.
[3] van Zijl, W J. 'Studies on Diarrhoeal Disease in Seven Countries', contained in *Bulletin of the World Health Organization* 35 (1966), pp 249-261.
[4] Rosenberg, Charles E. *The Cholera Years: The United States in 1832, 1849, and 1866* Chicago: University of Chicago Press, 1962.

The evidence provided by the history of the evolution of disease patterns since 1800 clearly signals:

a) that the synchronous recessions of incidence/virulence in tuberculosis, measles, scarlet fever, diphtheria, whooping-cough, cholera, typhoid fever and dysentery came about totally outside orthodox medicine's scope of influence; and

b) that in part this recession may be attributed to contemporaneously improved housing, better sanitation and sounder nutrition, though this cannot explain the fact that poliomyelitis remained unmitigated everywhere (for which no prophylactic nosode was available), nor that a recession did occur in overpopulated South American areas and in India (despite appalling housing, sanitation and nutrition, as ever, whereas nosodes were and are in widespread use there).

It seems to suggest itself that by default this astounding regression might only be attributable to the long-term prophylactic effects of homoeopathic nosodes, the effects of which are evidently also passed on to subsequent generations. Yet not all homoeopaths share this assessment, by any means. (See 'Euthenic (Nosode) Treatment', 'Insect (and Related) Remedies', 'Isopathy', 'Miasma', 'Prophylactic Treatment' and 'Vaccinosis'.)

Impotence

Refer to this under 'Emotional and Intellectual Reactive States and Some "Mentals"'.

Incompatible

● **Said of things that can not be mixed.**

Incongruous or mutually intolerant; unsuitable, for whatever reason, to be mixed, or perhaps just remotely combined, with another substance. For example, the blood of a group B donor may not be administered to a group A recipient, without resulting in an undesirable reaction: the two types of blood are said to be incompatible. (See 'Antidote', 'Complementary Remedies' and 'Inimical'.)

Individualization

● **Is to particularize medicine for any one patient.**

The hallmark of good homoeopathic practice. To paraphrase James Tyler Kent (1848-1916), in homoeopathy one sick person is to be cured, not some abstraction with a generic disease label. All major endeavours in homoeopathy promote individualization: the drug testing (proving) which records extremely individual responses (not averages); the method of drug selection for a particular patient – by its distinguishing characteristics (not the common symptoms); the homoeopathic disease identification (ipso facto also the drug-of-choice identification), which looks for the most unusual peculiarity among the symptoms of the personal disease process in the individual patient concerned (never for aggregates); and the drug reaction elicited, i.e. the curative response in each individual's distinct dynamic healing effort. (See also 'Classical Homoeopathy', 'Combinations of Homoeopathic Drugs', 'Disease and Drug Action in Homoeopathic Congruity', 'Headache', 'Homoeopathic Practice' and 'Therapeutic Science'.)

Infancy, Homoeopathic Remedies in

Infancy is the earliest period of extra-uterine life. It is also referred to as babyhood, and taken to end around the attainment of the age of two years. Certain conditions and ailments prevail during this time.

Donald Foubister, in his *Tutorials on Homoeopathy* (Beaconsfield: Beaconsfield Publishers Ltd, 1989, on pp 45-90) provides guidelines in this area in the section 'Homoeopathy and Paediatrics' covered in six informative chapters.

Infection

See 'Antibiotic', 'Antiseptic' and 'Miasma'.

Inflammation

● **A hot, swollen, painful, red area of reaction in the body.**

A fundamental, though complex dynamic process involving cytological and histological changes that occur in affected blood-vessels and adjoining tissue, activated by injury or provoked by a biological, physical or chemical agent (or a combination of any of these). This disease process may include morphological changes and destruction of inimical material. Its five cardinal homoeopathic indications are dolor (pain), calor (heat), rubor (ruddiness), turgor (swelling) and functio laesa (impaired function). With functiotropic (pathotropic) homoeopathic application of remedies, it is only necessary to find a drug capable of setting up these reactive signs, in the same manner and at the same spot, as presented by the symptoms. Inflammatory reactions feature particularly prominently in the following major remedies: Aconitum napellus (particularly liver inflammation), (Atropa) Belladonna (indurations following inflammations), Colchicum autumnale (joint or bowel inflammations), Cuprum metallicum, Ferrum phosphoricum album and Sulphur. In organotropic prescribing, the undermentioned medicines might well be considered in inflammations of:

Bladder – Chimaphila umbellata, Epigea repens, Eupatorium purpureum, Sabal serrulata

Bowels – Colchicum autumnale, Hydrastis canadensis
Brain – Veratrum viride
Eyelids – Apium virus, Argentum metallicum, Hepar sulphuris calcareum
Eyes – (Artemisia) Abrotanum
Genito-urinary mucosa – Cantharis vesicator
Heart – Bryonia alba
Lungs – Veratrum viride
Mouth – Kali chloratum
Stomach – Antimonium crudum, Argentum nitricum
Testicles – Cannabis sativa, Cantharis vesicator
Tonsils – Baryta carbonica, Hepar sulphuris calcareum
Tongue – Acidum nitricum, Hydrastis canadensis
Uterus – Kali hydriodicum
Veins – Hamamelis macrophylla, Vipera communis

Generally quick-acting in inflammatory conditions are the insect (and related) remedies (see entry under this).

Examples of syndetic pointers to two homoeopathic medicines:

Inflammation of joints with excessive hyperaesthesia, often in a patient who has developed an excessive sensitivity to the smell of cooking – Colchicum autumnale

Once inflammations cease, if followed by convulsions or delirium – Cuprum metallicum
(See 'Irritability'.)

Infusion

● **A medicinal brew.**

Prepared by plant material being steeped in freshly-boiled water. Used on rare occasions as an *ad hoc* homoeopathic remedy when the plant material happens to be at hand but the prepared remedy is not, as, for instance, soaking the lint with stinging nettle infusion in burns when Urtica urens is unavailable.

Inhalation

● **Medicine that can be breathed into the nasal passages, the throat, the bronchioles and lungs.**

Homoeopathic medicinal agents carried in volatile form. An example mentioned in 'Emergencies – Homoeopathic Treatment' is Adrenalinum 3CH atomized spray dispensed from a nebulizer hand pump. (See also 'Olfactory Medicines'.)

Inherited Factor(s)

See 'Lamarckism' and 'Miasma'.

Inimical

● **Hostile.**

Adverse; used in the materia medica to describe such homoeopathic drug effects under specified circumstances. Whereas the word 'antidotal' is used to describe a competing homoeopathic reactive propensity, the word 'inimical' is generally reserved for the description of a tendency to induce an opposing reaction. (See also 'Antidote', 'Complementary Remedies' and 'Incompatible'.)

Injurious Treatment

See 'Allopathy', 'Epistemological Assumptions in Homoeopathy', section 1 (Dermatitis Medicamentosa), 'Homoeopathized Allopathica', 'Isopathy', section on Isotherapeutic Agents, 'Jaundice', under Sulfanilamidum as a homoeopathic drug, and 'Miasma'.

Insect (and Related) Remedies

An important group of homoeopathic drugs (with which are generally also included the arachnida, myriapoda, crustacea, gorgoniaceae, merostomata, myriapoda and spongiae). These remedies together offer a very rich choice of symptom-complexes and they are, moreover, generally quick-acting. Their range of reactive effects is markedly in the areas of inflammatory and immune responses, as well as on the nervous system. Principal remedies are: Aphis chenopodii glauci (aphid), Apis mellifica, Apium virus (bee and its venom), Aranea diadema, Aranea ixobola, Aranea scinencia (spider), Astacus fluviatilis (crawfish), Badiaga (Spongilla fluviatilis) (fresh-water sponge), Blatta americana, Blatta orientalis (cockroach), Bombyx processionea (procession moth), Buthus australis (Prionuris scorpion), Cantharis vesicator (spanish fly), Cimex lectularius (bedbug), Coccinella septempunctata (ladybird), Coccus cacti (cochineal infesting cactus plant), Corallium rubrum (Gorgonia nobilis zoophytes), Culex musca (Mosquito), Dermatophagoides pteronyssinus (house-dust mite), Doryphora decemlineata (potato bug), Formica rufa, Acidum formicum (ant and its acid), Homarus (lobster), Latrodectus katipo, Latrodectus mactans (spider), Limulus cyclops (king-crab), Mygale lasiodora cubana (large black Cuban spider), Oniscus asellus (cellar-worm), Pediculus capitis (head louse), Scolopendra morsitans (centipede), Scorpio (scorpion), Spongia tosta (common sponge, roasted), Tarentula cubensis, Tarentula hispanica (tarantula), Theridion curassavicum (orange spider), Trombidium muscae domesticae (red acarus [parasitic mite] of the fly), Vespa crabro (European hornet), Vespa maculata (American hornet) and Vespa vulgaris (wasp).

Dynamized insect secretions belong, strictly speaking, to the sarcodes of animal origin (see under 'Isopathy').

Insect Stings and Bites

See 'Emergencies – Homoeopathic Treatment'.

Insoluble Substances

See "Bioavailability" and 'Colloid'.

Instructions to Patients

See 'Homoeopathic Practice', section Precautions.

Instruments for Remedy Preparation

See 'Utensils of Homoeopathic Pharmacy'.

Insurance Companies – Actuarian Index of Homoeopathy's Success

The London Life Assurance Office issued this statement in 1865:

> 'Persons treated by the homoeopathic system enjoy more robust health, are less frequently attacked by disease, and when attacked recover more speedily than those treated by any other system. . . . With respect to the more fatal classes of disease, the mortality under homoeopathy is small in comparison with that of allopathy [= orthodox medicine]. . . . There are cases not curable at all under the latter system which are perfectly curable under the former; finally, . . . the medicines prescribed by homoeopathists do not injure the constitution, whereas those employed by allopathists not infrequently entail the most serious, and in many instances, fatal, consequences'.[1]

The Homoeopathic Mutual Life Office of New York stated publicly that during the period 1870 to 1879, inclusive, it had sold 7927 life-policies to followers of homoeopathy and 2258 to others, and that whereas there had been 84 deaths in the first category (= >1.06%), there had been 66 in the second (= <2.93%). This meant that the claims risk for non-homoeopathic patients was shown to be considerably higher, in fact, precisely by a factor of 2.765 and that this actuarially justified the lower premiums charged to the followers of homoeopathy.[2]

Confidence in homoeopathy had grown to such a degree that from then onward life-insurance companies in the USA began to take on homoeopaths as accredited medical examiners, even though homoeopathy's view on

---

[1] Quoted from *American Homoeopathic Observer*, II (1865), p 288 by Dr Harris Livermore Coulter, medical historian, in his scholarly work *Divided Legacy: A History of the Schism in Medical Thought;* Washington: Wehawken Book Company, 1973, vol III (*Science and Ethics in American Ethics: 1800-1914*), pp 304-305.
[2] Quoted from *Public Opinion*, XXXVI (1879), p 430 by Harris Livermore Coulter, ibid., p 305.

pathology diverged significantly from that of orthodox medicine.[1] It was the profit-motivated life-insurance companies and their actuaries that provided the best assessment, in terms of dispassionate mercenary standards applied in a liberal economic and social environment, to homoeopathic treatment relative to any concurrently competing form of treatment (allopathic, Eclectic, osteopathic). Clearly homoeopathy came out way ahead of the others.

Internalization of Disease

See 'Miasma'.

International Homoeopathic League

Liga Medicorum Homoeopathica Internationalis; founded in 1925 by Dr Pierre Schmidt of Switzerland and Dr J Thuinzing of the Netherlands to provide a forum for homoeopathic practitioners, pharmacists, researchers and other homoeopathic scientists. The League meets at least once biennially. In 1955 it celebrated the bicentenary of Hahnemann's birth with a Jubilee Congress in Stuttgart, FRG, and in 1975 it celebrated its own fiftieth anniversary in Rotterdam, the Netherlands, where the League had originally been inaugurated.

On 12th October 1987 a large number of French homoeopaths, pharmacists, dentists, surgeons and veterinarians, motivated in part through impatience at what was perceived as entrenched scientific inertia, broke with the Liga and formed a rival body, the Organisation Médicale Homéopathique Internationale (International Homoeopathic Medical Organization). They were immediately joined by many non-French homoeopaths, including leading contingents or individual delegates from Argentina, Belgium, Brazil, Canada, India, Italy, Mexico, Portugal, Spain, the UK and the USA, who became founder members (though some of these preferred to retain their Liga membership concurrently). The OMHI, which publishes a journal, held its first international congress in Rome from 27th to 30th April 1988.

International Homoeopathic Medical Organization

See 'International Homoeopathic League', from which it broke away in 1987.

Ionization

Dissociation into ions, occurring when an electrolyte is dissolved in water. To ionize is to form ions by separating atoms, molecules, or radicals, or by adding or subtracting electrons from atoms by weakening the electric attractions in

---

[1]Coulter, Harris Livermore, ibid., p 304.

a liquid, particularly water. Ionization by collision is the removal of one or more electrons from an atom by its collision with another particle (e.g. an a-particle or another electron). The Swedish physicist and chemist, Svante Arrhenius (1859-1927) discovered electrolytic dissociation for which he received the Nobel Prize in 1903. He also studied toxins and antitoxins, antigens and antibodies, wrote the *Textbook of Cosmic Physics* and *Theories of Chemistry*, while also maintaining a lively interest in astrophysics. According to Arrhenius the object of homoeopathic dynamization was to reduce all substances designed for therapeutic use to 'a state of approximately perfect solution or complete ionization, which is fully accomplished only by infinite dilution'.[1] This stimulated the scientific quest in physics to discover whether the pharmacological message was not perhaps carried in the water molecules of the diluent present in all ultramolecular potencies. (See 'Drug Preparation' and 'Potency'.)

Iridology

Study of the markings, lacunae, laminae, fibrae, changes in colour, variations in textural density, irregularities, etc. in a patient's iris during the course of systemic disease. This technique of disease monitoring was originated by the Hungarian Ignaz von Peczely (1826-ca. 1902), an orthodox medical practitioner of Egervar (near Budapest). His first iris chart was only published in 1886 (in Vienna), although for nearly thirty years prior he had painstakingly observed what he called 'nature's record' in the iris. Iridology is not part of homoeopathy, though a few homoeopaths employ it as a diagnostic indicator.

Irritability

Has three meanings:

1 The property of a protoplasm, or nerve, or muscle, enabling it to respond to a stimulus: in fact, an integral component of the homoeopathic response mechanism;
2 The emotional potential of reacting to a stimulus immoderately;
3 The reactive state of tissues in response to trauma or an intrusive attack: being incipient inflammation (refer to this entry and to 'Disease and Drug Action in Homoeopathic Congruity', section 1 Generic Similarity, where the homoeopathic relationship of inflammation to irritant is set out).

   As a symptom component:

   In its second meaning, it is a homoeopathic 'mental'; and in its third meaning, it features in the homoeopathic drugs listed under 'Inflammation'.

[1]Arrhenius, Svante. Quoted by Stuart Close (1860-1929), Professor of Homoeopathic Philosophy at New York Homoeopathic Medical College (1909-1913), in *The Genius of Homoeopathy*, New York: Boericke and Tafel, 1924, p 212.

Examples of syndetic pointers to two homoeopathic medicines, relative to its second meaning:

In the patient with genito-urinary complaints, who is exacting, very irritable, difficult to please and can easily fly into a rage – Lilium tigrinum

A patient who is intensely irritable, then quickly laughs, is very restless and obstinate, suffers from spastic constipation, and has painful, hot, ulcerated patches on the tongue, also on its underside – (in miasma: an anti-psoric of wide range) – Sanicula aqua

Isopathy

● **The use of the 'same' (iso-) instead of the 'similar' (homoeo-) as medicines for curing disease.**

Treatment of disease by means of the presumed exopathic or endopathic causal agent, or by a product of the manifestation of the same disease; also the treatment of a diseased organ or a disturbed function by a non-pathological secretion or excretion from a 'similar' organ, or from the pathognomonically-associated tissue, of a plant or animal, believed to be capable of inducing a reactive state in the patient, although isopathy has never conducted Hahnemannian provings.

Sometimes, inaccurately, also taken to mean the treatment of a diseased organ by an extract made of a similar organ from a healthy animal not thought to be capable of producing a full drug picture in a proving, which is, therefore, never attempted, and which therapeutic approach, properly, is termed 'Organotherapy', for which there is a separate entry.

Isopathy's doctrine is summarized in the dictum: 'Aequalia aequalibus curantur', an unabashed imitation of the formulation of the law of similars. The fact that its remedies have never undergone provings, has made its claims, from the homoeopathic viewpoint, seem unsubstantiated and, hence, unsustainable.

Isopathy occupies a position of considerable ambiguity in homoeopathy. Many homoeopaths, from Hahnemann down, have been nonplussed by what is seen to be its sophistical rationale; yet quite a number of very prominent homoeopaths of recent years have failed to take up a firm position *vis-à-vis* Isopathy, as, for instance, Hans-Heinrich Reckeweg of the FRG and Othon André Julian of France. On the one hand Isopathy has been roundly condemned by some as a self-defeating therapeutic approach which is derived from an illogical oversimplification; yet, on the other, some have hailed it as one of the most fruitful concepts in homoeopathic therapeutics. This, within the context of its history and seen in the light of experimental evidence, is discussed more fully later in this entry.

A representative overview is offered of the areas where, everyone agrees, Isopathy's strong impact has substantially broadened the base of homoeopathy.

There are four classes of remedy that were introduced into homoeopathy thanks, in no small measure, to Isopathy's powerful influence. These are: the nosodes, the sarcodes, the isotherapeutic agents, and the extemporaneously prepared auto-isopathics.

The classified descriptions of a random selection of some of the homoeopathic remedies in these categories will help to exemplify the measure of their considerable influence as a remedy group. Clearly the remedies in the first two categories all have a fully developed drug picture quite like the other remedies in the materia medica of homoeopathy, and, equally, they are not seen as automatically curative (as held by Isopathy) in the diseases from which they were derived. In fact, the clinical evidence of the last one and a half centuries has tended to support this. On the contrary, a principal function of these remedies in homoeopathy is to stimulate a suppressed disease to manifest all its symptoms: a latent chronic miasma can be activated by the corresponding remedial nosode. The situation with regard to the last two categories is not quite as clearly definable in terms of homoeopathy, but is explained in the respective sections below.

1 Nosode

A nosode is a remedy, homoeopathically prepared from disease products, with its own full, distinct drug picture. (In France, and, indeed, practically in the whole francophone area, this word has been officially displaced by the word 'biothérapique', with an unaltered meaning.)

There are nosodes

(i) of plant origin:

Nectarianium (Cancer of trees; nectaria ditissima)
    homoeopathic basis: clinical provings by Bra and Chausse, 1900.
Secale cornutum (Spurred rye; a fungus called ergot)
    homoeopathic basis: toxicological evidence of spurred-rye disease and very extensive clinical provings.
Ustilago maidis (Maize-smuts; basidiomycetes fungus growing on zea mais)
    homoeopathic basis: proved by Roullin, 1830 and re-proved by Burt and Hoyne, 1872.

(ii) of animal origin:

Ambra grisea (Greyish pathological secretion from the intestine of the sperm whale)
    homoeopathic basis: proved by Hahnemann and Count von Gersdorff, 1827.
Hippozaenium (Extract of catarrhal discharge from horse's nares in glanders or farcy)
    homoeopathic basis: clinical provings by Garth Wilkinson and Drysdale, 1873.

Hydrophobinum (or Lyssinum) (Prepared from saliva of a rabid dog)
    homoeopathic basis: proved by Constantin Hering, 1833.

Oscillococcinum (Discovered accidentally during the 1930s by Dr Joseph Roy;
    in a 200CK potency of an autolysate prepared from Barbary duck heart and
    liver [Anas Barbariae hepatis et cordis extractum] containing, it was
    incorrectly thought, a bacterium, oscillococcus, associated with influenza-
    like states; Roy's spurious bacterial theory has some foundation in that his
    belief that game fowl are a prime reservoir for human influenza 'viruses'
    has been proved correct; hence the classification as a nosode rather than
    a sarcode);

homoeopathic basis: its reliability in treating influenza, over some seven
    decades, is the reason that, around 1981, it became, and has since remained,
    the most widely used influenza treatment in the whole of France.
    Homoeopathy could hardly have produced a more impressive, and
    consistent, clinical proving, with success rates in clinical usage reported in
    various population samplings ranging between (approximately) 80 and 90
    per cent, whenever the remedy was taken within 48 hours of the onset of
    disease symptoms. Furthermore, placebo-controlled clinical research has
    been conducted on a significant scale. Patients undergoing treatment with
    antibiotics or anti-inflammatory orthodox drugs were excluded; patients,
    taken at random, were included if they consulted a physician not later than
    48 hours after onset of an influenzal syndrome; patients were classified
    according to the criteria of age, sex, duration of the syndrome, whether
    smoker or non-smoker, and whether or not on self-medication: half received
    Oscillococcinum 200CK and half received a look-alike placebo. On the
    eighth day these patients were reassessed by their physicians. The over-all
    post-treatment account was:

	Oscillococcinum	Placebo
Shivering	85.7%	57.1%
Stiffness	72.5%	41.9%
Rhinorrhoea	44.4%	33.2%
Nocturnal cough	44.8%	31.0%
Diurnal cough	68.4%	34.3%
Fever	79.1%	40.0%

The remainder, making up to 100, is made up of the percentage of the
population which felt that the symptoms had remained unchanged or had
become aggravated. The patients were also asked to make their own assessment
concerning the effectiveness of the treatment:

Treatment considered as:	Oscillococcinum	Placebo
a failure	20%	62%
a success	80%	38%

A mathematical analysis validates, at an elevated degree of significance, this homoeopathic remedy's usefulness in influenzal syndromes, most particularly where fever, shivering and stiffness are concerned. There was a rerun of this experimental assay (refer to Experimental Evidence below).

(iii) of morbific microbial or viral origin:

Lueticum (or Luesinum, Syphilinum) (Spirochaeta pallida in syphilitic chancre exudate)
  homoeopathic basis: original pathogenetic experimentation by Hering 1834, full proving by Swan, 1880.
Tuberculinum Residuum (from filtration of the bovine stock of mycobacterium tuberculosis)
  homoeopathic basis: proved by O A Julian, 1960/61.
Variolinum (trituration of matter from smallpox vesicle; the DNA-poxvirus)
  homoeopathic basis: fragmentarily proved by Fincke and Swan, 1871 and subsequently clinically proved by Fellger on several hundred unvaccinated people and by Compton Burnett, who established that vaccination (i.e. 'inoculation' with the live virus of cowpox) subsequent to the administration of Variolinum 6CH will not easily take, even when such vaccination is repeated: the scratches tend to heal up immediately and do not smart or itch at all. [Perhaps this is a concrete expression of: (i) the homoeopathic stimulus to the production of agglutinins and (ii) the action on the opsonic index that well-indicated homoeopathic remedies have been demonstrated as consistently inducing in patients, by Charles Edwin Wheeler, MD, BS, BSc (1868-1946). These evident immunizant effects seem to have provided the stimulus for the fruitful exploration of other 'isopathic' areas within homoeopathy (such as Bowel Nosodes, Allergen potentization, Auto-isopathics, etc.).]

(iv) of pathological humoral origin [meaning, in disease: from blood, serum, calculi, sputum (especially of bronchorrhoea), squamae and transudate (of eczema, impetigo, etc.), leukorrhoea, smegma, the serous fluid (of ascites and hydrocele), pus and from cerebro-spinal (cephalorrhachidian) fluid, though, in this category, never from the patient's own products]:

Melitagrinum (Squamosa of eczema capitis)
  homoeopathic basis: proved by Skinner, 1893.
Psorinum (Sero-purulent matter of scabies vesicle was used by Hahnemann; the epidermoid efflorescence of pityriasis by Gross [a champion of Isopathy's cause])
  homoeopathic basis: proved by Hahnemann, 1828 and by Griesselich, 1832.
Septicaemium (Attenuations from contents of septic abscess)
  homoeopathic basis: proved by Swan, 1873.

(v) of non-lactose fermenting bowel organisms:
See separate entry under 'Bowel Nosodes'.

2 Sarcode

A sarcode is a remedy, homoeopathically made from preparations, or derivatives, of healthy plant, animal or human secretions, excretions or special ('related') tissue products, with its own full, distinct drug picture. (In France, and, therefore, practically in the whole francophone area, such a dynamized remedy is referred to as an 'opothérapique', or, where hormonal secretions are used, as an 'hormonothérapique', occasionally, somewhat loosely, as an 'organothérapique', although the latter, strictly speaking, designates a substance used in 'Organotherapy' (see this entry); this last-mentioned therapeutic approach, however, is not Isopathy.

There are sarcodes

(i) of plant origin:

Guaiacum (Gum resin of lignum vitae)
   homoeopathic basis: proved by Hahnemann, Hartmann, Langhammer and Tenthorn, 1828).
Terebinthina (Oleic exudation of pine trees)
   homoeopathic basis: proved by Hartlaub and Trinks, 1824).

The many proven alkaloidal, glycosidal, saponinate and similar plant extracts in the materia medica fall into this category too (see 'Alkaloid').

(ii) of animal, or human, origin:

Acidum deoxyribonucleicum (DNA)
   homoeopathic basis: placebo-controlled proving by O A Julian, 1970/72.
Acidum ribonucleicum (RNA)
   homoeopathic basis: placebo-controlled proving by O A Julian, 1970/72.
Acidum sarcolacticum (Does not exist independently: is the dextro-rotary isomer of lactic acid in the muscular fluids)
   homoeopathic basis: proved by W Griggs of the Hering Laboratory, Philadelphia, 1940.
Adrenalinum (Trituration or tincture of neurohormone of the medulla of the human glandula suprarenalis)
   homoeopathic basis: proved by the students of the New York Homoeopathic College under the direction of Dr V L Getman, 1904.
Calcarea carbonica (or Calcarea ostrearum) (Trituration of the middle layer of oyster shells)
   homoeopathic basis: proved by Hahnemann, 1826.
Cervus campestris (Trituration of the fresh hide and hair of the Brazilian Deer)
   homoeopathic basis: proved by Mure, 1890.
Cholesterinum (Trituration of cholesterin)
   homoeopathic basis: the joint work of Wilhelm Ameke, Compton Burnett,

Swan and Yingling, spanning four decades, produced the full drug picture by 1908.

Colostrum (First mammary secretion after childbirth)
homoeopathic basis: clinical proving by Bell, 1893.

Corticotrophinum (A.C.T.H. or adrenocorticotrophic hormone, a hormonal polypeptide, containing 39 amino acids, obtained from the anterior lobe of the porcine hypophysis, where it is formed in the basophil cells)
homoeopathic basis: proved by Templeton, 1952/53.

Folliculinum (Oestrone; the natural hormone secreted by the ovaries)
homoeopathic basis: extensive clinical provings by De Mattos, 1955/63 and very significant experimental work, described in detail at the end of the entry under 'Constitutional Type'.

Helix tosta (Trituration of toasted snail, i.e. of the molluscous body without the calcareous shell)
homoeopathic basis: clinical proving by W H Leonard, 1898.

Lac felinum (Cat's milk)
homoeopathic basis: pathogenetic experiments by Swan, 1893.

Pepsinum (Proteolytic ferment found in the gastric juice)
homoeopathic basis: clinical provings, quoted by Clarke, 1900.

Pulmo vulpis (Trituration of fox's lung)
homoeopathic basis: clinical proving by Eduard von Grauvogl, 1877.

Pyrogenium (some authorities prefer Pyrexin, since it is not a mere fever-producer, as Pyrogenium signifies; also known as Sepsin) (A product of chopped lean beef in water that was allowed to stand and decompose in the sun for 18 days)
homoeopathic basis: introduced by Drysdale, 1880; its use was greatly propagated by Compton Burnett's publication of 'Pyrogenium in Fevers and Blood-poisoning' in 1888; it was eventually proved by Sherbino, 1894.

Saccharum lactis (Milk-sugar; lactose)
homoeopathic basis: proved by Swan, 1892. Hahnemann chose Saccharum lactis as the chief vehicle of homoeopathic remedies, because it is the most nearly inert substance he could find. But experience and pathogenetic experimentation have shown that no substance is absolutely inert, whether attenuated (dynamized) or not. In other words, homoeopathy maintains that there is no such thing as an absolute placebo. In placebo-controlled clinical trials, the use of, say, Saccharum lactis is, therefore, regarded as a relative placebo.

Thyroidinum (Tincture prepared from entire thyroid gland)
homoeopathic basis: Original provings in 1962 by S K Gosh of Calcutta; double blind provings by Panos, Rogers and Stephenson under the auspices of the Research Committee of the American Institute of Homoeopathy, 1963/64.

Urea (Carbamide; the chief solid [white, crystalline] constituent of the urine of mammals)
homoeopathic basis: clinical proving by Prof Mauthner, 1854 and

subsequently by Compton Burnett.

All the potentized ophio-toxins (venomous secretions of snakes) as well as all other comparable remedies, based on animal-secretions (collectively, of porcupines, insects, arachnids, molluscs [besides the snail] and sea-dwellers [additionally to oyster shells]) also belong into this category of homoeopathic drug.

3 Isotherapeutic Agents

These are homoeopathized allopathica and homoeopathized hazardous industrial substances, as well as potentized allergens.

There are:

(i) Homoeopathized Allopathica (Tautopathics):

(See separate entry under this, and also refer to 'Tautopathy'.) These are homoeopathic remedies made from toxic medicines, to be used either to stimulate a chronic iatrogenic disease condition (a category of chronic miasma) to manifest all its symptoms, or simply in the standard homoeopathic manner of total disease-to-drug symptom similarity. The most frequently prescribed of the recently-proven homoeopathized allopathica with full, established drug pictures, generally elicited in placebo-controlled pathogenetic experiments, are:

BCG (Bacillus Calmette-Guerin vaccine, VAB, Vaccin Attenué Bilie)
Chloramphenicol
Chlorpromazinum
Corticotrophinum (A.C.T.H.)
Cortisonum and the Corticoids
Haloperidolum
Levomepromazinum
Maleatum of Perhexilinum (Pexidum)
Penicillinum
Phenobarbitalum
Sulfanilamidum
Sulfonamidum
Thioproperazinum

(ii) Homoeopathized Hazardous Industrial Substances:

Because any of these may bring about a reactive disease state and may even cause a chronic miasma to develop, what was said under Homoeopathized Allopathica above applies, *mutatis mutandis,* in this sub-section. A good many of these substances have full, established drug pictures of long standing, such as Iodium (proved by Hahnemann) or Niccolum (proved by Nenning). A pertinent discussion of the issues involved here will be found under Dermatitis Medicamentosa in 'Epistemological Assumptions in Homoeopathy', section 1.

(iii) Potentized Allergens:

Acarus Scabiei, the itch mite, has been medically implicated in 'scabies' since 1683, when a physician of Leghorn, Italy, described how slaves there carefully removed them from each other's skin, using needles. Linnaeus and Wichmann also drew attention to this mite some time before Samuel Hahnemann formulated the fundamentals of the homoeopathic concept as such.[1] Hahnemann was well aware of the existence of this itch mite when he described psora (a general term used in his time to denote a whole series of diverse skin ailments). Psora, according to Hahnemann, is a constitutional defect produced by the suppression of itching skin manifestations, leading to an interference with that organism's reactive force and the consequent production of chronic disease. His prime anti-psoric remedy is Sulphur, but he was also among the first to prove Psorinum, being potentized sero-purulent matter from the scabies vesicle (a Nosode of Pathological Humoral Origin, in section 1(iv).) Once again Hahnemann's unfailing intuition seems to have guided him, because two close relatives of Acarus Scabiei are the dandruff eating house-dust mite, Dermatophagoides Pteronyssinus, and its cousin, the flour-product consuming house-dust mite, Dermatophagoides Farinae. Both of these are important sensitizing components of house-dust, clearly implicated in the aetiology of some types of allergic rhinitis, eczema, bronchial asthma and a number of other disease conditions, and, quite like Psorinum, dynamized Dermatophagoides Pteronyssinus (or house dust mite) has become a homoeopathic remedy. It is not an Isopathic, but a homoeopathic, remedy for the same reasons set out by Hahnemann relative to Psorinum.[2] In the same manner and for similar reasons air-borne pollen have been potentized, since these are implicated in seasonal hayfever. For both these homoeopathic remedies good experimental work has been done in Scotland, at the Glasgow Homoeopathic Hospital in the 1970s and 1980s. Countless other allergens, besides, have been prepared as homoeopathic remedies along identical lines.

4 Auto-isopathics

These are ad hoc dynamizations extemporaneously prepared from the same patient's own products, such as blood, calculi, cephalorrhachidian (cerebro-spinal) fluid, excretions, extravascular fluid, exudates, hair (crinis), liquor amnii, lymph, menstruum, pus, secretions, seminal fluid, serum, smegma, sputum, squamae, synovia, tissues, toe- or fingernails (onyx, unguis), transudates, ventricular fluid or urine. This must remain an experimental area in homoeopathy, because obviously no provings are possible. The rationale underlying the use of these patient-own remedies is, that in these various

---

[1] Ameke, Wilhelm. *History of Homoeopathy: Its Origins and Conflicts,* originally published in German in Berlin, 1884, English rendering, London: Gould, 1885, p 69.
[2] Hahnemann, Christian Friedrich Samuel. *The Chronic Diseases, Their Peculiar Nature and Their Homoeopathic Cure,* translated from the second enlarged German Edition, 1835, Philadelphia: Boericke and Tafel, 1904, p 152.

secretions, excretions, fluids and tissues, there are very likely to be the body's own antidotal agents, similar in reactive potential to the disease, by which they were overwhelmed. With potentization (dynamization) their particular character will become enhanced (though they cannot become stronger) and that fact alone may give the organism a second chance to beat off the disease.

On pages 1480-1482, volume III of *A Dictionary of Practical Materia Medica* John Henry Clarke, MD (Holsworthy, Devon: Health Science Press, 1977) lists some evidence for Urinum (potentized patient-own urine) as a homoeopathic remedial agent, adding that 'urinotherapy is practically as old as man himself', and suggesting that 'the symptoms of uraemia may be taken as a pathogenesis of Urinum'. Evidence from the thirteen case-books in which Hahnemann's treatment of patients in Paris during the last eight years of his life are recorded, makes it clear that he used a remedy that he called 'Auto' at fairly regular intervals which seems to have been an *ad hoc* dynamization of an auto-isopathic psorinum, which, by virtue of potentization had an altered state and was no longer idem but really a simillimum, as he maintained for quite a long time (see footnote 5 to section 56 in the fifth edition of the *Organon*).

History of Isopathy

Before its full emergence under homoeopathy's aegis, Isopathy has a proto-history. There is the age-old urinotherapy referred to in the preceding paragraph. In Chinese Medicine preventive variolization was achieved, over centuries, by using the powder of the dried smallpox pustules as snuff. Amerind Folk Medicine in Columbia has, also for centuries, successfully used the macerated liver of a venomous snake as an 'anti-venom serum' for that snake's poisonous bite. Pliny the Elder (ca. 23-79 AD) in his scientific encyclopaedia *Natural History* stated, *inter alia,* that the saliva of a rabid dog, if taken in drink, will guard against rabies. Dioskorides Pedanios (first century AD), in his *De Materia Medica,* regarded as authoritative for sixteen centuries, said, 'where the disease is, there is the remedy' and recommended, among such other things, the application of crushed scorpion precisely where the scorpion had stung. Paracelsus (1493-1541), for example, recommended Fel Tauri (bull's bile) for hepatic cirrhosis. Oswald Croll, in *La Chimie Royale et Pratique* (French version, Paris, 1633) described as unfailingly curative for excessive menstrual bleeding, 3 or 4 drops of the same blood (always the most clear blood, he advised) given to the patient to drink – without her knowledge, though. Robert Fludd, called the Researching Jesuit of Ireland, writes in his *Philosophia Moysaica* (Goudae, 1638 p 149), ' . . .the worms eliminated by the organism, dried and powdered and given internally, destroy the worms. The sputum of a patient suffering from phthisis cures, after appropriate [spagyric method of] preparation, phthisis. The spleen of man, having undergone a particular [spagyric] preparation, is a remedy against an enlarged spleen. The stone formed in the bladder and in the kidney cure and dissolve such a stone.' A few years later Athanasius Kircher, in his work *Magna Sive De Arte Magnetica* writes, '. . . the spider's bite will be cured by the application of a spider, the scorpion's sting by the application of the scorpion, the poison of a rabid dog is drawn out of the body by the fur of the same dog.' (The English saying about 'the hair of the dog that bit' stems from Kircher.) In his treatise on poisons (*In Mundus Subterraneus,* Amsterdam, 1645) Kircher affirms: 'Ubi morbus, ibi etiam medicamentum morbillis opportunam' (where the disease is, there also is its proper remedy). In the same century, Lady Montague, wife of the English ambassador to the Ottoman Empire, had her child inoculated in Istanbul (Constantinople) by the extract of variolic pus. Prof Phillipus Netter of the Doge Republic of Venice in 1718, in his *Fundamenta Theoretica Medicinae Agentis* (vol II, p 646) wrote that he used the dry pus of a plague bubo for the treatment of bubonic plague. Francis Home of Edinburgh, Scotland, in his *Homoeo-medical Facts and Experiments* (London, 1754) told how he used the blood of a patient suffering from measles against that disease. Of course, Edward Jenner (1749-1823) was well aware of these developments, when 42 years later (in 1796) he began his variolizations with live cowpox vaccinations and arm-to-arm inoculations with lymph vaccine.

It is evident that Isopathy, as a medical method, reaches back into antiquity and was very widely known. In no sense can it be held that it was only a whimsical deviation from the homoeopathic norm. It was, however, only in the 1830s, after homoeopathy had been successfully established, that Isopathy made a concerted attempt to usurp homoeopathy's position as the new total medico-philosophical system, ready to displace existing medical orthodoxy.

Jenner's vaccination showed that cowpox (the artificial disease) was able to protect beforehand from smallpox (the real disease, whenever that might strike). It was the homoeopathic principle in action: in the eyes of many, homoeopathy was seen to be triumphantly effective. However, it was too dangerous a technique. Many died from Jenner's inoculations, because these infected them with fatal cases of cowpox as well as with other serious diseases, most often syphilis, either from the serum or from the non-sanitary instruments employed. Constantin Hering (1800-1880) began to look for ways to replace Jenner's cowpox vaccination. He was quite aware that Jenner operated within the law of similars and that vaccination was not an Isopathic treatment 'per aequale'.

Hering did valuable experimental work, from 1828, on the pathogenetic effects of snake venoms, demonstrating, for instance, that the 1CH potency of (Trigonocephalus) Lachesis produced a set of symptoms similar to those produced by the snake's bite, yet milder in degree. He decided that it was worth experimentally investigating the age-old claims concerning the benefits of using a rabid dog's saliva (in 1833), or material from smallpox scabs and many venoms and other disease products. In each case he conducted proper pathogenetic experiments (provings) that produced full drug pictures. In doing this experimental work Hering became the precursor of men like von Behring, Niehans, Koch and Pasteur, but he also provided the initial spark for the Isopathic euphoria which immediately followed.

The homoeopathic veterinarian Johan Joseph Wilhelm Lux (1776-1849), editor of the review *Zooaiasis* (the first veterinary periodical devoted to homoeopathic treatment of animals), who had done so much for homoeopathy since 1823, published his *Isopathik der Contagionen* (Isopathy of Contagions, Leipzig: Christian Heinz Kollmann, 1833). In it he explained how he came to be convinced of Isopathy's efficacy. The boss of the Hungarian Agricultural Society of Raab (now Györ) in the Dual Monarchy had asked him by letter for the best homoeopathic medicine against Lues bovum pestifera (rinderpest, German Löserdürre) and against Anthrax (infectious splenic fever, German Milzbrand). Because Lux did not yet know the specific homoeopathic remedies for these veterinary epidemics, and because he did not want to leave homoeopathy open to the charge of fragmentariness, he wrote back, 'All contagions carry, in their substance even, the means of their cure.' He then advised that a dynamized drop of blood from the cow infected with anthrax and a potentized drop of nasal mucus from the cow with rinderpest be administered to the respective animal patients, although he had never yet performed such veterinary experiments before. At that moment modern Isopathy sprang to life, with Lux regarded as its originator. Others soon followed. In *Isopathik der Contagionen* he set forth the principle 'Aequalia aequalibus curentur'; he called for the dynamization of the 'known' morbific agents (e.g. scab in sheep; tinea galli – a fungal infection involving chiefly the combs of turkeys and chickens; tinea in other animals; scabies of man; the pus of syphilis; the blood of the spleen of animals suffering from anthrax; the fluid taken out of the vesicles of Marochetti in hydrophobia; the faecal contagion of cholera; the lymph of plague; etc.) and for the potentization of all sorts of excretions and secretions of man and animals (e.g. bladder stones; faecal matter; the sweat of feet; saliva of epileptics, etc.). The most ardent supporters of Lux and Isopathy, who were also men of influence, were six doctors:

Attomyr (Pressburg, Austria [now Bratislava, CSFR]), physician-in-ordinary to Margrave Czakyf von Lentschau;

Gross (Leipzig, Saxony), one of Hahnemann's original group of Drug Provers and from 1836 co-publisher with Stapf of what since 1822 had been the first homoeopathic periodical, *Archiv für die homöopathische Heilkunst;*

Herrmann (Salzburg, Austria), homoeopath who wrote persuasively in the *Allgemeine Homöopathische Zeitung* about the 'medicinal power of substances of homonymous organs' (1844, vol XXVII, p 187) and published *Die wahre Isopathie* (The true Isopathy, Augsburg, 1848);

Jolly (Istanbul, Ottoman Empire), homoeopathic dentist;

Theuille (Moscow, Russia), a homoeopath who 'isopathized' leprosy and bubonic plague there, claiming in the *Archiv* (1837, vol VI, p 102) to have obtained numerous cases of cure;

Weber (Kassel, Hessen), homoeopathic veterinarian and councillor in the Court of Hessen; he published *Der Milzbrand, und dessen sicherstes Heilmittel* (Anthrax, and its surest Remedy, Leipzig: Reclam, 1836); he had trials, supervised by the Hessen health authorities (where he was a senior figure himself), in which Isopathic treatment of anthrax was compared to the orthodox veterinary treatment of the day: the latter came off rather badly.

These men, in turn, were followed by many others. There was a flood of books and professional articles about Isopathy. Eventually, many years later, this culminated in a book on Isopathic 'pharmacology' (see below).

Doctrinal pronouncements on Isopathy were:

'To cure a diseased organism, it is necessary that the organism be not universally ill, that there are still some parts that are healthy, and that one uses then an identical or analogous morbid agent, but in a relatively minuscule dose, to induce in the healthy parts of that organism some reactive powers, mediated by the nervous and circulatory systems, in order to stimulate a reversal in the diseased part, and to assist with the disburdening of . . . the morbid agent.' (Dr Denys Collet, a Dominican priest-doctor)

'The Isopathic medicines represent the simillimum par excellence, the faithful image of the morbid state of the moment and they may be successful where homoeopathy hesitates or fails even with the exact medicine. It is a powerful adjuvant of a well-conducted homoeopathic treatment. The possibilities of the Isopathic method exceed what is generally thought possible. An Isopathic medicine is a perfect image of the individual who has supplied its stock, that is to say, it contains the simillimum of which any materia medica cannot furnish the equivalent by the application of the law of similars.' (Dr G Dano)

Dr H Hager published a book in Germany (Ernst Günther, 1861):

Medicamenta Homoeopathica et Isopathica Omnia ad id tempus a medicis aut examinata aut usu recepta

This book lists many of the possible Isopathic preparations in use by then. Here is a very small representative selection:

Albinum: white excrements of constipated dog
  (for such a constipated pet)
Alveolinum: pus of dental alveolus
  (for infected empty tooth sockets, after extraction)
Balanorrhinum: mucilagenous fluid secreted in gonorrhoea from the penis
  (for gonorrhoea)
Boviluinum: mucous fluid flowing from nose and throat of cattle during
  rinderpest
  (for rinderpest)
Brossulinum: syphilitic exudate – pus of chancroid ulcer
  (for syphilis)
Cholelithinum: biliary calculus
  (for gall stone)
Condylominum: total condyloma
  (for condylomata)
Helinum: foot corn
  (for foot corn)
Humaninum: human stool
  (for whatever is abnormal about the patient's stool)

Lachryminum: tears
  (for grave conjunctivitis)
Leukorrhinum: abnormal vaginal discharge
  (for abnormal vaginal discharge)
Mastocarcinominum: pus of breast cancer
  (for breast cancer), etc.

Hahnemann, at first, adopted a benignly ambivalent attitude to Isopathy. In 1833, in the fifth edition of the *Organon,* in footnote 5 to Section 56 he wrote: 'A fourth mode of employing medicines in diseases has been attempted to be created by means of Isopathy, as it is called – that is to say, a method of curing a given disease by the same contagious principle that produces it. But even granting that this could be done, which would certainly be a most valuable discovery, yet, after all, seeing that the virus is given to the patient highly potentized, and thereby, consequently, to a certain degree in an altered condition, the cure is effected only by opposing a simillimum to a simillimum.' However, by 1842 (when he compiled the sixth edition of the *Organon*) he had become adverse to it, as is clear from the altered, and much longer, footnote (renumbered as 63). Since this edition did not appear until 1921 it cannot have contributed to the decline of Isopathy during the nineteenth century. The substance of this footnote is discussed under 'Epistemological Assumptions in Homoeopathy', section 1 (in the paragraph before the Collation on Dermatitis Medicamentosa).

But Isopathy also met with outspoken antagonism among the homoeopathic elite. Johan Ernst Stapf, the co-editor (with Gross) of the *Archiv für die homöopathische Heilkunst,* and its founder in 1822, as well as having been its able sole editor from then for fourteen years, was the first to point out the crucial differences between a homoeopathic nosode and an auto-isopathic preparation.

Dr Auguste Rapou attacked Isopathy strongly in his *Histoire de la Doctrine Médicale Homéopathique* (History of the Medical Doctrine of Homoeopathy, 2 volumes, Paris: Bailliere, 1847, pp 176 and 203).

Genke, a homoeopathic veterinarian, is quoted by Dr P W Ludwig Griesselich in his *Handbuch zur kritischen Studie der Homöopathie* (Manual for the Critical Study of Homoeopathy, French rendering, Paris: Bailliere, 1848). He pointed out that, from experience, prolonged and repeated trituration would destroy rather than enhance any of the properties of most normal contagions. Griesselich, himself a man of pronounced individuality, unintimidated courage and a very agile mind, though not averse to sarcodes and nosodes (he used Psorinum homoeopathically), openly condemned Isopathy in *Hygea,* the periodical he edited from 1834 to 1848 (vol III, p 327): 'What is called Isopathy in recent times . . . is only a subject of confusion, a superficial analogy [that is] incomprehensible.' And further on: 'A development of that question seems to us absolutely superfluous. Mere audacious opinion raised to a law based on misconception does not deserve to be aired publicly, rather, it is fitting that one should guard oneself against such an abominable madness. The positive facts that serve as foundation for Isopathy are small in number and are all easily brought back to the principle of homoeopathy.' Such was the influence of Griesselich over his contemporaries, that this man's judgement, more than anything else, decided the fate of Isopathy as an independent medical system. It faded and soon blended into the general background of homoeopathy where it has remained since, though not without continuing to exert profound influence. Notable examples of this are: the serum therapy of Emil A von Behring (Nobel laureate 1901 for this), the fresh cell therapy of Prof Paul Niehans (appointed Professor at the Vatican's Pontifical Academy for this, 1954, to succeed Sir Alexander Fleming), the tuberculin preparation used in the diagnosis and treatment of tuberculosis by Robert Koch (Nobel laureate 1905 for this), and, perhaps most striking of all, Louis Pasteur's method of veterinary immunization: against anthrax with an attenuated anthrax bacillus culture (from 1877) and against hydrophobia with an attenuated rabies virus in a suspension (of dried infected rabbit's spinal cord) (from 1882). These men owe an immense (usually unacknowledged) debt to the Isopathic pioneers in homoeopathy of at least half a century earlier, as well as to the continuing clinical evidence of sarcodes and nosodes, both in homoeopathic veterinary and in homoeopathic human medicine.

In the twentieth century, when Isopathy experienced a vigorous revival to its present semi-autonomous status within homoeopathy once more, the main developments, briefly, were:

Fr (Dr) D Collet published *Isopathie* (Paris: Balliere, 1898): 'If the real medicine should be an agent that is similar to that of the disease, nothing is more similar to the agent of the disease than the agent itself.'

Dr L Kruger (of Nimes) published *Isopathic and Harmonic Therapeutics: Viruses and Venoms as Internal Remedies* [title anglicized] (Paris: Balliere, 1899).

Dr Antoine Nebel (of Lausanne) conducted a full pathogenetic experiment (proving) on Robert Koch's tuberculin preparation, in 1901.

The Dean of the Hering Medical College and Hospital, Chicago, USA and its Professor of Materia Medica, Henry C Allen, published *The Materia Medica of the Nosodes* (Philadelphia: Boericke and Tafel, 1910; 576 pp).

Dr Leon Vannier launched the monthly journal *L'Homéopathie Française* in 1912 and from the very first issue regularly promoted Isopathy, referred to by him as Isotherapy. He strongly favoured the use of auto-isopathics in homoeopathy and linked the constitutional (morphological) types, as classified by his mentor, Antoine Nebel (see 'Constitutional Type'), to specific nosodes. Similarly with the chronic miasmata: the Hahnemannian specific remedies tended to be replaced by specific nosodes (see 'Miasma') by him:

Chronic Miasmata	Hahnemannian	Nosode
Psoric Miasma	Sulphur	Psorinum
Sycotic Miasma	Thuja occidentalis	Medorrhinum
Luetic Miasma	Mercurius	Lueticum

Chronic Miasmata	Hahnemannian	Nosode
Tuberculinic Miasma	Calcarea carbonica	Tuberculinum
	or Phosphorus	of one or
	or Stannum	other variety

From 1927 Vannier used what he called Sanguineous Autotherapy, meaning treatment with auto-isopathics made from the patient's own blood stock. He published *Deux Années de Pratique Isothérapique* (Two Years of Isotherapeutic Practice, bulletin of Société d'Homéothérapie de France, 1929) and L'Autothérapie Sanguine (Sanguineous Autotherapy, bulletin of le Centre Homéopathique de France, 1936, 2nd fascicle, p 584).

Dr Jules Roy published *Les Règles de l'Isothérapie Sanguine* (The Rules Governing Sanguineous Isotherapy, bulletin of Laboratoires Homéopathiques de France, 1929, p 135): 'Isopathia Homoeopathia Maxima Est' (Isopathy is the Foremost Homoeopathy, he wrote in *L'Homéopathie Française*, 1928, p 259).

Dr J M Munoz conducted a very interesting study on 'The Modification of Parameters of Patients' Blood through Isotherapy and the Use of Homoeopathic Medicines' (published in *La Revue Française d'Homéopathie*, 1933, vol IX, p 516).

Dr S Fortier-Bernoville conducted a systematic enquiry on the use of sarcodes, nosodes and auto-isopathics by homoeopaths in France. The result was: all homoeopaths were found to use sarcodes and nosodes; while almost half of them used auto-isopathics (*L'Homéopathie Moderne*, 1936, nos. 4 & 6).

Fortier-Bernoville himself extolled Artificial Phlyctenular Autotherapy [phlyctenae are small blisters, such as are made by first degree burns]; he would artificially provoke a phlyctenous eruption with cantharidin paste, and then draw that patient's auto-isopathic stock from the resulting phlyctenula (nodule of lymphoid cells with an ulcerated apex); he anecdotally reported cures with this method of auto-isopathic treatment in cases of Parkinson's disease, multiple sclerosis, herpes zoster, migraine and rheumatoid arthritis.

From then on there has been an ever-increasing interest in the francophone area in auto-isopathics: gastric juices in gastritis; leukorrhoea in metritis; venous blood in migraine; 1st-day menstrual blood in hypermenorrhoea and metrorrhoea; and much else began to be generally used. Curiously, some doctors even began to employ auto-isopathics in complex form, where several of the patient's own products are (redundantly?) combined.

Dr P Brotteaux published *L'Homéopathie et l'Isopathie* (Paris: Peyronnet, 1947) wherein the second section of the book is devoted to Isopathy, which, he said, is the culmination of the search for the true simillimum in homoeopathy ('Facts superabundantly prove that the real law is that of identity, the law of similars is a mere approximation' and elsewhere he stated that 'Homoeopathy is an approximation of Isopathy'); failures in Isopathic treatments, he expounded, do not invalidate the Isopathic principle, but point to the fact that the necessary antidotal component is sometimes absent in the secreta and other disease products used as stock, possibly due to the organism's efforts to react to other noxious stimuli such as anaesthetics, toxic medicines, coffee, alcohol, cocoa, analgesics, nicotine, etc.

Dr Pierre Schmidt, co-founder of the Homoeopathic League in 1925, in his translation from German to French of the sixth edition of *The Organon,* in 1952, defined the Isopathic remedies there as follows (Glossary, p 20): 'Application of an attenuated dose of a pathogenous product for curing the disease of which it is the result. If it is used after having been experimented with on healthy humans, it becomes a homoeopathic Nosode.'

Dr Othon André Julian published *Materia Medica der Nosoden* (Ulm: Karl F Haug Verlag, 1960 [only in 1962 did an edited French version of it appear in the author's home country]), which gave this section of homoeopathy a considerable impetus in the German-speaking area. The homoeopaths Reinhold Voll and Helmut Schimmel relied heavily on it in their electro-acupuncture and electro-organometry procedures (see 'Bio-Electronic Regulatory Medicine'), as did the homoeopath Hans-Heinrich Reckeweg for his antihomotoxic therapy (see 'Homotoxicosis'). All of them made very extensive use of sarcodes, nosodes and isotherapeutic agents, and they developed a big following, also outside the borders of the FRG, particularly with the publications of *Medikamententestung, Nosodentherapie und Mesenchymentschlakungstherapie* by R Voll, 1965 and *Ordinatio Antihomotoxica et Materia Medica* by Hans-Heinrich Reckeweg, 1974, which meant that these remedies were suddenly in very big demand.

Similarly, the increasing use of auto-isopathics spread beyond the francophone area. Dr R Parrot published the authoritative *Isothérapie dans sa Forme Individuelle* (Individual Isotherapy, Paris: Doins, 1967) which materially contributed to that spread, by competently updating his readers on the state-of-the-art in auto-isopathics.

Dr O A Julian published the English version of his *Treatise of Dynamized Micro-Immunotherapy* [term coined by him to describe, collectively, the entire Isopathic therapeutic section within homoeopathy] (poorly translated from the original French; first Indian edition, New Delhi: Jain Publishing Co, 1980).

Leslie J Speight published *Homoeopathy and Immunization* (Saffron Walden: Health Science Press, 1982) in which the following are, primarily, recommended as prophylactic homoeopathic medicines:

Varicella against Chicken Pox
Diphtherinum against Diphtheria
Rubella against German Measles
Influenzinum against Influenza
Morbillinum against Measles
Parotidinum against Mumps
Scarlatinum against Scarlet Fever
Variolinum or Malandrinum against Smallpox
Typhoidinum against Typhoid Fever
Pertussinum (Coqueluchinum) against Whooping Cough

Kathleen Priestman edited unpublished notes by Douglas Borland under the title *Homoeopathy in Practice* (Beaconsfield: Beaconsfield Publishers Ltd, 1982) where chapter 14 deals with 'The Use of Four Nosodes' – Lueticum (Syphilinum), Medorrhinum, Psorinum and Tuberculinum.

Donald Foubister in *Tutorials on Homoeopathy* (Beaconsfield: Beaconsfield Publishers Ltd, 1989) on pages 91 to 109 covers Scirrhinum and some Carcinosinum varieties [he had previously published his proving of Carcinosinum in 1958]; on pages 139 and 140 is a report of his pilot trial of the 'Osteoarthritic Nosode'.

To meet a steeply rising demand, the following eight homoeopathic pharmaceutical concerns, though not the only ones by any means, became the big suppliers of sarcodes, nosodes and isotherapeutic agents, most of whom would also dynamize any substance for a homoeopathic practitioner (for specific isotherapeutic, or ad hoc auto-isopathic, use):

Biologische Heilmittel Heel GmbH
Postfach 729,
D-7570 Baden-Baden,
Germany

Laboratoires Dolisos
62 rue Beaubourg,
F-75003 Paris,
France

Laboratoires Boiron
20 rue de la Libération,
F-69110 Sainte-Foy-lés-Lyon,
France

A Nelson & Co Limited,
5 Endeavour Way,
Wimbledon,
London SW19 9UH
UK

Pascoe Pharmazeutische Präparate GmbH
D-6300 Giessen,
Germany

Staufen-Pharma GmbH
D-7320 Göppingen,
Germany

Wala-Heilmittel GmbH
D-7325 Eckwälden, Bad Boll,
Germany.

Serocytotherapy – a Self-Contained Approach

The only branch of Isopathy that has not been properly reabsorbed into homoeopathy is so-called Serocytotherapy. This derivative of Isopathy was originated by Dr Jean Thomas (1902-1977), who first experimented in the early 1930s in Columbia with an analogue to the Bacillus Calmette-Guerin 'Vaccine' (BCG). Intradermal injections of this in lepromatous patients produced a dermal reaction histologically similar to that of leprosy, whereas similar injections in tuberculin-negative healthy children produced a picture characteristic of tuberculosis. The possibility of detecting by this means the presence of active leprosy in the early stages suggested itself to him and also the possible value of 'vaccination' in determining the effectiveness of treatment, because after intensive and successful therapy the characteristic lesion would not develop at the site of Thomas' 'inoculation' (all this was reconfirmed nearly a quarter of a century later by other researchers: *Arch. Derm. Syph.*, Chicago, 1954, vol LXX, p 631 and *Trop. Dis. Bull.*, 1955, vol LII, p 274). His outstanding scientific work led to this Frenchman being awarded the Chair of Pathological Anatomy at the University of Cartagena, in Bolivar, Columbia.

Some years later he joined his mentor, Prof Hibert, to become Head of the Laboratory of the Sacred Heart Hospital in Shanghai, China. Here he experimented with isoserum treatment first of all, but he also investigated the effects of using immune-antisera produced in horses specifically in reaction to ground and homogenized tissue cultures that had been injected into the horses. He might take cells from a cancerous cervix, inject these into a horse repeatedly over a period of time, where they induced the production of antibodies; he would then find that the 'anti-cancerous-cervix' anti-serum impeded the proliferation of certain malignant cells in a culture medium. His experiments with healthy tissue yielded similar results. For instance, an 'anti-human-skin' anti-serum he later found assisted in intensive care for patients who were badly burnt. Moreover, it had a clearly favourable effect on the evolution of skin grafts. Later the various anti-sera were lyophilized (freeze-dried) and homoeopathically dynamized (to a low potency) by the originator's son, Pascal Thomas of Lausanne, Switzerland.

These anti-sera potencies are administered either in the form of suppositories or injectables. Controlled experiments have shown that these dynamized anti-sera are both safe and therapeutically effective, particularly in the fields of rheumatology and immunology. Despite this anti-sera potencies have so far not been accepted by the vast majority of homoeopaths into their armamentarium, largely because unfounded claims were unfortunately made by some practitioners to the effect that Serocytotherapy is a rejuvenating and/or sexually revitalizing treatment. Since 1976 a sixty-four page scientific journal appears each month under the title *Cytobiological Review* (Ott-Verlag, Thun, Switzerland) devoted to this area of schismatic homoeopathy, cellular research and to Organotherapy (see entry under the last mentioned).

Experimental Evidence

Homoeopathy seems to accept the concept that some undefined component with an assumed dynamically antidotal effect is very probably present in a patient's disease products, and, with obvious modifications, has brought Isopathy's doctrinaire claims back on to a more sound scientific basis within homoeopathy.

The two experiments summarized under 'Constitutional Type' serve to demonstrate the effectiveness of isotherapeutic agents; precisely the same can be said of the third and fourth experiments given under 'Lithotherapy'.

O A Julian took conditioned rats and established that a certain ponderable dose of Thuja occidentalis perturbed the psychic equilibrium of these animals, in that they were shown to have lost their conditioning. However, those rats that had a dose of Thuja occidentalis 9CH administered had their psychic equilibrium re-established together with the restoration of their conditioning.

Prof A Cier, Dr Pharm Jean Boiron and Miss C Vingert published 'Effets preventifs d'Histamine 7CH et de Poumon Histamine 7CH sur les souris sensibilisées par Haemophilus Pertussis' (*Annales Homéopathiques Françaises*, 1968, p 180 ff). Sensitization of mice to the gram-negative bacterium Haemophilus Influenzae-Murium were used to determine the preventive effect induced by Histaminum 7CH and Pneumo-Histaminum 7CH (the latter obtained from bronchial smooth muscle). In vivo, a real protective effect was observed in that there was tolerance to the serous dispersal of histamine, identical with that observed in the non-sensitized controls. Examinations in vitro seemed to show that there was a difference between Histaminum 7CH and Pneumo-Histaminum 7CH in that the latter showed activity whereas the former did not appear to do so.

Prof G Netien, Dr Pharm J Boiron and A Marin carried out a very successful series of experiments demonstrating the effect of potencies of Cuprum Sulphuricum 15CH on the growth of plants previously poisoned by copper sulphate. (*British Homoeopathic Journal*, 1966, vol LV, no 186.) A very interesting aspect that emerged from these experiments was that, whereas the previously sub-intoxated plants were uniformly spurred into impressive growth by the homoeopathic dynamization of the very poison previously used on them, the control plants, that had not been exposed to any prior sub-intoxation, by contrast, seemed to remain unaffected by the copper sulphate in potency. That seems to confirm homoeopathy's tenet as set out under 'Altered Receptivity in Disease'. This concept was first put forward by the famous French physiologist Claude Bernard (1813-1878; Bernard's duct puncture, Bernard's canal and the Bernard-Horner syndrome are named after him). He was sympathetically inclined toward homoeopathy and wanted to warn against the simplistic interpretations to which some enthusiastic homoeopaths gave voluble expression: 'It has been known for a long time that any medicine will not act on the patient in quite the same manner as on a man in good health.'

Isopathy has, however, also had its experimental failures. G T Lewith, P K Brown and D A J Tyrell reported a controlled study of the effects of an isopathic

30CH dilution of influenza vaccine on antibody titres in man (*Complementary Medical Research*, Autumn 1989, vol III(3), pp 22-24). There were no significant or consistent increases in titre against any of the three dynamized viruses (H3N2, H1N1 and B) used in the vaccine.

There was the rerun of the Oscillococcinum 200CK trial in influenza-like illnesses (referred to earlier under section 1) (ii) – Nosode of animal origin). The large scale, double-blind, placebo-controlled clinical trial by J P Ferley, D Zmirou, D d'Adhemar and F Balducci has been published (*British Journal of Clinical Pharmacology*, March 1989, vol XXVII(3), pp 329-335). It covered 478 patients diagnosed, purely clinically, as suffering from an influenza-like illness by 149 general medical practitioners. This was during an epidemic in the French Rhône-Alpes area when there was the A H1N1 strain of influenza virus implicated. Patients who had previously been immunized against influenza, with any local infection, or with some immune deficiency were excluded. Only those were entered where the first manifestation of illness had occurred less than 24 hours prior, who had a rectal temperature of 38 degrees Celsius or above and who showed at least two of the following symptoms: shivers, stiffness, headache, and lumbar or articular pain. Patients randomly received Oscillococcinum 200CK (237 of them) or look-alike placebo (241 patients). Recovery criterion was set at: rectal temperature less than 37.5 degrees Celsius, with complete resolution of the said five cardinal symptoms.

Result after 48 hours:

	Oscillococcinum 2000K	Placebo	Statistical significance
Patients fully recovered	17% (40% of these had recovered at or before 36 hours) (68% of these were aged 30 yrs or less) (52% of these were classified on entry as moderately or mildly ill)	10%	$p = 0.03$ X2 tcst
Patients using no other treatment for pain or fever during trial	50%	41%	$p = 0.04$
Patients judged treatment efficacious	61%	49%	$p = 0.02$

J

Jahr's Description of Symptom Concentricity

See 'Therapeutic Science'.

Jahr, Georg Heinrich Gottlieb (1800-1875)

This eminent homoeopath was born in the village of Neudietendorf, near Erfurt, Thuringia (now part of Germany), a son of a Moravian family. The homoeopathic pharmacist of that village first aroused his interest in this scientific medicine. As a result, he later contacted Dr Karl Julius Aegidi (five years his senior) in Düsseldorf under whom Jahr, a qualified teacher, began to study Hahnemann's works. Thereafter he moved to Coethen to become, for eight months, Hahnemann's literary assistant, because, through his qualification, he was well suited to the task. It was he who completed the second, much enlarged, edition of Hahnemann's *Chronic Diseases* (see 'Chronic Disease') and laid the foundations of a repertory, and an encyclopaedia of symptoms. The amazing speed with which he was able to work led Hahnemann to chide him for his hastiness.

His competence in homoeopathy, though without formal training, was such that Hahnemann nonetheless recommended him to Princess Frederica of Prussia in Düsseldorf to replace Dr Aegidi, whom she had recently dismissed. So Jahr became his former mentor's successor, without yet having had any academic medical training. This made his position as Royal Physician rather tenuous, since the embittered Dr Aegidi had also begun to conspire against him.

In February 1835 he eventually decided to resign from this appointment in order to go to Bonn to study medicine formally. He financed his studies through the sale of his *Handbook of Data for Correctly Choosing Homoeopathic Remedies – from The Homoeopathic Medicines of Today in Their Primary and Secondary Effects Derived from Sick-bed Experience*. This 476-page work, complete with a good systematic, alphabetical repertory, was highly regarded and was soon translated into both French and English, because it contained, for the first time, all of the 143 remedies that had thus far undergone homoeopathic Hahnemannian provings. There were some complaints, notably from Dr David Roth of Paris (see 'History of Homoeopathy before 1900', under France), that the book was superficial, yet with the benefit of retrospective clinical experience since, it has become clear that the remedies and their effects were succinctly and lucidly described by Jahr. After qualifying he moved to France which appealed so much to him. There Minister Guizot granted him permission to practise medicine without having to submit to any further examinations, exactly as he had done for Hahnemann before him (see 'History of Homoeopathy before 1900', under France).

By his prolific literary output for homoeopathy (he published 258 works), Jahr did more than any other person, after Hahnemann, to propagate this medical method. He also edited and produced two homoeopathic journals in French:

1) with Dr Simon from 1842 to 1845 *Annales de la Médecine Homéopathique;* and
2) alone from 1861 to 1865 *L'Art de Guérir.*

Poetry constituted his non-homoeopathic literary pursuit: in 1850 he published a small anthology and in 1865 there appeared a poetical rendering of the Psalms and of the Book of Job by him.

He kept in close touch at all times with Hahnemann in Paris, never deviating from the originator's ideas, though at times this led him into journalistic controversies with the more pragmatic Griesselich (see 'History of Homoeopathy before 1900', under Germany, and 'Isopathy', under History of Isopathy).

It was Jahr who, together with Simon Felix Camille Croserio, was called by Mme Hahnemann on the day of Hahnemann's death. It was, in fact, these two men who signed as witnesses on Hahnemann's death certificate.

Jahr's major conceptual contribution to homoeopathy was the observation that patient susceptibility to a drug conforms to the rule that the clearer and more positively any finer, or peculiar, or even any characteristic symptoms of a remedy are evident in a patient, the higher the degree of receptivity that may be anticipated to that medicine, and, hence, the higher the potency of choice is likely to be. Jahr further observed that while there is no change in a drug's homoeopathicity as it is taken from crude substance, through the low potencies, beyond Avogadro's number, to the high potencies, there is a subtle change along the way. It is not in the drug's strength or weakness: it is in the development of the drug's peculiarities (away from the commoner symptoms), or as Jahr described it, 'a mere gathering of quality', as it rises in the scale of dynamizations. (See 'Epistemological Assumptions in Homoeopathy', section 5, 'Homoeopathic Laws, Postulates and Precepts', section 10, and 'Therapeutic Science', referring to Jahr's description of symptom concentricity.)

Among his very many thought-provoking writings, his major works are:

Manual of Homoeopathic Medicine (four volumes) (1836)

Elementary Concepts of Homoeopathy (1839)

New Manual of Homoeopathic Practice (1841)

Jahr's Symptom Codex: A Digest of Symptoms (1845)

New Homoeopathic Pharmacopoeia (1850) (remained the profession's standard reference work for a long time, and is still viewed as the ultimate source reference today)

Alphabetical Repertory of Skin Symptoms (1850)

Jahr's Clinical Guide and Pocket Repertory (1850)

Nervous Derangements and Mental Disease (1855)

The Homoeopathic Treatment (1856)
The Venereal Diseases (1868)
Forty Years of Practice (1869).

This famous homoeopath, throughout his thirty-five years in Paris had a busy practice. Despite his successful career, he had a generous disposition and was public-spirited enough to be engaged for a number of years in the later 1860s at a public hospital, without pay. Although this endeared him to people generally, it did not help him, when in 1870, with the outbreak of the Franco-Prussian War, he was expelled from France. His pro-Prussian sympathies certainly erased all his qualities in the minds of his French hosts. At that time Germany achieved national unity by gathering together, under the hegemony of militarist Prussia, the scattered German-speaking principalities and kingdoms that were not under the Hapsburg dominion of the Viennese Dual Monarchy. His patriotic pride was fired by this German development and he published a poem entitled, 'To Germany. A Commemoration on the Foundation of its new Empire, 1871.' Needless to say, this did not endear him to many people outside the Prussian sphere of influence. In fact, it ushered in the saddest part of Jahr's life. The degree of his patriotic fervour can be gauged by the fact that though he was, by then, without financial means of his own, he used all the proceeds from the sale of his poem to help wounded German soldiers.

After his expulsion from France, he moved to Brussels in Belgium, but the Belgians were piqued and refused him permission to practise medicine, despite his almost forty years in active practice, and with an immense literary output in that field behind him. He then moved to Germany, about which he still fondly held romantic misconceptions. There he had come to be regarded as a virtual foreigner and was cold-shouldered. He also found it too difficult, now at 71 years of age, to begin building up a practice in competition with young, keen and agile homoeopaths.

Disillusioned with the newly created German Empire, he returned to Belgium and lived at various times in Luik (Liège), Brussels and Ghent, sometimes in the most indigent circumstances, though he never complained or became a burden to anyone. Finally the society running the Dispensaire Hahnemann issued an appeal to all the homoeopaths of Belgium to procure a yearly salary for Jahr, just enough to save him from direst necessity. But on the 11th July, 1875 a compassionate fate finally put an end to his want, which had been palliated only by the extreme paucity of his needs in life.

Jaundice

A reactive symptom, very occasionally with a grave prognosis, characterized by a staining yellow of:

a) the excretions (particularly urine) with bile-pigment;
b) some secretions (sweat, and the milk of mothers who are nursing may be slightly tinged);

c) the entire integumentum (body covering);

d) the sclera (white of the eyes); and

e) some deeper tissues.

This symptom is an example of how homoeopathy looks in depth at any presenting disease picture, and is not merely an exercise in superficial symptom matching, as some of its detractors would have it.

The homoeopathic significance of this symptom varies with many concomitants, such as degree of jaundice, age of patient, past history and medication, and other symptoms which may be present (e.g. pyrexia, hepatomegaly, enlarged gall-bladder, anaemia, splenomegaly, reticulocytosis, pancytopenia, abdominal discomfort, albuminuria, and cholaemic symptoms). These, in addition to the peculiar or striking symptoms that normally guide the homoeopath's choice, will have to be taken into account to arrive at the correct, and therefore effective, homoeopathic remedy. As a symptom component, it features in:

	Extract of the relevant pathogenetic highlights from the materia medica
Bryonia alba	associated with hepatalgia >from lying on right side;
(Matricaria) Chamomilla	from a fit of anger or a severe fright;
Chelidonium majus	associated with yellow stools and pains under angle of right scapula;
Chionanthus virginica	associated with hepatic congestion, as with obstruction of the common bile-ducts, constipation, greyish-white stools (lack of stercobilin), bilious temperament or arrested menses;
Chloramphenicol (Chloromycetinum)	associated with haematemesis, anorexia, diffuse abdominal pains, cholera-like syndrome, pancytopenia, dyspnoea, catarrh of the mucous membrane of the duct and/or of the duodenum and/or of the pancreas, involving the ampulia of Vater;
Chlorpromazinum	associated with painful hypogastric colic, stubborn constipation, liver enlarged and sensitive, atony of the urinary bladder, diminution of blood platelets, eosinophilia, acquired haemolytic anaemia, or agranulocytic angina;
Convolvulus duartinus (Ipomoea)	associated with a skin of dry appearance despite cold sweats, bilious yellowish-green vomit, hiccoughing, soft orange-yellow stools, rectal tenesmus, and/or distended abdomen, cholecystitis or viral icterus;

Crotalus horridus   associated with albuminuria, blood disorgan-
                                   ization and/or viral hepatitis (such as Yellow
                                   Fever);
Dolichos pruriens   associated with severe irritation;
Guatteria guameria   associated with hepatitis, conjunctival jaundice
                                   with photophobia, biliary lithiasis and inflam-
                                   mation of the gall-bladder, epigastric pain
                                   <from movement;
Hirudo medicinalis   associated with haemolytic crisis, chills, fever,
                                   nausea, vomiting, pain in abdomen or back,
                                   splenomegaly, urine red or black, suicidal
                                   impulses;
Iodium   associated with chronic lupoid hepatitis, without
                                   obstruction of the larger bile-ducts;
Mercurius solubilis   with catarrh in bile-ducts and an inability to lie
   hahnemanni   on the right side;
Phosphorus   associated with malignant parenchymatous
                                   jaundice as in acute yellow atrophy (known as
                                   von Rokitansky's syndrome);
Sulfanilmidum   associated with allergenic, and toxic (miasmatic)
                                   liver reactions to orthodox drugs;
Thyroidinum   in Icterus Neonatorum accompanied by vomiting.

Other significant medicines that may be considered are:

Acidum nitricum   with hepatalgia
Aconitum napellus   with hepatalgia
Arsenicum album   from mercurial intoxation
(Matricaria) Chamomilla   rage/anger may be a cause
Cinchona officinalis   from malaria with bilious diarrhoea
Iris versicolor   from biliary deficiency
(Trigonocephalus) Lachesis   pronounced yellowness
Mercurius vivus/sol.
   hahnem.   after Aconitum napellus
Natrum sulphuricum   anger may be a cause
Nux vomica   with costiveness and sensitivity in liver region
Ptelea trifoliata   with post-prandial liver problems

Examples of syndetic pointers to two homoeopathic medicines:

Where solid unreasoning fear overwhelms the jaundiced patient with
   symptoms of inflammation and great pain in liver area – Aconitum
   napellus
In the jaundiced patient, who loved meat, suddenly turned vegetarian, with
   hepatic and gastric symptoms worse after meals, and hyperaemia of the
   liver – Ptelea trifoliata

(See 'Miasma', relative to the pathogenesis given above under Sulfanilamidum.)

Jenichen, Julius (1787-1845)

An equerry and homoeopath from Wismar, Grand Duchy Mecklenburg, whose life tragically ended in suicide, and who is said to have been the first to employ very high potencies. He took dynamizations higher than anyone had done before him, initially as far as to the 2500th, 8000th and the 16000th centesimal potencies. For this he was, however, repudiated by Hahnemann.[1] Others also disapproved of his very high potencies. Richard Hughes, for instance, wrote, 'Jenichen purported to produce the 60000th potency. Dr Dudgeon has shown that, working five hours a day, and allowing a second for each shake, it would take him five weeks to raise – according to his method – a single drug to this height' and further, 'Jenichen's preparations, which first broke ground in the new field, are now believed to be simply succussions of an ordinary attenuation without further dilution – ten of such shakes being reckoned as producing a potency one step higher in the scale'.[2] The characteristically dry Dr R E Dudgeon cruelly remarked that fortunately Jenichen shot himself when he reached that potency [the 60000th] or there would be no telling what heights he might have reached.[3] (See also 'Potentizing Method'.)

---

[1] Haehl, Richard. *Samuel Hahnemann: His Life and Work*, two vols, London: Homoeopathic Publishing Co, 1922, vol I, p 326.

[2] Hughes, Richard. *A Manual of Pharmacodynamics*, sixth edition, London: Leath and Ross, 1893, p 104.

[3] Dudgeon, R E. *Theory and Practice of Homoeopathy*, London: Leath and Ross, 1854, p 355.

K

Kali

Kalium; potassium; an alkaline metallic element, symbol K, occurring abundantly in nature, as well as in the homoeopathic materia medica, yet, in both instances, always in combination, as salts.

Kent, James Tyler (1849-1916)

This influential US homoeopath, who started out in his medical career as an adherent of the Eclectic School of Medicine, was born into a large Baptist family in Woodhull, New York. He married his first wife, Ellen, but she died very soon afterwards (in 1872) at 19 years of age. He graduated at the early age of nineteen years with a Ph.B. from Madison (now Colgate) University; two years later he had an AM degree from the Bellevue Medical College. Then he undertook postgraduate study for two courses at, and graduated from, the Eclectic Medical Institute of Cincinnati, Ohio. At 26 years of age he set up in practice as an Eclectic physician in St Louis, Missouri. He built up a reputation as a good writer and soon established himself as a distinguished member of the Eclectic National Medical Association. His conversion to homoeopathy came about through an astonishing recovery under homoeopathy of his alarmingly deteriorated second wife, Lucy H. Kent, who could not be cured either Eclectically or by orthodox medicine. Thereupon he resolved to study homoeopathy with the man who had cured his wife, Dr Richard Phelan. That was during 1878 when Kent was 29.

He was an ardent 'high-potency' practitioner and became leader in the USA of the group following that tradition, at the end of the nineteenth century, after the death of Carroll Dunham (1828-1877) and Adolph Lippe (correctly, Adolphus Count zur Lippe-Weissenfeld [1812-1888]). He emphasized the role of 'mentals' in deciding on any homoeopathic medicine, he resolutely advocated the 'single' remedy, and was emphatic that the homoeopath was always to wait until all improvement had ceased before repeating the indicated drug dose. He taught that for any chronic problem the 200CH potency or higher should be used to resolve it. He did more than anyone to keep combinations of homoeopathic drugs at a relatively moderate level of public accessibility, but more significantly, almost single-handedly he brought homoeopathy back from the state of philosophical hybridization it had reached by 1900 with homoeopathic prescriptions based on pathology alone. He founded the Society of Homoeopathians, for the like-minded. The large number of antagonists, particularly in France, were soon to refer to his followers as 'the Kentist Sect', dismissing references in the literature to Kent as so much hagiography. Yet he and his followers remained undeterred.

After Kent was widowed a second time, he married once more. His third wife was Dr Clara Louise Toby Kent (1856-1943), through whom he came to be a Swedenborgian, which so markedly influenced his homoeopathic views. He was appointed professor of Materia Medica at the Homoeopathic Medical College of St Louis, which post he held from 1881 to 1888. He then became professor of Materia Medica and Dean of the Post-Graduate School of Homoeopathy in Philadelphia. These positions he held from 1890 to 1899. He occupied the chair of professor of Materia Medica at the Hering Medical College and Hospital, Chicago from 1903 to 1910. A most inspiring teacher, he moulded some of the best-known homoeopathic minds of the earlier twentieth century, among whom were the likes of Douglas Borland (1885-1960), Sir John Weir, GCVO (1879-1971) and indirectly both Margaret L Tyler (1857-1943) and Pierre Schmidt (1894-1987). Ten years after the demise of Richard Hughes (champion of low-potency prescription guided by both pathology and semiology, but with a preference for the former), i.e. in 1912, the second edition of Kent's *Lectures on Homoeopathic Materia Medica* was reviewed in the British Homoeopathic Journal (April 1912, no. 2, pp 28-29) with these ambivalent words that still showed the strong influence of Hughes:

'Dr Kent has his own way of looking at things . . . He approaches the materia medica almost exclusively from the clinical standpoint. His descriptions of the medicines sum up his experiences of them as gathered at the bedside or in the consulting room. He makes no attempt to be exhaustive, but aims to focus attention on the salient characteristics of each drug and to drive these home by picturesque description, and to fix them in the memory by frequent repetition. As a rule nothing is said about dosage, but when a dose [meaning 'potency'] is recommended it is in a high attenuation. The pathogenic aspect is but little noticed, consequently the homoeopathic relationship between the drug and the diseased states for which it is recommended is not displayed. . . . It was no doubt thought unnecessary to spend time in proving homoeopathic relationships to those already convinced of the rule "similia similibus" and willing to take those relationships for granted. The suggested use of the drug goes in most instances far beyond the strict application of its pathogenesis and presupposes a reference to a schema and repertory which include many purely clinical symptoms. An attempt is also made to define the type of constitution for which a given drug is most suitable . . . Evidently the author considers this a point of great importance, and we fully agree with him, but for the sake of accuracy in prescribing, the characteristics of the drug disease [meaning here 'pathology' experimentally induced in the healthy by the drug] would be required to be most carefully defined in a large number of instances or by many observers before they could be accepted as indicative for patients. The book is illuminating and most valuable to the clinician, but it will be seen that it is not meant for everybody. It would not be a suitable work to place in the hands of a student who is tentatively finding his way . . . to the homoeopathic methods of treatment. He would miss the homoeopathic connexion between drug and disease. It would be far better to give him a volume of Dr Hughes' *Pharmacodynamics* [originally published in 1880] where the pathogenesis of each drug is displayed and its homoeopathicity to its clinical applications clearly demonstrated. Hughes should be the text-book for the beginner, Kent will be invaluable as a supplement . . . Perhaps some day we shall have a materia medica which will combine the good qualities of each, but we may have to wait long, since its production will require a union of different orders of mind.'

An acute miasma scarlatina in his youth is said to have left a chronic miasma of post-infective dyscrasia causing a kidney ailment that ultimately killed him in 1916. Bright's disease is listed as the cause of death on his death certificate. His major writings include:

Repertory of the Homoeopathic Materia Medica (1877)

[this popular reference work comprises 1464 pages (including various instructive monographs on aspects of repertorization); it was extensively revised by Kent's widow, Clara Louise, from 1939 to 1943, and thereafter again up to 1961 by two unnamed leading authorities on homoeopathy to bring it into conformity with the major standard materia medica texts of T F Allen, C Hering and J H Clarke]

What the Doctor Needs to Know in Order to Make a Successful Prescription (1900)

Lectures on Homoeopathic Philosophy (1900)

Lectures on Homoeopathic Materia Medica (1904)

New Remedies, Clinical Cases, Lesser Writings, Aphorisms and Precepts (1926)

Addenda and corrigenda to Kent's masterly *Repertory of the Homoeopathic Materia Medica* are being published to this day.[1,2] Sir John Weir and Margaret L Tyler wrote the instructive booklet *Repertorizing* (London: The British Homoeopathic Association, 1912, 24 pages) to assist those who might be bewildered by the stupendous tome of 1423 pages that make up the core of Kent's Repertory. Margaret L Tyler also wrote *A Study of Kent's Repertory* (Ashford, Kent: Headley Brothers, 1914, 19 pages) with deep sympathy for the daunting volume, in which she said, in her inimitable way, on page one, 'Kent's Repertory is such a maze,' as part of an explanation for writing it. (See also 'Tyler, Sir Henry James (1827-1908)'.)

Key-Note

● **Representative characteristic.**

In music, the first (i.e. lowest) note of the scale of any key, which forms the basis of, and gives its name to, that key. Such a note becomes the fundamental tone around which an entire piece of music is accommodated. In homoeopathy analogous use has regularly been made of a number of musical terms. For example, a patient may tell of 'being out of tune', or the homoeopath may speak

[1] Schindler, M. 'Nachträge zu den Ischias-Rubriken im Kentschen Repertorium' (Annexure to the Sciatica Rubrics in Kent's Repertory), *Zeitschrift für Klassische Homöopathie*, Jan/Feb 1990, vol XXXIV(1) pp 25-27 is an example of the addenda.

[2] Eppenich, H. 'Mittelverwechslungen im Repertorium von Kent' (Erroneous Transposition of Remedies in the Repertory of Kent), *Zeitschrift für Klassische Homöopathie*, Jan/Feb 1990, vol XXXIV(1), p 24 is an example of the corrigenda.

of the 'tone' of the organism or a muscle. In standard homoeopathic practice the term 'key-note' signifies any of the following: pivotal symptom complex; sum and substance of the drug (or disease) picture; leading characteristic(s); however, in pathological prescribing in homoeopathy it may refer to the pathognomonic symptom of a symptom complex (syndrome).

In 1868 the US homoeopath Henry Newell Guernsey (1817-1885) published his book *The Key-Note System*, giving details of the concept as first taught and practised by him, designed to facilitate drug diagnosis. He was wrongly accused of being in conflict with homoeopathy's prescription requirement of drawing on the totality of symptoms, or at least of falling short of that ideal, by arrogating exclusive preference to one leading symptom only. In fact, he did not teach that the key-note of the case alone was to be met by one sole key-note of the remedy, whilst all other features of case or medicine were to be ignored. Guernsey's key-note was simply to be either the predominating symptom or the syndetic feature which readily directs attention to the totality. Therefore, in homoeopathy the key-note's function is merely suggestive.

Soon after H N Guernsey, Adolphus Lippe (1812-1888) published *Key-Notes* [and Red Line Symptoms] of the Materia Medica (part given in parentheses is an augmentation compiled in the 1970s from Lippe's writings in homoeopathic journals worldwide during the third quarter of the nineteenth century – now also incorporated in his republished book [Calcutta: A Bagchi Publishers, no year of publication, ca. 1979]).

In 1898, the homoeopath E B Nash (1838-1914) called the key-notes the 'Leaders in Homoeopathic Therapeutics', as the title of his book indicates.

The Canadian Henry C Allen (1837-1909), Professor of Materia Medica at the Hering Medical College and Hospital, Chicago, USA, wrote a few years before his death:

> 'The life-work of the student of the homoeopathic Materia Medica is one of constant comparison and differentiation. He must compare the pathogenesis of a remedy with the recorded anamnesis of the patient; he must differentiate the apparently similar symptoms of two or more medicinal agents in order to select the simillimum. To enable the student or practitioner to do this correctly and rapidly he must have as a basis for comparison some knowledge of the **individuality** of the remedy; something that is **peculiar, uncommon,** or sufficiently **characteristic** in the confirmed pathogenesis of a polychrest remedy that may be used as a pivotal point of comparison. It may be a so-called "key-note", a "characteristic", the . . . central modality or principle – as the aggravation from motion of Bryonia alba, the amelioration from motion of Rhus toxicodendron, the furious, vicious delirium of (Atropa) Belladonna, or the apathetic indifference of Acidum phosphoricum – some familiar landmark around which the symptoms may be arranged in the mind for comparison. Something of this kind seems indispensable to enable us to intelligently and successfully use our voluminous symptomatology'.[1]

[1] Allen, Henry C. *Key-notes and Characteristics with Comparisons of Some of the Leading Remedies of the Materia Medica including the Nosodes,* Third Edition, Philadelphia: Boericke and Tafel, 1910, Preface to the First Edition, p 5.

In 1924 Stuart Close (1860-1929) described a medicine's key-note as the "Genius of the Remedy". Genius, in this sense, being the dominant influence, or the essential principle of the remedy which gives it its individuality'.[1]

Kinesics

Study of bodily motion as wordless communication.

Kinesiology

Study or science of movement, including the active and passive structures involved. The phrase 'applied kinesiology' was first coined (ca. 1972) by some chiropractors (Dr Goodheart *et al.*) to describe manually performed ergometric assessments following proximate, but not necessarily contiguous, exposure to substances suspected of provoking reactions in the subject. This is not part of homoeopathy, although a small number of homoeopaths use this procedure as a diagnostic aid.

Knerr, Calvin B (1847-1940)

US homoeopath who from 1879 to 1891 worked as co-editor, with Prof Carl Gottlieb Raue, Karl ('Chas') Mohr and the author's son, Walter E Hering, almost entirely posthumously on Constantin Hering's ten volumes of *The Guiding Symptoms of our Materia Medica*. His other major writings include:
Coup de Soleil
Knerr's Repertory
Drug Relationship

Korsakovian Dynamization (Potentization)

Method of homoeopathic drug potentization (dynamization), denoted by the symbol K, introduced in Russia in 1829 by General von Korsakoff. The Hahnemannian method of drug processing requires the use of a fresh phial at each liquid potency stage. In the Korsakovian method, however, just one and the same phial is used throughout an entire dynamization series, requiring less effort, expenditure and storage space. But this method has proved to be inaccurate in one important respect as it introduced considerable variations in the rate of molecular deconcentration in potencies. (See 'History of Homoeopathy before 1900' under Russian Empire, and more particularly 'Potentization Methods', where the method's inconsistency is explained.)

Küchler, Johanna Leopoldine Henriette (1764-1830)

Maiden name of Hahnemann's first wife. (See 'Hahnemann, Christian Friedrich Samuel (1755-1843)'.)

[1] Close, Stuart. *The Genius of Homoeopathy*, New York: Boericke and Tafel, 1924, p 154.

L

Laboratory Equipment

See 'Utensils of Homoeopathic Pharmacy'.

Labour

Delivery; process of childbirth at the normal termination of pregnancy, which is preceded by dilation of the os uteri, and involves the expulsion of a foetus from the uterus accompanied by the complete dilation of the cervix, and is followed by the more or less complete extrusion of the membranes and placenta. Homoeopathic remedies that show marked functiotropism in labour and have been demonstrated to improve the efficiency of this process include:

Caulophyllum thalictroides
Cimicifuga racemosa
Mitchella repens
Rubus idaeus
Trillium erectum.

(See 'Combinations of Homoeopathic Drugs' for pertinent experimental evidence.)

Lamarckism

● **Sees organic evolution as being due to inheritable changes come about in an individual owing to habit, tendency and the environment.**

Postulates that newly acquired characteristics may become hereditable to descendants, whether as an adaptive function of systemic effects (vitalism) or as an outcome of use or disuse (neo-Darwinian evolutionary theory). This is denied by those who hold the alternative view, representing the rigid orthodoxy inherent in the mechanistic theory of Mendelian Inheritance.

Jean-Baptiste P A Lamarck (1744-1829), the French botanist, zoologist and biological philosopher, is the originator of this theory. He had a strong influence on the work of Charles Darwin (1809-1882), the celebrated English biologist and evolutionist, who accepted Lamarck's theory (it was the latter-day Darwinians of the twentieth century who denied it). Lamarck was Professor of Botany at the Jardin des Plantes in Paris from 1792. In 1809, the year of Darwin's birth, he published *La Philosophie Zoologique* in two volumes, which contained this theory as the basis of the evolution of life on earth; his contemporaries virtually ignored his teachings completely. Hahnemann, also one of his contemporaries, only arrived in Paris six years after Lamarck's demise and there is no evidence that any contact existed between the two innovators, although Hahnemann's concepts concerning miasmata seem to follow Lamarckist lines. (See 'Genetic Assimilation', 'Heredity', 'Homoeosis', 'Miasma' and 'Mnemism'.)

Lanolin

See 'Adeps Lanae'.

Latent Disease, Latency

See 'Miasma'.

Laterality

Right or left dominance of some members (arms or legs), of certain organs, of the cerebral cortex, or of disease manifestations, and of the curative action of corresponding homoeopathic drugs. For example, Iris versicolor, Nitrum (saltpetre, potassium nitrate) and Lycopodium clavatum all have a predominantly right-sided action, whereas a curative predisposition favouring the left side is evident in the following drugs: Colchicum autumnale, (Trigonocephalus) Lachesis and Rhododendron chrysanthum.

Latin Aphorisms in Homoeopathy

Short pithy definitions of concepts, as well as truths of general import, and phrases of special relevance in homoeopathy (and other medical disciplines), are traditionally captured in Latin apophthegms. A translation is given for the ones in more common use, with a textual reference if applicable.

a posteriori – reasoning based on experience, proceeding inductively from effects to cause, from actions to laws, and the like; opposed to *a priori*

a priori – reasoning independent of experience, based only, deductively on principles of reason; opposed to *a posteriori*

ab ovo usque ad male – from exultation right down to wretchedness

aequalia aequalibus curantur – the same cures the same (see 'Isopathy'.)

aude sapere – dare to know (see 'Hahnemann, Christian Friedrich Samuel (1755-1843)', under Hahnemann's Contribution to Science and his Impact on the Practise of Medicine.)

cessat effectus cessat causa – remove the effect and you remove the cause, meaning when the effect ceases, the disease (the cause of the effect) has also ceased

concordia discors – harmony in discord

contraria contrariis curentur – let the adverse (symptoms) be cured by their contraries (see 'Hahnemann, Christian Friedrich Samuel (1755-1843)', under The Rationalist Medical Tradition.)

ex nihilo nihil fit – from nothing, nothing comes (see 'Determinism'.)

in manu vis medendi – in the hand is the power of healing (see 'McTimoney Chiropractic'.)

Isopathia Homoeopathia maxima est – Isopathy is the foremost homoeopathy (see 'Isopathy', under History of Isopathy.)

magis venenum, magis remedium – more poison, greater remedy

materia peccans – disease-inducing substance

mutatis mutandis – things being changed that have to be changed; an adverbial phrase meaning simply 'with the obvious, necessary changes'

mutato nomine de te fabula narratur – change but the name, and it is of you the story tells

natura sanat – Nature heals (see 'Hahnemann, Christian Friedrich Samuel (1755-1843)', under The Empirical Medical Tradition.)

naturam expellas furca, tamen usque recurret – if you drive Nature out with a pitchfork, she will soon find a way back

nihil in intellectu nisi prius in sensu – nothing in the intellect was not first in the senses (see 'Hahnemann, Christian Friedrich Samuel (1755-1843)', under The Empirical Medical Tradition.)

nil mortalibus ardui est – nothing is too arduous for mortal men

nil prodest quod non laedit idem – no thing improves which is not also harmed at the same time

non inutilis vixi – I have not lived in vain (see 'Hahnemann, Christian Friedrich Samuel (1755-1843)', under The Empirical Medical Tradition.)

omne similia similibus confirmatur – everything similar is confirmed by (in) the similar (see 'Hahnemann, Christian Friedrich Samuel (1755-1843)', under The Empirical Medical Tradition.)

post hoc, ergo propter hoc – subsequent to this, therefore, because of it (see 'Guiding Symptoms of the Materia Medica' and 'Post Hoc, Ergo Propter Hoc'.)

primum non nocere – above all, not to injure (see 'Hahnemann, Christian Friedrich Samuel (1755-1843)'.)

salus aegrotis suprema lex – the health of the patient is the highest law

similia similibus curentur – let likes be cured (or treated) by likes (see 'Homoeopathic Laws, Postulates and Precepts', section 1)

simplex, simile et minimum – simple, similar and least (see 'Classical Homoeopathy'.)

stans pede in uno – without effort

tolle causam – remove the cause; or seek out the cause

ubi morbus, ibi etiam medicamentum morbillis opportunam – where the disease is, there also is its proper remedy (see 'Lux, Johan Joseph Wilhelm (1776 – 1849)'.)

vis concili expers mole ruit sua – force without mind falls by its own weight

vis medicatrix naturae – the healing power of Nature (see 'Dynamis', 'Homoeostasis' and 'Vitalism'.)

Law of Bioenergetic Drug Action

See 'Homoeopathic Laws, Postulates and Precepts', section 2.

Law of Homoeopathic Efficacy

See 'Homoeopathic Laws, Postulates and Precepts', section 3.

Law of Quantity and Dose

See 'Homoeopathic Laws, Postulates and Precepts', section 4.

Law of Similars

See 'Homoeopathic Laws, Postulates and Precepts', section 1.

Law of Stimuli

See 'Homoeopathic Laws, Postulates and Precepts', section 5.

Laws of Nature

Order of the regularities found in Nature.

In the sound tradition of Empirical medicine, in which homoeopathy is firmly rooted, the laws of nature are not generally seen as eternal imperatives (firmly embedded in Rationalism's deterministic and ultimately fideistic theories), but as no more than human constructs that refer to certain regularities observed and described by scientists (and unobtrusively sustained by Empiricism's probabilioristic theories). The French mathematician and astronomer Pierre Simon Marquis de Laplace (1749-1827) showed how large numbers of events can behave in a typical way, even when the individual events may seem to be unpredictable (e.g. the laws of chance in gambling, or, more recently, the patterns of chaos).

The evident predictability of some of these observable regularities of nature serves as an objective basis for the modelling of a scientific form of medicine, which necessarily leads to its practice by the homoeopathic method, whereas the disregarding of which manifestly leads to the entrenchment of aimless revisionalism in medical practice. Moreover, without such reliance upon the observed regularities, there should be no basis whatever for the principle of objective reproducibility. This probabiliorism is the essential foundation underpinning the self-consistent scientific method in homoeopathy.

As is the case in all biological laws (e.g. Mendel's Law in genetics), the Law of Similars is a secondary, as opposed to a fundamental, law. It seems that the majority of homoeopaths believe that the primary laws, to which this law may be reduced, are timeless and transcendent, rooted in a sort of meta-universe of mathematical relationships to the four observed forces, which between them account for the behaviour of everything in the universe (i.e. gravitational, electromagnetic, weak-nuclear, and strong-nuclear forces). Two mathematicians, the Soviet Union's Alexander Friedmann (in 1924) and France's Georges Lemaitre (in 1927) were ignored when they forespelled the later, so-called De Sitter-Einstein universe which contemplates a single mathematical description of the entire known universe utilizing relativity and differential geometry. Through it the laws of nature have a mathematical expression at present, and by virtue of the property of covariance that expression is the same for all observers no matter what their state of motion or acceleration.[1]

In the future, propelled by the mathematics of the quantitive understanding of chaos, computer-assisted in iterative processes, performing, say, 10^{12} arithmetical operations per second will change the mathematical description of the physical world, yet this presents no epistemological problem to Empirical science, relying, as it has always done, on the results of observed phenomena. For the moment, however, these mathematical relationships are seen as dependable (though not as indefinitely immutable), while the concrete universe remains physically undefined. This curious inversion of the everyday perspective is exactly the world view of quantum theory that is espoused by nearly all physicists of today, who are concerned with so-called fundamental physics.

There is, by now, a quantum theory for most branches of classical Newtonian physics (which had sought reality in the material [solid particle] state of the universe at each instant). Now there is even quantum cosmology, one interpretation of which postulates a selection principle that is said to have come into existence with the universe and then brought into being the laws that are suited to the maintenance of the life impulse and consciousness. The majority of homoeopaths seems to ally itself to this world view, seeing the selection principle as consonant with, or analogous to, homoeopathy's own similia principle, and 'the life impulse and consciousness' as essentially synonymous with homoeopathy's dynamic force (immanent organizing [life] principle). In turn, the origin of the life principle and consciousness is seen in quantum cosmology in terms of oscillations and resonance, which, of course, is not merely the measurable stuff of quantum theory and its formulae, but is also the polemical stuff over the defence of which homoeopathy has fought a quixotic paper war for so long.

It is generally agreed that all scientific evidence appears to indicate that there is an immeasurable universe, consisting of space almost totally devoid of matter, yet replete with radiation. Most of what infinitely little there is of actual matter is in a state of frenetic motion, and, in turn, an infinitesimal part of that is living matter, of which a negligibly small part, and only very recently, was endowed with consciousness.

[1]Kerzberg, Pierre. *The Invented Universe: The Einstein-De Sitter Controversy (1916-1917) and The Rise of Relativistic Cosmology,* Oxford: Clarendon Press, 1989.

The German physicist and Nobel Laureate, Werner Karl Heisenberg (1901-1976), whose development of the theory of quantum mechanics dominated the twentieth century's development of nuclear and atomic physics since 1925, said, 'Die Vorstellung von der objektiven Realität der Elementarteilchen hat sich also in einer merkwürdigen Weise verflüchtigt' (The concept of an objective reality inherent in elementary particles, therefore, has strangely evaporated).[1] The Welsh mathematician and philosopher, Earl Bertrand Arthur William Russell (1872-1970), declared that it gradually seemed as though matter, like the Cheshire cat, was becoming more and more transparent by degrees, until nothing now remained of it but its smile, evidently in amused mockery of those who still believe in its existence.[2]

Sir Karl R Popper (born 1902, Vienna), the philosopher of natural science, maintains that it is only man's critical appraisal which permits the establishment of any new hypothesis. This only becomes possible if the new hypothesis appears to represent an improvement over all those preceding it. What is expected of a new hypothesis, Popper says, before it may supplant an earlier one, is the following:

1) the new hypothesis must be able to solve those same problems at least as efficiently as were solved by its predecessors;

2) the new hypothesis must render predictions deducible, which are not yielded by the older theories; these should preferably be predictions that contradict those of the older theories, wherein might lie a noteworthy scientific breakthrough.

Popper further says that point 1 is a necessary safeguard to prevent regression, but that point 2 is optional though worthwhile because it is revolutionary.[3] Homoeopathy clearly solves the problems of medical therapeutics much more efficiently than other hypothesis of medical practice and, in contrast to any of the older medical theories, it makes possible universal predictions, particularly in the area of prognosis. This does represent a revolutionary scientific breakthrough in the practice of medicine proper.

What seems to be required of the scientist investigating homoeopathy is an open-mindedness that would permit the kind of mental reversal Aristotle (ca. 384-322 BC) spoke of in *Metaphysics* [983a11]: 'The acquisition of knowledge must lead to a state of mind exactly opposite to that in which we originally began our search . . . For it must seem strangely perplexing to anyone who has not yet realized that it is possible for something to exist, though it cannot be measured, not even by the smallest unit.' (See also 'Epistemological Assumptions in Homoeopathy', 'Philosophical Premise of Homoeopathy' and 'Radiant State of Matter, Theory of'.)

[1] Heisenberg, Werner Karl. 'Das Naturbild der heutigen Physik', *Universitas*, vol. IX, 1954, p 1158.
[2] Russell, Earl Bertrand Arthur William. 'Mind and Matter' in *Portraits from Memory*, New York: Simon and Schuster, 1956, p 145.
[3] Popper, Sir Karl R, and Sir John C Eccles. *Das Ich und sein Gehirn*, Munich: R Piper GmbH & Co KG, 1982, pp 188-189.

Life Force

See 'Dynamis' and 'Laws of Nature'.

Life Principle

See 'Dynamis' and 'Vitalism'.

Liga Medicorum Homoeopathica Internationalis

See 'International Homoeopathic League'.

Like Remedy

Similar remedy; simillimum (also similimum); the drug indicated in a certain case, because, when given to a healthy person, it is able produce the symptom complex most nearly approaching that of the diseased patient in question.

Lilienthal, Samuel (1815-1891)

US homoeopath who, though born in Munich, Kingdom of Bavaria (now part of Germany), graduated at the New York Homoeopathic Medical College and Hospital for Women, where he later held the post of professor of Gynaecology and physician to the New York homoeopathic dispensary for twenty years. He was editor of the *North American Journal of Homoeopathy* from 1870 to 1885, and during 1874 also of the *New York Journal of Homoeopathy*. His most outstanding contribution to homoeopathic scientific literature is the comprehensive, accurate and perennially useful reference work entitled:

Homoeopathic Therapeutics (commonly known as *Lilienthal's Therapeutics;* New York: Globe Printing House, 1878, 1154 pages).

His other major writings include: *Treatise of Diseases of the Skin* (1876)
Works on the Materia Medica (1886)
Hereditary Insanity (1886)
Aetiology of Tuberculosis (1887)

Linctus

Lincture; syrupy medicinal preparation (e.g. a cough mixture) that was originally intended to be licked up with the tongue, as the term suggests.

Liniment

Embrocation; liquid homoeopathic preparation for external application, most commonly by friction to the skin, or as an application to the gums. (See 'Externally Applied Homoeopathic Drugs'.)

Lippe, Adolphus (1812-1888)

After Constantin Hering, this nobleman was the most outstanding homoeopath in the USA. His full name was Adolphus Graf zur Lippe-Weissenfeld. He was born on the family's estate near the old town of Görlitz, lower Silesia, Electorate of Saxony (now part of eastern Germany) and studied law in Berlin, Prussia. Thereafter he migrated to the USA and studied medicine there at Allentown Homoeopathic Academy, Pennsylvania. After graduating he was associated with the Hahnemann Medical College, Philadelphia, for the remainder of his life. There he became a friend both of Constantin Hering (1800-1880) and of Carl Gottlieb Raue (1820-1886, professor of Special Pathology and Therapeutics). In fact these three men were members of the teaching staff in 1865, at the time when the widowed Melanie Hahnemann entered into unsuccessful negotiations with the Faculty of the Hahnemann Medical College, asking for an extraordinarily large sum of money for her late husband's manuscript of the sixth edition of the *Organon*.

Lippe was the most forceful polemicist of the period on the advantages of high-potency prescribing, and was always on the side which opposed the UK's Richard Hughes and the USA's Charles J Hempel, who wanted to re-interpret homoeopathic therapeutics through the elaborations derived from the science of pathology (see entries under the names of both men, and 'History of Homoeopathy before 1900', section United Kingdom). Lippe's major polemical contribution in that field was:

'The Relation of Homoeopathy to Pathology and Physiology' (*Transactions of the Pacific Homoeopathic Medical Society*, I (1874-1876), pp 160-166).

Other major writings include these books:

What is Homoeopathy?

Key-Notes [and Red Line Symptoms] of the Materia Medica

(part given in parentheses is an augmentation compiled in the 1970s from Lippe's writings in homoeopathic journals worldwide during the third quarter of the nineteenth century – now also incorporated in his book by the publishers)

Text-Book of Materia Medica.

In 1880 his son, Constantin Lippe, published the Repertory to the More Characteristic Symptoms of the Materia Medica which he dedicated to his namesake, Constantin Hering.

Lithotherapy

Literally means rock-therapy. Popularized by the French homoeopath Max Tétau, this therapeutic approach relies on the dechelating effect of low homoeopathic potencies (usually 8DH) of geological material (rocks and naturally occurring minerals). Most of these remedies have not undergone any homoeopathic provings, although clinical observations extending over about fifteen years (mainly in France), seem to indicate lithotherapy's relative efficacy. Its thirty-three remedies are administered, normally, in perlingual oral ampoules. Their main indications are:

1 Adulares – Prostatic adenoma
2 Apatite – Vertebral osteoarthrosis
3 Azurite – Hypertension
4 Barytine – Cerebral arteriosclerosis
5 Betafite – Parasitic infections and pre-diabetes
6 Bornite – Anti-infectious and anti-inflammatory agent
7 Chalcopyrites – Inflammatory rheumatism and paradontoses
8 Conglomerate – Dry and weeping eczema, various skin disease manifestations
9 Diopside – Tetany and remineralization in adolescent and child
10 Galena – Some pre-diabetic states
11 Garnierite – Allergies of all types
12 Glauconia – Asthenia, tetany and neurovegetative imbalance
13 Green Jasper – Biliary diskinesia
14 Haematite – Anaemia and hypotension
15 Iron Pyrites – Recurrent colibacillus infection
16 Lazulite – Hepatic insufficiency and cramping pains in lower limbs
17 Lepidolite – Depressive states
18 Lithium Tourmaline – Tranquillizing action in depressed states
19 Monazite – Hypoglycaemia and cancerous diathesis
20 Native Gold – Anti-inflammatory agent, increase in body's general powers of resistance
21 Native Silver – Analgesic, anti-inflammatory agent
22 Obsidian – Cervical osteoarthrosis
23 Orpiment – Coxarthrosis
24 Pink Sandstone – Constipation and atonic functional colonic disease
25 Pyrolusite – Aphthous ulcers and allergies of all types
26 Quadratic Feldspar – Generalized osteoarthrosis
27 Rhodonite – Insomnia
28 Saccharoid Marble – Gastritis, peptic ulcer and gastric ulcer
29 Stibnite – Chronic bronchorrhoea, bronchiectasis and emphysema
30 Trachyte – Spasmodic and whooping cough
31 Ulexite – Recurrent rhinopharyngitis and aphthous ulcers
32 Uraninite – Anti-parasitic agent
33 Versailles Chalk – Senile osteoporosis and decalcification

The indications here are only given in terms of pathological entities that are totally alien to the homoeopathic idiom, and by this fact alone, unfortunately, the whole therapeutic approach is flawed in the eyes of many homoeopaths. To some degree Bach's Flower Remedies and the Tissue Salts of Schüssler's Biochemic Medicine had been presented to homoeopathy in a similar way, and neither Bach nor Schüssler had conducted any homoeopathic provings on their remedies. Despite these shortcomings, homoeopathy adopted both these sets of remedial agents. It remains to be seen whether lithotherapy will ever be granted the same distinction.

Lithotherapy aims at normalising the patient's metabolic pathways that may be disturbed by a blockade of enzyme catalysis due to a chelation, that is an inactivation of the metal ions so essential for metabolic activity. The saturation of the air with sulphur and other chelating molecules, and the presence in foodstuffs of traces of pesticides, fertilizing agents and insecticides as well as the later additives, such as sequestrants, result in an excessive intake of chelates, often with severe metabolic consequences which this therapeutic approach aims to correct.

Experimental Evidence

Dr Menetrier demonstrated the anti-infectious and anti-inflammatory effects of copper gluconate 5DH in patients with various viral disorders, including influenza, brought about by the resulting dechelation of trapped copper ions.

Miss L Wurmser and Prof Lapp, in two separate placebo-controlled trials, demonstrated the significantly increased excretion of both arsenic and bismuth, eliminated from guinea pigs in their urine, after the prior administration of a large but non-toxic dose of either arsenic or bismuth. The eliminatory effect was brought about in each case by the injection of Arsenicum Album 7CH or Bismuthum 7CH, respectively. Distilled water was injected as placebo.

Prof A Cier and Dr Mouriquand similarly demonstrated the urinary excretion of arsenic and antimony in two comparable experiments on pigeons, while measuring the variations in vestibular chronaxic index. Six weeks after the subintoxication, Arsenicum album 7CH, in the one trial, and Antimonium 7CH, in the other, were injected, while distilled water was injected as placebo into the control group. In the birds that received the homoeopathic potencies the chronaxia returned to normal in a few days and arsenic, or antimony, respectively, was again found in the excreta in proportion of from 12-17% of what had been known to have been fixed in the body. The birds that received the placebo remained unchanged for at least 60 days from the subintoxication, with the chronaxia returning to normal only after 90 days.

In controlled studies involving the excretion of radioactive antimony, in experiments on rats, it was shown that under the influence of the ultramolecular (sub-physiological) potency of 15CH of the same radioactive antimony a marked increase in its excretion could be measured.

Dr Max Tétau asked, 'Why not use the complete, naturally occurring minerals and rocks, rather than the isolated metalloid or chemical substances, as, after all, homoeopathy has always preferred to make its mother tinctures from the complete plant material rather than from an alkaloid, a saponin or a resin?' He justifies lithotherapy's selection of mineral substances, relative to the indications listed, by pointing to the fact that there is a crystalline structural analogy between the mineral and the chelate from which the metal ion is to be liberated. As an example: It is because the chelating complexes entrapping calcium and phosphorus have a crystallographic structure belonging to the quadratic system, and not to the hexagonal system, that in the treatment of osteoarthrosis of the vertebral column and in senile osteoporosis, dynamized quadratic feldspar, and not triclinic feldspar, is used, in addition to potentized Apatite, which is phosphate of calcium, containing ions of carbonate, fluoride, chloride and/or hydroxyl, the major constituents of bones and of teeth. For homoeopathy this could just prove to be too uncomfortably reminiscent of the doctrine of signatures (see 'Anthroposophical Medicines'). The best and most consistent results appear to be obtained with the 8DH potency.

LM Potencies

Quinquagenimillesimal or 50-millesimal dynamizations. (See 'Potentizing Methods'.)

Loschmidt's Number

See 'Avogadro's Number'.

Lotion

Lotio; a wash; a class of pharmacopoeial preparations which are liquid dispersions or deconcentrations (of miscibles), generally intended for external application. Oil-in-water suspensions (i.e. involving immiscibles) are referred to as emulsions.

Low Potency Prescribing

Some homoeopaths, engaged in busy practices, find they cannot spend more than 15 minutes with each patient. During this time they are obviously unable to elicit the totality of symptoms on which to individualize the prescription, as they know they ought to. So they begin by treating the symptoms 'low' (i.e. functiotropically, or pathotropically, with low dynamizations, which means with potencies ranging from Θ to 6DH or 3CH). They will have the patient call back a few times, during which time they gradually build up a picture of mentals and generals and so on, over several consultations. Only then do they come in with the 'high' total remedy (i.e. with a single remedy in a high potency). Such practitioners say there is less risk of contamination among low potencies. They also maintain that patients who are newcomers to homoeopathy initially find it easier to relate to such a method of drug-to-ailment homoeopathic treatment. They point out, additionally, that at first Hahnemann also worked with low potencies (in fact from 1793 to 1828, i.e. for as long as 35 years). Moreover, they feel that it is very close to the principle of 'homoeopathic drainage' (detoxication) initiated by the French. Finally they emphasize that it makes for easy comparative efficacy evaluations when homoeopathic organotropic remedies can be compared for effectiveness with orthodox remedies that are similarly targeted in the same patients' illnesses. These opinions and the issues they raise above are expressed in an article by Duncan M Cameron in The British Homoeopathic Journal.[1]

The great apologist for homoeopathy during the first half of the twentieth century, Charles Edwin Wheeler (1868-1946), had the following to say on this subject in his lecture delivered on 8th October 1937 in the Great Hall, British Medical Association, Tavistock House, London: 'Many – most homoeopathists use very small, actually infinitesimal, doses but the principle of homoeopathy is applicable with any range of dosage. Hahnemann tested it and confirmed his belief in it for ten years with doses not far removed from those of ordinary practice and no scholar needs reminding that homoeopathic does not mean infinitesimally small.'[2]

Ian Mckinlay Burns' illuminating article 'The Value of Low Potencies' is featured in full by Kailash Narayan Mathur.[3] Burns tells of his training in Scotland at the Glasgow Hospital and Dispensary where he gathered the impression that all genuine homoeopaths used the range of 30CH, 200CH, 1M to 10M dynamizations, and not really below the 30CH. Although Dr Mitchell of St Annes-on-Sea, whose assistant he later became, introduced him to the 9CH potency, he remained convinced that 30CH was the 'low' potency of choice. He confined his reading to Kent and Allen, and had a great deal of clinical success with the high potency range he was using. Finally he was appointed physician to the Manchester Homoeopathic Clinic in England, and took over an old-established homoeopathic practice in that city. He was flabbergasted when he discovered that his predecessor, who had been fifty-four years in the practice and had been Senior Physician to the Clinic, had rarely used any potency higher than 3DH, but regularly used potencies lower than that or had simply employed mother tinctures. He had even alternated his remedies and continued their use over quite prolonged periods of time, day in and day out. This, to Burns, at the time, was absolute heresy. What was even more surprising was that the predecessor was, in fact, something of a homoeopathic legend who had apparently been achieving excellent results with all kinds of illness over the years, and had absolute confidence in his remarkable method of choosing and applying the medicines. Burns has recorded many cases and the corresponding prescriptions. Here are two:

1) Lady with a renal calculus, radiographically confirmed; he told her the medicine would make the stone come away as gravel inside three months; before the three months were up she was free from pain and brought the promised gravel in a jar to the practice. Rx: Berberis vulgaris 3DH & Urtica

[1] Cameron, Duncan M. 'Low Potency Prescribing', *British Homoeopathic Journal*, vol XLI, no 2, April 1951, pp 77-87.

[2] Wheeler, Charles Edwin. 'A Hundred Years of Homoeopathy', London: *The British Homoeopathic Association*, 1937, p 4.

[3] Mathur, Kailash Narayan. *Principles of Prescribing: Collected from Clinical Experiences of Pioneers of Homoeopathy*, New Delhi: B Jain Publishers, 1981, pp 645-654.

urens Θ, in alternation each day for the entire period of treatment.

2) Gentleman, aged 62, with bronchial asthma, resistant to all Orthodox medical treatment; Arsenicum album 30CH – no effect. Rx: Nux vomica 1DH 15 drops in half a glass of water, of which 5ml half-hourly, to be reduced to three-hourly. He was relieved within the hour and by next morning all spasm had gone. For the next twenty years he had Nux vomica 1DH handy and would occasionally take it at the slightest sign of a wheeze. He was never again seriously troubled with asthma and died at 82 from a cerebral haemorrhage.

Other medicines were	Conditions cleared up
Pulsatilla nigricans 3DH bid	Asthma, nasal catarrh, greenish discharge;
Arnica montana 3DH tid	Blind boils on scalp, limbs and trunk;
Sulphur 3DH bid	Skin rough, thickened over whole body, intense itching, bleeds on scratching;
Ledum palustre 3DH tid	Recent harmorrhage into vitreous humour, and hence blind;
Pulsatilla nigricans 3DH bid	Nasal catarrh and frontal sinusitis;
Kali bichromicum 3DH bid	Sinusitis with thick greenish discharge;
Bryonia alba 3DH bid	Osteoarthritis.

Further remedies that were very successfully prescribed very low are:

Kali sulphuricum, Hepar sulphuris calcareum, Mercurius solubilis hahnemanni, Mercurius corrosivus, Apis mellifica, Antimonium crudum, Arsenicum iodatum, (Atropa) Belladonna, Sulphur, Urtica urens, Hydrocotyle asiatica, Acidum fluoricum, Cimicifuga racemosa, Ruta graveolens, Rhus toxicodendron, Rhododendron chrysanthum, guaiacum officinale, Chelidonium majus, Causticum, Acidum benzoicum, Terebinthina, Hamamelis macrophylla, Carbo vegetabilis, Secale cornutum and Spigelia anthelmia.

The patients often expected Burns to continue prescribing what they had been given by his predecessor. So he too slipped into low potency prescribing. Actually he began to mix high and low potencies often in the same patient with great success by his own account. He says, 'I firmly believe in the efficacy of the higher "dilutions", but I am convinced that we cannot afford to neglect any area of homoeopathic prescribing which may benefit our patients, or which may be of value in research'.[1]

(See 'Detoxication', 'Drainage', 'Mother Tincture', 'Pathotropism' and 'Potency'.)

Low Potency Solution

See 'Dose'.

Lucretius (Titus Lucretius Carus) (ca. 99-55 BC)

See 'Philosophical Premise of Homoeopathy'.

[1] Loc cit.

Lues Venerea

Syphilis. (See 'Miasma', under Luetic Miasma.)

Luetic Miasma

See 'Miasma'.

Lux, Johan Joseph Wilhelm (1776-1849)

The pioneer in veterinary homoeopathy who later became the father of modern Isopathy (refer to this entry). He was born the son of a veterinarian at Oppeln on the river Oder in the Prussian province of Upper Silesia (now Opole, Slask, Poland). He studied veterinary medicine at the Civil Veterinary School of Berlin (1800) and thereafter human medicine and natural sciences some thirty years after Hahnemann at the University of Leipzig (Lux graduated from there in 1805).

His earlier writings include: *Characteristics of Rinderpest Epidemics*, Leipzig, 1803; his translation of Tolnay's *Artis Veterinariae, Compendium Pathologicum*, 1808; *The Rights of Shepherds*, 1815 (pointing out pertinent conditions of injustice; this earned him some opprobrium in the circles of power, where he was afterwards referred to as a 'rotten head' [= seditionist infecting others with bad ideas]); *New Method to Check a Rinderpest Epidemic* (an analysis of the teachings of Marshall Ferrand), Leipzig, 1809; and *The Popular Compendium on Domestic Animals*, 1819.

In 1823 he introduced homoeopathic treatment for animals with immediate success. He founded a number of homoeopathic societies, and on the 14th October, 1832 he dedicated to Hahnemann the first volume of his veterinary review *Zooaiasis*. Lux possessed an amiable and courageous personality which helped him to win over many of a constant flow of numerous adversaries. He is also known to have had a passionate interest in pomology, the science and practice of fruit-culture.

In 1833 he had his *Isopathik der Contagionen* published by Kollmann in Leipzig. In it he first set out his theory that every contagious disease contains within itself the trigger for its own cure. Hering said he believed that the contemporaries of Lux in homoeopathy actually underestimated the significance of that man's contribution to homoeopathy at the time, which led to the unfortunate neglect in reprinting much of his published work. Hering showed his bias toward this form of treatment when in 1833 he wrote, 'whatever scourge arrives from the Orient, the remedy will reach us at the same time'.[1] The part played by Lux in the Isopathy movement within homoeopathy is detailed in 'Isopathy', under History of Isopathy.

In 1974 the American Institute of Homoeopathy published the following statement, reflecting the extent to which Lux is seen as an apostate there even

[1] Hering, Constantin. *Bibliothèque Homéopathique* II (1833), p 107.

to this day: 'There has been and still is widespread confusion about the relationship between isopathy and the homoeo concept. Many see them as essentially identical. Nothing could be more erroneous. Lux, the father of isopathy, taught that the physician had only to identify the physical cause of the condition which, when done, automatically yielded the appropriate remedy. The physician had only to administer some of the substance which was the disease cause. The homoeo-discipline, on the other hand, does not concern itself with the real or presumed physical or chemical cause of the disease. Its operative data are the total symptom complex exhibited by the reacting organism (i.e. the disease process) and the pathogenesis of the drug of choice, as demonstrated by repeated testing over many decades. These two symptom patterns must be matched together on the basis of similarity. There is a far closer relationship between isopathy and immunology, a relationship which is more than implied by the phrase, "nosological relationship".'[1]

[1] Baker, Wyrth P, Allen C Neiswander and W W Young. *Introduction to Homoeotherapeutics,* Washington: American Institute of Homoeopathy, 1974, chapter on Principles and Methodology p 4, footnote.

M

M. A. P.

A homoeopathic combination remedy composed of three moulds: Mucor (from decaying vegetable matter), Aspergillus (found in soil, faeces and on fruit, converting starch to fermentable sugars) and Penicillium (common mildew). This most useful mixed homoeopathic preparation is often mistakenly referred to as 'mixed autumn pollens' (incorrect construction put upon the moulds' acronym), not least because it is often astonishingly effective against hayfever-like symptoms, with itching eyes, sneezing, catarrh, prickly throat, wheezy chest, and a dry irritating cough.

Maceration

Process in which a drug of organic origin is steeped in a liquid, with or without some application of heat, until the tissues become softened and the soluble matter contained in the cells has been dissolved. (See also 'Percolation'.)

Macroscopy

Examination of objects with the naked eye; hence 'macroscopic'.

McTimoney Chiropractic

Developed and taught by John McTimoney in the UK from 1972, it is a non-diagnostic variant of Chiropractic technique on humans where palpatory examination only (without x-ray) leads on to a gentle form of manipulation; it also provides an adaptation of such manipulation for the treatment of animals. Its motto is: 'in manu vis medendi' (in the hand is the power of healing). The objective of McTimoney Chiropractic is to help the body realign itself, thereby to restore correct nerve function, resulting in pain relief and improved health. As an adjunctive modality the homoeopath may find McTimoney Chiropractic complementary to homoeopathic treatment.

Magistral

Magistralis (Latin). Denoting a pharmaceutical solution, tincture, or other medication prepared extemporaneously according to a homoeopath's prescription, as distinguished from an officinal preparation. (See also 'Officinal'.)

Magnetic Field Therapy

Biomagnetism; magnetotherapy. Proponents of this therapeutic approach have long held that all materials, including organic molecules and tissues, are susceptible to magnetism and that this can be employed to stimulate a dynamic curative response. In fact, it has recently been confirmed that some organic (carbon-based) molecules, arranged in a regular way to form solids (with the spins of all unpaired electrons spontaneously aligned pointing unidirectionally), are themselves able to act as magnets; moreover, it has also been shown that all materials are, in fact, magnetic.[1] Most materials in a magnetic field are repelled. This is known as diamagnetism which is quite weak and interacts with an external field. Hahnemann, in sections 286 and 287 of the *Organon of Medicine,* said magnets and electricity could be used curatively, especially in disease states involving 'abnormal sensations and involuntary muscular movements'. (See 'Acupuncture', 'Electrotherapy', 'Naturopath' and 'Radiant State of Matter, Theory of'.)

Massage Therapy

Employs stroking, friction, kneading, percussion, rolfing, pinching, vibration, gelotrypsy, passive muscle stretching and joint articulation, as well as specific pressure exertion, singly or in any combination, as a method for therapeutically manipulating the body. This is a naturopathic treatment which is complementary to homoeopathy. Hahnemann in section 290 of the *Organon of Medicine* recommends it, in moderation, particularly for a chronic invalid because it will 'restore the tone of the muscles, and blood and lymph vessels.' He also ascribes a certain 'mesmeric influence' to massage. However, great caution is to be exercised with the use of essential plant oils in massage (as in aromatherapy, a variant of massage therapy) because these will act homoeopathically, or may even produce a proving, in the patient.

Matching Three or More Guiding Symptoms

See 'Disease and Drug Action in Homoeopathic Congruity', under section 8.

Materia Medica

● **Contents of a reference book containing all the necessary information for the proper use of medicines.**

Deals with the origin, composition and properties, sometimes also the classification and reference source (authority), of medicinal agents. These properties include physical, chemical and biological, where appropriate

---

[1] Miller, Joel, and Arthur Epstein. 'Magnetism without Metals', *New Scientist,* 23rd June 1990, vol MDCCXXII, pp 52-56.

toxicological characters of the drug, as well as its reactive propensity as a homoeopathic therapeutic agent. Also the appellation of the academic subject, that treats of the origin and mode of preparation of drugs, their pathogenetically, toxicologically and clinically established characteristics and indications, the potencies used commonly, the preferred route of administration and dosage, taught at homoeopathic medical schools, usually elevated to the level of a department headed by a professor. (See 'Organization of Symptoms in Materia Medica' and 'Sources of Homoeopathic Drug Semiology'.)

Measures

See 'Abbreviations, Symbols, Weights and Measures'.

Measuring Glass

See 'Utensils of Homoeopathic Pharmacy'.

Mechanical Causes of Disease

See 'Causes of Disease'.

Mechanism of Physiological Response in Homoeotherapeutics

See 'Physiological Response in Homoeotherapeutics, Mechanism of'.

Medical Methodism

See 'Method'.

Medicine

Has three meanings:
  1) Remedy; drug; medicament.
  2) The non-surgical art of preventing, treating, or curing disease, according to various 'Schools'.
  3) Since Hahnemann, also the predictive science that treats of disease in all its relations.

Medicines

See 'Drug'.

Medico-Legal

Relating to both medicine and the law. In the nineteenth century homoeopathy in the USA was conspicuously in the forefront in establishing a clear relationship between its scientific perception of disease and health on the one hand and existing law and order on the other. For example, of the most profound significance in the 1880s for the ultimately accepted legal definition of insanity was homoeopathy's *Insanity in its Medico-Legal Relations* by A C Cowperthwaite, MD, Ph.D., LL D.

Homoeopathy's abiding influence during the last 25 years of the nineteenth century on US sanitary laws, concerning quarantines, vaccinations, sanitation, epidemics, and the establishment of dispensaries is outlined under 'Verdi, Tullio Suzzara (1829-1902)'.

More recently, the homoeopath Royal Copeland (was first the Health Commissioner of New York City, then Health Commissioner of New York State, then moved to US Senate) introduced and piloted the well known 1938 Food, Drug and Cosmetic Act in its slow and tortuous five-year passage to the US statute books.

Memorizing Symptoms

See 'Key-Note'.

'Memory' Carried in Hydro-ethanol Solvent Used in Potentization

See 'Solvation Structures'.

Mental Illness, Homoeopathic Assessment of

Mental illness is a broadly inclusive term encompassing any of the following:

a) disease predominantly affecting the brain or central nervous system, with pronounced behavioural symptoms, e.g. acute alcoholism or senile dementia;

b) personality disorder, characterized by abnormal behaviour, e.g. paranoia or cyclothymia;

c) disorder of conduct, evidenced by socially deviant behaviour, e.g. compulsive pyromania or kleptolagnia.

In the *Organon*, section 218, Hahnemann advises the careful determination of the totality of physical symptoms that were present before the onset of any mental illness, to guide the homoeopath in the selection of the appropriate drug.

Mentals

Homoeopathic category of symptoms, relating to the mind; sometimes erroneously called 'mental symptoms', with the implication that they refer to psychiatric conditions, which they do not. Homoeopaths following in the tradition of Adolph Lippe, James Tyler Kent, Robert Gibson Miller, Margaret Tyler, Sir John Weir, Dame Margery Blackie and Pierre Schmidt rank the mentals consistently above all other symptoms, both in the selection of key-notes for drugs and in disease picture assessment. (See 'Disease and Drug Action in Homoeopathic Congruity', section 9.)

Mesmerism

Hypnosis; treatment by suggestion during an induced state of high influenceability in a patient. Autogenic training and autosuggestion (self-hypnosis) are self-help versions of mesmerism that can be taught to a patient. Hahnemann, in section 288 of the *Organon of Medicine* says of mesmerism: 'This curative force, often so stupidly denied . . . differs so much from all other therapeutic agents. It is a marvellous, priceless gift . . . to mankind by means of which the strong will of a well-intentioned person upon a sick one . . . can bring the vital energy of the healthy mesmerizer into another person dynamically.' Franz Anton Mesmer (1733-1815), an Austrian physician who developed this system of therapeutic suggestion, which he originally called Animal Magnetism, gave his name to the terms mesmerism and mesmerize.

Metal Remedies

Mineral remedies made from a particular category of non-gaseous chemical elements. Metals are characterized by opacity, and high thermal and electrical conductivity; the latter decreases with increased temperature, however. They are electro-positive elements that tend to lose electrons in chemical reactions rather than gain them. Their oxides, dissolved in water, yield alkaline solutions. Many metals are lustrous, malleable and ductile. Over three quarters of the known elements are metals, including some that are not readily thought of as such: antimony, beryllium, bismuth, lithium, magnesium, osmium, potassium and sodium. But the category excludes non-metallic elements that have, on occasion, been incorrectly referred to as metals, such as chlorine, iodine, phosphorus and sulphur. There is also an intermediate category of metalloids, where elements resemble metals in at least one aspect; thus arsenic, carbon, germanium, selenium, silicon and tellurium belong into this category on account of their electrical conductivity. For at least two millennia, from the time of the ancient Persians and Greeks, mercury, gold, silver, copper, tin, iron and lead were the object of alchemy's intensive experimental quest for ascertaining the constitution of matter and the essence of life. The alchemists were constantly seeking the virtues and qualities of these, and later of other metals, which could be applied to human benefit. By such processes as combustion, solution, evaporation and condensation in combination with salts, acids, alkalis and with substances such as sulphur, arsenic and sel ammoniac a great many metallic compounds were produced. By the time of Paracelsus (1493-1541), when other metals were being mined, a fairly large reservoir of experiential knowledge had been accumulated concerning the reactive effects on humans of many of such metallic substances. But it was the genius of Hahnemann that devised the trituration process making it possible to have insoluble metals in curative homoeopathic medicines in potentizable colloidal form (see 'Colloid'). A number of metals are represented in the materia medica only by their salts (e.g. uranium by Uranium nitricum, or potassium by the many Kali medicines). (See also 'Mineral Remedies' and 'Tissue Salts'.)

Metastasis

The moving of local manifestation of disease in accordance with Hering's Rule in disease intensification:

1) from the surface to the interior (e.g. eczema to asthma);

2) from the extremities to the upper parts of the body (as, for instance, seen in the many different arthritides that begin in the small joints); and/or

3) from the less vital organs to the more vital (this, for example, may be seen in action in mumps, if inappropriately treated, when the symptoms around the parotid gland will subside (the less vital organ) and the testis becomes affected (the more vital organ). (See 'Homoeopathic Laws, Postulates and Precepts', section 14, and 'Therapeutic Science'.)

Method

Unifying mode of procedure; the manner, system, or sequence of events of performing cognate actions, such as performing dietary manipulations, (surgical) operations, the carrying-out of experiments, making assessments, conducting provings, or the arrangement of entire therapeutic approaches. For example, 'Paracelsan method' has come to mean the use of chemical agents only, in the treatment of disease.

In a historical context it refers to the unvarying procedure in a regular systematic treatment taken to be proper for the cure of a specific case of illness (a named 'disease'). The method was laid down by the adherents of 'The School of Medical Methodism' in their Rationalist system of medicine. This is a variant of the dominant mechanistic philosophy. It began with the introduction into the practice of medicine of the atomic theory of Democritus (ca. 460-357 BC), which meant the acceptance into physiology of a corpuscular (atomistic) interpretation of organic activity. The corpuscles or atoms were believed to obey nothing but the laws of physics and hydraulics, thus banishing all vital spontaneity from organic activity. In recent times medical Methodism was propagated by Descartes in his *Treatise of Man* (1662), and by many prominent physicians of Hahnemann's day, including William Cullen (1712-1790), John Brown (1735-1788), Francois Joseph Victor Broussais

(1772-1838) and Francois Magendie (1782-1855). It was what Hahnemann perceived as Cullen's error, whilst translating the latter's *A Treatise on Materia Medica* from English into German in 1790, that led him to insert the famous footnote on page 114 of volume II bluntly contradicting the author about his views on intermittent and quartan fevers. And it was precisely this moment's insight which provided the spark that was to culminate in the development of self-consistent medical science, in the form of homoeopathy.

Miasma

- **A condition which may be acquired or inherited underlying chronic or recurrent disease states.**

(Plural: Miasmata) or anglicized to Miasm (plural: Miasms); means stain, defilement or taint, and describes a lingering, and sometimes hereditable, disposition due to an externally-induced disturbance of physiology following:

1 infection or contagion;
2 injurious medical treatment;
3 bad hygiene and/or environmental effects;
4 occupational hazards.

A miasma is a resulting stereotypical disease condition, sometimes heredotransmissible, that – on the one hand – may either be latent or active, and – on the other – acute or chronic. Nevertheless, it is always the result of both a maintaining cause (hence the lingering disposition) and an exopathic exciting cause (the noxious trigger). Hahnemann recognized that, among the entire mass of morbid phenomena in homoeopathy's symptomatology, there was a certain number of disease pictures of a fixed, recurring type, acquiring such uniformity by originating from a specific cause. (In homoeopathy a specific irritant will produce a recognizable disease picture.) To these recurring disease pictures he allocated one, or more, appropriate so-called specific remedy/ies, as being always applicable and usually indispensable for an effective cure. In 1806, in his *Medicine of Experience*, he wrote: 'We observe a few diseases that always arise from one and the same cause, e.g. the miasmatic maladies . . ., which bear upon them the distinctive mark of always . . . remaining diseases of a peculiar character; and, because they arise from a contagious principle that always remains the same, they also always retain the same character and pursue the same course . . . These few diseases, at all events those first mentioned (the miasmatic), we may therefore term specific, and bestow upon them distinctive appellations. Should a remedy have been discovered for one of these, it will always be able to cure it, for such a disease always remains essentially identical, both in its manifestations (the representatives of its internal nature) and its cause.' With regard to the 'contagious principle', Hahnemann, though not having the benefit of a microscope, in his usual intuitive manner, put forward an uncannily accurate explanation more than half a century ahead of Robert Koch and others who first discovered that different types of bacterium were associated with some types of infectious disease. He suggested in 1832 (*Lesser Writings,* p 758) that cholera, for instance, was caused by 'an enormous . . . brood of excessively minute, invisible, living creatures.'

Hahnemann's generalizations about the phenomena of disease also led him to regard epidemic fevers as a class of specific disease, distinct from the general mass of morbid phenomena that homoeopathy deals with every day (see 'Epidemiology'), where each epidemic has features of its own (the genus epidemicus), and since it always is the product of a single cause it will, in all individual cases, be amenable to one and the same specific remedy, the epidemic's simillimum. In developing his generalizations, Hahnemann laid the foundation of the systematics of disease aetiology, later named miasmatics.

His pioneering work in this area can be compared to that of his contemporary, the Baron George Cuvier, a naturalist and father of the science of paleontology (1769-1832) who, in pre-Lamarckian and pre-Darwinian zoology, reduced the animal kingdom to four fundamental classes. This classification the baron based upon the general characteristics of the animals' internal structure. The four classes were Vertebrates, Molluscs, Articulates and Radiates, which serves the purposes of animal classification perfectly well, even today. It was only the intellectual conformism imposed by the constraints of evolutionary theories of one shade or another that all but displaced his method of zoological classification.

Hahnemann's systematics primarily divides the active miasmata into acute and chronic diseases (*Organon of Medicine,* sections 73 and 78-80).

Acute Miasmata
Acute miasmata, for which Hahnemann felt that one or several constant (specific) remedies had been, or could be, found, comprise:

Autumnal dysentery; Bubonic plague; Cholera; Croup; Hydrophobia (rabies in man); Influenza; Malarial fever (ague); Measles; Miliaria rubra; Mumps; Scarlet fever; Water-colic of Lunenberg; Whooping-cough; Yellow fever.

He always added an 'etc.' to any such listing, and, indeed, others have been added since (e.g. Abortus fever, Amoebiasis, Diphtheria, Chickenpox, Rubella, Poliomyelitis, Smallpox, Typhoid, Typhus, etc.).

Miasmata Due to Bad Hygiene
In the active category Hahnemann makes a distinction between 'the true natural chronic diseases', the Chronic Miasmata, and those diseases that 'are inappropriately named chronic, which people incur who expose themselves continually to avoidable noxious influences.' Under the latter he includes addiction, dietary perversion, malnutrition, excessive exercise or worry, and unhygienic living conditions. In recent times homoeopathy has added the effects of environmental pollutants, as well as those due to radiopathic and/or

geopathic stress, to this category. Hahnemann prescribes an improved mode of living as essential for a cure. Notwithstanding this, certain recognizable disease entities, for which there may even be constant (specific) homoeopathic medicines, are in this group too. One example is goitre when induced by an unbalanced and excessive consumption of cabbage and/or rapeseed. For this the specific drug is Spongia tosta.

Chronic Iatrogenic Miasmata

These are brought on by injurious medical treatment, are discussed under 'Auto-immune Syndrome', 'Isopathy', the section headed Homoeopathized Allopathica, and under 'Epistemological Assumptions in Homoeopathy', section 1 dealing with Dermatitis medicamentosa. Hahnemann, of course, inveighed against this form of Chronic Miasma, and the reasons for its cause, in many of his writings. J Compton Burnett's Vaccinosis belongs here, too. So does the long-term damage produced in those who react to the pertussis vaccine (ably documented by Harris L Coulter & Barbara L Fisher in *DPT: A Shot in the Dark,* New York: Warner Books, Inc, 1986). The list of allopathic products capable of causing severe miasmatic reactions, often with pronounced long-term effects, is large and diversified. In addition to the products listed under the three entries mentioned above, a few more examples of such injurious medicines are: morphine and its derivatives, phenolphthalein, barbiturates, sulfbromphthalein, phenothiazine, the various Orthodox tranquillizers, dinitrophenol, pituitrin, hydralazine, the anti-rabies 'vaccine', and many others (see also other allopathica mentioned below, under inherited miasmata).

Miasmata Arising from Occupational Hazards

These represent that vast section of lingering afflictions brought on by occupational exposure to metals, alloys, metallic compounds, salts, alkalis, acids, aromatic and aliphatic carbon compounds, as well as chemical and volatile irritants, toxicants and asphyxiants, the great majority of which have undergone homoeopathy's extensive pathogenetic experimentation (provings). One miasmatic example is chrome ulcers, that resemble punched-out holes but that show no tendency to malignant change, on the skin of a patient who has constantly been handling sodium bichromate as a colour worker for a number of preceding years. Another is the onset of mesothelioma (a rare malignant neoplasm) of the pleura in a patient who 33 years previously had been exposed to asbestos (crocidolite) dust in the ambient air for four weeks in the course of his occupation as a mining engineer.

Classical Chronic Miasmata

In addition to any occupation-, pollutant-, or drug-induced miasma or the miasma of a post-infective dyscrasia (e.g. a post-viral syndrome), Hahnemann (in *Chronic Diseases* and the *Organon*) provided a broad, fundamental classification of chronic disease stereotypes, like Cuvier did in his animal systematics. The chronic diseases were classified into three broad rubrics by him and named after the characteristic skin changes occurring in the initial stage:

1 luetic (or syphilinic) miasma – where chancres, ulcers in the skin and mucosa are the changes – the miasma of destruction;
2 sycotic miasma – where condylomata appear and proliferative mucosal and skin changes take place – the miasma of excess;
3 psoric miasma – where scabious, eczematoid or similar itch inducing skin changes occur – the miasma of deficiency. To these Antoine Nebel and Henry C Allen first added a fourth of equal importance:
4 tuberculinic (or pseudo-psoric) miasma – where body-sweats and weight-loss are the accompanying signs – the miasma of exhaustion. The tuberculinic miasma is really a combination of the taints of the luetic and psoric miasmata: the destruction of the former in cavitation with the exudative element of the latter; hence its alternative label, the pseudo-psoric miasma. To these Leon Vannier finally added a fifth of comparable significance to the other four:
5 oncotic (or cancerinic) miasma – where changes in body odour, unusual discharges, intumescences, changes in warts and/or moles, sallowness of hue affecting the skin, and sores that refuse to heal, occur – the miasma of adaptive failure.

There are Hahnemannian specific remedies as well as nosodes to which each of these five fundamental conditions is amenable, either singly, or in alternation, or in some sequence, with other homoeopathic medicines:

Chronic Miasmata	Hahnemannian	Nosode
Luetic miasma	Mercurius	Lueticum
Sycotic miasma	Thuja occidentalis	Medorrhinum
Psoric miasma	Sulphur	Psorinum
Tuberculinic miasma	Calcarea carbonica	Tuberculinum
	or Phosphorus	of one or other
	or Stannum	other variety
Oncotic	Lapis albus	Nectarianinum
	or Aurum muriaticum	or Carcinosinum
	natronatum	or Scirrhinum

An explanatory contrast between Chronic and Acute Miasmata by means of two prototypical examples:

	Chronic	Acute
Miasma	Syphilis	Scarlet fever
	(Miasma luetica)	(Miasma scarlatina)
Transmission	Congenital	Infection
	or by contagion	

	Chronic	**Acute**
Infective phase	Life-long	Brief; but sometimes a carrier state may persist for a long time
Duration	Life-long	Five to ten days
Spontaneous recovery	Impossible	Possible
Disease metastasis	In phases, from outside to inside (chancre to tabes dorsalis)	Uniformly, from inside to outside (inflamed throat and furred tongue to exanthema)
Presenting form	Extremely varied (e.g.: chancre, oral lesions, lymphadenitis, maculopapular eruption, arthralgia, bone lesions, cardiovascular syphilis, neurosyphilis, locomotor ataxia, gummata, atrophy of optic nerves, necrosis of nasal and jaw bones, etc.)	Uniform progression (sore throat, high fever, halitosis, tongue covered with heavy white fur on first two days, then peels leaving smooth red strawberry tongue, a salmon-pink flush over entire body except circumorally, really being a profuse pinpoint papular rash that peels 3 to 5 days later)
Complications if untreated	Tissue destruction, dystrophy and dystonia	Sequellae include: cervical adenitis, acute otitis media, mastoiditis, septic arthritis, empyema, pneumonia, septicaemia, in the medium term; and latent glomerulonephritis (with or without an acute haemorrhagic episode) and/or rheumatic fever, in the longer term
Specific drug	Mercurius	(Atropa) Belladonna)
Nosode	Lueticum	Scariatinum

Miasmata of Post-Infective Dyscrasias

From the above example it can readily be understood how very common a miasma of post-infective dyscrasia may be. A young patient's mother who might, for example, say that her son 'has not been well since he had scarlet fever eleven years ago', is unknowingly alluding to this miasmatic category.

Concerning the occasional hereditation of the five Chronic Miasmata, with any other conditions of miasmatic origin subsumed here, homoeopathy has vast clinical experience in effectively arresting this hereditary effect. To mention a random selection (with the likely miasma type in parentheses): heredodegeneration (iatrogenic), heredoataxia (sycotic or luetic), heredolues (luetic), heredotuberculosis (tuberculinic), and a number of heredoimmunity (psoric) conditions have been shown to respond to well-indicated miasma-specific homoeopathic drugs. It is evident that the Oncotic Miasma is likewise subject to true hereditability. It is known, for example, that a woman whose mother and/or sisters have had breast cancer is at risk approximately two times more than average. Similarly, brain tumours and sarcomas occur more frequently than expected in the siblings of children with these tumours. When an identical twin has childhood leukaemia, the probability that the other twin will develop the disease within two years of the date of diagnosis of the first is about one in five, which is far greater than the rate for the general population, or even for adopted siblings who have shared the same environmental influences. A rare cancer of the eye, bilateral retinoblastoma, for instance, also runs in consanguinous families. The chances that a patient who might have been non-homoeopathically cured of this kind of cancer will have a child afflicted with it are statistically known to be very high indeed, whereas the statistical incidence has been anecdotally reported to drop to that of the rest of the population when appropriate miasma-specific homoeopathic treatment intervened. Apart from the hereditability of the five Chronic Miasmata, examples of other miasmatic teratogenic (heredomiasmatic) effects are evident – only or overwhelmingly – in the offspring. These congenital effects are caused by such other (non-Chronic) miasmata in the parentage, as are selectively outlined here:

1) Induced by injurious medical treatment, the latent parental miasmata which produce congenital anomalies in their offspring later extend to – e.g. cranial defects from aminopterin; hypoplasia of the nose from warfarin sodium; yellow fluorescence of the teeth from tetracycline; masculinization of the external genitalia of infant girls from progestins; phocomelic deformities from thalidomide; clear cell carcinoma of the cervix and/or infertility in the adult daughters from diethylstilboestrol; etc.

2) Induced by radiopathic stress, the latent parental miasmata which produce congenital anomalies extend to – e.g. a variety of malformations and other defects in a large proportion of human infants after the ionizing radiation produced by the atomic bomb explosions in Japan in 1945; the very large number of seriously deformed calves and piglets (headless, or without eyes, limbs or ribs) reported to have been born during the first nine months of 1988

limbs or ribs) reported to have been born during the first nine months of 1988 in the Narodichi district 50 km southwest of Chernobyl, Ukrainian SR, where on the 26th April 1986 the then most serious nuclear accident in history had taken place; the leukaemia contracted by children whose fathers had worked at Sellafield (formerly Windscale) atomic plant in Cumbria, UK where they were known to have been exposed to radiopathic stress prior to conception of the miasmatically afflicted children, etc.

3) Induced by an infection, the acute maternal miasmata which produce congenital anomalies extend to – e.g. the very mild acute miasma Rubella (German measles) having disastrous embryopathic effects, such as cardiac defects, hearing loss, congenital glaucoma and other eye defects, spastic diplegia, autism and delayed psychomotor development; the even milder acute miasma Cytomegalic Inclusion disease and Salivary Gland Virus disease both having disastrous effects on the offspring; the Acquired Immune Deficiency Syndrome (AIDS) having a potentially lethal effect on such a miasmatic's unfortunate offspring; etc.

4) Induced by environmental pollutants, the latent miasmata which produce congenital anomalies extend to – e.g. cerebral palsy from inorganic mercury ingested by parent(s) through fish from polluted waters; the statistically seemingly heightened leukaemia risk in children of parents consistently exposed to a certain minimum dosage of electro-magnetic pollution (e.g. as produced around high-tension cables); etc.

5) Induced by occupational or similarly extensive exposure, the latent parental miasmata, which are thought to be producing observed inherited effects, seem empirically to extend to a whole range of reactive states, related to each of which an altered state of receptivity would have been passed on, in the Lamarckian sense, to a descendant – e.g. any phototoxic or photosensitive reaction, whether topical or oral, in an offspring of someone known to have been exposed as undermentioned, is strongly suspected as resulting from a transmitted photosensitivity miasma that would need to have been latent in at least one of the parents. The exposure by the parent to agents such as any of the following could have provoked the evident inherited hypersensitivity:

- Antiseptics (e.g. Bithionol, Tetrachlorsalicylanilide)
- Diuretics (e.g. Thiazides and related Sulfonamide compounds)
- Coal tar derivatives (e.g. Anthracene, Acridine, Phenanthrine, Pyridene)
- Sunscreening Agents (e.g. Digalloyl triolaete, Aminobenzoic acid)
- Tranquillizers (e.g. Chlorpromazine [Thorazine])
- Antibiotics (e.g. Demethylchlortetracycline hydrochloride [Declomycin])
- Antihistaminics (e.g. Promethazine hydrochloride [Phenergan hydro-chloride])
- Antifungals (e.g. N-butyl-4 chlorosalicylamide [Jadit], Griseofulvin)
- Antibacterials (Sulfonamides)
- Oral Hypoglycaemics (e.g. Chlorpropamide [Diabinase], Tolbutamide [Orinase]

- Anti-vitiligo treatment (e.g. Furocoumarins [also found in perfumes])
- Tannic Acid products
- Cosmetics (and their diverse components, notably collagen, orris root, and the oxidizing agents employed for skin bleaching purposes consisting of mercury, resorcin and salicylic acid)
- Soap (containing, say, tetrachlorsalicylanilide [TCSA] or tribromosalicylanilide [Carbolic/coal tar])
- Perfumes (also included in creams, powders, hair preparations, depilatories, soaps and deodorants).

There are considerable variations in contemporary approaches to miasmatic prescribing:

1) The Argentinian Tomas Pablo Paschero (born 1904) considers miasmata to be of environmental rather than inherited origins, whereas his compatriot Dr E A Masi considers that disorders of a spiritual nature make for deep-seated and as such also hereditable miasmata. Both believe that patients will only need one remedy and that this will never change throughout the patient's life.

2) The Mexican Proceso Sanchez Ortega (born 1919), probably the most respected living homoeopath of all Latin America, says that, though he agrees with Dr Paschero about miasmata being environment-induced and feels that the hereditary aspects may be totally ignored, several different remedies frequently have to be used, before the patient can be cured, treating, in his words, each layer as it presents, rather like peeling an onion.

3) The majority of the world's homoeopaths, however, differ from the prevailing Latin American positions, in that they uphold the broader Hahnemannian tenets on miasmata. They observe that certain toxic factors produce very particular patterns of disease, making familial medical histories important to be projected both into the past and into the future, because the elimination of both inherited and hereditable toxic factors means improvement now as well as sparing the future generation the resulting debilitation. Although Ortega's ignoring of the hereditary aspect is not accepted generally outside Latin America, his views on clearing a patient's problems layer by layer have gained much ground in recent years and have gone far towards introducing into homoeopathic miasmatic prescribing more and more pluralism and the use of complex remedy combinations (more particularly for acute miasmata), as well as increasing venturesome clinical experimentation with nosodes and sarcodes.

Hahnemannian miasmatic tenets recognize latent miasmata that may have been incubated during acute miasmatic episodes, following which there may remain behind latent post-infective dyscrasias (e.g. so-called subclinical post-viral syndromes). Through pollution of the atmosphere and food, certain other subclinical conditions may develop that are, in fact, latent miasmata too. After some immunizations there may be latent vaccinoses. Through suppressive treatment a condition that was never cured may be pushed deeper; though the patient may become or remain superficially symptom-free, a lingering latent miasma will very probably then have been established that could, at any time, be stimulated to transform itself into its chronic-active (symptomatic) phase.

The latent versions of the five chronic miasmata are generally free of the overt characteristic skin changes associated with the active forms. Yet there are then other, equally clear, indicators that the homoeopath will take into account, the most obvious of which would be aspects of the patient's history. The World Medical Association has recently acknowledged what homoeopathy had long maintained, namely that apparently healed childhood tuberculosis can be reactivated later when the host is debilitated or his/her immunity diminished, e.g. in diabetes mellitus, alcoholism, malnutrition, etc.[1] In their latency, each of the five broad miasmatic categories then becomes the phylum in homoeopathy's singular taxonomy where the class, order, family, genus, and ultimately the individual species of disease is determined by the patient's own unique illness pattern. It is in such cases that pluralism in prescriptions is common, linked to the layer-by-layer approach initiated by Ortega.

Of significance is that a miasma is always a disturbance of physiology, an organic taint, a disease condition, or an affliction suffered by an individual, but it can never be synonymous with the concept 'epidemic' as such. That is not to say miasmata may not, occasionally, reach epidemic proportions. Orthodox Medicine now employs the words 'miasma' and 'miasmata' occasionally, but has placed an inaccurate construction upon its homoeopathic meaning. In Orthodox nomenclature it is erroneously taken to mean 'Noxious effluvia or emanations regarded as the cause of various epidemic diseases.' This has led to a further malapropism in Orthodoxy: 'Miasmology: The science that deals with air pollutants and aerosols in general, and especially in relation to human health.' (*Stedman's Medical Dictionary*, XXIInd edition, Baltimore: The Williams & Wilkins Co, 1973, p 781.)

Experimental Evidence

A series of investigations demonstrating convincingly the inheritance of acquired characteristics, in the Lamarckian sense, subsequent to controlled sensitizing exposure in previous generations was carried out by C M Waddington in his laboratory in the early 1950s.[2,3,4] He used fruit-flies that were subjected to abnormal stimuli in their earlier stages of life, some of which consequently showed abnormal development, and this acquired abnormality was hereditable to subsequent generations of fruit-flies. In one experiment, young pupae whose larvae were transforming into fruit-flies were exposed to

[1] Gillibrand, Ivan M. Editorial, *Journal of the World Medical Association*, vol XXXVI, no 3, May/June 1989, pp 33 & 34.

[2] Waddington, C M. 'Selection of the Genetic Basis for an Acquired Character' *Nature*, 1952, vol CLXIX, pp 278-279.

[3] Waddington, C M. 'Experiments in Acquired Characteristics' *Scientific American*, 1953, vol CLXXXIX, pp 92-97.

[4] Waddington, C M. 'Genetic Assimilation of the Bithorax Phenotype' *Evolution*, 1956, vol 10, pp 1-13.

a heat of 40 degrees Celsius for four hours. Some of the emerging flies lacked cross-veins in their wings. In a second study, eggs that were three hours old were exposed to ether fumes for 25 minutes. Some of the fruit-flies that ultimately emerged developed a double thorax with a second set of wings attached to it. In both experiments the abnormal fruit-flies were selected as parents of the next generation, which was again exposed to the same stimulus. This was repeated for a number of generations. With each successive generation an ever higher proportion of fruit-flies showed the abnormal characteristics. After as few as eight such generations, matings by these fruit-flies gave rise to offspring that showed the abnormality even in the absence of the initiating stimulus. So-called genetic assimilation had occurred, which in the mainstream of homoeopathic thought is considered as an occasional possibility in the processes of transmission of human miasmatic effects from generation to generation.

(Refer also to contrasting and/or complementary concepts under 'Constitutional Type', 'Disease', 'Epidemiology', 'Epistemological Assumptions in Homoeopathy', section 4 and 'Humoral Pathology in Prescribing'. See entries under 'Allergy', 'Altered Receptivity in Disease', 'Auto-immune Syndrome', 'Chronic Disease', 'Diathesis', 'Environment', 'Foods as Health Problems', 'Heredity', 'Homoeosis' and 'Lamarckism'.)

Miasmatics

Science of miasmatic disease; subject taught at homoeopathic medical schools; was usually elevated to the level of a department headed by a professor. (See 'Miasma'.)

Miasmology

See 'Miasma'.

Microscope

Instrument that gives an enlarged optical image of an object or substance, invented by the Dutchman Z Janssen in 1590. The term denotes a compound microscope, since the simple microscope is no more than the magnifying glass used for very low magnification. In 1903 the Hungarian Zsigmondy and the Austrian Siedentopf, jointly, invented the ultramicroscope with which it became possible to view particles hitherto too small to be seen by the compound microscope, e.g. fog or smoke particles. Even this instrument was not capable of showing the aggregate of atoms or molecules of an insoluble substance present in a finely dispersed state in a homoeopathically prepared colloid (upward from 8DH potency), by the method invented by Hahnemann, and the scientific reality of which was generally dismissed as an absurdity until fairly recently. When in 1940, the Germans Ruska and von Borries produced the Siemens electron-microscope, with which it was possible to discern actual molecules for the first time, Hahnemann was conclusively vindicated on this point. (See also 'Colloid' and 'Utensils of Homoeopathic Pharmacy').

Midwife

Accoucheuse; a woman who practises the art of assisting other women in childbirth, which practice is referred to as midwifery. The term, which means the same as obstetrics but is very much older, is derived from the Middle English 'mid', meaning 'with', and 'wif', meaning 'woman'. (See 'Labour', 'Obstetrics and Homoeopathy'.)

Mineral Remedies

An important group of homoeopathic drugs with a special affinity for the organs and with a wide range of effects, notably in the areas of energy reserves, skin ailments and afflictions of the alimentary tract. Those mineral remedies that are insoluble, like the metals, are made soluble by a method discovered by Hahnemann (see 'Colloid'). The group includes Antimonium, Phosphorus, Silicea and Sulphur, which are all very important remedies. Among the very active mineral acids in this group are Acidum aceticum, Acidum benzoicum, Acidum fluoricum, Acidum nitricum, Acidum oxalicum, Acidum phosphoricum, Acidum sulphuricum, Acidum sulphurosum and Kali aceticum. Also included are the various mineral salts, among which some of homoeopathy's most deeply acting remedies are to be found, like Arsenicum album, Kali bromatum, Kali carbonicum, Kali sulphuricum, Magnesia phosphorica and Natrum muriaticum. (See also 'Lithotherapy', 'Metal Remedies' and 'Tissue Salts'.)

Missionary School of Medicine

Founded in 1903 by Dr Edwin A Neatby (1858-1933), and being affiliated to the British Faculty of Homoeopathy, it offers intense three-months' full-time training to Protestant missionaries unable to take normal full homoeopathic medical training. This continues to prove invaluable to those who are stationed in remote areas and whose spiritual work frequently has to compete for followers with shamanism which nearly always also provides large elements of ethnomedical healing, along with religious cults, to the local community. The School's syllabus covers:

Anatomy; Physiology; Basic Nursing Procedures; Primary Health Care; Dentistry; Environmental Hygiene; Eye Diseases; Tropical Diseases; Nutrition; Homoeopathy; Elementary Medicine; Homoeopathic/Medical Terminology; Microscopy; Obstetrics; Anaesthetics; First Aid; Paediatrics.

In all subjects there is both theory and practical work (the latter at Royal London Homoeopathic Hospital). The Tropical Child Health Unit, Institute of Child Health, London University offers a vast array of facilities as well as its tape/slide library to the students of the Missionary School of Medicine.

Mnemism

Mnemic hypothesis; Semon-Hering theory. This is occasionally employed in polemic support of certain miasmatic phenomena. It postulates that stimuli (irritants) leave engrams (definite traces) on the protoplasm of plants or animals, and when such stimuli are repeated persistently they induce a biological habit which endures after the stimuli have ceased, and that such habits are capable of being transmitted with engrammed germ cells to the descendants. (See 'Lamarckism' and 'Miasma'.)

Modalities

● **Factors that qualify a particular symptom.**

Symptomatic attributes or conditions in respect of sense experience, manner or quality, that are associated with: times of day, seasons, periodicity, thermic and/or meteorological factors, motion, locality, laterality, volitional actions, position, kinaesthesia, pressure, perception, touch or other sensations. They are usually expressed as changes, viz. either ameliorations or aggravations, e.g.: an itching nettlerash is better for being washed with cold water in the early morning, but gets worse from the warmth of the bed at night. However, phrases like 'brought on by' or 'altered into such-and-such a state by' may also describe modalities. Virtually all homoeopaths regard modalities as strongly indicative symptom components, that are important in deciding in favour of the use of one homoeopathic drug over another. The syndetic pointers to a number of homoeopathic medicines given in this Dictionary are often based on modalities qualifying the particular symptom of the entry concerned. In this regard, the entries under 'Chilliness', 'Discharges from the Body', 'Fever', 'Inflammation', 'Irritability', 'Jaundice', 'Mouth, Peculiar Taste in', etc. may serve as examples. (See 'Disease and Drug Action in Homoeopathic Congruity', section 3, and 'Syndetic Pointers'.)

Modifying Factors in Disease

May contribute to ill health by impeding the organism's dynamic curative effort. They include deficiency, excess, mal-elimination of toxins, malabsorption of nutrients, or their toxic contamination, as much as psychogenic, geopathic, ante-natal, climatic or infective stresses. Any one of these burdens may be of considerable significance, and must be identified, and if possible eliminated, before or during homoeopathic treatment. (See 'Environment', 'Foods as Health Problems', 'Homoeosis', 'Miasma', 'Nutritional Equipoise' and 'Vitamin'.)

Molecule

Smallest particle of any kind of matter – element or compound – which can exist in a free state while still preserving the character of that kind of matter. The homoeopathic conundrum thrown into sharp relief under the entry for 'Atom' applies here also (refer to that entry).

Monograph

Treatise on a single homoeopathic drug, or on one subject, or even on one class of objects, such as a habitat, a species, a genus, or a larger group of plants, animals, minerals, toxins, etc. bound together by some element of affinity or concatenation.

Morphological Characteristics

See 'Constitutional Type'.

Morphological Imbalance

See 'Idiosyncrasy'.

Morphology

Treats of the characteristic configuration or the structure of living organisms. (See 'Constitutional Type'.)

Mortar and Pestle

The most frequently used utensils in small-scale comminution. Different kinds of mortar and pestle have specific utilities in preparing or grinding different materials, the efficiency of which depends largely on the extent of contact between the surfaces of the head of the pestle and the interior of the mortar. In homoeopathy porcelain, glass or semi-vitrified pottery ware is employed for mortars and pestles, but not metal, wood or marble. For the grinding and mixing operation, when homoeopathically triturating, it is important that pestles be not interchanged, but remain paired off with the mortars to which each belongs. A mortar and pestle set, once used for preparing one homoeopathic drug, should not be used for the preparation of any other, unless the contact surfaces have first been reground or reglazed. (See also 'Cleansing of Utensils and Sterilization' and 'Utensils of Homoeopathic Practice'.)

Mother Tincture

The symbol for this is Θ (theta). It is the drug solution (alcoholic, hydroalcoholic, aqueous or glyceric) prepared in accordance with homoeopathic pharmacopoeial standards from the corresponding original succus or other soluble base constituent of the medicine. In preparing the homoeopathic mother tincture (in significant contradistinction to either the phytotherapeutic or the allopathic mother tinctures), the quantity of the original drug and the vehicle are proportioned, with very few exceptions, in such a way that it should represent one tenth (1/10) of the original drug: thus, in fact, Θ=1D. The historical reason for this is that in 1940 the Government of the USA appointed a Pharmacopoeia Committee which in 1941 recommended a uniform drug strength of 10% for all preparations, except for a few. The Homoeopathic Pharmacopoeia of the US of 1941 incorporated these recommendations, which were soon adopted elsewhere too.

Mother Tinctures and Solutions of other than 10% Drug Strength:

Acidum hydrocyanicum (2% Solution of the acid with an equal volume of alcohol fortis)	1/100
Acidum picricum (Solution in alcohol fortis)	1/100
Ambra grisea	1/100
Ammonium aceticum (Solution)	1/100
Arsenicum album (Solution)	1/100
Bromium (Solution)	1/100
Cactus grandiflorus	1/20
Calcarea caustica (Solution)	1/1000
Causticum (with an equal volume of alcohol fortis)	1/2
Chlorinum (Solution)	1/1000
Crotalus horridus (Solution, in glycerinum)	1/100
Croton tiglium	1/100
Cuprum aceticum (Solution, in aqua destillata)	1/100
Elaps corallinus (Solution, in glycerinum)	1/100
Glonoinum (Solution)	1/100
Kali arsenicosum (Solution)	1/100
Kali chloricum (Solution, in aqua destillata)	1/100
Kali permanganicum (Solution)	1/100
Mephitis mephitica putorius	1/100
Mercurius cyanatus (Solution)	1/100
Moschus moschiferus	1/20
Phosphorus	1/667
Sulphur (in alcohol fortis)	1/5000

This effectively means that the vast majority of mother tinctures and solutions (of 10% strength) have their lowest available potency at the 2D level. The ones with the 1/100 strength, being equivalent to a 2D deconcentration, have their lowest available at 3D, while the ones with the 1/1000 strength, that are equivalent to a 3D deconcentration, have theirs at 4D. Very commendably this introduced, half a century ago, a considerable safety factor into the use of mother tinctures, solutions and lowest potencies into homoeopathy. This safety factor, which is both convenient and absolutely error-proof, is often over-looked in appraisals of the safety of homoeopathic remedies in the very low potency range.

Experimental Evidence

Many mother tinctures (perhaps between thirty and forty) are frequently used by homoeopaths in a manner where the patient's reaction leads one to infer a concomitant bacteriostatic effect, additional to the principal healing stimulus. Ronald W Davey, John M Grange and others have published two studies[1,2] clearly demonstrating the preventive and inhibiting effects by 73 homoeopathic mother tinctures (further diluted 1:20 to obviate the non-specific inhibitory effect of the ethanol component) on the pathogenic action by 20 strains of microbial organisms. These latter included Staphylococcus aureus (MRSA), resistant to virtually all known orthodox 'antibiotics', and a strain of Pseudomonas aeruginosa regarded by orthodox medicine as multi-drug resistant, as well as Klebsiella pneumoniae, also particularly resistant in orthodox treatment. In addition to 48 diluted homoeopathic mother tinctures proving to be 'broad-spectrum antimicrobials' (of which 9 demonstrated activity against all three strains of Pseudomonas and 4 against Klebsiella pneumoniae) another 25 were shown to be 'antistaphylococcal agents'. The investigators stated (p 3 of later study) that 'the level of activity of some tinctures was similar to that of Fleming's original broth cultures of Penicillium.[3]

Tests for drug interactions (within the given study context) were also undertaken on twelve tinctures in all combinations as mixtures of equal parts of any two of them. Such assays were designed to show whether the observed effect of two medicines in combination is additive, synergistic, antagonistic or unchanged, compared to that of either separately. It is significant that five pairs produced a clear synergistic effect, by at least doubling their cumulative effectiveness, while one pair (Hydrastis canadensis with Eucalyptus globulus) showed an antagonistic effect, in that together their effectiveness was half that of Hydrastis alone, and a quarter that of Eucalyptus alone. It may well be that some of these effects are being unwittingly exploited by the low potency homoeopathic combination remedies. (See also 'Combinations of Homoeopathic Drugs', 'Dose', 'Expression' and 'Potency'.)

[1]Grange, John M, Ronald W Davey and S K Jonas. 'A Study of the Bacteriocidal and Bacteriostatic Effects of Preparations Derived from Plant Material Used in Herbal and Homoeopathic Medicine', *Complementary Medical Research*, August 1987, vol II, 2, pp 135-140.
[2]Davey, Ronald W, Julia A McGregor and John M Grange. 'Screening Tests for Antibacterial Substances in Plant Extracts', *Complementary Medical Research*, January 1990, vol IV, 1, pp 1-7.
[3]Fleming, Sir Alexander. 'On the Antibacterial Action of Cultures of a Penicillium with Special Reference to Their Use in the Isolation of B Influenzae', *British Journal of Experimental Pathology*, 1929, vol X, pp 226-236.

Mouth, Peculiar Taste in

As a common homoeopathic symptom component it features prominently in a large number of drugs, 85 of which are selected here. This exemplifies one small aspect of homoeopathy's abundant symptom matching capacity:

Aesculus hippocastanum	coppery
Agricus muscarius	sweet taste, yet saliva bitter, smell as of horse-radish
Aloe socotrina	bitter-sour
Alumina	sweet-sour saliva with musty smell
Ammonium carbonicum	dry, metallic-sour
Anhalonium lewinii	nauseating, woolly, insipid
Antimonium crudum	salty
Antimonium tartaricum	fatty feel, bitter-salty taste, insipidity of food
Apocynum androsaemifolium	honey-like
Arnica montana	bitter, salty
Aurum metallicum	milky taste
Baptisia tinctoria	flat, slightly bitter
Bismuthum	sweetish-metallic
Borax veneta	loss of taste
Bryonia alba	(see below)
Cadmium sulphuratum	first sweetish, then bitter and burning
Calcarea carbonica	abundant sour salivation
Capsicum annuum	foul, like putrid water
Carbo vegetabilis	of blood
Causticum	greasy, rancid
(Matricaria) Chamomilla	bitter regurgitations
Chelidonium majus	bitter, pasty
Chlorpromazinum	chalky, yeasty
Cinchona officinalis	bitter, though food tastes salty
(Erythroxylon) Coca	dry, peppery sensation, lost all appetite
Cocculus indicus	coppery
Coffea cruda	delicate, of hazel nuts, or sweet almonds
Cuprum metallicum	strong metallic, with salivation
Cyclamen europaeum	putrid
Digitalis	sweetish, fetid saliva
Euonymus atropurpurea	pasty, dry
Euphorbia amygdaloides	stinging and peppery at back of throat
Euphorbia lathyris	acrid taste with musty odour
Fagopyrum esculentum	taste of ingesta after meals, foul taste in mornings
Ferrum muriaticum	insipid
Graphites	of rotten eggs, much salivation, urine-like smell from mouth

Gymnema sylvestre	astringent, mildly bitter-acid, with loss of taste for both sugar and bitters
Hepar sulphuris calcareum	ptyalism, longing for acids, and tasteless eructations
Histaminum hydrochloricum	heat and itching in the mouth
Hydrastis canadensis	flat, peppery
Iberis amara	dry, bitter-peppery
Ignatia amara	regurgitation of bitter serous matter
Indole	of putrefaction
Kali carbonicum	foul, slimy with much salivation
Kali sulphuricum	insipid, pappy
Lacticum acidum	coppery
Ledum palustre	mouldy
Lemna minor	foul
Lobelia inflata	acrid, burning, mercurial
Lycopodium clavatum	dry, malodorous
Magnesia carbonic	sour, with bloody saliva and hawking up pea-coloured fetid particles
(Hippomane) Mancinella	of blood, very bitter
Mercurius cyanatus	styptic, metallic, disagreeably bitter
Mercurius corrosivus	salty, or very bitter
Mercurius vivus and Mercurius solubilis Hahnemanni	coppery
Natrum muriaticum	saliva salty, loss of taste and smell
Natrum phosphoricum	sour eructations, each producing mouthfuls of food
Natrum sulphuricum	slimy mucus taste
Nitricum acidum	bloody with foetor oris
Nitroso-muriaticum acidum	coppery
Nux vomica	sour, nauseating
(Oenanthe) Phellandrium	cheese-like or clam-like, water has sweet after-taste, but beer tastes bitter
Phenobarbital	bitter, morning nausea
Oleum animale	sour, fatty feeling on palate
Petroleum	mawkish, reminiscent of garlic
Phosphoricum acidum	tongue swollen, dry, tasting of viscid, frothy mucus
Phosphorus	sour, particularly after meals
Pimpinella saxifraga	earthy, acrid, burning
Piper methysticum	sweet, then piquant and sharp, then pappy and tasteless
Plumbum metallicum	risings, with sweetish taste of food
Podophyllum peltatum	cannot distinguish sweet and sour, everything has a putrid taste

Pulsatilla nigricans	greasy
Pulsatilla nuttaliana	flat bitter-rough, changing to sweetish vinegar-like
Pyrogenium (Pyrexinum)	fetid
Rheum palmatum	sour-smelling salivation
Rhus toxicodendron	greasy-sweetish
Sabadilla	copious accumulation of sweetish jelly-like saliva
Selenium	sweetish, disagreeable taste after smoking tobacco
Sepia officinalis	salty, putrid
Stannum	sourish-bitter, with acid saliva
Sulphur	bitter
Trifolium pratense	taste of drug in mouth which disgusts patient
Trillium cernum	greasy
Yohimbinum	disagreeable metallic
Yucca filamentosa	of rotten eggs
Zincum metallicum	of blood

Examples of syndetic pointers to one homoeopathic medicine:

In a patient, often unusually susceptible to the cold, dry East wind, whose bitter taste and inclination to vomit is aggravated by motion but relieved by the frequent drinking of cold water – Bryonia alba.

Mustard Gas

$(ClCH_2CH_2)_2S$. (See entry under 'Nitrum cum Sulphuri Praecipitati et Carboni' where the homoeopathic experiments of 1943 on mustard gas are referred to.)

N

Nash, E B (1838-1914)

This US homoeopath's particular influence derives largely from an important 501-page publication, entitled:

Leaders in Homoeopathic Therapeutics.

This classic originally appeared in 1898 and because it found great favour amongst homoeopaths it went through four editions in the short span of fifteen years. In it he displays an uncanny ability to fasten upon the mind of the reader the salient characteristics, the key-notes, of each homoeopathic medicine. More than ninety years later this still remains a frequently consulted, convenient ready-reference manual. Other major writings by him include:

Testimony of the Clinic
How to Take the Case
Regional Leaders
Leaders in Sulphur
Leaders in Respiratory Organs
Leaders in Typhoid

Natural Order

In botanical and zoological classification, the division just above family and just below class (sometimes also subclass and/or superorder) is order (sometimes also suborder and/or infraorder); below family the classifications are, in descending order, genus and species. Natural order is generally given in materia medica entries where applicable.

John Henry Clarke (1853-1931) said,

> 'The Homoeopathic Materia Medica consists potentially, we may say, of anything and everything that may be found in the universe. Man himself epitomizes the universe, and nothing in the universe can therefore be said to be unrelated to him. It is his business to find out the indications for the uses of the substances at his command, and the methods in which they are to be prepared and applied. Some of them he has discovered, and the substances thus rescued from the unknown constitute the Homoeopathic Materia Medica as it is at present developed. . . . [By knowing which natural order remedies belong to, will enable those who refer to the Materia Medica to understand] the order of their natural kinship. Readers will be able to discover how far natural relationship and clinical relationship correspond so far as the Homoeopathic Materia Medica at present extends.'[1]

[1] Clarke, John Henry. *A Clinical Repertory to the Dictionary of Materia Medica*. Bradford, North Devon: Health Science Press, 1979, Part V, p 325.

Naturopath

Heilpraktiker; practitioner of natural therapeutics skilled in the diagnosis of illness, deficiencies and physical defects, and their treatment and prevention by making use of physical forces and natural agents, as well as by supporting or harnessing the patient's own life forces. According to the UK's General Council and Register of Naturopaths naturopathy is a therapeutic system which has four principal hallmarks:

i)   it seeks to facilitate and promote the body's inherent physiological self-healing mechanism;
ii) it recognizes the uniqueness of each patient;
iii) it always attempts to establish and treat the cause of a condition, not merely the end effect; and
iv) it always requires that the whole person be treated, not just the local area which may be affected.

The naturopath makes use of supportive physical forces and agents such as light, water, air, thermal effects, magnetism, earth, electricity or vibration; and harnesses the patient's own life forces more directly with massage, through rest, by exercise, by stimulating reflexes, by making dietary prescriptions or by employing the patient's own heterostatic capacity.

The naturopath may achieve alterative therapeutic effects by any of the following approaches: actinotherapy, bioresonance-therapy, colonic irrigation, cryotherapy, cupping, electrotherapy, exercise, rest, remedial dance therapy, heliotherapy, hydrotherapy, magnetic induction therapy, massage therapy, megavitamin therapy, olfactory sympathicotherapy, pattern and visualization therapy, pelotherapy, phototherapy, plant juice therapy, reflex and zone therapy, remedial diets and fasting, rolfing, sound and ultrasound therapy, thalassotherapy, traction, and/or the identification and correction of influences due to geopathology. There is a minority of naturopaths that has experimentally ventured upon other therapeutic approaches, such as chromo-, crystal-, orgone-, or polarity-therapy, in addition to the traditional naturopathic treatment. With the possible exception of megavitamin therapy, these approaches to treatment may, by and large, be in harmony with homoeopathy and are, therefore, often considered as complementary.

A naturopathic physician is defined by the US Department of Labour *Dictionary of Occupational Titles*, 1965, 3rd edition, vol. I, Definition of Titles, Numeric Code 079.108 (Medical Services). From this it is evident that in the USA there has, in recent times, been a tendency to place a much broader construction upon the word 'naturopathy', so that there it is now sometimes taken to mean a medley of both adjunctive therapies (i.e. non-diagnostic modalities, e.g. hypnosis) and full medical practices (i.e. total therapeutic systems, e.g. homoeopathy). That blurs the obvious distinction between the adjunctive therapies (such as listed in the paragraph above) and autonomous, full medical disciplines, including the practices of such as a chiropractor, a homoeopath, an osteopath, a phytotherapist (herbalist) or a practitioner of Oriental Medicine. The attempt to roll all these functions into one single linguistic unit would appear to be a semantic implausibility. In any event homoeopathy certainly wishes to distance itself from such a conglomerate of therapeutic modalities and practices, because of the diversity of rules, and on account of some conflicting treatment approaches, as well as owing to the prevalence of 'group treatment' of diseases which relies on the standard non-homoeopathic disease classification system, and, not least because a tendency could arise to prescribe coercive or physiological medications as a result of doctrinal cross-contamination.

Neatby, Edwin A (1858-1933)

English homoeopath who first worked in general homoeopathic practice and later specialized in gynaecology at the London Homoeopathic Hospital. In 1903 he founded the Missionary School of Medicine (refer to this entry). He co-authored two significant homoeopathic books:

A Manual of Homoeotherapeutics (with T Stoneham)

A Manual of Tropical Medicine and Hygiene (with his uncle, Thomas Miller Neatby, who had been an active supporter of the views on pathology of Richard Hughes (refer to the entry 'Hempel, Charles Julius (1811-1879)').

Negative General Symptoms

Absence of certain striking or customary features of disease manifestations as a general symptom of a case. Examples are: fever without thirst, coldness with aversion to being covered, hunger without appetite, or an exanthematous disease without appearance of the eruption. Such uncustomary symptom deficiencies are highly significant in the homoeopathic drug diagnosis, specifically for the individualization of any case of disease.

Nettlerash

Hives; urticaria. (See 'Allergy' and 'Emergencies – Homoeopathic Treatment' under Angioneurotic Oedema.

Neural Therapy

Has been employed in Europe since early in the twentieth century. It aims to restore the resting potential of $+9$ mV in chronically depolarized cells of impaired function, by injecting small amounts of xylocaine or procaine, which carry a higher electrical charge. This often leads to the swift restoration of proper cellular function in a variety of neuro-muscular conditions. The approach is considered compatible with homoeopathic treatment by some, whilst it is regarded as inadmissible by other homoeopaths.

Neurosis

A state of tension or irritability of the nervous and/or emotional system; or functional nervous disease associated with no evident lesion. This is too broad a symptom category for homoeopathy to be a very useful remedy indicator for the homoeopath.

Neutral Substance

For pharmaceutical purposes, a substance which is neither alkaline (base) nor acidic. It should be noted that non-reactive substances in crude form (e.g. Silica) can, for homoeopathic purposes, become therapeutically highly active (non-neutral) when dynamized (potentized). Moreover, since homoeopathy has established (by pathogenetic experiment) that no substance would appear to be absolutely medicinally inert there cannot be a 'neutral substance' in any absolute, but at best only in a relative sense. (See 'Epistemological Assumptions in Homoeopathy', section 6.)

Nisus Formativus

The formative impulse. (See 'Dynamis' and 'Laws of Nature'.)

Nitrum cum Sulphuri Praecipitati et Carboni

Black Gunpowder; Carbon-sulphur-kali-nitricum. As a standardized mixture, and not a chemical compound, it is a remedy that is homoeopathic to septic conditions (abscess, acne, septicaemia, carbuncles, boils, septic tonsillitis, vaccinosis, infected cuts and bites). John Henry Clarke conducted an auto-proving with it in a 2DH potency. He published the results in August, 1915, referring to it, in those bellicose times, as the 'war remedy'. In fact, external events such as wars frequently influence the scientific development of homoeopathy. Another example is John Paterson's 'Report on Mustard Gas Experiments (Glasgow and London)', published in the *British Homoeopathic Journal* during the Second World War, on 25th January, 1943. In this double blind controlled trial using volunteers, Paterson demonstrated not only the prophylactic effects of a potency of mustard gas, but also its clear therapeutic effect after the application of the liquid gas. No large-scale benefit was ever derived from this investigation, as both sides in that conflict refrained from using any chemical weapons, and by the 1980s, during the Iraq-Iran War where mustard gas was first used again, the homoeopaths seemed to have forgotten Paterson's successful experiments of 45 years earlier.

Nocebo

See 'Epistemological Assumptions in Homoeopathy', section 6.

Noesis

An intellectual perception of the world.

Noetic

Science of the intellect. As an adjective: of, or pertaining to, or existing in, the intellect or mind; purely intellectual or abstract.

Nomenclature, Discrepancies in

Terms describing a few pharmaceutical vehicles have had their meanings transposed when they reached the English-speaking area. These differences have led to some confusion. It is important to note that what are labelled 'granules' internationally, are termed 'pillules' or 'pills' by English-speakers, whilst what are internationally referred to as 'globules' or 'globuli' are known to English-speakers as 'granules'. (See 'Granules' and 'Pillules'.)

Dynamization, as used by Hahnemann, means potentization. This is true internationally, except that in French the word 'dynamisation' has become synonymous with succussion. This has led to serious misapprehensions, when, at times, very low deconcentrations were given a potency number that actually referred to the number of times it was succussed (with no corresponding serial deconcentrations).[1] (See 'Potentizing Methods'.)

Confusion often enters into international French/English communications surrounding the terminology concerning products of nosological and biological origin. Below, some of the terms and phrases are placed side by side:

English	French
nosode	Biothérapique (does not mean 'a biological')
sarcode	opothérapique
sarcode (of hormonal origin)	hormonothérapique
organotherapeutic (preparation)	organothérapique (though this is occasionally inaccurately used synonymously with 'opotherapique', meaning 'sarcode')
a term not generally used in English for 'medicine in minimal amounts', commonly applied to some homoeopathic combination remedies	oligothérapique

[1] Already complained of by Richard Hughes in *A Manual of Pharmacodynamics*, sixth edition, London: Leath and Ross, 1893, p 104.

English	French
biological (preparation)	médicament biologique
biological shield	écran thermique
biological warfare	guerre microbienne

Nosocomial

Referring to a new disorder, additional to a patient's original condition, acquired while being treated in a hospital, the Greek synonym for which is 'nosocomion'.

Nosode

Homoeopathically prepared remedy from disease products with its own full distinct drug picture. Homoeopathy recognizes five separate categories of nosode (these are fully described under 'Isopathy'). When this term is used in orthodox medicine it signifies a bacterine (i.e. a bacterial 'vaccine') said to enhance immunity. (See also 'Bowel Nosodes'.)

Nosodes in Miasmata, Use of

See 'Isopathy' and 'Miasma'.)

Nosology

Nosotaxy; the classification of ailments. Hence 'nosological'.

Nosopoietic

Pathogenic.

Nurse

Has two meanings, both as a verb and as a noun.
  Verb:
  1) To suckle an infant.
  2) To perform all the requisite offices in the care of disabled or diseased patients.
  Noun:
  1) Person who has the care of an infant or young child.
  2) Trained individual who has the care of a patient, performing all the requisite offices in relation to the toilet, personal hygiene, monitoring of vital signs (pulse rate, blood pressure, body temperature, etc.), giving of food and remedies under the direction of the homoeopath.

Nursery Age to Adolescence, Homoeopathic Medication from the

Well established remedies particularly suitable for infants, children and adolescents are often listed along with the most common ailments that may affect the paediatric patient. Since the bias of prescription is primarily pathotropic, low potencies are generally suggested in such listings, although this remains a matter of absolute discretion for the attending homoeopath. There are some medicines that may be applicable to be found under 'Externally Applied Homoeopathic Drugs'.

It seems appropriate to state the 'like' folk-method of applying heat locally to pain which is both safe and effective in severe pain in children. It involves heating lint or cotton wool next to the fire, and changing this frequently. Obviously this method is occasionally inappropriate should the pain be aggravated by heat. The entry under 'Fever' provides some other useful hints: a practical 'like' folk-method for profuse perspiration, and some important advice on diet and fluid regimen with feverish illness will be found there.

The most convenient form in which to administer homoeopathic medicines to children is probably in drop form that can be mixed in a quarter tumbler of spring water, stirred vigorously and given, either in teaspoonfuls, or from a feeding bottle to which a little warm water has been added. If granules (pillules, powders) are administered, they may be dissolved and administered in the same way, or, in older children, a dose thereof may be given dry under the tongue. The frequency of repetition will vary: a likely dosage regimen may be

severe symptoms + high temperature: one dose every half hour
as improvement sets in: one dose every two hours
as the symptoms begin to subside: one dose every four hours

(see also entry under 'Dose').

A current text-book on homoeopathic paediatrics is:

Homoeopathy in Paediatric Practice by Hedwig Imhäuser, translated from the German original into English by Sigrid Penrod (Heidelberg: Karl F Haug Verlag, 1988, 236 pages)

Donald Foubister in *Tutorials on Homoeopathy* (Beaconsfield: Beaconsfield Publishers Ltd, 1989) devotes chapters 6 to 11 [pages 45-90] to 'Homoeopathy and Paediatrics', where he provides much detailed and valuable advice.

Nutrient

Item of food, which may be either indispensable or non-essential for sustenance.

Nutrition

A function of living organisms which consists in the consuming and then metabolically assimilating substances whereby energy is produced and body tissues are built up. Also the study of requirements in terms of food and drink for: activity, growth, maintenance, repair and convalescence, lactation, gestation and reproduction. (See also 'Dietary Therapy' and 'Homoeopathic Practice'.)

Nutritional Equipoise

A prerequisite in homoeopathy for (a patient's) health. Always of concern to the homoeopath should be the following: the interactions of nutritional factors with a patient's biochemistry, physiology and anatomy, and how the clinical application of knowledge about such interactions, including the individual homoeopathic reactive effects, may be elicited; also how these can be used in the modulation of structure and function for the prevention and treatment of disease, as well as in the betterment of health. A comprehensive sourcebook on this subject is Melvyn R Werbach's *Nutritional Influences on Illness* (second revised edition, Tarzana, Ca: Third Line Press Inc, which was then published in the UK – Wellingborough: Thorsons Publishers Ltd, 1989, 512 pages). (See also 'Foods as Health Problems'.)

Nutritional 'Supplements' (Herbals, Vitamins, Minerals etc.)

Routine consumption, say, on a regular daily basis, of therapeutically active substances, generally on the flimsiest of pretexts – for instance, certain 'herbal' preparations – is deplored by homoeopathy. Sooner or later, reactive effects due to constant palliation, irritation (e.g. herbal laxatives) and/or suppression will become evident in the incautious consumer. (See also 'Phytotherapy'.)

O

Observation

Attentive examination of phenomena, with a view to a fuller homoeopathic appraisal of the patient's condition. The homoeopath seeks out, in each case, that which is peculiar, uncommon, characteristic or individual. To that end he records any striking statements made by the patient, he remains on the alert and constantly observant, before, during and after the physical examination, looking for unusual facial expressions, extraordinary physical demeanour, noting odours, clothing, hair, manners, complexion, gait, speech, foibles and whims, speech, tidiness, posture, movement, etc. He quietly observes also things like the amount of covering on the sick-bed, the degree of light and ventilation in the patient's room, his reactions to noise, the items of food and drink that are specially asked for, or that are left unconsumed, etc. The homoeopath also attaches great importance to the time-honoured surveillance in the tradition of Empirical medicine of the faeces, sputum, exudates, urine and of the vomit. In non-homoeopathic medicine this manner of patient-observation has all but disappeared, having been displaced by specialized diagnostic tests, isolating the practitioner from important body processes. (See also 'Diagnosis', 'Disease and Drug Action in Homoeopathic Congruity' and 'Questionnaire'.)

Obstacles to Treatment Response

See 'Homoeopathic Practice'.

Obstetrics and Homoeopathy

The term obstetrics is derived from the Latin 'obstetrix', meaning 'midwife' or 'the woman who stands by' the one giving birth. It is a branch of health care that deals with parturition, its antecedents, and its sequels. It is concerned, principally, therefore, with the phenomena and management of pregnancy, labour, and the puerperium, in both normal and abnormal circumstances.

The original excellent textbook on the subject, which is still well worth consulting, was written by a close friend of Hahnemann in Paris, Simon Felix Camille Croserio, entitled *Manual Homeopatico de Obstetricia*, Havana: Imprenta de A Graupera, 1855 (Calle Obispo 113, La Habana, Cuba for Bailly-Bailliere, Madrid, Spain). Six good contemporary homoeopathic reference works on this subject are:

1 *Homoeopathic Therapeutics, as Applied to Obstetrics* by Sheldon Leavitt, Professor of Physiology and Clinical Midwifery, Hahnemann Medical College and Hospital, Chicago, Illinois, USA. Calcutta: Haren & Brother, reprint 1962 [121 pages]. It is divided into three principal sections:
   i)   The Clinical and Pathogenetic Indications for Homoeopathic Remedies in Obstetrics;
   ii) A Clinical Repertory of Homoeopathic Therapeutics as Applied to Obstetrics;
   iii) The Index.
2 *Handbook of Practical Midwifery* by J H Marsden, New Delhi: Jain Publishing Co, reprint 1973 [327 pages]. It includes full instruction for the homoeopathic treatment of the disorders of pregnancy, and the accidents and any disease incident to labour and the puerperal state.
3 *The Accoucheur's Emergency Manual* by W A Yingling, MD, Ph.D., Member of the International Hahnemannian Association. New Delhi: Jain Publishing Co, reprint 1982 [323 pages]. It gives assistance in obstetric emergencies, at the bed-side, for appropriate remedy selection.
4 *Homoeopathy in Practice*, chapter 7 [pages 75-90] entitled 'Obstetrics and Some Gynaecological Conditions', by Douglas Borland – edited by Kathleen Priestman. Beaconsfield: Beaconsfield Publishers Ltd, 1982.
5 *An Obstetric Mentor* by Clarence M Conant, Calcutta: Roy Publishing House, second reprint 1970 [159 pages]. It is a handbook of homoeopathic treatment during pregnancy, parturition and the puerperal period, having additionally drawn worldwide on homoeopathic authorities, viz. the published works on midwifery by the following: Guernsey, Richardson, Croserio, Jahr, Hale, Ludlam, Eaton, Eggert, Ostrom and the files of *The Homoeopathic Journal of Obstetrics* (USA).
6 *Homoeopathie in Frauenheilkunde und Geburtshilfe* by Erwin Schlüren, Heidelberg: Karl F Haug Verlag, 1980, 211 pages. It is divided into ten convenient thumb-indexed sections.

(See also 'Antenatal Homoeopathy', 'Euthenic (Nosode) Treatment', 'Gynaecology' and 'Pregnancy'.)

Occupational Disease

Miasma through damage produced in the course of patient's occupation. (See 'Miasma'.)

Officinal

Officinalis (Latin). Denoting a chemical, a succus, a solution, a tincture or other medication held in stock in a generally accepted prepared form, usually as laid down in a homoeopathic monograph or pharmacopoeia. This is distinguished from a magistral preparation. (See also 'Magistral'.)

Ointment

Salve; unguentum; a semi-solid vehicle for homoeopathic substances intended for external application. Different bases used as such a vehicle have varying functions. An oleaginous base will keep the remedy in prolonged contact with the patient's skin while, at the same time, having an emollient effect: it acts as an occlusive dressing. A water-soluble, or greaseless, base will only contain water-soluble homoeopathic substances. A water-in-oil emulsion base will permit the incorporation of aqueous homoeopathic solutions. An oil-in-water emulsion, or cream base, on the other hand, may contain Adeps lanae [anhydrous lanolin], Paraffinum mollum album (or flavum) [white (or yellow) petroleum jelly], and/or waxes. (See also 'Cerate', 'Cetaceum', 'Paraffinum mollum album [or flavum]' and 'Vehicle'.)

Old Age Home

Asylum for the aged; institution for the housing and care of geriatrics. A large number of such institutions, that very successfully provided only homoeopathic treatment to its resident aged, was in existence in the USA before 1920. (See 'Gutman, William' and 'History of Homoeopathy before 1900', section on United States of America.)

Oleum Amygdalae

Almond oil; the fixed oil expressed from the seeds of the bitter almond. This should not be used uncritically as a homoeopathic vehicle (e.g. as base for an ointment for chapped hands, as is sometimes recommended), because Amygdala amara has its own proven homoeopathic drug picture which should correspond to the patient's condition, if it is to be effective. (See 'Vehicle'.)

Oleum Olivae

Olive oil; the fixed oil expressed from the ripe fruits of Olea europaea. It is a pale, slightly greenish yellow oil with a faint odour and a bland taste. It is slightly soluble in alcohol and miscible with acetone, chloroform, ether and light petroleum. Its weight per ml 0.910 to 0.913 g. Sterilized by heating for one hour at 150 degrees Celsius. Although, in relative terms, it can be said to have no intrinsic medicinal qualities, it may be given by rectal injection (0.5 to 6.0 ml warmed to about 32 degrees Celsius) to soften impacted faeces; externally it is an emollient, employed to soften the skin and crusts in eczema and psoriasis, and as a non-medicinal lubricant for massage (see 'Massage Therapy'). Oleum olivae is stable and has similar properties to Teel oil, and is used interchangeably with this in the preparation of liniments, ointments and soaps. In liniments it is generally one part medicine to nine parts Oleum olivae. (See 'Vehicle'.)

Olfactory Medicines

For several years from 1832 Hahnemann experimented with olfaction as a route of medicinal administration. This idea of the effectiveness of smelling, or rather inhaling, homoeopathic medicines came to him as a result of the following interesting assumption (in which he also displays his intuitive understanding of both the medicinal pathway from the mucous membranes in the upper region of the nasal cavity, and the nature of cholera): 'Above all other drugs Camphor possesses the property of speedily killing by its vapour the most minute animals of a low order. Consequently, it will be able to kill most speedily, and to annihilate the cholera miasma (which most probably exists because of a murderous organism, undetected by our senses, which attaches itself to a man's skin, hair, etc., or to his clothing and is thus transferred invisibly from man to man).' In his correspondence with Boenninghausen, and elsewhere, he repeatedly mentions the healing effect achieved through smelling medicines. On the 28th April, 1833 he wrote to Boenninghausen saying that he and his assistant, Dr Gottfried Lehmann (1788-1865), had for nine months treated all their patients by letting them only smell their medicines, with very good results. Subsequently, in paragraph 248 of the *Organon,* he suggests smelling homoeopathic drugs in liquid form (in a small vial, containing, say, between 3 and 5 ml) whenever apparent aggravations manifest themselves, in order thereby to obviate these. He stipulates there: 'the medicine which is to be used by olfaction every two, three or four days, . . . also must be thoroughly succussed eight to ten times before each olfaction.'

The use of olfactory medicines in diverse forms has been maintained by a small number of practitioners. A recent exponent is the Frenchman Jean-Pierre Willem who refers to a naturopathic variant as 'la sympathicothérapie nasale', describing it as 'une médecine d'urgence, d'action rapide, aux effets immédiats et spectaculaires' (a medicinal emergency measure, quick acting with immediate and spectacular effects).[1] In a verbal communication (Paris, January 1990) with the author Dr Willem pointed out that primates were observed to be in the habit of breaking off and gently crushing leaves and other parts of plants, to then sniff them seemingly for their 'health-restorative' effects. The Swede Patrick Störtebecker and other investigators have demonstrated the direct pathway for transport of inhaled metal fumes (e.g. mercury from dental amalgam) from the oro-nasal to the cranial cavity (i.e. the atomic particles settle on the mucous membranes in the upper region of the nasal cavity, whence they are transported directly to the brain and the hypophysis) via the olfactory nerves, or the valve-less cranial venous system that provides an open pathway from the oro-nasal cavity to the intracranial cavity.[2,3] This direct nose-brain pathway

---

[1]Willem, Jean-Pierre. *Guide des Médecines Harmoniques,* Saint-Amand-Montrond: Editions Robert Jauze, 1986, pp 160-163.

[2]Störtebecker, Patrick. 'Dental Significance of Pathways for Dissemination from Infectious Foci', *J Can Dent Assoc,* 1967, vol XXXIII, pp 301-311.

[3]Störtebecker, Patrick. *Mercury Poisoning from Dental Amalgams: A Hazard to Human Brain,* Stockholm, Störtebecker Foundation for Research, 1985.

bypasses the general arterial bloodstream and the liver's detoxifying processes. The same pathway is applicable to other materials too (like toxins, amino-acids, and even micro-organisms),[1] besides metals.[2]

Olive Oil

See 'Oleum olivae'.

Oncotic Miasma

Cancerinic miasma. (See also 'Miasma'.)

Operation

Action of a medicinal agent; also any surgical procedure.

Opposite Action of Large and Small Doses

See 'Homoeopathic Laws, Postulates and Precepts', section 5.

Opsonic Index

Opsonin is an antibody that combines with a specific antigen to sensitize it in such manner as to make it more readily engulfed by phagocytes (phagocytosis). This is known as opsonization. A certain amount of opsonin is always found in the serum, normally, ready to protect in this manner against unwanted, common micro-organisms. Other categories of opsonin are only produced in reaction to specific stimulation, either during disease or in response to the secondary homoeopathic drug effect, as was shown by studies undertaken by Charles Edwin Wheeler (1868-1946). Wheeler could report that Arsenicum album 'appears to be almost a general stimulant to phagocytosis, Veratrum viride raises the opsonic index to Pneumococcus, Phosphorus to that of the Tubercle bacillus, Hepar sulphuris calcareum that to Staphylococcus aureus, and Baptisia tinctoria increases the agglutinating power to Bacillus Typhosus'.[3] Margaret L Tyler (1875-1943) quotes Wheeler from his *Case for Homoeopathy*: 'There is no scepticism in regard to the next experiment. In typhoid fever the body develops a substance which is not normally present in it, called agglutinin; which causes the typhoid bacilli to clump together, and forms a stage in the defence mechanisms against the disease. If healthy people

[1] Störtebecker, Patrick. 'Mercury Poisoning from Dental Amalgam through a Direct Nose-Brain Transport', *Lancet,* May 1989, vol XXVII, part 1(8648), p 1207.

[2] Perl, D P, and P F Good. 'Uptake of Aluminium into Central Nervous System along Nasal-Olfactory Pathways', *Lancet,* 1987(i), p 1028.

[3] Wheeler, Charles Edwin. *An Introduction to the Principles and Practice of Homoeopathy,* Rustington, Sussex: Health Science Press, 1971, pp 35-36.

take the drug Baptisia persistently, they develop (more or less according to individual susceptibility) this agglutinin in their blood.'[1]

The opsonic index is expressed as a numerical value representing the relative quantity of opsonin in the blood of a patient with an infectious acute miasma. It is calculated as follows:

$$= \frac{\text{Phagocytic index of normal serum}}{\text{Phagocytic index of test serum}} = \frac{1}{X}$$

Optometrist

Refractionist who, after determining the condition of refraction of the media of each eye, fits spectacles, if required, to correct visual defects. Homoeopathy regards optometry as an adjunctive health care service.

Order

See 'Laws of Nature' and 'Natural Order'.

Organic Clock

Homoeopathy views disease as a corrective process. Its presenting symptom picture changes with time. The same is true of drug pictures elicited in pathogenetic experiments (provings), except that many of these have a fixed diurnal pattern of troughs of aggravation, or particular effectiveness (this is known as 'medicine time'). Research findings (developed beyond the pioneering work by Forsgren[2] into the phases of the liver metabolism) link the phases of the liver metabolism to these recorded homoeopathic drug effects, although this is certain to be only a partial explanation.

Here follows a selection of prominent drugs which produce changes, aggravations or ameliorations diurnally at the times shown. The complementary correspondence between the known biological changes (briefly indicated in the right column below) on the one hand, and the 'medicine times' and 'drug effects' for each remedy as per the materia medica on the other is remarkable. This underscores the overall cohesiveness of homoeopathic science. The following list is an adaptation of one similar produced by Gerhard Köhler in his excellent handbook (see footnote 2 below).

Arsenicum album	01h00	Capillary contraction at its most pronounced; lowest level of cardio-vascular output;

[1] Tyler, Margaret L. *Homoeopathic Drug Pictures*, Rustington, Sussex: Health Science Press, 1970, p 111.
[2] Köhler, Gerhard. *The Handbook of Homoeopathy: Its Principles and Practice*, translated from German, Wellingborough: Thorsons Publishing Group, 1986, p 57.

Acidum benzoicum	02h00	Lowest level of kidney
Acidum nitricum	02h00	function, hence highest level
		of unelimitated waste
		products in blood and other
		body fluids;
Ammonium carbonicum	03h00	Pulmonary circulation at its
Antimonium tartaricum	03h00	lowest point, with venous
Kalium carbonicum	03h00	return sluggish;
Aurum metallicum	04h00	Critical switch at this time in
Chelidonium majus	04h00	the metabolism from the
Lycopodium clavatum	04h00	absorptive, constructive,
Nux vomica	04h00	assimilatory, to the
Podophylum peltatum	04h00-08h00	retrograde, destructive,
Sulphur	04h00-08h00	dissimilatory phase; the
		rhythms of cellular
		chemotaxis are superseded
		by those of the reticular
		system of the brain and the
		autonomic nervous system
		as also by the secretory
		programme of the entire
		glandular system;
Aloe socotrina	05h00	Entero-absorption of lipids is
Podophyllum peltatum	as above	progressively reducing from
Sulphur	as above	this time;
Eupatorium perfoliatum	06h00-08h00	Gradual rise of body
Podophyllum peltatum	as above	temperature, as is normal in
Sulphur	as above	homoithermal organisms,
		begins then;
Ailanthgus gladulosa	08h00	
Chininum arsenicosum	08h00	
(Daphne) Mezereum	08h00	
Carbo vegetabilis	08h00	Disorders of thermal
Kali carbonicum	09h00	regulation become evident
Melilotus alba	09h00	from this time;
Melilotus officinalis	09h00	
Natrum muriaticum	09h00	
Stannum metallicum	09h00	
Baptisia tinctoria	10h00	
Wyethia helenoides	10h00	
Argentum nitricum	11h00	The dissimilatory phase of the
(Nanthex) Asafoetide	11h00	metabolism ends at this
(Trigonocephalus) Lachesis	11h00	time, often associated with

Natrum carbonicum	11h00	pronounced hypoglycaemia;
Sulphur	11h00	
Zincum metallicum	11h00	
Eugenia jambos	12h00	
Moschus moschiferus	12h00	
Fulsatilla nigricans	12h00	
(Gonolobus) Condurango	13h00	Maximal biliary secretion from
Sarsaparilla	13h00	about this time;
Chelidonium majus	13h00-14h00	
Chelidonium majus	as above	
Clematis erecta	14h00	
Ptelea trifoliata	14h00	
Conium maculatum	15h00-18h00	
(Citrullus) Colocynthis	16h00	Switch at this time in hepatic
Crotalus horridus	16h00	rhythms to nocturnal phase;
Lycopodium clavatum	16h00	
Podophyllum peltatum	16h00	
Pulsatilla nigricans	16h00	
Thuja occidentalis	16h00	
Causticum	17h00	Peak of body temperature at
Chelidonium majus	17h00	this time, as is customary
Chincona officinalis	17h00	for homoiothermal
Graphites	17h00	organisms;
Helleborus niger	17h00	
Tuberculinum	17h00	
Argentum nitricum	18h00	
Hepar sulphuris calcareum	18h00	
Nux vomica	18h00	
Silicea	18h00	
Ambra grisea	19h00	Decrease of body temperature
Lycopodium clavatum	19h00	is normal at this time;
Rhus toxicodendron	19h00	
Sulphur	19h00	
Baryta carbonica	20h00	
Elaps corallinus	20h00	
Muriaticum acidum	20h00	
Phosphorus	20h00	
Aconitum napellus	21h00	
Bryonia alba	21h00	
(Cephaelis) Ipecacuanha	22h00	Pulse rate and blood pressure
Phosphorus	22h00	at their lowest levels, hence
		decreased circulatory output
		then;

Aralia racemosa	23h00	
(Atropa) Belladonna	23h00	
Rumex crispus	23h00	
Argentum nitricum	24h00	At this time capillary
(Trigonocephalus) Lachesis	24h00	contraction proceeds.

B S Luke's *Remedies Round the Clock and Medicine Time* (Berhampur: Swadheen Press, 1979, 83 pp) and Cyrus M Boger's *Times of the Remedies and Moon Phases* (reprint, New Delhi: Indian Books and Periodicals Syndicate, 1972, 168 pages) may serve as handy and detailed reference works on this subject.

Organisation Médicale Homéopathique Internationale

See 'International Homoeopathic League'.

Organismic Field

At any level of holistic structural complexity, a region of dynamic, physical and/or energetic influence constituting a holon, which, together with other holons, composes part of a larger whole. All such organismic fields are organized in many-layered nested holarchies. In 1967 Arthur Koestler proposed the concept holon as denoting a whole that, simply, is capable of being part of a larger whole. In the cosmology consonant with homoeopathy's assumptions such organismic fields, seen as ever-ascending holarchic components, would cover: atoms, molecules, cells, tissues, organs, biological systems (e.g. the respiratory or the vascular system), individuals, cultures, ecosystems, planets and galaxies, to mention the most obvious. In fact, the entire cosmos can be seen as an organismic field, as opposed to a machine (the view of the mechanistic theory). The English scientist James Lovelock CBE put forward the idea that the earth can be viewed as a self-regulating biological organism. This, the so-called 'Gaia hypothesis', could also be said to describe an organismic field, or a holon. (See 'Dynamis', 'Epistemological Assumptions in Homoeopathy', 'Laws of Nature' and 'Vitalism'.)

Organization of Symptoms in the Materia Medica

Since Hahnemann's *Materia Medica Pura* (six volumes, published 1811-1821) the schemata for this have not altered greatly. Constantin Hering's *The Guiding Symptoms of Our Materia Medica* (ten volumes, Philadelphia: Estate of Constantin Hering, 1879-1891) is representative of the order of symptom arrangement in the nineteenth century. Symptoms were ranked in forty-eight categories in the following sequence:

| 1 Mind | 3 Inner Head |
| 2 Sensorium | 4 Outer Head |

5	Sight and Eyes	27	Cough
6	Hearing and Ears	28	Inner Chest and Lungs
7	Smell and Nose	29	Heart, Pulse, Circulation
8	Face	30	Outer Chest
9	Lower Part of Face	31	Neck and Back
10	Teeth and Gums	32	Upper Limbs
11	Taste, Speech, Tongue	33	Lower Limbs
12	Inner Mouth	34	Limbs in General
13	Palate and Throat	35	Rest, Position, Motion
14	Appetite, Thirst and Desires	36	Nerves
15	Eating and Drinking	37	Sleep
16	Hiccough, Nausea and Vomiting	38	Time
17	Scrobiculum and Stomach	39	Temperature and Weather
18	Hypochondrium	40	Fever
19	Abdomen and Loins	41	Attacks
20	Stools and Rectum	42	Locality and Direction
21	Urinary Organs	43	Sensations
22	Male Sexual Organs	44	Tissues
23	Female Sexual Organs	45	Touch/Injuries
24	Pregnancy and Parturition	46	Skin
25	Voice, Larynx, Trachea	47	Constitution, Stages of Life
26	Respiration	48	Relationship

Representative for the early part of the twentieth century is John Henry Clarke's *A Dictionary of Practical Materia Medica* with its accompanying *Clinical Repertory* (three volumes, London: The Homoeopathic Publishing Co, 1900-1904). Symptoms were ranked in thirty-one categories in the following simplified sequence:

	Clinical Descriptions	13	Stool and Anus
	Characteristics	14	Urinary Organs
	Relations	15	Male Sex Organs
	Causation	16	Female Sexual Organs
1	Mind	17	Respiratory Organs
2	Head	18	Chest
3	Eyes	19	Heart, Pulse, Arterial Tension
4	Ears	20	Neck and Back
5	Nose	21	Limbs
6	Face	22	Upper Limbs
7	Teeth	23	Lower Limbs
8	Mouth	24	Generalities
9	Throat	25	Skin
10	Appetite	26	Sleep
11	Stomach	27	Fever
12	Abdomen		

Representative for the last quarter of the twentieth century is Frenchman Othon André Julian's *Materia Medica of New Homoeopathic Remedies* (English translation, Beaconsfield: Beaconsfield Publishers Ltd, 1979). Symptoms were ranked in terms of the following schema:

General
Mind
  Psychological
  Nervous
  Sleep
  Endocrine
Digestive System
  Mouth, Tongue, Pharynx
  Stomach, Intestines, Abdomen
Circulatory System
  Thermoregulation
Respiratory System
  Throat
  Lungs, Pleura
Sense Organs
  Nose
  Eyes
  Ears
Urogenital System
  Urinary
  Male Genital
  Female Genital
Locomotor System
  Upper Limbs
  Lower Limbs
  General
Skin
Biological Disturbances
  Chemical
  EEG, ECG, EMG
Modalities
  Aggravation
  Amelioration
  Laterality
Positive Diagnosis
  [meaning diathesis, state – like upset libido, or constitutional type]
Differential Diagnosis
  [meaning similar but different drug diagnoses, by comparison with related remedies]
Clinical Diagnosis
  [cognate standard disease entities].

(See 'Materia Medica' and 'Pathogenetic Experiment'.)

Organon

● **Hahnemann's analysis of the elements of medical practice systematically set out in one book by that name.**

Means 'organ' in Greek; organum (in Latin); a morphic unit; any structurally united collection of cells that is normally capable of coherently exercising a specific life-furthering function for the benefit of the greater whole – the individual body (e.g. such functions as: respiration, sensing, reproduction, digestion, secretion, etc.).

When written with an initial capital letter, it usually refers to the *Organon of the Rational System of Medicine* by Christian Friedrich Samuel Hahnemann (1755-1843). He took the title for his magnum opus from two renowned men: from Aristotle (ca. 384-322 BC), whose work *The Organon*, as the compendium of his logical treatises, is taken to be the instrument and basis of all reasoning, and from Francis Bacon, Lord Verulam and Viscount of St Albans (1561-1626), whose brilliant *Novum Organum* furnished a better mode of investigation of the truth underlying nature than the scholastics had done before him.

Hahnemann's *Organon* is a conceptual unit of the universal systematics of medicine, known as homoeopathy, which has been confirmed by coherent empirical observation and experiment. It sets out with great succinctness homoeopathy's consistent philosophy, the rules of scientific medical practice as applied to the patient, and the general natural laws of similitude and cure, as well as the principles derived therefrom. After the first edition there appeared medical orthodoxy's *Anti-organon* that railed against the homoeopathic medical discoveries. This was written by Professor Dr Heinroth of Leipzig, but it only managed to weaken orthodoxy's claim to a scientific foundation. The *Organon* soon became, and has remained, a medical classic, despite the later unsuccessful attempts in many orthodox quarters to smother it in silence.

The first edition of Hahnemann's *Organon* was published in Leipzig in 1810; the second in that city in 1818; the third in Coethen in 1824, which was translated into French by Ernst Georg Freiherr von Brunnow; the fourth also in Coethen in 1829; the fifth also in that city in 1833, which was translated into English by Dr R E Dudgeon who subsequently revised his own translation of this edition as late as 1893; and finally Hahnemann had completed the sixth edition in Paris by the 20th February, 1842 according to a letter he addressed to Mr Schaub, at his publishers' address in Düsseldorf, Rhineland, West Prussia. In each of these editions Hahnemann introduced further refinements to his coherent medical systematics. However, the sixth edition was not released for publication by Hahnemann's widow, nor by her heirs, until early in 1920. It was then that Hahnemann's best-known biographer, Dr Richard Haehl, with the aid of a fairly substantial sum of money from Professor William Boericke of the University of San Francisco, salvaged the original manuscript of the sixth edition of the *Organon* from the Ruhr area whilst this was being wracked by violent revolutionary disturbances.

Hahnemann's French widow had to flee from her country during the Franco-Prussian war in 1870 on account of her German surname. She left with the Hahnemanns' adopted daughter Sophie (née Bohrer) and son-in-law, Dr Karl Baron von Boenninghausen, and they all settled in his father's estate at Darup near Münster in the Ruhr area. They took all Hahnemann's manuscripts (including the thirteen case-books of Hahnemann's last eight years of practice in Paris) with them and this is where they remained for the next half century. Excerpts from, and references to, the *Organon* in this Encyclopaedic Dictionary, unless otherwise indicated, are taken from or refer to the sixth edition.

A copy of Hahnemann's *Organon* is indispensable on the bookshelf of every serious student of medicine. Anne M Clover has written *Homoeopathy Reconsidered: A New Look at Hahnemann's Organon* (London: Victor Gollancz Ltd, 1989, 128 pages) in which she carefully re-appraises the therapeutic systematics definitively laid down by Hahnemann.

Organotherapy

Treatment of disease by dynamized preparations made from animal organs corresponding to those afflicted in the respective patients. An example would be the administration of potentized pig's liver in a case where cirrhosis of the human patient's liver was evident. This 'similarity' (pig's liver to patient's liver) is erroneously thought to be somehow homoeopathic. Moreover, because of the superficial similarity to homoeopathic medicines in the pharmaceutical production process which such remedies undergo, these medicines are sometimes prescribed as a complementary medicinal therapy by some homoeopaths (particularly in the francophone area). To prescribe potentized animal Kidney (Ren) in nephritis or dynamized animal Skin (Cutis) in eczema cannot be described as homoeopathic prescribing.

This is an outgrowth of what was a popular theory in medicine stretching back over a long period prior to Hahnemann. Nonetheless, he did not incorporate it into homoeopathy.

Organotherapeutics is to be clearly distinguished from the truly homoeopathic sarcodes (discussed in detail under 'Isopathy') and also from the prescribing of homoeopathic remedies organotropically (see 'Organotropism').

An authoritative text-book on the subject is *L'Organothérapie diluée et dynamisée* by Drs Claude Bergeret and Max Tétau (Paris: Librairie Maloine SA Editeur, 1971 [240 pp]). (Refer also to 'Nomenclature, Discrepancies in' regarding the unfortunate ambiguity in French surrounding the word 'organothérapique'; see also the entry 'Rademacher, Johann Gottfried (1772-1850)'.)

Organotropism

Predilection or affinity for certain organs. For example, Phosphorus has a potent action upon the liver.

Low potencies are generally organotropic, often constraining the homoeopath's choice at such a potency level to search amongst remedies with the appropriate organ affinity. Organotropism is not to be confused with Organotherapy for which there is a separate entry. (See also 'Aetiotropism', 'Drainage', 'Pathotropism' and 'Rademacher, Johann Gottfried (1772-1850)'.)

Orificial Surgery

See 'Surgery'.

Orphanage

Asylum for parentless children; institution for the housing and care of orphans. A large number of such institutions, that very successfully provided only homoeopathic treatment to its resident children, was in existence in the USA before 1920. (See 'History of Homoeopathy before 1900', section on United States of America.)

Ortega, Proceso Sanchez (born 1919)

Mexican homoeopath, who is regarded by many as the most eminent of Latin America. His work has contributed considerably to a broadening of the concept of chronic miasmata within homoeopathy. This is discussed under the entry for 'Miasma'. His major literary work on that subject has been translated into English, under the title:

Notes on the Miasms or Hahnemann's Chronic Diseases (New Delhi: National Homoeopathic Pharmacy, for Libraria de la Homeopatia de Mexico AC, 1980, 295 pages)

(See 'Miasma.)

Orthodox

Holding opinions currently accepted as correct; in accordance with the right practice or doctrine as authoritatively laid down at the time, especially in theology or medicine. In the latter case it is used to describe mainstream medicine in the Rationalist tradition which is of a deterministic and/or fideistic character or quality, and brooks no deviation from its established system.

Orthoptics

Study of faulty binocular vision with particular emphasis on defects in the action of the ocular muscles and on improper visual habits, coupled to treatment principally involving the retraining of the ocular muscles. (See 'Bates' Method of Eyesight Training'.)

Osmosis

Phenomenon of the passage of certain solutions and fluids through any porous substance, or through a membrane.

Osteopathy

Method of diagnosis, prevention and treatment of ailments, primarily by physiomedical means, based on the principle that much of the pain and disability which man suffers stems from abnormalities in the function of body structures as well as damage to these by degeneration, trauma, inflammation, or any other structural change. Osteopathy recognizes abnormal function, in the absence of pathology, as a common, or even likely, cause of symptoms. Like homoeopathy, it also maintains that the human body is constantly striving toward self-sufficiency and self-correction. It is a form of treatment that is complementary to homoeopathy.

Oxygenoid Constitution

See 'Constitutional Type'.

P

Pack

Bundled, wrapped or tied lot of articles or goods. In hydropathy it means wrapping the patient in a sheet or blanket, where the former is most often wet. Also referred to as 'wickel'[1] (this, the 'wet body pack', is described in some detail under 'Fever'). This process with a sheet wrung out of cold water is a 'cold pack' (preferred in fever-chills); when wrung out of hot water it is a 'hot pack' ('homoeopathically' suggested by pronounced pyrexia). As opposed to these 'wet packs', a 'dry pack' is the enwrapment of a patient in dry, warmed blankets for the purpose of inducing profuse perspiration. (See also 'Diaphoresis' and 'Naturopath'.)

Paediatric Remedies

Well established homoeopathic medicines which are particularly suitable for infants, children and adolescents for the most common ailments, hygienic problems, acute miasmata and symptom complexes that are known to affect young patients.

A current text-book on homoeopathic paediatrics is:

Homoeopathy in Paediatric Practice by Hedwig Imhäuser, translated from the German original into English by Sigrid Penrod (Heidelberg: Karl F Haug Verlag, 1988, 236 pages)

Moreover, Donald Foubister in *Tutorials on Homoeopathy* (Beaconsfield: Beaconsfield Publishers Ltd, 1989) devotes chapters 6 to 11 [pages 45-90] to 'Homoeopathy and Paediatrics', where he provides much valuable advice.

Pain

An impression on the sensory nerves causing – to a varying degree – physical discomfort, distress, suffering, or, in severe instances, agony. It is triggered in the patient by a disease-induced physiologic dysfunction, or by injury. In either event, it serves as a signal to the sufferer that a destructive process being dynamically countered by the organism is in progress. This, in turn, means it is a very widely encountered symptom component in the total disease picture of patients. The fact that James Tyler Kent in his *Repertory of the Homoeopathic Materia Medica* lists over 100 types of pain sensation with references to corresponding homoeopathic drugs, is proof of its almost universal presence

[1]Garten, M O. *The Natural and Drugless Way for Better Health,* West Nyack, NY: Parker Publishing Co Inc, 1969, pp 181-183 [Wickel is the German for 'bandage'].

in disease. Dr M T Santwani in his *Pain: Types, Significance and Homoeopathic Management* (New Delhi: Jain Publishing Co, 1980) provides a useful table of 78 types of pain sensation, alphabetically from 'aching', 'bearing down' and 'benumbing' to 'wrenching', 'wringing' and 'writhing' pain sorts. In addition to enumerating alongside the homoeopathic remedies chiefly having that type of pain in their pathogeneses, frequently reconfirmed since by clinical usage, he provides the precise meaning for each of the adjectives that describe the sensations of pain. He also gives a listing against each entry, where he gives a likely version of the sensation just as this might be phrased by a patient, in the current English idiom.

In the light of the regular presence of pain in most disease states, in one non-unique form or another, this common sensation can only be regarded as a 'generality'. The homoeopathic drug that corrects the condition provoking the pain will, simultaneously, be the drug to cure the pain. Such a well-indicated drug may often be found through the modalities of the pain and its modifying factors. (See 'Modalities' and 'Pain Relief Methods in Homoeopathy'.)

Pain Relief Methods in Homoeopathy

As a rule, pain sensation in homoeopathy is treated as any other symptom would be, namely as a part of the patient's presenting totality. The significance of pain, within that totality, as a remedy indicator increases with the greater distinctness of the modalities of pain and the presence of distinct modifying factors. However, there are occasions (e.g. in terminal illness; or when symptoms are too sketchy and the pain too violent) when pain relief becomes the primary homoeopathic object. Then a functiotropic, organotropic or pathotropic approach becomes the appropriate homoeopathic avenue of treatment.

A selection of the more outstanding agents promoting anodynia in a fairly general way are listed here, together with their algesiogenic-pathological keynotes and tentatively suggested potencies (only to be used under professional supervision and with proper care, as a few may become lethal in quantity, – and some of the indicated potencies have recently become illicit, or at least difficult to obtain, in a number of countries):

Acidum phosphoricum	Pains of cancer (potency: 1CH);
Arnica montana	Bruised pains (potency: 3CH to 30CH; locally, mother tincture, but never applied hot or for broken skin);
Aurum metallicum	Bone pains (potency: 3CH to 30CH, the latter for increased blood pressure);
(Atropa) Belladonna	Congestive, throbbing pains and spasms of involuntary muscle, biliary colic (potency: 1CH to 30CH);

Betonica officinalis (Stachys betonica)	Neuralgias, gastric pains, nervous tension (head)aches, pains from sinus and catarrhal congestion (dose: 4ml of mother tincture);
Bryonia alba	Myalgia, pain in joints, teeth, trachea and torticollis, pains < by slightest motion, > by lying on painful side (potency: 1CH to 12CH);
Cactus grandiflorus (Selenicereus spinulosus)	Acts on cardiac and arterial muscle fibres particularly, is homoeopathic to pains associated with constrictions and congestions in circular muscular fibres, prosopalgia (trigeminal neuralgia) (potency: mother tincture [made from flowers] to 3CH – higher in nervous palpitation);
Cataria nepeta	Abdominal pains (dose: 10 drops of mother tincture in water);
Dioscorea villosa	Remedy for many kinds of pain, it ranks with the polychrests in this aspect in the materia medica, but has a very special affinity for painful affections of abdominal and pelvic viscera (potency: mother tincture to 3CH);
Echinacea purporea	Pain from: corrosive burns, frost-bite, electrical burns, Röntgen ray (X-ray) burns, radiation burns (locally applied moist dressings or compresses with mother tincture);
Eupatorium perfoliatum	Aching pain in bones with soreness of muscles, sore inflamed nodosities of joints, painful dropsical swelling (potency: mother tincture to 3CH);
Euphorbia heterodoxa	In its use allopathically as an external application in cases of cancer it always produced the most excruciating pains: conversely in homoeopathic attenuations it alleviates the burning pains of cancer, which is both the key-note and in fact its principal indication for employment (potency: 3CH to 6CH);
Euphorbium officinarum	Pains of cancer, burning pain in bones (potency: 3CH to 6CH);
Hoitzia coccinea	Pains of cancer of the uterus (adjuvant treatment: 2DH orally and simultaneous vaginal douches of a decoction of 10%); [1]
Hypericum perforatum	Pains from injured nerves (potency: mother tincture to 3CH internally, or mother tincture

[1] De Legarreta, Manual M. *Patogenesia de Cinco Medicinas Introducidas en la Materia Medica Homeopatica para la Curacion del Tifo y Otras Pirexias,* La Veridad, Mexico City, 1911, under entry for Hoitzia coccinea, and in *North American Journal of Homoeopathy,* Vol I, 1907, pp 2444 ff.

	used externally for painful burns, neuralgias, puncture-wounds, post-operative pains, animal bites and street injuries);
Kalmia latifolia	Cardialgia in angina pectoris, rheumatoid neuralgia (potency: mother tincture to 6CH);
Ledum palustre	Pain as from punctures, pains shooting upward, eye-ache, haemorrhoidal pain, gouty nodosities (potency: 3CH to 30CH);
Magnesia phosphorica	Strong colic, painful membranous dysmenorrhoea, pains of stomach cancer, tic-douloureux (potency: 3DH in warm water);
Passiflora incarnata	Neuralgias and violent aches (particularly of the head, or associated with convulsions) (dose: 40–60 drops of mother tincture in warm water);
Pothos Foetidus (Ictodes foetida, Symplocarpus foetidus)	Chronic rheumatic pains; spasmodic pains, distressing soreness of physometra (uterine inflation and tension);
Piscidia erythrina	Neuralgic and spasmodic pains with nervous excitement, profuse sweat, insomnia (dose: 2ml of mother tincture in water);
Psoralea corylifolia (Babchi)	Pains of cancer, skin diseases and ulcers (may also be used topically);
Scutellaria laterifolia	Pains associated with neurologic and neuromotor (e.g.: epileptoid) conditions (dose: 2ml mother tincture in water);
Spigelia anthelmia	Shooting, tearing, stabbing neuralgia, ciliary neuralgia, stitches in diaphragm, eye-ache, periodically recurring headache beginning in cerebellum, pain in temporo-mandibular joint, earache, toothache, rheumatic pain (potency: 6CH for neuralgic symptoms alone, 2CH if these are accompanied by inflammatory symptoms);
Verbascum thapsum	Neuralgia affecting zygoma, temporo-maxillary joints, ears, joints of lower extremities, abdominal pain far down extending to sphincter and which it causes to contract (dose: mother tincture 5 drops, internally, or oleum to be instilled into meatus in otalgia).

Methods of pain relief offered by acupuncture, chiropractic, mesmerism, naturopathy and osteopathy are considered as complementary modalities to homoeopathy and these are seen as adjuvant therapeutic approaches, whereas coercive chemoanaesthesia is not.

Example of a syndetic pointer to a homoeopathic medicine:

Where septic conditions, abscesses, wounds, etc. are painful or very sensitive to touch, but if it feels grateful under the cold tap, or is relieved by cold generally – Ledum palustre

(See also 'Contra-indication against Administering Simillimum', 'Douche' section Teeth and Gums, 'Emergencies – Homoeopathic Treatment', 'Externally Applied Homoeopathic Drugs', 'Headache' and 'Pain'; the question of the use of palliatives [enantiopathic medicines] in homoeopathy is briefly discussed under 'Hempel, Charles Julius (1811-1879)'.)

Palliation

Mitigating or reducing the severity of symptoms, usually by the employment of enantiopathic medicines. (See 'Allopathy', 'Pain', 'Pain Relief Methods in Homoeopathy' and 'Phytotherapy'.)

Palpate

To examine and perceive by touch; to feel and press with the fingers and the palms of the hands in order to assess: the degree of resistance offered by tissue areas tested; the outline of organs or tumours of the abdomen; the heart beat or the vibrations in the chest; the local temperature variations on body surfaces; the extent of articular mobility of joints, or crepitation in them; variations in characteristics of muscles; the sounds elicited by percussion; and/or the reactive involuntary movement, or functioning of a part, in response to a manual stimulus applied peripherally. Hence 'palpable' means perceptible to touch, evident or plain.

Panacea

● **Cure-all.**

Panchrest; a non-homoeopathic concept for a remedy claimed to be curative of all illnesses. (See also 'Polychrest'.)

Paracelsus, Philippus Aureolus (1493-1541)

See 'Philosophical Premise of Homoeopathy' and 'Spagyric'.

Paraffinum Mollum Album (or Flavum)

Vaselinum album (or flavum); white (or yellow) petrolatum; white (or yellow) petroleum jelly. (See 'Ointment'.)

Parallelism

Term used to describe the state of coextensive correspondence existing, amongst others, between the like actions of disease and a drug on a healthy organism, leading to the curative collimation that is homoeopathy. (See also 'Homoeopathicity'.)

Parallels in Symptom Modalities

See 'Disease and Drug Action in Homoeopathic Congruity', section 3, and 'Modalities'.

Paralogism, Homoeopathy Accused of

See 'Post Hoc, Ergo Propter Hoc'.

Parietal

Relating to the wall of any hollow organ or cavity.

Particulars (Symptoms)

Symptoms that relate to organs or parts of the patient (stomach, back, genito-urinary, mouth, etc.). (See 'Generals' and 'Particulars' (Symptom Types)'.)

Partisanship within Homoeopathy's Diverse Conventions

At any given time in the twentieth century there have been three major currents of conformity within homoeopathy. Though uniform therapeutic goals are pursued by all three, based on a common doctrinal principle, they represent, nonetheless, three distinct conventions of homoeopathic observance. They could be said to constitute three parochial orthodoxies in constant speculative competition with one another. These three correspond, largely, to three linguistic spheres of influence:

a) the Anglo-Saxon sphere – where the orthodox method of homoeopathic practice is seen as unswervingly following the repertorial style of James Tyler Kent and his spiritual successors;
b) the Francophone sphere – where the ubiquitous morphotypological school is viewed as the only homoeopathic orthodoxy;
c) the Teutonic sphere – where the bias toward 'clinicopathologic homoeopathy' is construed as the true homoeopathic norm.

Although there is intolerant orthodoxism evident in some quarters of all three factions, the majority of homoeopaths, though supportive of one or other group, avoid open partisanship and display a mature latitudinarianism.

Paschero, Tomas Pablo (born 1904)

Argentinian homoeopath of considerable international stature who emphasized environmental rather than inherited origins for miasmata, believing that the psychogenic and other effects thus miasmatically induced in a patient are of such enduring character, that the patient will only need one remedy and that this may never change throughout the patient's life. Of special importance is his paper, entitled:

The Mental Symptoms in Homoeopathy (1975: transactions International [LMHI] Homoeopathic Congress)

(See 'Miasma'.)

Patent and Proprietary Medicines

See 'Eclipse of Homoeopathy (1920-1965)', 'History of Homoeopathy before 1900', sections on UK and USA, and 'Simmons, George Henry (1852-1937)'.

Paterson, Elizabeth (1907-1963)

See 'Paterson, John (1890-1954)'.

Paterson, John (1890-1954)

Glaswegian homoeopathic researcher who, together with his wife Elizabeth, took up the pioneering work on the 'Bowel Nosodes' that had been begun by Edward Bach (1886-1936). They worked for a time with Thomas M Dishington and Charles Edwin Wheeler. John Paterson succeeded the former as physician at the Mount Vernon Children's Hospital in Glasgow, Scotland. The Paterson couple worked together diligently on their research for 26 years, and Elizabeth continued alone after she was widowed, until 1963. They concluded that

1 the non-pathogenic bowel flora undergoes definite changes in disease, which might entail the flora turning pathogenic;
2 the balance of bowel flora is disturbed in disease;
3 similar changes are also observed in drug provings.

Bach had held that the non-lactose fermenting rods were closely associated with the chronic miasma 'Psora', and John Paterson postulated that the chronic presence of gram-negative diplococcus was directly related to the chronic 'Sycotic' miasma. His major writings include:

Sycosis and Sycotic Co. (Paterson) (1933)

Some Bacteriological and Clinical Aspects of Rheumatism (1933)

Psora and Sycosis in Relation to Modern Bacteriology (1936)

Lecture Demonstration Showing the Technique in the Preparation of the Non-Lactose Fermenting Nosodes of the Bowel and the Clinical Indications for their Use (1936)

The Role of the Bowel Flora in Chronic Disease (1948)

The Bowel Nosodes (1949)

The most complete bibliography extant of the bowel nosodes of Bach and Paterson is that compiled by Francis Treuherz.[1] (See 'Bowel Nosodes'.)

Pathogen

Any substance causing disease.

Pathogenesis

Production, development, or mode of origin of:
    either disease (morbific) processes,
    or drug reactions.

Hence, 'pathogenetic' may signify either disease-inducing or nosopoietic, respectively. (See 'Pathogenetic Experiment'.)

Pathogenetic Experiment

Proving (transliteration of the German 'Prüfung', meaning test or assay). Homoeopathy views disease as a dynamic process and not as an entity, though it sees the direct, producing causes of disease as entities. It also holds that the action of any disease-producing substance is always modified by the specific condition (state) of an individual organism at the time. Such condition is always determined by a myriad of factors, ranging – almost panoramically – from the individual's genetic constitution (see also 'Adaptiveness'), through nutrition (see also 'Dietary Therapy' and 'Foods as Health Problems'), to environmental influences (see also 'Environment' and 'Miasma'). The same applies to drug action and any reaction thereto (see also 'Altered Receptivity in Disease').

No-one could ever predict with certainty the exact effect of a drug on every individual in a given population sample. To be able to approximate that, a way had to be found to assess fully the anticipated effects of a drug on individuals in all their diversity. Hahnemann attacked the problem from an altogether new angle. He was the first to investigate exhaustively the subjective effects of drugs on individual, healthy human organisms, then collating all subjectively and objectively assessed responses. His method for obtaining such detailed pathogenetic information has not changed, except that additional placebo control has become customary in the second half of the twentieth century. In accordance with the three rules concerning potencies in provings (see 'Homoeopathic Laws, Postulates and Precepts', section 10) the substance is given in different dynamizations (potencies) or physiological strengths to

[1]Treuherz, Francis. 'A Bibliography of the Bowel Nosodes of Bach and Paterson and the Flower Remedies of Bach', *British Homoeopathic Journal,* vol LXXVII, April 1988, pp 112-116 [copies available from author: Flat 2, 18 The Avenue, Brondesbury Park, London NW6 7YD].

groups of healthy volunteers, the provers, over a set period. The provers note in their diaries (the so-called day-books) any signs and symptoms that develop, such as any changes in temperament, or in intellectual acuity, or fatiguability, or tussive irritation, or thermalgesia, or absolutely any other altered state(s). At the end of the assay period all this information is ordered, where prominent or frequently occurring effects are given most importance. This information is augmented by known toxic effects of that homoeopathic medicinal agent, as well as by other effects: for instance, as observed in a clinical and/or veterinary setting, where it may clear up symptoms unexpectedly. By this method are gathered the 'proven' phenomena, being the sum of the peculiar or specific properties or characteristics of drugs generally, as well as the subjective data established by many provers individually.

A great volume of such drug effects was determined in this manner and then permanently recorded in the materia medica. These records span almost 3000 homoeopathic medicines. Periodically drugs undergo re-provings, because the subjective nature of their effects alters in accordance with changed environmental influences (e.g. modern pollution levels). Being indirectly monitored are these and comparable new influences as they affect individual provers. (See 'Hempel, Charles Julius (1811-1879)', section on "Cyclopaedia of Drug Pathogenesy", 'Organization of Symptoms in Materia Medica' and 'Sources of Drug Semiology'.)

Pathological Predisposition

Proneness to a recurrent physical condition; this often points to the constitutional drug. Examples are: varicose veins (Pulsatilla nigricans), boils (Sulphur), attacks of bronchitis (Phosphorus), constipation (Nux vomica), multiple exostoses and frequent sprains (Calcarea fluorica). (See 'Constitutional Type'.)

Pathological Prescribing

See 'Drainage' and 'Pathotropism'.

Pathological Remedy

See 'Drainage' and 'Pathotropism'.

Pathology

Deals with the development of abnormal conditions, as well as the varied functional and structural changes that result from the disease process. In a disease which is curable through the use of drugs, the homoeopath will never base his prescription simply on the pathological findings (the phrases in common homoeopathic usage, 'pathological prescribing' and 'pathological remedy', have quite a different meaning, explained under 'Drainage'). As impeccably argued by Coulter, the place which pathology occupies in homoeopathy is, nonetheless, important for four reasons:[1]

a) Pathological findings can make it possible to distinguish those cases that are likely to respond to drug treatment from those where, say, hydrotherapy, manipulation, nutritional adjustment, electrotherapy or surgery may be preferable.

b) Pathological investigations can identify an epidemic disease process (cholera, typhoid fever) at an early stage, enabling the correct remedy that is specific to the particular genus epidemicus to be administered. Similarly, pathological tests can name an acute miasma (malaria, scarlet fever, whooping cough) permitting the immediate selection of the specific acute miasmatic remedy.

c) Knowledge based on pathological findings delimits the symptoms of the patient's altered dynamis from those symptoms which are only a secondary consequence of some gross structural alteration (e.g. 'micturition frequency', if produced by the mechanical pressure of a tumour impacted in the pelvis, would not help to make the correct choice of remedy as the symptom does not express the dynamic disharmony of the disease process itself, but is secondary to a disease product. It would be promptly relieved by the surgical excision of the tumour).

d) Through pathological investigations it is possible to divide cases with a favourable prognosis from those with a grave prognosis. When abnormal conditions and changes due to the distortions and misdirections produced by the disease process are very far advanced, and certain vital organs have been irreparably damaged, the use of a deep-acting simillimum may hasten the demise of the patient. In such cases the simillimum is strictly contra-indicated and only remedies with a superficial action, or palliatives, are indicated.

(See also 'Diagnosis', 'Disease', 'Disease and Drug Action in Homoeopathic Congruity', 'Drainage', 'Epistemological Assumptions in Homoeopathy', 'Hempel, Charles Julius (1811-1879)', 'Miasma' and 'Pathotropism'.)

Pathotropism

This refers to a homoeopathic drug's affinity for a particular category of pathological process. An example would be the use of Ferrum phosphoricum at the commencement of an acute inflammation throughout the body. Prescribing such a remedy under such circumstances would justify both the remedy and the prescribing to be qualified by the adjective 'pathological'. Further examples would be, say, the prescribing of Ruta graveolens for epicondylitis (tennis elbow), or Arnica montana for bruising, or shock after injury.

[1]Coulter, H L. *Homoeopathic Medicine*. St Louis: Formur Inc Publishers, 1975, pp 45-47.

To illustrate this peculiarly homoeopathic idiom, a short list of pathological remedy selections applicable, for example, to a patient with jaundice is provided here. Jaundice as a reactive symptom, very occasionally with a grave prognosis, is characterized by a staining yellow of:

a) the excretions (particularly urine) with bile-pigment;
b) some secretions (sweat, and the milk of mothers who are nursing may be slightly tinged);
c) the entire integumentum (body covering);
d) the sclera (white of the eyes); and
e) some deeper tissues.

The homoeopathic significance of this symptom varies with many concomitants, such as degree of jaundice, age of patient, past history and medication, and other symptoms which may be present (e.g. pyrexia, hepatomegaly, enlarged gall-bladder, anaemia, splenomegaly, reticulocytosis, pancytopenia, abdominal discomfort, albuminuria, and cholaemic symptoms). These, in addition to the peculiar or striking symptoms that normally guide the homoeopath's choice, will have to be taken into account to arrive at the correct, and therefore effective, homoeopathic pathological remedy. As a symptom component, jaundice features in:

Relevant pathogenetic highlights from the materia medica:

Bryonia alba	associated with hepatalgia > from lying on right side;
(Matricaria) Chamomilla	from a fit of anger or a severe fright;
Chelidonium majus	associated with yellow stools and pains under angle of right scapula;
Chionanthus virginica	associated with hepatic congestion, as with obstruction of the common bile-ducts, constipation, greyish-white stools (lack of stercobilin), bilious temperament or arrested menses;
Chloramphenicolum (Chloromycetinum)	associated with haematemesis, anorexia, diffuse abdominal pains, cholera-like syndrome, pancytopenia, dyspnoea, catarrh of the mucous membrane of the duct and/or of the duodenum and/or of the pancreas, involving the ampulla of Vater;
Chlorpromazinum	associated with painful hypogastric colic, stubborn constipation, liver enlarged and sensitive, atony of the urinary bladder, diminution of blood platelets, eosinophilia, acquired haemolytic anaemia, or agranulocytic angina;

Convolvulus duartinus (Ipomoea) — associated with a skin of dry appearance despite cold sweats, bilious yellowish-green vomit, hiccoughing, soft orange-yellow stools, rectal tenesmus, and/or distended abdomen, cholecystitis or viral icterus;

Crotalus horridus — associated with albuminuria, blood disorganization and/or viral hepatitis (such as Yellow Fever);

Dolichos pruriens — associated with severe irritation;

Guatteria guameria — associated with hepatitis, conjunctival jaundice with photophobia, biliary lithiasis and inflammation of the gall-bladder, epigastric pain < from movement;

Hirudo medicinalis — associated with haemolytic crisis, chills, fever, nausea, vomiting, pain in abdomen or back, splenomegaly, urine red or black, suicidal impulses;

Iodium — associated with chronic lupoid hepatitis, without obstruction of the larger bile-ducts;

Mercurius solubilis hahnemanni — with catarrh in bile-ducts and an inability to lie on the right side;

Phopshorus — associated with malignant parenchymatous jaundice as in acute yellow atrophy (known as von Rokitansky's syndrome);

Sulfanilamidum — associated with allergenic, and toxic (miasmatic) liver reactions to orthodox drugs;

Thyroidinum — in Icterus Neonatorum accompanied by vomiting.

Other significant medicines that may be considered are:

Acidum nitricum — with hepatalgia
Arsenicum album — from mercurial intoxation
Cinchona officinalis — from malaria with bilious diarrhoea
Iris versicolor — from biliary deficiency
(Trigonocephalus) Lachesis — pronounced yellowness
Mercurius vivus/sol. hahnem. — after Aconitum napellus
Natrum sulphuricum — anger may be a cause
Nux vomica — with costiveness and sensitivity in liver region
Ptelea trifoliata — with post-prandial liver problems

Examples of syndetic pointers to homoeopathic medicines when these are selected pathologically are:

Where solid unreasoning fear overwhelms the jaundiced patient with symptoms of inflammation and great pain in liver area – Aconitum napellus

In the jaundiced patient, who loved meat, suddenly turned vegetarian, with hepatic and gastric symptoms worse after meals, and hyperaemia of the liver – Ptelea trifoliata

(See 'Miasma', relative to the pathogenesis given above under Sulfanilamidum.)

William H Burt's concise *Physiological Materia Medica* (Third edition reprint, New Delhi: Jain Publishing Co, 1978, 992 pages) provides one of the older, but comprehensive, reference works for this, the functiotropic, and the organotropic, therapeutic approaches. (See also 'Aetiotropism', 'Disease and Drug Action in Homoeopathic Congruity', 'Drainage', 'Organotropism' and 'Therapeutic Science'.)

Peculiar or Unusual Symptoms

See 'Homoeopathic Practice'.

Pellets

See 'Pillules'.

Pelotherapy

Pelopathy; naturopathic and/or hydropathic treatment of disease by means of mud baths and packs. (See 'Naturopath'.)

Percolation

Process of extraction of the soluble portion in solids where the liquid menstruum (solvent) is permitted to trickle down through a comminuted or ground mass of these solids, to be immediately filtered slowly through some porous material and then collected.

Perfume

A (blend of) standardized aromatic essence(s) obtained from plant or animal material; lately more frequently chemically synthesized. There are about seventy-five primary aromatics standardized in perfumery, most of which originate from starting material found in the homoeopathic materia medica. This means that perfumes, similar to the oils of aromatherapy, are able to elicit reactive responses in those within olfactory reception. For this reason, most homoeopaths insist that no perfume (eau de toilette, etc.) be worn by their patients, and that medication be not contaminated by such scents. (See 'Homoeopathic Practice' section Precautions; for 'Aromatherapy' see 'Massage Therapy'; refer also to 'Olfactory Medicines'.)

Periodicity

Pattern of recurrence at regular, measurable intervals; generally denoting in homoeopathy recurrent exacerbations, ameliorations, paroxysms, and the like, evident in the process of disease or drug action. (See 'Organic Clock'.)

Perlingual

Through or by way of the tongue, and tongue area; the most favoured administration route for homoeopathic medication.

Pessary

Medicated vaginal suppository; also an appliance introduced into the vagina to correct any uterine displacement.

Pestle

See 'Mortar and Pestle'.

Petroleum Jelly

See 'Vaselinum Flavum'.

Pharmacochemistry

Pharmaceutical chemistry.

Pharmacodynamics

Relates to drug action and organic reaction in a living organism. Richard Hughes (1836-1902) is the author of *A Manual of Pharmacodynamics* (London: Leath and Ross, sixth edition 1893) which originally appeared in 1867 under the title *Manual of Homoeopathic Practice for Students and Beginners*. This was changed to its later title with the publication of the third edition in 1875-6. That written work had a significant part to play in the fateful symptomatology-pathology dispute within homoeopathy. It subtly prepared many for the idea that pathology (which deals with the results and products of the disease process) is really part of the homoeopathic method of drug selection (whereas that method concerns itself with the disease process proper). (See 'Hempel, Charles Julius (1811-18790)', 'Hughes, Richard (1836-1902)', 'History of Homoeopathy before 1900', sections on UK and USA, 'Simmons, George Henry (1852-1937)' and 'Therapeutic Science'.)

Pharmacognosy

The term was originated by one of the German students in 1815, (C A Seydler, of Halle an der Saale), by combining the Greek 'pharmakon' (drug) and 'gnosia' (study) [less correctly, some say, 'gnosis' (knowledge)], to describe an applied science that is a branch of materia medica. It records the physical characteristics of drugs particularly in their natural or unprepared state, then it deals with the biologic, biochemical and economic features as well as the sources of crude plant and animal drugs.

Moreover, it also deals with their natural constituents as well as their derivatives. As examples:

a) In the case of the Foxglove, not only its leaf, Digitalis Purpurea [authority: Hahnemann],[1] but also the isolated glycosides, Digitalinum [authority: Bëhr][2] and Digitoxinum [authority: Kopfel][3] are to be studied by pharmacognosy in homoeopathy.

b) In the case of the Glandula Suprarenalis, not only the extract of the gland as such, Adrenalinum [authority: Getman],[4] but also the isolated cortico-suprarenal hormone, the sarcode Cortisonum [authority: Templeton][5] is to be studied by pharmacognosy in homoeopathy.

Pharmacography

Treatise on, or description of, drugs.

Pharmacological Message

By means of mechanical energy (trituration or succussion) the pharmacological message of the original drug is imparted to the molecules of the diluent used in homoeopathic preparations. These molecules surround the original drug molecules in so-called solvation structures, which are 'three-dimensional polymers'. The energy applied between deconcentration stages

[1] Hahnemann, C F S. *The Chronic Diseases, their Peculiar Nature and their Homoeopathic Cure*, translated from the second enlarged German edition of 1835 by Prof Louis H Tafel, Philadelphia: Boericke and Tafel, 1904, pp 671-692.

[2] Allen, T F. *The Encyclopaedia of Pure Materia Medica*. Ten volumes. New York: Boericke and Tafel, 1874-1879, vol III, pp 75-92.

[3] ibid., pp 121-123.

[4] Allen, H C. *The Materia Medica of the Nosodes*, Philadelphia: Boericke and Tafel, 1910, pp 1-5.

[5] a) Stephenson, J. *Hahnemannian Provings. A Materia Medica and Repertory*, Bombay: Roy Publishing House, 1963, pp 38-40.

  b) Templeton, W L. *British Homoeopathic Journal*, 1956, vol XLV, pp 89-97.

induces the replication of these shape-encoded inter- and intra-molecular structures, which keep being passed on to successive potencies long after the original shape-imparting molecule of the original drug has been diluted away. (See 'Drug Preparation', 'Potency', 'Potentizing Methods' and 'Solvation Structures'.)

Pharmacology

Science of medicines; deals with drugs, their sources, nature, appearance, chemistry, biochemical effects, physiological assimilability, bioavailability, toxicity, biodisposability, teratology, application and action in potency (in terms of homoeosis – as a rule, diminished vital action in disease calls for low potencies, while increased vital action responds better to high dynamizations): all this against the general background of the three fundamental homoeopathic pharmacological concepts of:
  a) similarity
  b) contrariety
  c) proportionality.

Pharmacopoeia

Authoritative reference work containing monographs of medicines and other therapeutic agents, specifications for the sources of, and standards for the strength and purity of, base substances and mother tinctures, formulae and methods of preparation of these substances and their derivative potencies, as well as descriptions of processes for the testing of starting materials. Under the entry 'Potentizing Methods' homoeopathic pharmacopoeias widely regarded as authoritative are listed. (See 'Potentizing Methods' for the description of some of the prescribed processes.)

Pharmacy

Shop in which, by (or under the control of) a pharmacist, medicines are stocked, or prepared, and either dispensed against practitioner prescriptions, or simply sold over-the-counter; branch of materia medica that (i) treats primarily of the preparation and dispensing of homoeopathic drugs and other substances, and (ii) is further concerned with the collection of raw materials, their identification, preservation, and mutual inimicality or compatibility as drugs administered in proximity to one another.

Phenomenological Method of Treatment

The homoeopath takes his orientation from observed individual phenomena, relative to each prover or patient. Hence, homoeopathy is said to employ a phenomenological method of treatment, in contradistinction to a symptomatic method of treatment which homoeopathy usually condemns.

Philiston of Locri (ca. 415-360 BC)

See 'Humoral Pathology in Prescribing.'

Philosophical Premise of Homoeopathy

The four paradigmatic tenets which constitute the philosophical bedrock of homoeopathy are summarized thus:

1 The ways of nature are ultimately harmonious and knowable to man, because effects follow causes in unbroken succession.
2 To every action there is an equal and opposite reaction: that is, action and reaction are ceaseless, equivalent and reciprocal.
3 Matter and force (energy) are essentially interchangeable and their transformations continuous.
4 Matter-force is indestructible and persistent, and infinitely divisible, so that there is no lower limit to the quantity of action necessary to effect any change.

The principle of equivalence of mass and energy (in the third proposition), for which there has since been proof provided, was only fully enunciated in 1905 in Berne, Switzerland, by Albert Einstein (1879-1955), the German-born physicist, as part of the Theory of Relativity.

The second proposition was originally stated by Sir Isaac Newton (1642-1727), the English physicist, mathematician and natural philosopher, in his Third Law of Motion: 'When two bodies interact, the forces exerted by each body on the other are equal and opposite'. Analogous to this is homoeopathy's Law of Bioenergetic Drug Action (see 'Homoeopathic Laws, Postulates and Precepts', section 2): 'Action and reaction are equal and opposite', meaning the action of a drug and the reaction of the targeted organism are, at the same time, similar (equal) and antidotally stimulatory (opposite).

The fourth proposition's second part was first formulated by Pierre Louis Moreau de Maupertuis (1698-1759), the French mathematician, naturalist, scholar and pre-Darwinian evolutionist, in his Axiom of Least Quantity: 'The quantity of action necessary to effect any change in nature is the least possible'. What he had announced as a law soon became an axiomatic principle of natural science. Based on this, the US homoeopathic philosopher, Bernhardt Fincke (1821-1906), who first enunciated the principle of assimilation (see 'Homoeosis'), formulated the Posological Rule of Least Action (see 'Homoeopathic Laws, Postulates and Precepts', section 6): 'The rule of least action (maxima minimis), an essential complement of the Law of Similars (similia similibus), and always co-ordinating with it, prescribes that the decisive momentum is always a minimum, frequently an infinitesimal'. This refers to the minimum functional dose, and in practical terms, to a homoeopathic drug's distinctive preparation and application, both of which govern the remedial agent's curative properties and action with systematic predictability.

Prior to 1796, when Hahnemann's *Essay on a New Principle for Ascertaining the Curative Power of Drugs* appeared, there is a long list of eminent physicians that had maintained (certainly, some of them more forcefully or explicitly than others) that drug-similars might or ought to be used in disease; meaning the employment of medicines which promote and aid (assist in developing) the body's inherent self-healing effort. These men discounted as therapeutically irrelevant the causal assumptions derived from elaborations in the other sciences, and refused to base their therapeutics on such (Rationalist) elaborated, often a priori, knowledge. Symptoms were simply viewed by them as signs of the curative process which was to be aided in medicine.

[Elizabeth Danciger has written an absorbing study of the historical roots of homoeopathy entitled *The Emergence of Homoeopathy: Alchemy into Medicine* (London: Century Hutchinson Ltd, 1987, 117 pages). She places this scientific culmination of medical systematics – homoeopathy – in the context of its antecedent sources, some of them remote, among which she includes Islamic alchemy, the neo-Platonism of Paracelsus, the Hermetic-Cabalistic tradition, the diverse tides of Renaissance science, Cartesianism, the Enlightenment, and other pre-homoeopathic philosophical currents. That work was, however, not consulted in the preparation of this entry.]

The most famous names in medical history are among the homoeopathic proto-historical (Empirical) group (– Empiricism's guiding dictum is 'nihil in intellectu nisi prius in sensu' [see 'Latin Aphorisms in Homoeopathy']):

Hippocrates (ca. 460-ca. 377 BC), in the writings attributed to the man who is called the Father of Medicine, was the first on record to point out the homoeopathic principle that like cures like; he and those around him placed medicine on a scientific foundation, freeing it from superstition, and gave sound and shrewd descriptions of many disease conditions. He is also considered as the author of the Hippocratic oath. Named after him still are Hippocrates's bandage, cap, and cord, and Hippocratic facies, fingers, nails, and succussion.

Herakleides of Tarentum (around 280 BC), was the first to write very articulate commentaries on all the Hippocratic works; he pursued pharmacological research which produced such valuable material that all succeeding medical writers worked with it, including the influential theoretician Claudius Galen (ca. 130-201 AD).

Herophilos of Chalcedon (in 3rd century BC), one of the first recorded to dissect the human body, described the brain, noting cerebrum and cerebellum, gave his name to the cerebral sinus (torcular Herophili), clearly distinguished between nerves, tendons and blood vessels; he named the duodenum and the prostate gland; he used gymnastics and dietary treatment empirically, and introduced counting the pulse against a water-clock. He accurately described a variety of pulse rhythms, and he is one of the great botanical pharmacologists of antiquity.

Serapion of Alexandria (around 240 BC), together with Herophilos of Chalcedon was founder of the Empirical School of Medicine; he called himself the first 'non-dogmatist' physician. He relied on experiential evidence to guide him to the very effective use of similars: for instance, of sharp, stimulating and dilating ointments in the throat area in cynanche (collective term for gangrenous pharyngitis, Ludwig's angina, tonsillitis, quinsy), or astringent plant remedies in epilepsy that would actually restrict the parts that were most agitated, which others (the 'dogmatists') had vainly sought to relax.

Lucretius (Titus Lucretius Carus) (99-55 BC), was a great Roman poet and philosopher with the most extraordinary insight; though no physician himself, his influence was of profound (though little recognized) significance to medical Empiricism right up to the present day and continues so to be. His life-work is contained in six volumes comprising a single poem *De rerum natura* ('The Nature of Things', i.e. 'The Nature of the Universe') which is in hexameter of the most vivid language and imagery, written with the consummate skill of a master versifier (he inspired Tennyson's romantic poem 'Lucretius' in the nineteenth century). Philosophically Lucretius used the premises of Epicurus (342-270 BC) as his springboard (Epicureanism taught that virtue should be followed because it leads to happiness in this life, that there is no hereafter with death simply being the end of life, that the gods have no interest in, nor relation to, human affairs, and that the universe is a system of atoms organized into patterns and structures). Lucretius lived as a near-recluse, nauseated both by the carnage of the civil wars and by the scramble for wealth and power that was fast debilitating the Roman republic; in his writing he maintains a rigidly logical form but is fired by the passion of his own cogent common-sense convictions. In the first three books he lucidly sets out and systematically demonstrates certain of his basic principles:

nothing is created out of nothing;

nothing is ever annihilated;

the universe consist of an infinitude of minute, indestructible particles called atoms;

atoms have no properties except distinctive sizes, weights and shapes;

all other properties of material objects as perceived (e.g. warmth, scent, colour, etc.) only result from the impact on human sense organs of any given variety of atom combinations;

there is an infinity of empty space through which atoms eternally fall with a spontaneous declination (meaning 'swerve') in their downward path, which results in the formation and organization of the clusters evident in the surrounding void (the lifeless atom-stream is seen to blossom into the inexhaustible variety and splendour of the perceptible universe);

all atomic accretions (e.g. earth, water, sky [air]) are destructible;

the individual immortal soul is a figment, but there is an intrinsic freedom in nature, which is the basis for the humans' freedom of will and capacity for making judgemental choices.

In the other three books these principles are applied to the explanation of a diversity of phenomena:

to sight, hearing, to the other three senses and to sex in Book IV;

to cosmogony, to plant, animal and human evolution, and to human society and culture in Book V;

to natural phenomena such as lightning, magnetism, and volcanoes in Book VI.

Underlying his whole exposition is the evergreen Empirical postulate that the only source of knowledge is sense perception; this is seen as an infallible source since it is verifiable just as it is repeatable; he takes the medical Empirical position ('nothing can be considered good medicine that counters the curative effort as expressed by the organism's evident symptoms') to its inevitable universal application when he makes it clear that he views his physical doctrines as providing a solid base for his ethical construct that nothing is good except what seems 'good' (meaning agreeable) to the organism's senses. With Epicureanism, he identifies pleasure with good and pain with evil, and holds that atomic disequilibrium is bad (and pain-inducing on an organic level) but the readjustment to atomic equilibrium is good (and experienced as an accompanying sensation of pleasure on an organic level). In the long run, he and Epicurus say though, the highest good lies not in bodily pleasure *per se* but in establishing the maximum of equilibrium (absence of pain) in a state called 'ataraxia', meaning imperturbability, to be fostered by temperance, retirement from public life, freeing oneself of dependencies, the renunciation of power, wealth, and other lusts, and through the furtherance of the pleasures of the mind such as, above all, true friendship. He was highly sensitive to all suffering and to all beauty, and he believed, in a callous and salacious age, that if men were once delivered from their ignorance, from which sprang their groundless superstitious fears and fruitless desires, that this would enable them to enjoy a life of true felicity in unruffled detachment, where they could be ever vividly aware of the satisfying sense of that omnipresent equilibrium to be savoured exquisitely in everything that one touched, heard, saw, smelled or tasted; his genius in this context is memorably expressed in his imaginative portrayal of 'primitive man' (Book V), whilst his great sensitivity is exemplified by the intensity of his sympathy with a cow bereaved of her calf (Book II, 352-366). Moreover, his clear perception of individual constitutional idiosyncrasies he expressed in his saying 'One man's meat is another man's poison', which has gained access to the idiomatic repertoire of most European languages; the parallels are obvious between the disdainful attitude consistently meted out to Empirical medicine by Rationalist (mainstream, orthodox) medicine, and that of the (mainstream, orthodox) philosophy of Rationalism in all its variations unceasingly attempting to smother or belittle Lucretius' Epicureanism.

a) For Christian apologists, moulded by orthodox theology, his positive doctrines were stamped as blasphemous and perverse, leaving him from about the third century AD with very little influence during the entire Middle Ages.

b) In 1473 the first printed edition of his poem surfaced, which suddenly found many imitators and admirers of his poetic style, but he was not begun to be taken seriously as a thinker until the seventeenth century, when his poem's signal effect of opening people's minds to new ways of seeing 'the nature of things' were noted (cf. Bacon, Boyle, Cervantes, Columbus, Copernicus, Galileo, Kepler, Newton, Shakespeare, *et al*). Matters turned very much in his favour at a time when sense-perceptible experiments, measurements and calculations were replacing discursive speculation; he was taken to have provided a new model of the universe which made a surprisingly suitable framework for virtually all the newly discovered scientific facts; many were influenced more strongly than they realized by his Epicureanism, since they freely borrowed many of their technical terms from that era of antiquity; yet whilst the mechanics of the universe could be drawn along such lines, the rest of Lucretius' inferences were scornfully dismissed by uncomprehending men who were either orthodox Christians or at least devout deists.

c) In more recent times there is abundant evidence that Lucretius left his impress on the minds of an entire range of Europeans, notably Goethe, A E Housman, Edmund Spenser and Voltaire, but though they admired him as a poet their Rationalist preconceptions made them incapable of seeing anything but precocious childishness in his philosophy and science; on prudential grounds his Book IV, which also deals with sex, became a target for furiously cruel satires on the folly of lovers; as recently as the nineteenth century a sharp distinction was regularly made by commentators between his genius as a poet and the silliness of his theme, saying in all seriousness that he had cast about for some inconsequential subject on which to exercise his great art, picking the Epicurean philosophy to please his patron, the praetor Gaius Memmius; in 1864 H A J Munro introduced an edition of this poem thus: 'To Lucretius the truth of his philosophy was all-important,' adding, 'To us on the other hand the truth or falsehood of his system is of exceedingly little concern except insofar as it is thereby rendered a better or worse vehicle for conveying the beauties of his language and the graces of his poetical conceptions'; it is only in very recent times that there has begun to emerge a view of the universe in which he would feel at home.

Almost twenty-one centuries – from the century BC to the present – was the time it took for Lucretius' science and philosophy to cease to be labelled as absurd; even on the level of incidentals do his theories fit the present view of reality well: for example, he contrasts the smooth atoms of fluids with the interlocked atoms of steel (Book II, 391-397 and 444-450) which corresponds with currently accepted knowledge about molecular structure, or his much laughed-at description of the occasional unpredictable 'swerve' of an individual atom's path from the straight course, which he associated with human free will, is compatible with the principle of indeterminacy recognized by the physicists of today; Lucretius' special significance, however, for Empiricism generally, and for homoeopathy in particular, is his whole answer to the challenge of existence: a sincere, courageous vision that produced a full working model – **constructed from the data of the senses alone** – of the universe, of human society, as well as of any individual response.

Aulus Cornelius Celsus (25 BC-50 AD), was a Roman of the patrician class, who defied Roman social convention by becoming a physician, which, for patricians, was considered beneath their status. His literary output was encyclopaedic and greatly advanced for his time: he favoured dissection of cadavers, presenting clear though brief anatomical descriptions; his description of malarial fevers cannot be surpassed, and his view that fever was an effort on the part of nature to combat and eliminate morbid material from the body exactly forespelled the homoeopathic teaching of one and three quarter millennia later (he felt able to say, 'Give me a drug that will produce a fever and I'll cure every illness'). He advised that snake venom be extracted by sucking as it was not lethal when swallowed, though it would be when absorbed into a wound (pathogenetic experiments in homoeopathy by Constantin Hering and others have since established this as true); he described an operation for crushing stones in the bladder (lithotomy), as well as amputations and trepanation (removal of part of the skull), and plastic surgery for the repair of the nose, ears and lips. He addressed the subject of treatment of fistulas, ulcers, tumours, wounds, fractures, hernias, dislocations, bone decay and necrosis; he discussed ligatures and devised effective methods for stopping haemorrhages. He has given his name to Celsus's area, chancre, kerion, operation, papules, and vitiligo; his repute was still so high fifteen centuries after his death that Theophrastus Bombastus von Hohenheim adopted the name Paracelsus (= 'surpassing Celsus') under which he appears below in this entry.

Pliny the Elder [Gaius Secundus Plinius] (ca. 23-79 AD) wrote *Naturalis Historia* in 37 books, in thirteen of which he describes a great number of medicinal plants and drugs, as well as commenting on medical customs of his time: for instance, he complained that the orthodox practice of his day, 'Methodism, reducing the whole of medicine to the discovery of causes, made it a matter of guesswork' (book XXVI, no. vii).

Dioskorides Pedanios (in 1st century AD), naturalist and military surgeon, travelled extensively with the army of Emperor Nero from 54 to 68 AD, studied 'military' diseases and collected and identified some 600 different medicinal plants; this he published in his *De Materia Medica*; this work remained the authoritative materia medica for sixteen centuries in the Arab, Greek and Latin sphere of influence. Many of the names he gave to plants are still used today; his concise botanical descriptions, often including habitat and distribution, were very accurate; he is considered one of the founders of botanical science; his extensive experience led him to the observation he captured in the phrase 'where the disease is, there is the remedy also'.

Sextus Empiricus (around 200 AD), was an able physician and eminent philosopher; almost 500 years after the founding of the Empirical School by Herophilos and Serapion (see above) this man appeared as one of the six most prominent philosophers of Skepticism, telling his medical followers to avoid giving logical explanations of phenomena; instead he emphasized the description of symptoms. His general philosophical thesis was that man cannot know independent reality but only the state of his own mind (he applied this universally, saying we cannot know whether God exists, because our minds cannot attain any absolute truth). It is this man's name and his teaching of the philosophical system of Skepticism (rather than Empirical medicine), which is totally dismissive of all knowledge (obviously in medical practice as well), that has produced a lingering slur on Empirical Medicine by association with the man's name, even though Empirical Medicine is founded on experiential evidence as a clear guide to successful treatment.

Paul of Aegina (607-690) an eclectic surgeon of Byzantium, philosophically in harmony with medical Empiricism, wrote the *Epitome* of surgery in seven volumes in which lithotomy, trepanation, surgery of the eye, tonsillectomy, and amputation of the breast are fully described.

Philippus Aureolus Paracelsus (1493-1541) so greatly admired Celsus of the first century AD that he adopted the name Paracelsus to replace his real name Theophrastus Bombastus von Hohenheim; he revolutionized the sciences of chemistry and medicine, being regarded as the father of modern experimentalism in both; he contributed substantially to pre-homoeopathic pharmacy, pharmacology and especially to proto-homoeopathy, amongst many other things, through his interest in minerals and miners' occupational diseases which he developed in the Tirol (Austria): he taught the use of similar remedies and foreshadowed the concept of the occupational miasma of homoeopathy in his extensive writings (particularly on zinc, cobalt, bismuth, the alums, and the vitriols); he also anticipated Arthur Koestler's 'holon' concept in his teaching that the organism is one whole, all of whose parts interact and intercommunicate, the smallest part of which contains everything which is found in the largest and that the same is true of the organism in relation to the universe as a whole ('microcosm' and 'macrocosm' are the terms coined for this); he has also been credited with the discovery of hydrogen in the course of his (al)chemical experimental work.

Girolamo Cardano (1501-1576) [also known as Geronimo; full name gallicized and anglicized to Jerome Cardan; also occasionally teutonized to Hieronymus Kardaun] is one of the greatest physicians of sixteenth century Europe; a genius, whose activities were manifold, he was a principal figure of the High Renaissance in Milan, Pavia and Bologna; because of his omnicompetent and penetrating intellect, as well as his positive attitude toward knowledge he became, like Leonardo da Vinci (though never attaining the latter's stature), a versatile leader in the transition from the mediaeval to the modern world; he was also profoundly steeped in mathematics, philosophy, literature and natural science. He received his medical degree at the University of Padua in 1526, but because of his illegitimate birth he had difficulty in gaining admittance to the College of Physicians; in 1536 he published his first book of note which was a scathing attack on the medical practices of the members of the board, yet three years later he was admitted to practice; he soon became the rector of the College and then the most sought-after physician in all Europe; the only offer to go abroad that he accepted was to travel to Scotland to treat Archbishop Hamilton's serious asthmatic condition there. He published most of his mathematical output in *Ars magna* in 1545, where (i) he was first to structure some algebraic fundamentals in what has since become a *sine qua non* for modern algebra, in which (ii) he also set out a systematic theory of equations, including some calculations with imaginary numbers, and in which (iii) he genially provided the key for the solution of equations of third and fourth degree (referred to as Cardan's Formula). This amazing physician, moreover, gave his name also to several intricate inventions that are still much in use today: (i) the Cardan Mount (gimbal mount for compasses, gyroscopes and other navigational equipment), (ii) the Cardanic (flexible drive) shaft, and (iii) the Cardan (universal) joint; together with Benvenuto Cellini (1500-1571) and Michel de Montaigne (1533-1592) he is credited with having been first to introduce the autobiographical form as an innovation into modern literature. In his written self-portrayal he, the physician, first classifies all the attributes of man, thereafter he weaves his own peculiarities into the autobiographical text under each head, covering physical, intellectual and moral details about his own life, thereby imaginatively re-affirming his individuality magnified through his unquestionable powers of self-examination. His books on popular science *De rerum varietate* (Of the Variety of Things) and *De subtilitate rerum* (Of Subtle Things) appeared in many editions; he made the first attempt to create a theory of probability in his book on gambling *De ludo alea* (On Games of Chance); he published his prime medical work in Pavia in 1566 under the title *Ars curandi* (The Art of Curing) in which he introduced many novel ideas that subsequently withstood his opponents' onslaughts very well In this work he clearly sets out as an incontestable fundamental the Empirical aphorism:

'omne similia similibus confirmatur'

(Everything similar is confirmed by [in] the similar).

In medicine, as in everything else, he applied his powerful mind, and his lectures as professor of medicine in Pavia and Bologna always attracted large numbers of students. In 1570, after eight years as professor of medicine at Bologna, he was arrested there by the Inquisition on vague charges (it was rumoured, at the instigation of orthodox medics [at the time orthodoxy, in its Rationalist speculations on methods on which to base therapy, was moving from the Galenic 'logical categories of contraries' toward Iatrochemistry, Iatromechanism and Iatromathematics, these being the medical emulations, respectively, of the state of chemistry, hydraulics and mathematics of the day]), and although he received a fairly lenient sentence, he was forbidden to publish any more; the last six years of his life he spent in Rome in a vain attempt to gain a pardon. His son, also an Empiricist physician of note, was put to death in 1560 after having been accused of poisoning his wife (it was again rumoured that orthodox physicians bore false witness against him).

Thomas Sydenham (1624-1689), called the 'English Hippocrates' did research study at the famous Montpellier University (France) (see entry below, under Georg Ernst Stahl) and received the degree of Doctor of Medicine from Cambridge University; a great clinician who brought a fresh approach to Empirical medicine, he believed that illness is itself a kind of cure (an attempt by the body to get its vital healing forces back to normal). He always emphasized personal observation and the use of simple similar remedies (he was opposed to polypharmacy); he insisted on the best possible care for every patient and held that symptoms were just nature's way of throwing off morbific matter, for the patient to recover; he employed similars in non-medicinal therapeutics as well: he introduced the cooling method in the treatment of smallpox (rejecting the diaphoretic treatment generally in use then), he treated patients with intermittent fever by sweating them out (while others prescribed refrigerants), he prescribed a life in the open for phthisis (others kept such patients indoors). He was one of the first known to administer iron in anaemia, is reported to have given fish liver in rickets, definitely gave cinchona in ague (malaria), and mercury against syphilis (the obvious but unconscious homoeopathizing is remarkable); he clarified the categorical difference between a symptom and an illness (e.g.: a headache is a symptom that may be there for many reasons, from influenza to excessive alcohol consumption, the symptom-inducing illness) and his perception of infectious disease was far in advance of his time. He made a special study of epidemics in relation to seasons, years, ages and reintroduced the Hippocratic idea of 'epidemic constitution'; in 1651 he was the first to describe rickets; in 1666 he published his *Treatise on Fevers;* he defined and classified the fevers, chorea, hysteria, smallpox, malaria, the venereal diseases, and distinguished clearly between gout and acute rheumatism, discussing pathology and therapeutics. His radical new methods angered and alienated the influential orthodox physicians of that period (who collectively subscribed to the Iatrochemical doctrine, by then in vogue, of prescribing acids and alkalis to neutralize the organism that was diagnosed to be suffering from one or other such chemical excess), yet Sydenham had a staunchly loyal following of important patients and counted as his close friends people like the liberal philosopher John Locke ([1632-1704] founder of philosophical Empiricism: 'all knowledge is derived from experience')[1] and the Hon Robert Boyle (established 'Boyle's Law: 'volume of gas varies inversely as the pressure upon it, provided temperature be

---

[1]The other two great English liberal philosophers of Empiricism, who had the profoundest influence on the eighteenth and nineteenth centuries, were: Locke's direct intellectual heir, David Hume (1711-1776), a celebrated historian besides, who made philosophical skepticism within Empiricism respectable once more; and The Bishop of Cloyne, George Berkeley, DD (1685-1753), who propounded that the only things that are real are our ideas of what is presented to our senses, which forespelled homoeopathy's view that sense-perceptible symptoms and signs are the only real determinants of a patient's disease.

constant'). He gave his name to Sydenham's laudanum, and Sydenham's chorea (also called St Vitus' dance).

Georg Ernst Stahl (1660-1734), a physician and chemist, emphasized the role of the 'Anima Sensitiva' (= homoeopathy's dynamis) as motivating all activities of the human body, including the curative effort; treatment, generally by similars, sometimes by specifics, was only to be supportive of the Anima; he stands at the beginning of the modern Vitalist movement in Empiricist medicine. He developed the phlogiston theory, in which he postulated a substance of negative mass that would have to be given off by a substance when it underwent combustion to account for the increase in mass of the ash over the starting substance. His concept of the Anima Sensitiva remained influential in the Medical School of Montpellier (France) until the end of the nineteenth century (Montpellier Empiricism advocated unadulterated observation and therapy based on experience only, regarding itself as faithful to Hippocrates, thus the portal superscription on one of the University's main buildings: 'Hippocrates, olim Coensis, nunc Monspaliensis' [Hippocrates, previously of Cos, now of Montpellier]. Moreover, Montpellier Empiricism spread to Paris after the 1789 revolution; and Dr d'Amador, Montpellier's professor of medicine, became a strong and open supporter of homoeopathy from the 1830s). The phlogiston theory was ultimately abandoned in the 1780s when Antoine Laurent Lavoisier (1743-1794 [when he was executed on the guillotine]) demonstrated that uptake of oxygen was involved in all combustion, which accounted for the ponderal discrepancies accurately noted by Stahl.

Giorgio Baglivi (1668-1707), as professor of theoretical medicine, surgery and anatomy in Rome, combined Hippocratic precepts with those of the ancient Empirics, and then reconciled these with the doctrines of Bacon; he fundamentally reformed medical practice through his profoundly influential book *De praxi medica ad priscam observandi rationem revocanda* (Rome, 1696: 2 vols) in which he declared (p 200) that no medicines were to be prescribed at the outset to avoid disturbing the natural course of disease, or preventing the healing crisis from coming on, or transforming acute diseases into chronic ones. Anticipating Hahnemann he urged greater attention to the 'peculiar and constant' symptoms and to ignore the 'common' ones; he accepted the use of acupuncture in medical practice (p 237) which had then just been brought to Europe for the first time; he maintained that a productive medical method would yield 'knowledge, not opinion' and criticized orthodox Galenism for sterile non-inventiveness. He was censorious of professional arrogance in medical men, and disapproving of their infatuation with baseless hypotheses (Methodism was beginning to become fashionable in orthodoxy then); but he was also critical of the one-off, anecdotal experiences of some Empirics, calling (p 172/3) for a scientific, 'a rational Empiricism, an Empiricism made literate, uncovered by method and not by chance, fertilized in the intellect, based on daily exploration of the facts of disease'. In other words, he yearned for what Hahnemann was to introduce into medicine.

John Hunter (1728-1793), a distinguished Scottish biologist, practical surgeon, obstetrician and physiologist, was a skilled dissector and an exponent of the comparative method in anatomy; he organized a museum; he owned a private printing press and was his own publisher; he experimented with embryological monsters, keeping his own menagerie of these; he studied fossils, and did significant investigations of animal behaviour; he was the first to trace the ramifications of nasal and olfactory nerves, to describe the descent of the testes in the foetus, and to prove the importance and function of the lymphatic system through studies on animals. He studied coagulation of blood, formation of pus and gunshot wounds; in physiology he was a Vitalist, believing that the dynamis (vital force, living principle) exists prior to physical structures; his operation for popliteal aneurysm remains a classic; he was the first to draw up 'Principles of Surgery' for this independent discipline (in 1790 he became surgeon-general). He strongly believed in personal investigation by the physician to obtain first-hand knowledge (he actually inoculated himself with syphilitic matter to study the development of syphilis at first hand); he rejected the a priori methods of orthodoxy that relied on physics, chemistry, astrology or signatures to provide rationalist constructs that determined therapeutics. As he had never received formal training in medicine, but had brilliantly learnt it from astute observation and practice, he became and remained an enthusiastic apostle of the experimental method of Empirical medicine, with which this profoundly original man affected Edward Jenner (1749-1823) who from 1770, after completion of his apprenticeship, was a pupil in the house of John Hunter (see 'Isopathy'). In 1786 Hunter published his *Treatise on the Venereal Disease* in which he first put forward a number of the essential fundamentals incorporated later by Hahnemann in his concept of drug provings (three years later Hahnemann published his *Instruction for Surgeons Respecting Venereal Diseases* in which he acknowledges Hunter's book in twenty-three references); the major share of the credit for the discovery of the drug proving (pathogenetic experimentation) must thus accrue to Hunter. He had similarly advanced ideas in many other areas: for example, he pointed the trail for Darwin ninety years later when he was first to note that the embryo passed through a series of stages in each of which it variously resembles some lower creature, or, another instance was when he put forward perfectly precise views, that have retained their validity to the present time, concerning the nature of geological change (his papers on geology were only published some time after his death, because a friend, wanting to protect Hunter's scientific reputation, drew attention to the then unheard-of opinion in the papers that made the earth much older than the accepted 6000 years). Hunter's enormous contribution to homoeopathy's proto-history is summarized briefly in his views:

i) A patient's constitutional predisposition is of profound importance – not everyone is equally susceptible (he speaks of 'the aptness of the living principle to be irritated by a . . . cause').[1]

---

[1] Hunter, John. *Works* in 4 vols, London: Longman, 1837, vol II, p 150.

ii) No (part of any) organism is simultaneously capable of being diseased in two ways (he speaks of the 'principle that no two different fevers can exist in the same constitution, nor two local diseases in the same part, at the same time').[1]

iii) Medicines neither act on a 'disease', or on its 'poison', by chemical neutralization, nor do they act through any form of evacuation they may induce in the patient, but only by their 'stimulating power' on the diseased organism; any medicine (no inkling of similarity here) will introduce an artificial irritation acting upon the constitution, which may extinguish the existing incompatible irritation, as these are unable to co-exist.[2]

iv) The effects of medicines might often be confused with the symptoms of disease, so he warns against the administration of more medicine than is necessary,[3] although it was left to Hahnemann to take this to its ultimate conclusions by discovering the similarity principle, and hormesis, the biphasic action of drugs.

v) Hunter was the first to make the observation that infection depends upon the quality of the poison, never on its quantity, clearly distinguishing between the two,[4] forespelling homoeopathy's concept of effective communication of medicinal power as always being dependent upon quality, rather than crude quantity; he also noted that a patient recently cured of an infection is, for a time, much harder to re-infect,[5] anticipating the long-lasting curative effect inherent in well-indicated homoeopathic drugs, as well as the isopathic concept in prophylactic homoeopathy.

Contribution by Christian Friedrich Samuel Hahnemann

One serious defect impeded the complete evolution of scientific medicine within the paradigm of medical Empiricism beyond this point: the lack of an exact and serviceable theory of drug action. Hahnemann completed this:

i) Through trials on the healthy (pathogenetic experiments, drug provings) he clearly identified a phenomenon for which he coined the word 'Arzneikrankheit', meaning 'drug disease', because this artificial disease is fully comparable to 'normal disease', where the symptoms are indistinguishable from the effects brought on by a morbific agent as in disease though they are a healthy organism's reaction to the drug. In other words, a dual effect is in evidence, where two different circumstances (the 'natural' disease and the drug response or 'artificial' disease) produce identical effects.

ii) Experiment and observation further led him to the discovery of hormesis, the biphasic action of medicines; in his *Essay* of 1796 he wrote, 'medicines have more than one action: the first a direct action which gradually changes

[1] Ibid., pp 131-132.
[2] Ibid., p 455.
[3] Ibid., p 470.
[4] Ibid., p 142.
[5] Ibid., p 165.

into the second (which I call the indirect secondary action). The latter is generally a state exactly the opposite of the former'.[1]

The uniform pattern that emerged, which Hahnemann was the first to describe, showed that where there was a palpable similarity between the patient's disease symptoms and the primary symptoms of the drug, the disease irritation would always reliably be extinguished, because the later secondary symptoms of the drug, which are the patient's appropriate reaction to it, will overwhelm and annihilate that disease provided the organism's reactive capacity is adequate.

Hahnemann's reliable technique for establishing and applying 'similarity', through the system of homoeopathy, had suddenly produced for the lacuna in Empirical medicine an analytical relationship between the disease process and drug action, that has yielded the only self-consistent scientific therapeutics with consistently predictable results.

Hahnemann's discovery, being in harmony with other natural laws and principles (and particularly proposition 1) at the beginning of this entry), dramatically and permanently removed homoeopathic therapeutics from the realm of the purely speculative, that doggedly confounds all other medical systems. In Hahnemann's own words (preface to the second edition of the *Organon*) this had elevated it to 'a pure science of experience' quite like 'physics and chemistry'.

Moreover, Hahnemann contributed in yet a different way to scientific therapeutics, from the viewpoint of Rationalist Medicine. In 1623, the Italian scientist Galileo Galilei (1564-1642) averred that science is concerned only with primary qualities – only those of the external world that could be weighed and measured. Secondary qualities and their assessment – as, for instance, in the perception of beauty, the comprehension of meaning, the determining of value, or the experience of love – fell outside the realm of science. Fourteen years later, the French author, mathematician and philosopher, René Descartes (1596-1650), who ironically is probably best known for the dictum: 'Cogito, ergo sum' [I am thinking, so I exist], relegated the conscious mind to the position of scientific inconsequence. He did this by espousing Galileo's doctrines in his (unpublished) book *Le Monde,* and later, less blatantly in his (published) *Discours de la Méthode, Meditationes de prima philosophia* and *Principia philosophiae,* as well as by stating in these three books that there are two radically different kinds of substance. The first, physical or extended substance (res extensa) has length, breadth, depth and can therefore be measured and divided. The second, thinking substance (res cogitans) is unextended and indivisible. The external world, of which the patient's body is a part, was confined to the first category, while the internal world of the mind belonged for ever to the second. That was to make the former objective and the latter

[1] Hahnemann, Christian Friedrich Samuel. *The Lesser Writings of Samuel Hahnemann* Collected & translated by R E Dudgeon. New York: Radde, 1852, p 266-267.

subjective, leading to the permanent exclusion of subjective experience from the reductionists' external world.

Subsequent scientific models, which reached into the very recent past, could lead only to hypotheses that remained devoid of consciousness. For example, the recent reductionist models of a patient's consciousness, as conceived by orthodox psychiatry, would attempt to explain subjective experience only mechanistically, as an aspect of brain function alone. Thus, for example, a transcendent state of mind, during which the world may be experienced as all-embracing love, would need to be ascribed to a temporal lobe dysfunction, or anger might only be explained as the sudden transmission of neural impulses in the amygdala-hypothalamic structures of the brain.

Hahnemann, about 150 years after Galileo and Descartes, clearly grasped the attendant difficulties for medicine inherent in such a one-sided dogma. He repeatedly stated his 'totality of symptoms concept', which explicitly made subjective experiences and objective phenomena inseparable and co-extensive in any given patient. His enlightened conception of psychodynamics is summarized in sections 210-230 of the *Organon*. His use of the words 'dynamis' and 'vital force' can leave no-one in any doubt about precisely where he stood relative to the non-material aspects of disease and its cure. He understood, with the foreboding of genius, that the acceptance (as it ultimately was by Rationalist Medicine) of the dominant model put forward by Galileo and Descartes would inevitably lead to perceptions which were both scientifically inappropriate and misleading. Clearly, the homoeopath cannot help but use a subjectively contaminated mental model to assess the patient before him, just as any non-homoeopathic practitioner cannot ever avoid doing. This makes the independent objective external world in the context of medicine fictional. Equally, a patient, or prover, devoid of consciousness would be reduced to a mere caricature of him- or herself and the scientifically accurate remedy could never be homoeopathically matched under such circumstances.

Homoeopathy takes as its data in each case both the so-called objective phenomena and the subjective experiences, without attempting to make any distinction between them. That becomes its particular guiding symptom combination. As a scientific system it is consistent within itself in that it requires the matching of that particular combination of symptoms with a comparable model in its materia medica. There is a predictable curative-reactive relationship between the 'natural disease' of the patient and the 'artificial disease' recorded in the materia medica, provided these are properly matched and the natural disease is within reversible limits.

The therapeutic science of homoeopathy proceeds as does reductionist science: Anew with each patient it sets up a hypothetical sub-set within the whole homoeopathic theory; each administration of a properly matched medicine tests the whole theory upon which homoeopathy rests; certainly it also probes the homoeopath's ability to chose well-indicated remedies, allowing for falsification and reselection. A true science is cumulative and has an unchanging base. In the full sense described here, homoeopathy is a true science, as defined by Sir Karl Popper (born Vienna, 1902), the philosopher of science.[1]

Phobia

Unfounded or morbid dread. The word is used as a suffix in combination with terms expressing the object of dread. Phobias in all their diversity feature in the materia medica.

Phosphoric Constitution

See 'Constitutional Type'.

Phosphoro-Sulphuric Constitution

See 'Constitutional Type'.

Phototherapy

Naturopathic treatment of disease by means of light rays; part of the large category of actinotherapy. (See 'Actinotherapy' and 'Naturopath'.)

Physical Characteristics

See 'Constitutional Type'.

Physicalistic Theory

Materialism. (See 'Vitalism'.)

Physiological Dose

● **Substantial dose.**

The word 'physiological' may be used to qualify the action of a drug when given to a healthy person, as distinguished, for instance, from its 'therapeutic' action when so used, or, at the other extreme, from its effects in a 'toxicological' dosage. By logical extension 'a physiological dose' was generally considered to mean the quantity that was given to a healthy prover in a pathogenetic experiment, as opposed to 'a therapeutic dose' reserved for the patient. Since the patient's dose in homoeopathic practice almost always turns out to be potentized, i.e. is highly deconcentrated (perhaps infinitesimally so), it follows

[1] Popper, Sir Karl R, and Sir John C Eccles. *Das Ich und sein Gehirn,* Munich: R Piper GmbH & Co KG, 1982, pp 140, 146, 156 and 157.

that in common usage, the phrase 'physiological dose' came to mean the opposite of therapeutic, and became synonymous with a ponderal quantity, i.e. one that is materially substantive.

Physiological Response in Homoeotherapeutics, Mechanism of

An authority on medicinal therapeutics, Solis Cohen, quoted in the 1974 Addendum to the Homoeopathic Pharmacopoeia of the United States,[1] maintains:

1 Drug effect depends on the physiological reaction of the body in contact with the drug.
2 Drugs develop no new power or quality in the body.
3 Drugs add no new energy but merely increase or hinder its liberation.
4 Drugs may provoke latent potentialities and deflect the lines of projection of the vital forces.

This expounds upon homoeopathy's vitalist position on the issue. To achieve what is described by Cohen, homoeopathy routinely employs the monophasic reactive effect of Arndt-Schulz. This aims for and relies on the reaction contributed by the living organism alone, not on any direct drug action. To explain: Hahnemann discovered that any drug given to a sick or healthy person has a biphasic action, termed hormesis. This means it will produce two distinct symptom patterns – the one is the immediate coercive effect of the drug, the other, the organism's reaction, which, broadly speaking, is the opposite of the first. Moreover, the phrase 'drug effect' would more fittingly be applied to orthodox (coercive) pharmacotherapeutics, rather than to any homoeopathically elicited curative effort in an organism. The physiological mechanism of this lies in exploiting the sensitized body's response to an incitant agent (the homoeopathic drug) as may, for instance, be detected by the afferent fibres of the central nervous system, or show itself in altered basophil degranulation, or, as suggested by Sheila and Robin Gibson,[2] in facets of the metabolism in prostaglandin synthesis, just as in a multitude of other physiological ways.

Experimental Evidence
A series of successful basophil degranulation experiments concerning histamine release are mentioned in outline under 'Epistemological Assumptions in Homoeopathy', section 5: Base Drug – Ultramolecular Dose. However, histamine release happens at the end of a reactive chain of events made up of more than a dozen metabolic stages and there are strong

[1]American Institute of Homoeopathy. *Compendium of Homoeotherapeutics – Addendum to the Homoeopathic Pharmacopoeia of the US,* Falls Church, Va: American Academy of Homoeotherapeutics, 1974, pp 16-17.
[2]Gibson, Sheila and Robin. *Homoeopathy for Everyone,* Harmondsworth, Middlesex: Penguin Books Ltd, p 153.

indications that the homoeopathic stimulus could engage the response mechanism much earlier in this process, and that the observed dye-induced changes in the above experiments may only be the result of achromia due to, say, previously altered intracellular pH. Professor Jacques Benveniste has since reported[1] that he was conducting fresh experiments using machine-made potencies, that all tests were double blind in triplicate, that results were expressed as absolute numbers of cells (not as percentages) and that seven laboratory workers routinely achieved positive results (statistically significant).

The following experiment shows not only the physiological mechanism of the reactive effect brought about by a low potency homoeopathic medicine on the capture of neurotransmitters, but it also serves as a clear example of the reversal of the primary direction of drug response, leaving only the secondary, more or less opposite, reactive effect, when any drug is taken from the ponderal to the potentized form. That means from the normal biphasic to the monophasic state as used by homoeopathy. Example:

'A Study of the Action of Gelsemium Sempervirens upon the Capturing of Neurotransmitters by Synaptosomal Preparations of Various Fractions of Rats' Brains'.[2]

Mental disease may, amongst other things, readily be linked to abnormal functioning of specific mediator systems in the cerebro-spinal system. It was, therefore, decided to adapt modern techniques in testing the reactive effect of Gelsemium sempervirens (Jasminium virginianum), a medicine which homoeopaths classically use in cases of distress and anxiety, because of its ataractic homoeopathic effects. Gelsemium sempervirens is an extremely poisonous plant which strongly affects the central nervous system. Its toxicological symptomatology is muscular cramps and quiverings, with incoordination, followed later by paralysis. The work was carried out under the scrutiny of Professor Henri Pacheco at his laboratories at the National Institute of Applied Sciences in Lyon. He, a Professor of Chemical Biology, had been vociferous in his condemnation of homoeopathy's 'meretricious claims', prior to this series of experiments. He was to become a powerful advocate of homoeopathy subsequently.

The study observed the action of Gelsemium sempervirens (mother tincture and potencies) in the preparations of rats' brains upon the synaptosomal capturing of three of the main mediators: norepinephrine (1-noradrenaline), dopamine (Θ-hydroxytyramine) and serotonin (5-hydroxytryptamine). This was shown to be a very precise 'in vitro' method, which made it possible to postulate and to measure modifications occurring on the pre-synaptic level, even when these were insubstantial. It was found to be a reliable model for

---

[1] Reilly, David Taylor. 'Zentrum zur Dokumentation für Naturheilverfahren – Homöopathie im Brennpunkt: Hazy Reflections from Essen', quoting Prof J Benveniste in his report on the conference 14th-15th October 1989, *Complementary Medical Research*, May 1990, vol IV, no 2, pp 51-53.

[2] Research Committee of the Liga Medicorum Homoeopathica Internationalis, General Secretary to the. *Aspects of Research in Homoeopathy*, vol I, 1983, reporting the work of Jean Boiron, J Abecassis and P Belon. Sainte-Foy-Les-Lyon: Editions Boiron, 1984, section III, pp 39-50.

'in vivo' phenomena: when nerve cells are crushed, the nerve ends form vesicles called 'synaptosomes' which have the same properties as those of an intact neuron. Cerebral localization of the noradrenergic, serotoninergic and dopaminergic routes are well known. Furthermore, it is well established that signals are transmitted at the synapse, from one neuron to another, by means of neurotransmitters. These are neurochemicals which are liberated and then proceed to act upon specific receptors in the second neuron before being partially re-collected and metabolized. When a nerve impulse reaches the first neuron there is a synthesis of neurotransmitter from a precursor amino-acid (such as, for instance, tryptophan to serotonin – under the effect of an enzyme [tryptophan-hydroxylase], tryptophan is transformed into 5-hydroxy-tryptophan, which under the influence of a second enzyme [tryptophan-decarboxcylase] becomes serotonin). The neurotransmitter is then stored inside the neuron in vesicles (synaptosomes, or neurosomes). When the nerve influx reaches the termination of the neuron the vesicle bursts, releasing the neurotransmitter, thereby raising its concentration level in the synaptic space. In this manner the neurotransmitter comes into contact with a receptor whose specific active sites (proteins) undergo a temporary deformation creating a new electrical potential that again sets off the nervous impulse, now flowing through the second neuron. If a 'blocking' product is introduced, this attaches itself to the receptor blocking the active sites. Thus the nerve influx cannot reach the second neuron (such as, for instance, at peripheral neuroeffector junctions [motor end-plates, or autonomic ganglia] where the receptors of acetylcholine may be blocked by bungarotoxin, a substance that has been isolated).

Most orthodox psychopharmacological interference with a neuro-transmitter's metabolism acts in one of three ways:

a) upon the amino acid precursor (tryptophan for serotonin, or tyrosin for dopamine and for norepinephrine);
b) upon the enzyme reactions governing the neurotransmitter's precursor;
c) upon the release mechanism of the neurotransmitter.

The action of a certain neuroleptic (imipramine hydrochloride) and a central nervous system stimulant (amphetamine) of orthodox pharmacology are, however, thought also to have an effect on the neurotransmitter capturing level, besides other interference, of the sort given above.

It should now be restated that when a nerve impulse passes, it liberates a neurotransmitter (a chemical mediator) whose action on fixing itself onto a post-synaptic receptor brings about a new electrical potential, allowing the nerve impulse to carry on into the second neuron. Not all of the neurotransmitter will be spent in this way, however. Because nature is thrifty it will retrieve a part of the quantity of that released neurotransmitter, while the balance will be metabolized. This salvaging of the neurotransmitter is called 're-uptake' or simply 'capture'. It is the amount of neurotransmitter thus re-captured that by way of feed-back retroactively regulates the finely tuned pre-synaptic receptors to determine the quantity of neurotransmitter to be available immediately subsequently. It is precisely here that the Gelsemium sempervirens has been shown to have its effect.

In a 10^{-2} deconcentration this homoeopathic agent causes a very strong inhibition of norepinephrine, dopamine and serotonin re-uptake in all fractions of rats' brains, localized in the cortex, the hypothalamus, the brain stem and the mesencephalon (midbrain), thereby correspondingly affecting the pre-synaptic receptors. With potencies ranging up to 10^{-5} the capturing of the three neurotransmitters in the various cerebral fractions remains somewhat inhibited. Yet as the potencies move higher, on the level from 10^{-7} to 10^{-11} the inhibiting effect has ceased, and in its stead a slight but significant activation of this capturing is evident, particularly of dopamine in the cortex, and of norepinephrine and serotonin in the mesencephalon. This is a clear 'reversal of the usual direction of response' with the increased potency level. Injections of Gelsemium sempervirens tincture 'in vivo' have likewise had an altering effect on the capture of neurotransmitters, proving that it was neither quickly catabolized in the peripheral area, nor unable to pass the haematomeningeal barriers.

The results confirm that the tincture of Gelsemium sempervirens and certain of its potencies have a demonstrable reactive effect, evincing hormesis, i.e. a pattern that conforms to the biphasal action of drugs first described by Hahnemann in 1796[1] and later formalized as the Arndt-Schulz law. The physiological mechanism of this is clearly identifiable, as it measurably alters the re-uptake of neurotransmitters in a predictable manner, namely by the inhibition hereof in the very low potency range, and by its activation in the more elevated potencies. Plainly the results also mean that this particular homoeopathic drug has an effect on nerve impulses. Finally, there is nothing to prevent the conclusion being drawn that the physiological mechanism observed in these phenomena is linked to the known therapeutic effect of homoeopathic Gelsemium sempervirens, or its effect on provers as recorded in the materia medica.

A mature theoretical framework within which experimental investigations in this area might be undertaken was recently proposed by Fritz-Albert Popp, a distinguished biophysicist, with an abiding interest in homoeopathy and its relationship to physics and other natural sciences has, *inter alia,* been consistently involved, both theoretically and experimentally, since the 1970s in investigations into high homoeopathic potencies. He published some half dozen papers on the subject during the course of about fifteen years up to 1990. The Government of the FRG showed its profound respect for him by appointing him as supervisor of some of its research on that topic.

In a paper[2] he presented a unifying scientific hypothesis that might serve as a framework for a great deal of homoeopathic experimentation. He first

[1] Hahnemann, Christian Friedrich Samuel. 'Essay on a New Principle for Ascertaining the Curative Power of Drugs, and Some Examinations of the Previous Principles', *Hufeland's Journal,* 1796, vol II, parts 3 & 4, pp 391-439 and 465-561.
[2] Popp, Fritz-Albert. *British Homoeopathic Journal,* 1990, vol LXXIX, pp 161-166.

examined several existing theories critically, then extracted from these what little to him seemed tenable and colligated with this three phenomena that are frequently linked with (the interpretation of) a homoeopathic medicinal response, viz:

i)   the placebo effect ('non-substantial' interactions induced in some way 'informationally';

ii) hormesis (biphasic medicinal dose/response action);

iii) the exquisitely receptive sensitivity of living systems.

He then scrutinized the resultant concepts.

He began by challenging the currently prevailing orthodox view of the placebo effect as exclusively targeting the belief-system in a non-substantial interaction, and of drug action as only targeting the biochemical system in a substantial interaction. He rebutted this 'either-or' position. Clearly, drugs can affect the psychic response, just as psychological states (e.g. stress, frustration, fear, elation) will distinctly alter the pattern of biochemical products in an organism. He, by contrast, felt logic demanded the construction of a more comprehensive gradation of the effects involved:

Field	Specificity to Substance	Biological Significance	Delocalization/ Interaction distance in cms
Nuclear physics	very high	low	10^{-12} to 10^{-8}
Molecular physics/chemistry	relatively high	moderate	10^{-8} to 10^{-7}
Homoeopathy	moderate	high	10^{-7} to 10
Psychology	low	very high	10 to 100

Here, instead of the conventional 'either-or' position, he offered a model of a continuous transition from substantial interactions to non-substantial ones. With decreasing substance specificity and simultaneously increasing delocalization, the 'informational' aspect of the interaction (i.e. the biological significance) gains importance in contrast with purely chemical (substantial, local) specificity, which decreases.

Moreover, with increasing delocalization the Arndt-Schulz law comes into its own (this refers to the reversed biological effects in various ranges of concentration of the same medicinal agent, in other words, the biphasic dose response described by Hahnemann). Popp's presentation accords well with homoeopathy's simile principle and potency rule, and is, furthermore, supported by recent evidence[1] on changes in water structure (e.g. solvation

[1](a) Resch, Gerhard. 'Solvation Structures', transactions of the XXXII International Homoeopathic Congress held 5th-11th October 1977 by the Liga Medicorum Homoeopathica Internationalis, New Delhi: Vigyan Bhawan, pp 113-116

(b) Hüttenrauch, R and Fricke, S. 'Veränderung der Wasserstruktur durch Gelbildner', *Pharmazie*, 1987, vol XLII, p 635

(c) Berezin, A A. 'Isotopic 'Lattice Ghosts' as a Possible Key to Memory Effects in Water', personal communication from Centre Européen de Recherche Nucléaire (F Caspers) to F A Popp quoted in *British Homoeopathic Journal*, 1990, vol LXXXIX, p 166.

cages, clathrates, 'lattice ghosts') through interaction with solutes when succussed.

Popp pointed out that biochemistry lacked this homoeopathic dimension and it was, on that account, unable to make predictions relative to the simile principle and the mechanism of the Arndt-Schulz law. Instead it usually attributed unexplained mechanisms to complex reactivities of receptors and enzymes. Popp went on to assert that a non-linear allosteric reaction (feedback) at low substance deconcentrations can, evidently, not be explained by biochemistry. He, further, pointed out the highly significant fact that with the deconcentrations normally used in homoeopathy, synergetic biological effects appear. These were, for instance, clearly observed in the FRG Government experiments with formaldehyde up to higher potencies, and in others.[1]

He dismissed a biochemical interpretation of homoeopathy as misdirected, quite like the placebo hypothesis earlier.

Popp also linked the extraordinarily high sensitivity of biological systems to homoeopathic efficacy. In the said paper he confined himself to thermodynamic aspects of 'electroreception' to introduce a model of homoeopathic efficacy. He attempted to show that the sensitivity of biological systems could not be described in terms of biochemistry. It was, instead, based on deviation from thermal equilibrium, with sensitivity and sickness as coupled phenomena. Here, too, his formulae demonstrated that a non-local event is decisive for the description of health: the pattern of the manifold excited states in the biological system (translations, spin states, rotations, vibrations, electron excitations) determined the spectral sensitivity, the transparency and regulatory activity within the system, as well as the 'behaviour' in terms of health and disease.

Popp stipulated that a theory of homoeopathy would need to describe in a consistent manner (i) the simile principle and (ii) the potency rule, including high potencies, so as to present an integral model of homoeopathy on which convenient experimental investigations could (and should) be mounted. He stated that most, if not all, extant hypotheses of homoeopathic efficacy were defective. For example, the mere postulation of the memory function of water failed to address the question of the memory time of water which depends on thermal dissipation. How could thermal dissipation be avoided to such an 'unbelievably' long extent (for weeks, or even years)?

He then went on to posit the assumption that coherent states might account for the efficacy of homoeopathy both in the biological system as well as in the medicinal agent. [Coherence = opposite of randomness in physics, especially with reference to radio, light, acoustic waves, laser beams, or wave interaction.] This assumption accords well with the fact that the simile principle and the potency rule reflect certain physical properties of coherent states. It seemed that even Jahr's symptom concentricity axiom relative to the rule of efficacy of homoeopathic potencies could be reduced to this same assumption. Popp

[1] Popp, Fritz-Albert. *Bericht an Bonn*, Essen: Verlag für Ganzheitsmedizin, 1988.

presented his new model of the mechanism of physiological response in homoeotherapeutics as a platform from which to launch experimental investigations. Popp concluded this significant paper[6] with the following words:

'According to E del Guidice,[1] the Goldstone theorem alone provides a sufficient condition of coherent states, as soon as certain symmetry-breaking takes place by the process of succussion. We showed in 1978 that the introduction of a momentum operator into the Hamiltonian of the dilution describing the succussion procedure favours considerably the creation of coherent states. [Hamiltonian = a post-Newtonian mathematical function concerned with the motion of a system, external forces and kinetic energy.] Their [the coherent states'] lifetimes are in the order of 10^7, or even higher. ... the high number of non-thermal bosons introduced by mechanical shaking [succussion] provides relatively long decay times, when dropping the quasi-thermal occupation probabilities. [Boson = fundamental nuclear particle described by Bose-Einstein statistics, having angular momentum 'nh', where 'n' is an integer and 'h' is Planck's constant.] In addition, with progressive relaxation, the decay will turn (by the change of its exponential decay law into a hyperbolic one) more and more into the stable subradiance regime, which has been postulated by Dicke, and which is now experimentally verified.[2] Consequently, our model does not only describe the simile and the potency rule on the basis of coherent states. It also makes it possible to propose a clear physical mechanism (phonons of the succussion frequency), which provides coherent states of sufficiently long life-times, as soon as Dicke's theory and the high sensitivity of biological systems are taken into account. [Phonon = quantum of thermal energy in acoustic mode for lattice or clathrate vibrations: the interaction of such energy with matter reduces to that between phonons and atoms.] As a result we are able to cite and propose experiments which help to examine the hypothesis.'

Despite Popp's deprecation of a biochemically based approach to homoeopathic experimentation, exactly such an approach was intensively investigated for four years from 1986. The work covered the effects of high and low homoeopathic dynamizations (potencies) of pure, single, chemically well-defined basic substances on systems of cellular function in animals with which an affinity was suspected, i.e. specifically mast cells, lysosomes and zinc-dependent enzymes. The homoeopathic agents and their potencies included orally administered aqueous potencies and/or lactose tablets of: Adrenalinum, Arsenicum album, Calcarea carbonica, Ferrum phosphoricum, Histaminum hydrochloricum, Kali cyanatum, Phosphorus, Silica, Sulphur, Zincum aceticum and Zincum metallicum, in dynamizations of 4DH, 6DH, 8DH, 12DH, 30DH, 60DH, 200DH and 1000DH. In April 1990, the results were published,[3] relative to which the authors chose to refrain from making

[1]del Guidice, E and Preparata, G. 'A Collective Approach to the Dynamics of Water', *MITH* 89/10, Geneva: Library of the Centre Européen de Recherche Nucléaire.
[2]Crubbellier, A and Pavolini, D. 'Superradiance and Subradiance II', *J Phys B At Mol Phys*, 1986, vol XIX, p 2109.
[3]Harisch, Günther, and Michael Kretschmer. *Jenseits vom Milligram: Die Biochemie auf den Spuren der Homöopathie* [Beyond the Milligram: Biochemistry on the Trail of Homoeopathy], Berlin/Heidelberg/New York: Springer-Verlag, 1990, 138 pages.

making any therapeutic extrapolations in print. The reason given by the investigators, Michael Kretschmer and Günther Harisch, for their quest was that all the experimental results in homoeopathy so far, without also having examined the biochemical aspect fully, would never permit of comprehensive conclusions about homoeopathy.

The results as published, amongst many other things, show identical effects whether aqueous potencies or lactose tablets are administered. Here follows a very condensed extract of a few of the statistically significant results:

In mast cells – a consistently increased histamine release: most pronounced with Zincum metallicum in 4DH and 6DH, with Sulphur in 12DH and higher, with Phosphorus in 30DH and higher, with Histaminum hydrochloricum in 4DH and 30DH, Silica in 6DH, and Calcarea carbonica in 6DH.

In lysosomes – a broad increase of glycosidase and protease activity, except with Arsenicum album in 12DH by which alone this was surprisingly impeded; with Ferrum phosphoricum in 8DH there was, in fact, distinct activation of lysosomal proteases and corresponding effects in series of measured glycosidases, whilst there was also an evident reduction in mitochondrial oxygen consumption.

In zinc-dependent enzymes – The cytosolic enzyme alcohol-dehydrogenase showed some differences in circadian activity in addition to a measurably pronounced susceptibility to Zincum aceticum; the mitochondrial zinc enzymes showed pronounced differences in circadian activity in response to Zincum aceticum; the microsomal NADPH-cytochrome-P450-reductase (without direct zinc-dependence) showed a clear circadian variation in susceptibility in response to Zincum aceticum.

A few other highlights from this series of important experiments that can not be conveniently compartmentalized into subcellular systems:

Kali cyanatum Kali cyanatum 4DH and 30DH caused intensification of both mitochondrial respiration and succinic dehydrogenase; these same dynamizations also led to the activation of xanthine oxidase and of the microsomal NADPH-cytochrome-P450-reductase (do such effects indicate that Kali cyanatum 4DH and 30DH would increase the oxygen consumption of liver cells, thereby activating certain oxygen-dependent functions?).

Ferrum phosphoricum Polarographic chemical analyses demonstrated a significant reduction of mitochondrial oxygen consumption with Ferrum phosphoricum 8DH, 12DH and 30DH, while correspondingly impeding activity of the mitochondrial enzymes super-oxide dismutase and succinic dehydrogenase; there were measurable changes found in the concentration of the tripeptide GSH in the entire liver homogenate, with that variation pointing to a shift of the cellular thiol-disulfide functions provoked by Ferrum phosphoricum 8DH, 12DH and 30DH inclining toward the disulfide; there were only hints of alterations in the cytosolic glutathione-peroxidase activity, a GSH-dependent function, however; and only with the 8DH potency of Ferrum phosphoricum did the cytosolic part of glutathione-reductase sink significantly.

Adrenalinum Polarographic chemical analyses demonstrated a significant increase in mitochondrial oxygen consumption with Adrenalinum in potencies 4DH, 8DH, 12DH and 30DH, whilst the GSH concentrations fell significantly below those of the placebo-group; on the other hand, the clear increase of microsomal GSH-S-transferases were only produced by potencies 12DH, 30DH and 200DH, whereas the potencies 6DH, 12DH and 30DH provoked an increase of the cytosolic GSH-S-transferases.

This successful pioneering work has shown that biochemical investigation methods are well suited to demonstrating the effects of homoeopathic microdoses (whether ultra-molecular or not) on the level of the cellular metabolism. To Kretschmer and Harisch must go all the credit for methodically doing the primary experimental probing whereby they have opened up an important pathway that will surely be followed in much purposive investigation work to follow theirs.

This type of experimental work has furthered scientific knowledge about the detail of the mechanism of the physiological response induced by homoeopathic medicines. It cannot answer the questions 'Why is . . .?' or 'How is . . .?', but it certainly has answered some 'What happens . . .?' questions in homoeopathy. One might say that such results would be applicable within homoeopathic practice solely to the area of so-called pathological prescribing. It is, nonetheless, evident that the physiological response mechanism to the homoeopathic stimulus is quite as amenable as any other strange phenomenon in biochemistry to the methods of investigation proper to that branch of science. This is also in no way in conflict with the tenets of the Empirical tradition of medicine.

(See 'Altered Receptivity in Disease', 'Animal Experiments', 'Drainage', 'Epistemological Assumptions in Homoeopathy', section 10, 'Experimental Research in Homoeopathy', 'Heterostasis', 'Homoeopathic Laws, Postulates and Precepts', 'Homoeopathy', 'Homoeosis', 'Hormesis', 'Pathology', 'Pathotropism', 'Philosophical Premise of Homoeopathy', 'Potency', 'Potentizing Methods', 'Solvation Structures' and 'Veterinary Homoeopathy'.)

Physiology

Science that studies the manner in which healthy animal or plant organisms maintain their normal vital functions and processes.

Physiomedical Methods

● **Physical medicine: e.g. chiropractic, electro-therapy, hydropathy, physiotherapy, osteopathy, surgery, etc.**

The employment of physical rather than medicinal means of treating disease. In terms of Dake's Exclusion Synopsis, such physiomedical methods can never be related to the homoeopathic law of similars. (See 'Chiropractic', 'Electrotherapy', 'Homoeopathic Laws, Postulates and Precepts', section 16, 'Hydrotherapy', 'Massage Therapy', 'Naturopath', 'Osteopathy' and 'Surgery'.)

Phytopharmacon

A medicine made directly from plant material. See 'Phytotherapy'.

Phytotherapy

● **Medical herbalism.**

This term was coined by Dr Henri Leclerc (1870-1955) for what is also known variously by the older terms of herbalism, botanical medicine, herbal medicine, and (in 19th century USA only) as Eclecticism; this last, because it was a selective blend of Amerind herbal practice and European settler folk medicine. It is an Empirical system of medicine, as old as humanity itself, that employs plant remedies only (derived from trees, ferns, seaweeds, lichens or other vegetation) destined to support the healing life force. It uses only biogenetically produced plant source material, so as to retain the full synergistic potential for health restoration in each of its readily assimilable herbals (also known as phytopharmaca [singular: phytopharmacon] meaning 'phytopharmacological agent'). In phytotherapy remedies are most frequently administered internally, but these may also be employed as poultices, lotions, compresses, embrocations, in herbal baths (phytobalneotherapy) and/or employed in phytodietetic therapy, where plant products, with a recognized direct therapeutic action, may be introduced into the patient's regular diet, for example, infusions drunk either as a preventive measure, or to assist a deficient organic function.

Phytotherapy is to be found in all cultures of the world. For instance, it is a cardinal component of Oriental Medicine (of which some other components are acupuncture, tuina, diet and environmental correction). In Occidental Medicine its written record reaches indirectly from Imhotep (around 2780 BC), the Egyptian scholarly priest-physician, who was also the creator of man's first large stone monument, the Step Pyramid of Sakkara. Many of those who are famous in homoeopathy's proto-history (refer to the pen sketches in 'Philosophical Premise of Homoeopathy') have abundantly added to that record. Probably the most remarkable phytotherapist during the Middle Ages was the Benedictine Abbess St Hildegard of the Rupertsberg Convent (near Bingen, Germany) (1098-1179), who was a medical botanist of some stature, a poet, a mystic, author of religious works, and an incisive social critic. She was gifted with clairvoyance and visions throughout her life and used her gift of prophecy to denounce hidden ecclesiastical abuses and evil deeds. It would appear she used the same gift to guide her, unfailingly, it was said, in the correct use of medicinal plants for those who needed treatment. Curiously, the Catholic Church, many of whose corrupt and dangerously powerful ecclesiastics she had exposed and denounced, reveres her as a Saint – not because the Abbess was ever officially canonized, but on the Church's traditional obligation in canon law to submit to 'vox populi, vox Dei', on the lingering insistence of which the Abbess was allotted a yearly place in the Roman martyrology, on the 17th September, the day of her death.

There is a direct line of uninterrupted succession within Empirical Medicine of those who practised phytotherapy, but the therapy's weakness is precisely that of all of Empirical Medicine prior to Hahnemann, namely the lack of an acceptable, valid theory of drug action (which only Hahnemann provided). It is significant that whereas virtually the entire materia medica of phytotherapy has been homoeopathically proven (pathogenetically experimented upon), conversely by far the majority of medicines of plant origin first employed (and proven) by homoeopathy have, strangely enough, no place at all in phytotherapy.

Occidental phytotherapy experienced, in this century, a resurgence which led to a wide therapeutic dispersal in a rapid superficial spread. This was in response to a relatively uncritical popular acceptance. Yet neither the complex of cellular constituents, interacting with others and producing a synergistic (primary) action on the organism, nor the (secondary) curative-reactive – or what is simply, the homoeopathic – effect were investigated. Phytotherapists quite frequently seem to prescribe herbals, viewed superficially, in a way that could be compared to organotropic prescribing in homoeopathy. For example, Urtica urens (stinging nettle) is prescribed by phytotherapists for allergic eczema and to promote milk production in mothers, whereas the symptom picture in the homoeopathic materia medica shows that, in material doses on healthy persons, amongst other things, it arrests the flow of milk in lactating mothers and brings on itching and stinging patches on the skin of provers, pointing to its homoeopathic effectiveness in application. Another example might be the use by phytotherapists of Cineraria maritima, exactly like that of the homoeopaths, namely the plant's irritant juice as eye drops, which will first induce a low degree of hyperaemia, soon to be followed by the secondary, beneficially reactive effect that helps in many eye conditions such as, for instance, conjunctivitis.

Such resemblances repeat themselves practically with each herbal. These parallels and correspondences in indications are sufficiently numerous and striking that one must conclude that, although the two medical systems make use of plant materials in fundamentally different ways from one another, with the handing down through generations of the lore of the healing properties of herbs, an unconscious concretion of repeated curative phenomena, muted by legend, occurred which is palpably consistent with the law of similars. Phytotherapy has no way to recognize this, nor a formulated principle on which to predict therapeutic effect, because it does not test its plant materials' primary effects on healthy subjects first to record the ensuing guiding symptoms. This epistemological weakness gives phytotherapy, though it may *de facto* appear to be close to homoeopathy, no real reason to be regarded as anything other than a vestigial remnant of medical Empiricism, carried over from the period ante-dating homoeopathy, and has since become a 'vegetarian' form of orthodoxy. The latter, in its turn, derisorily labels phytotherapy as 'folk medicine' on account of precisely this defective *raison d'être*. Homoeopathy, on the other hand, through its experience with organotropic prescribing, believes that the effects achieved by phytotherapy must, of necessity, be more ephemeral than those achieved by homoeopathy with the same plant product, once this is dynamized and only when it has been homoeopathically fully matched to the particular symptom-syndrome of a patient.

Apparently bending to legislative pressures in various countries, phytotherapy is subjecting its plant remedies to the conventional tests of quality, efficacy and safety, as currently conceived within the enantiopathic pharmacological paradigm. It is striving to attain full validation of its claims, and to standardize, along the lines laid down by medical orthodoxy, the means of assessment of its performance. Homoeopathy sees this as partially misdirected for four reasons:

1 The safety tests, apart from possible animal cruelty aspects, are viewed as superfluous, since there is a proven fund of knowledge, in most cases established through use on patients over centuries, about any risk element(s) attaching to remedies. The same, *mutatis mutandis*, can be said of tests for efficacy claims, except that one should add that no phytotherapist worthy of the name would be fooled for long by the odd, rather fanciful claim that has, here and there, been included in the texts of some of the older 'Herbal Manuals'.

2 Historical precedent seems to show that any Empirical medical system approaching too close to the orthodox medical paradigm of the day is first rendered impotent and subsequently smothered. (The experience of homoeopathy in this regard, and the historico-philosophical reason for it, are analysed under 'Hempel, Charles Julius (1811-1879)' and under 'Simmons, George Henry (1852-1937)'.)

3 Since total curative effectiveness is, in reality, guided by a herbal's homoeopathic and not its enantiopathic indications, the results of such tests can only demonstrate the palliative (and not the ultimately curative) effects of the phytopharmaca so tested; moreover, as individual predispositions vary a great deal (see 'Altered Receptivity in Disease'), a possible first step towards monitoring the curative-reactive effect, might be with the aid of some 'single-case research designs', which are more adaptable while still offering experimental rigour in randomization and blind assessment.

4 The framework for current testing procedures has instilled in the minds of phytotherapists the disease classification as used by orthodox medical pharmacology, which, in turn, appears to have led a number of phytotherapists to prescribe on a herb-per-symptom basis, totally outside

the patient's constitutional context and altogether foreign to phytotherapy's original aim of supporting the dynamis.

The last two aspects, in particular, severely limit phytotherapy's value, at present, as a form of treatment complementary to homoeopathy. (See also 'Clinical Trials' and 'Epistemological Assumptions in Homoeopathy', section 7 concerning the spurious concept of the selective action of drugs.)

Pilules

Minute pills; pellets, more or less spherical in shape and made of pure beet sugar and/or cane sugar ($C_{12}H_{22}O_{11}$). They are hard and range in size from approximately the size of a mustard seed to a pepper corn. The sizes commonly employed are nos. 30, 40 or rarely 60, derived from the number of millimetres taken up by ten pillules lined up in a straight row. Homoeopathic use: Vehicle for dispensing the medicines with which they may have been impregnated. (See 'Dose', 'Nomenclature, Discrepancies in', 'Vehicle' and also 'Granules'.)

Placebo

● **Dummy medicine; sometimes also sham surgery.**

In homoeopathic practice, it refers to a non-medicated substance, that is relatively inert pharmacodynamically, sometimes administered to allow a previous remedy a prolonged period of action without undue medicinal interference, or to allow for the observation of a patient for a period without homoeopathic medication in order to arrive at the simillimum, or, perhaps, to contrast the effects of relative non-medication in controlled experiments with those of medication in two comparable groups of patients.

A number of other aspects to the placebo-concept within the homoeopathic paradigm were discussed by the Groupement Hahnemannien du Docteur Pierre Schmidt during a colloquium on that very wide subject ('Colloque sur Placebo') on the 27th and 28th November 1989 at l'Ecole d'Homéopathie Hahnemannienne, Dauphine-Savoie, France. The proceedings were published in the *Cahiers: Gr Hahnem Doct P Schmidt*, XXVII(6), pp 201-239. (See also 'Epistemological Assumptions in Homoeopathy', section 6.)

Plant Juice Therapy

Hybrid between folk medicine, phytotherapy and naturopathic dietary supplementation. Within the limits outlined under 'Foods as Health Problems' it may be compatible with homoeopathy, provided the attending homoeopath is first made aware of what plant juice is to be administered to the patient.

Plaster

Semi-solid waxlike preparation, a.k.a. emplastrum in massa, which, once warmed, can be spread on, and at body-temperature is adhesive to, the skin. Also a fabric or other material made to be adhesive to the skin to keep small dressings in position. Its uses include: protecting excoriated parts; the holding of wound-edges apposite to one another; to apply homoeopathic drugs to the surface to elicit their reactive effects (see 'Externally Applied Homoeopathic Drugs'), or for the support of sprained parts (e.g. a sprained ankle). The term also describes the technique of the application of such material.

Non-homoeopathic (namely allopathic) applications of plasters are medicated with irritants, rubefacients, vesicants, etc. that are designed to 'counter-irritate', redden or blister the skin. Plasters in use in orthodox pharmacy in this last-named category are impregnated with substantive doses of one of the following: Belladonna, Cantharides, Capsicum, Colophony (see 'Resin'), Diachylon (Lead monoxide oleate), Ferric oxide, Lead (Plumbum), Melilotus, Mercury, Mustard (Sinapis), Resin, Salicylic acid or Soap.[1]

Poison

Toxin; substance injurious to health or dangerous to life, whether applied externally, taken internally, or exposed to environmentally. Homoeopathy regards the distinction between 'poisons' and 'non-poisons' as spurious, because it is not a matter of a substance's essence but merely one of its quantity. Hahnemann said that no substance is poisonous if taken in its proper dose.[2]

Politics and Homoeopathy

See 'History of Homoeopathy before 1900', 'Medico-Legal', 'Simmons, George Henry (1852-1937)' and 'Verdi, Tullio Suzzara (1829-1902)'.

Pollution

See 'Drainage', 'Environment' and 'Miasma'.

Pollution-free Starting Material

Utmost care has always to be taken in the preparation of homoeopathic medicines. Original substances must be free of extraneous pollutants, whether

[1]The Council of The Pharmaceutical Society of Great Britain. *The Extra Pharmacopoeia Martindale,* vol I, 24th edition, 1958, London: The Pharmaceutical Press, pp 230, 352, 355, 356, 820, 847, 882 & 1378.

[2]Hahnemann, Christian Friedrich Samuel. 'Was sind Gifte, was sind Arzneien?' [What are Poisons, What are Medicines], 1806, *Journal der praktischen Heilkunde,* vol XXIV, part III, pp 40-57.

chemical, physical or biological, and the plants used must have been grown under pollution-free conditions. To achieve this, large homoeopathic pharmaceutical laboratories that are situated in areas that no longer enjoy a pollution-free atmosphere, install particle counters that monitor the carefully filtered air whilst medicines are prepared under a positive air pressure derived from a sterile compressed air supply. (See 'Mother Tincture', 'Potentizing Methods', 'Succus' and 'Utensils of Homoeopathic Pharmacy'.)

Polyclinic

Also policlinic; a nosocomial homoeopathic establishment, generally with a dispensary, where patients are treated, and may be studied, on an outpatient basis, for conditions of all kinds.

Polychrest

Remedy that is widely applicable because it is capable of producing a wide range of reactive symptoms in provers during pathogenetic experiments. It is often particularly useful in chronic illness because, through its broad spectrum of action, it normally affects all tissues of the patient's body in some degree. All the polychrest remedies have come to be considered as 'constitutional drugs' by the majority of homoeopaths, because the provings of these remedies have shown that certain persons, i.e. those of a particular morphological type, will produce a much fuller picture of the total symptomatology than others.

Sheila and Robin Gibson of the Glasgow Homoeopathic Hospital, whose homoeopathic clinical trials in rheumatology were the first to be published in the *British Journal of Clinical Pharmacology*,[1] have elsewhere made a suggestion as to how polychrests might be used in laboratory (in vitro) studies. They said, a 'potentially useful system for laboratory study could well be the various steps in prostaglandin synthesis. In view of the wide effects that defects in this metabolic system can have on the body, they may well be suited to study of the polychrests – that is, the remedies with a wide sphere of action'.[2] There is consensus among homoeopaths that the following, for instance, are polychrests: Arsenicum album, Baryta carbonica, (Atropa) Belladonna, Bryonia alba, Calcarea carbonica, Calcarea phosphorica, Carbo vegetabilis, Causticum, Cuprum metallicum, Ferrum metallicum, Ignatia amara, (Trigonocephalus) Lachesis, Lycopodium clavatum, Natrum Muriaticum, Nux vomica, Phosphorus, Plumbum metallicum, Pulsatilla nigricans, Sepia officinarum, Silicea and Sulphur. The following are less readily recognized as polychrests, which they undoubtedly are: Acidum nitricum, Aluminium

[1]Gibson R G, Gibson S L M, MacNeill A D, and Watson-Buchanan W. 'Homoeopathic Therapy in Rheumatoid Arthritis: Evaluation by Double-blind Clinical Therapeutic Trial.' *British Journal of Clinical Pharmacology*, 1980, vol IX, pp 453-459.

[2]Gibson, S and R. *Homoeopathy for Everyone*. Harmondsworth, Middlesex: Penguin Books Ltd, 1987, p 153.

metallicum, Calcarea silicica and Graphites. But only a minority of homoeopaths regard the following as polychrests: Aesculus hippocastanum (Edwin M Hale [1829-1899] in his *Specific Therapeutics of the New Remedies* of 1875), Lac caninum (Henry C Allen [1837-1909] in his *Materia Medica of the Nosodes,* republished Calcutta: Sett Dey & Co, 1958, p 46), and Sanicula aqua (John Henry Clarke [1853-1931] in the second part of vol II of his *Dictionary of Practical Materia Medica,* Bradford, Devon: Health Science Press, 1977, p 1091). (See 'Constitutional Type'.)

(See also 'Constitutional Type'.)

Polymer

● Complicated molecule that may be important in homoeopathic pharmacy in that the medicine-message could be shaken into the water-alcohol mixture used in the diluting stages of remedy preparation.

Substance (with an elevated molecular weight) made up of a chain (multiples) of identical, recurrent 'fundamental units' (molecules). They are produced in homoeopathy by successive 'consolidations' and 'adaptations', shaken into drug-specific shapes by the mechanical stimulus in potentization (refer to 'Potency' for experimental evidence). As all biological reactions are shape-specific, it may be of considerable significance that the potentization processes result in solvation structures of a diversity of particular shapes in the diluent of the medicine, as, indeed, they seem to do. (See 'Pharmacological Message', 'Physiological Response in Homoeotherapeutics, Mechanism of', 'Potency' and 'Solvation Structures'.)

Polymeric Structures in Potencies Peculiar to Each Drug

See 'Polymer' and 'Potency'.

Polypharmacy

The mixing of many drugs in a single prescription. (See 'Combinations of Homoeopathic Drugs' and 'Hahnemann, Christian Friedrich Samuel (1755-1843)'.)

Posology

Science of dosage; the branch of both therapeutics and materia medica that relates to the determination of the quantities and/or doses in which homoeopathic drugs are to be administered. It is not, strictly speaking, concerned with the choice of, or variations in, potencies (dynamizations) to be employed in any particular case. (See also 'Dosage', 'Dose', 'Dose Repetition' and 'Homoeopathic Laws, Postulates and Precepts', particularly sections 6, 7, 8 and 11.)

Post Hoc, Ergo Propter Hoc

Logical proposition setting out a type of fallacy, or paralogism, of which homoeopathy has been accused, specifically an error in reasoning that has the appearance of being sound. The proposition is always captured in this Latin phrase meaning 'subsequent to this, therefore, because of it'. Some superstitions are rationalized by precisely this fallacy: e.g. when being the thirteenth in a group, or the act of accidentally breaking a mirror are followed by misfortune, and it is taken that the misfortune is the inevitable result.

During the 1870s homoeopathy was confronted by its antagonists with the accusation that it was guilty of this paralogism by linking what might be no more than accidental similarity in symptoms produced in medicinal provings to those cured in sick patients by the same medicine.[1] It was, in large measure, this accusation which motivated Constantin Hering to compile the ten volumes of his *Guiding Symptoms* which became his successful rebuttal of this casuistry (he called it 'slander which was . . . flung at our School'). His monumental work comprises the symptoms of provings that had also been confirmed through cures from fifty years of homoeopathic records.

Harris Livermore Coulter, Ph.D., has written in some depth about this issue in *Divided Legacy: A History of the Schism in Medical Thought*, vol III *Science and Ethics in American Medicine*, Washington, DC: Wehawken Book Company, 1973, pp 171-172, 225, and 385.

(See 'Guiding Symptoms of the Materia Medica'.)

Postage Stamps and Homoeopathy

Three countries have issued postage stamps depicting either Hahnemann's bust or his profile:

1954 Brazil to commemorate the World Homoeopathic Medical Congress during October, held for the first time in that country; his bust is printed in a deep turquoise with a face value of 2.70 Cruzeiros.

1955 FRG to commemorate the Bicentenary of Hahnemann's birth at Meissen in the Electorate of Saxony on 10th April 1755; his bust is printed in a strong orange with a face value of 20 Pfennige and a surcharge of 10 Pfennige levied for a humanitarian charity, in harmony with the stamp's inscription 'Helfer der Menschheit' (Helper of mankind).

1977 India to commemorate the International Congress held for the second time in that country from 5th to 11th October by the Liga Medicorum Homoeopathica Internationalis at New Delhi; his profile is printed in black with a scroll below it containing the words: 'Cinchona bark was to Hahnemann what the falling apple was to Newton and the swinging lamp to Galileo', and alongside, with Hahnemann facing it, the Cinchona plant is shown in olive green; the stamp's face value is 2.00 Rupees.

[1] Hering, Constantin. *The Guiding Symptoms of Our Materia Medica* (10 vols), reprint New Delhi: B Jain Publishers, 1974, vol I (originally published 1879), Preface p 6.

The first homoeopath to be honoured by his country for outstanding contribution to science was Prof Licinio Athanasio Cardoso (1852-1926):

1952 Brazil to commemorate the centenary of his birth; his bust is printed in a deep blue-grey, with a face value of 60 Centavos.

The next philosopher-scientist to be so honoured was Sir J C Bose FRS. In his illustrated lecture on 'Drug Action and Response' to the British Homoeopathic Society on 23rd June 1926, he highlighted:

a) the varying reaction to the same drug in different individuals;
b) how certain chemical substances had a great effect in extremely minute doses;
c) that the crucial thing for the homoeopathic practitioner was to find the critical dose, while remembering that the critical dose for different persons is a great variable.

He showed how the Arndt-Schulz law operates in practice by demonstrating the lethal effect of Cobra venom in a dilution of one part in a thousand, by contrast with its extraordinary stimulant effect in a very high dilution.

On the role of the dynamis in effecting cure he said: 'There is the question of the power of resistance, the inner power that is what you are after. Drugs do not help you, except in helping you to get the inner power of resistance increased.'

Charles Edwin Wheeler (1868-1946) in the vote of thanks expressed his delight that such an eminent scientist should be giving such very conspicuous support to homoeopathy. Dr M Burford on that occasion asked whether it was not high time for homoeopathy to conduct systematic phytopathogenetic experiments (meaning provings on plants, as are done on humans) to enable scientific cures now also to be undertaken for all manner of plant maladies.

1958 India to commemorate the centenary of his (Boses's) birth; his bust is printed in a dark bronze-like shade with a face value of 15 naya Paisa.

Over the years many other prominent individuals associated with homoeopathy have been commemorated on postage stamps and homoeopathic events and anniversaries have often been announced by special postal cancellations (franking marks). These were collected and published in a 24-page illustrated booklet by Dr Diwan Harish Chand under the title *Stamped on My Memory, but Not Cancelled: Philately and Homoeopathy* (New Delhi: Universal Offset Printers, 1978).

Post-Infective Dyscrasia

See 'Miasma'.

Postulate on Biological Evolutionary Development

See 'Homoeopathic Laws, Postulates and Precepts', section 12.

Postulate on Disease Development, Dual

See 'Homoeopathic Laws, Postulates and Precepts', section 13.

Postulate on Posological Appropriateness

See 'Homoeopathic Laws, Postulates and Precepts', section 11.

Potency

● **The especially produced capability in a medicine to effect a dynamic stimulus in the appropriate patient.**

The stage of altered remedial activity to which a drug has been taken by means of a measured process of deconcentration, with succussion, or by trituration, of the medicinal substance, which is thus brought to a state of diminutive or infinitesimal subdivision. This process, if performed according to the prescribed mathematico-mechanical attenuation procedures for potentization (dynamization), increases both the physical solubility and the physiological assimilability of the drug, while also changing its therapeutic activity in its use as a homoeopathic remedy. In a broad sense the altered therapeutic activity of a homoeopathic medicine brought about by dynamization (the process of potentization) follows a constant rule, known as the 'Arndt-Schulz law'. The simple summary of this is that minute stimuli encourage life activity, medium to strong stimuli tend to impede it, and very strong stimuli to stop or destroy it. (See 'Homoeopathic Laws, Postulates and Precepts' section 5.)

Conventions differ slightly concerning the symbols used to signify potencies, for instance:

Where each stage of deconcentration is on the scale of 1:100 –

the 30th centesimal may be shown as either 30c or 30 or 30CH or C30; or

the 9th centesimal may be shown as either 9CH or C9 or 9c or 9; or

the 12th centesimal may be shown as either 12 or C12 or 12CH or 12c.

The symbol K sometimes features in this scale, denoting the Korsakovian method of potentization (see 'Potentizing Methods').

Where each stage of deconcentration is on the scale of 1:10 –

the 3rd decimal may be shown as either 3x or D3 or 3D or 3DH; similarly the 6th decimal may be shown as either D6 or 6DH or 6x or 6D.

Although the Korsakovian method of potentization is also used in this scale, particularly by self-dispensing homoeopaths when making up their own potencies, the symbol K seems to feature only very occasionally in this scale.

Where each stage of deconcentration is on the scale of 1:50000 –

the 1st LM potency is shown as 0/1;

the 2nd LM potency is shown as 0/2;

the 10th LM potency is shown as 0/10.

The very high deconcentrations, made in the USA by Boericke and Tafel, Philadelphia, and by Ehrhart and Karl, Chicago –

where the deconcentration is 10^{-2000} 1M;
where the deconcentration is 10^{-20000} 10M;
where the deconcentration is $10^{-200000}$ CM;
where the deconcentration is $10^{-2000000}$ MM.

The dynamizations that are usually readily available through laboratories and from pharmacies are:

In the francophone area: Θ, 3DH, 6DH, 4CH, 6CH, 9CH, 12CH, 15CH and 30CH.

In the teutonic area: Θ, 3DH, 4DH, 5DH, 6DH, 8DH, 10DH, 12DH, 15DH, 30DH, 60DH, 100DH, 200DH, 400DH, 1000DH and 2000DH.

In the English-speaking area: Θ, 1DH (1x), 1CH (1c), 3DH (3x), 6DH (6x), 12DH (12x), 6CH (6c), 30CH (30c or 30), 200CH (200), 1M, 10M and CM [in parentheses are the older Roman numerals used as written potency designations, which are still fully current in the English-speaking areas].

The infrequently used LM potencies are, theoretically at least, available everywhere.

Potencies other than those given above would normally have to be made up by pharmacists against prescription.

The altered state of remedial activity of a homoeopathic drug, as represented by its potency, may refer to any one of a variety of its pharmacodynamic aspects. For instance, many important properties which are not evident in a drug's crude state are only manifested in it in potency. Some exceptionally effective remedies in potency are inert in their crude state, some others are basically toxic substances that may become household remedies once homoeopathically processed into a potency. It is said that for every case there is an optimal potency just as there is a most similar remedy. As an approximate rule, diminished vital action in disease calls for low dynamizations, while increased vital action responds better to high potencies.

Henri Voisin undertook an extensive investigative study of the records of pathogenetic experiments[1] to assess, firstly, the elapsed time before particular reactions occur in provers, and, secondly, to ascertain what had already been established by clinical usage, namely that

low potencies are best suited to organic disease;
medium potencies are most effective for influencing function;
high potencies produce the best response with 'mentals'.

According to Dame Margery Blackie[2] factors that help the homoeopath to decide on his choice of potency are

a) the constitution of the patient, since some are so much more sensitive than others;
b) the nature of the homoeopathic drug, specifically whether it produces a sensitive proving or not;

[1]Voisin, Henri. *Die vernünftige kritische Anwendung der Homöopathie,* translated from French to German and published by Fritz Stockenbrand, Ulm an der Donau, 1960.
[2]Blackie, Dame Margery G. *The Patient, Not the Cure.* London: Macdonald and Jane's, 1976, p 96.

c) the nature of the illness, e.g. a gross tissue affection (like a peptic ulcer) calls for a very different potency to an interference with the metabolic processes of the body.

Gerhard Köhler[1] states that the lowest useful homoeopathic potency for drugs that are practically inert in the crude state usually corresponds to the 8DH, as it does for colloids and lithotherapeutic agents (see 'Colloid' and 'Lithotherapy'). He also maintains that highly toxic drugs only show alterative properties above their 'aggressive range', which is upward from about the 10DH.

Charles Edwin Wheeler[2] probably voices the experience of the majority of homoeopaths when he says that it is incorrect to state that high potencies are invariably more effective than low ones. It happens quite frequently that the high will relieve more effectively (would they have come into use otherwise?), but equally it happens that low potencies succeed after high ones have failed. It should always be remembered that a remedy, if well indicated in terms of the law of similars, would be homoeopathic even without recourse to a potency thereof, as exemplified by the occasional use of mother tinctures, whenever one of these happens to be the most appropriate form of the remedy for the particular case.

Wheeler[3] explains that Hahnemannian potencies from tincture or base drug to 3CH or 6DH are classified as 'low'; above that up to 12CH or 24DH as 'medium'; then above that up to 30CH or 60DH as 'high'; and beyond that as 'very high'. It is important to remember that the corresponding classification of Korsakovian potencies is totally different (as set out under 'Equivalents Established between 'K' and 'H' Potencies' and 'Potentizing Methods').

It has become accepted practice that lower potencies given in repeated doses are used as tissue remedies (in the sense of Wilhelm Heinrich Schüssler), as organ remedies (as held by J Compton Burnett), when prescribing on the basis of morbid anatomy (as recommended by Richard Hughes), in some acute diseases provided there is no irreversible tissue destruction, or for some intercurrent symptom which is not responding to the main remedy in a high potency, well indicated though it be. For chronic illnesses a cure can only be found in some remedy that will enhance the afflicted organism's central mechanism of defence and then usually in the higher potencies and in infrequently repeated doses.

In incurable and terminal illness the potency problem does not arise, for then the exact simillimum is contra-indicated and the homoeopath normally selects some palliative or 'Biochemic' remedy in a low potency to safeguard against severe aggravation and consequent death.

[1]Köhler, Gerhard. *The Handbook of Homoeopathy: Its Principles and Practice,* translated from the German by A R Meuss, Wellingborough: Thorsons Publishing Group, 1987, pp 145-146.
[2]Wheeler, Charles Edwin. *An Introduction to the Principles and Practice of Homoeopathy.* Rustington: Health Science Press, 1948, p 22.
[3]ibid., p 15.

Homoeopathy distinguishes between two kinds of effect produced by drugs. All doses yield secondary symptoms (the organism's reaction), whereas perceptible primary symptoms (the drug's coercive action) are produced only by relatively large doses. Smaller doses and infinitesimal potencies of well-indicated remedies yield no undesirable primary symptoms but only the gradual restoration of health through the stimulation of the patient's own reserves of vital energy (dynamis). In his 1796 *Essay* Hahnemann mentions 'moderate' doses, and three years later he first announced the principle of the infinitesimal dose, the continued use of which was justified ultimately by experience.[1] Many enthusiastic homoeopaths in Hahnemann's day were taking the potencies ever higher. In 1829 Hahnemann laid down a rule that all homoeopathic medicines were to be diluted and potentized up to the thirtieth centesimal (30CH), and not beyond it, in order to have 'a uniform mode of procedure in the treatment of all homoeopathists' so that 'when they describe a cure' anyone 'can repeat it as they do, and' all homoeopaths effectively 'operate with the same tools'.[2,3] He certainly did not always follow this rule himself; his introduction, late in life, of the 'LM potencies' *de facto* legitimizes that particular form of high potencies.

This rule was, and has remained, in conflict with homoeopathy's principle of professional individualism, previously greatly emphasized. Although some homoeopaths strictly adhered to this instruction from 1829 onward, others reserved their right to determine the medicinal potencies of daily use as seemed best to them. This split in attitude has remained to the present day. For example, in France where homoeopathic medicines are officially recognized and included in the French Pharmacopoeia it is illegal (except in some pre-existing proprietary formulae, like 'Oscillococcinum 200') to potentize beyond the 30CH in deference to this rule. The German-language area is beginning to show signs of tending in the same direction, although no fixed limit has been set there. By contrast, in the English-speaking part of the world there is a strong inclination to favour potencies from the 30CH upward.

Since Avogadro's number (a.k.a. the Loschmidt limit) has been passed at 12CH, or more accurately at 23DH, at which stage no molecule of the original medicinal substance can statistically be expected to remain in the dynamization, though two centuries of clinical experience has solidly established the curative efficacy of the potencies higher than that, the following question arises.

How Do Homoeopathic Potencies Accomplish This?
In an effort to arrive at an answer a long series of chemical, physical and biological experiments have been undertaken that have yielded repeatable,

[1] Haehl, Richard. *Samuel Hahnemann, His Life and Work.* 2 volumes. London: Homoeopathic Publishing Company, 1922, vol I, pp 311-312.
[2] ibid., p 322.
[3] Bradford, Thomas Lindsley. *The Life and Letters of Dr Samuel Hahnemann.* Philadelphia: Boericke and Tafel, 1895, pp 191-192.

statistically significant, objective evidence, pointing to the existence of a physico-chemical force-field in the potencies which is certainly carried forward into the ultramolecular dynamization stages. In default of any other explanation it has to be assumed that the prescribed methods of potentization consistently bring this about. It is astonishing with what astute perception Hahnemann answered this, because he had posed the same question to himself too. He said that if homoeopathic potencies remain active it was not merely because the procedure for dynamization must produce the most intimate mixture, but it was because the very manner of preparing homoeopathic medicines brings about a surprising physical change and an exchange in the medicinal material due to the trituration and succussion in the potentizing process.

Experimental Evidence

(Note: The mathematical equivalents for potency deconcentrations are $- 10^{-2}$ = 1CH; 10^{-3} = 3DH; 10^{-4} = 2CH; 10^{-5} = 5DH; 10^{-6} = 3CH; etc.)

1880	G Jaeger	Found that in human test subjects their reaction time was affected by potencies up to 10^{-400} of Aurum metallicum, Aconitum napellus, Natrum muriaticum and Thuja occidentalis;[1]
1923	L Kolisko	Showed that the growth of wheat is affected by soaking the seed in potencies from 10^{-15} to 10^{-30} of Copper salt, Antimony trioxide and Iron sulphate.
1928	H Junker	Conducted a well-controlled test of the effect of potencies of Orange juice 10^{-25}, Octyl alcohol 10^{-24}, Potassium oleate 10^{-26}, Atropine sulphate 10^{-26} and nonylic acid 10^{-24} and 10^{-27} on the daily changes in the growth of paramecia cultures. Significant changes were obtained.
1931	W E Boyd & J Paterson	Demonstrated that the Schick test for diphtheria could be changed from positive to negative through the oral administration of either Diphtherinum 10^{-402} or Alum precipitated toxoid 10^{-60}. This trial was not controlled, but the data are significant since the results of

[1] Stephenson, James H. 'A Review of Investigations into the Action of Substances in Dilutions Greater than 1×10^{-24} (Microdilutions)'. *Journal of the American Institute of Homoeopathy*, 1955, vol XLVIII, pp 327-335 (Quoted both by Jean Boiron, then Secretary-General to the Research Committee of the Liga Medicorum Homoeopathica Internationalis in *Aspects of Research in Homoeopathy* vol I, 1983, p 76, and by Harris L Coulter in *Divided Legacy: a History of the Schism in Medical Thought* in 3 vols; vol III, Washington: Wehawken Book Company, 1973, p 493.) These, and other experiments, are described there with full bibliographical references.

		change from Schick positive to Schick negative were more than twelve times the accepted rate of spontaneous change.
1932 to 1936	W Persson	Tested the effect of various potencies of Mercuric chloride on the rate of fermentation of starch by ptyalin (salivary amylase) and of the effect of a number of other potentized substances on the lysis of fibrin by pepsin and trypsin. In the starch experiment, which was well controlled, he obtained a sinusoidal curve showing reactions to all potencies up to 10^{-120}, whereas none of the controls were affected abnormally. The results in the fibrin series of experiments were comparable.
1943	J Paterson	Demonstrated the effects of a potency of Mustard gas given prophylactically, as well as after application of the liquid gas in a double blind controlled trial.[1]
1948	L Wurmser & P Loch	Found that the wave-length of light was affected by potencies from 10^{-24} to 10^{-30} of Quinine sulphate, Aeschulus hippocastanum and Taraxacum dens leonis.
1951	M Gay	Showed variations in the dielectric constant (relative permittivity, or specific inductive capacity) of different series of dynamizations.[2]
1954	W E Boyd	At the end of a 15 year retest of Persson's starch experiments, overwhelming statistical evidence at the 10^{-60} potency level of the effects of Mercuric chloride on a starch-distase preparation could be published, completely confirming Persson's results.[3]
1958 1964	E Heintz	Studied certain physical constants of successive potencies for more than twenty years: he

[1] Paterson, J. 'Report on Mustard Gas Experiments (Glasgow and London)'. *British Homoeopathic Journal*, 24th January 1943.

[2] von Hippel, Arthur R. *Dielectrics and Waves*. Wiley, 1954. Comprehensive treatise from macroscopic and molecular approaches. Also Jean Boiron in public lecture 'Research in Homoeopathy', Johannesburg, RSA on 1981/02/19, and Philippe Belon in direct reference in his introduction to: *Aspects of Research in Homoeopathy, Volume I*. Published under the auspices of the Secretary-General to the Research Committee of the Liga Medicorum Homoeopathica Internationalis. Sainte-Foy-Les-Lyon: Editions Boiron, (English translation) 1984, p 10.

[3] Boyd, W E. 'Biochemical and Biological Evidence of the Activity of High Potencies'. *British Homoeopathic Journal*, 1954, vol XLIV, no 1, pp 6-44.

1970		could demonstrate the effects of potencies up
1973		to 10^{-18} on the behaviour of fish under controlled conditions.[1]
1963	J Boiron & Mlle Zervudachi	Showed the effects of potencies of Sodium hydrogen arsenate from 10^{-3} to 10^{-19} on the respiration of wheat coleoptiles.[2]
1966	Prof G Netien, J Boiron & A Marin	Showed the effect of potencies of Copper sulphate 10^{-30} on plants poisoned by copper sulphate.[3]
1965	Prof A Cier,	Demonstrated the influence of prior treatment
1967	J Boiron, J Braise & Mlle C Vingert	with Alloxan 10^{-18} on the subsequent diabetogenic action of crude Alloxan on mice, and also its use after injections of Alloxan.[4]
1975	M Aubin & J Bildet	Published the results of their studies of the effect of intraperitoneal injections of Phosphorus 10^{-14} and 10^{-30} on the liver enzymes of rats poisoned by carbon tetrachloride.[5]
1976	M Aubin, S Baronnet, P Bastide, G Burantin, J Chezaud & F Villie	Demonstrated the action of Arnica potencies on the dehydrogenase levels in the muscles of experimental rats undergoing exercise.[6]

[1] Heintz, E. 'Nouvelles expériences sur la mode d'action de dilutions successives: Vérification expérimentale de la loi d'Arndt-Schulz'. *IXe Assises Scientifiques Homéopathiques*, Vichy, 1970/05/29, pp 3-17. Also 'Measurement of the Movement of Fish and Other Animals in Response to Chemical Stimuli'. *Experientia*, 1958, vol XIV, p 155; *Comptes Rend. Acad. Sci.*, 1958, vol CCXLVI, p 1309; 1962, vol CCLV, p 2283; 1964, vol CCLVIII, p 3572; *Proceedings 28th Congress for Homoeopathic Medicine*, Vienna, 1973, p 191.

[2] Boiron, J, and Mlle Zervudachi. 'Action de dilutions infinitésimales d'arseniate de sodium sur la respiration de coleoptiles de blé'. *Annales Homéopathiques Francaises*, 1963, p 738.

[3] Netien, G, J Boiron and A Marin. 'Action de dilutions infinitésimales de sulfate de cuivre sur des plantes préalablement intoxiquées par cette substance'. *Annales Homéopathiques Francaises*, 1966, p 130.

[4] Cier, A, J Boiron, J Braise and C Vingert. 'Sur le traitement du diabète expérimental par des dilutions infinitésimales d'Alloxane'. *Annales Homéopathiques Francaises*, 1966. Also in English: 'Experimental Diabetes Treated with Infinitesimal Doses of Alloxan'. *British Homoeopathic Journal*, 1967, vol LVI, p 51.

[5] Aubin, M, and J Bildet. 'Etude de l'action de différentes dilutions homéopathiques de phosphore blanc (Phosphorus) sur l'hepatite toxic du rat'. *La Documentation Homéopathique, les Laboratoires Homéopathiques de France*, 1975, p 56.

[6] Aubin, M, S Baronnet, P Bastide, G Burantin, J Chazaud and F Villie. 'Action de diverses dilutions d'Arnica sur les taux de lactate deshydrogenase et de malate deshydrogenase du muscle de rats soumis a une épreuve d'effort'. *Proceedings at the XVth Assises Scientifiques Homéopathiques*, Dijon, 1976/04/30.

This and much other published experimental evidence[1] of potency action established that homoeopathic medicines in potency elicit a reactive response other than the placebo effect. Yet what needed to be investigated beyond that was the question: What really happens when solutions are serially potentized and what is it that gets carried forward into the ultramolecular stages? What is that 'surprising physical change and exchange in the medicinal material' that Hahnemann said dynamization brought about?

Was it electrolytic dissociation (see 'Ionization') as Nobel prize winner Svante Arrhenius had suggested at the beginning of the twentieth century? Or could it be that a specific inter- or intramolecular arrangement takes place in the solvent, whose molecules might surround those of the solute forming macromolecules, perhaps in the water component of the dilute alcohol used in potentization? It was E Heintz in 1941 whose pioneering work produced the first evidence for macromolecules by studying infra-red absorption patterns of homoeopathic potencies (succussed solutions) which indicated that polymers were produced in this way in the solvent.[2] There seemed to be a kind of clustering effect differing from drug to drug that gets carried over into the ultramolecular stages of potentization as a distinctive and stable impress. A large amount of work has been carried out to verify this hypothesis, the more so since such a phenomenon – as homoeopathy well knows – would have both theoretical and practical repercussions in physiology, physics and other branches of science. In 1965 G P Barnard, senior physicist at the National Physics Laboratory, Teddington, Middlesex, UK, and from 1967 to 1969 he and Dr James H Stephenson of New York, USA, investigated this aspect of homoeopathic potencies in their viscosity studies. Their findings suggested that the process of dynamization, of succussing and triturating the medicinal substance with the dilute alcohol, causes the solvent (there is also a great deal of water in the lactose of triturations) to become arranged into giant polymers (molecular aggregates), specific to its penetrative stimulant, the basic drug. Each polymer maintains a constant three-dimensional spatial pattern, the so-called solvation structures, from one potency into the next higher, and beyond the Avogadro limit.

The projected physics of this process can briefly be summarized thus: it is known that a diversity of patterns of crystallization appear in water (ice) under different barometric pressures; hence it suggests itself that at non-freezing temperatures (at which potentization is usually undertaken, of around 25 degrees Celsius) a variety of patterns of polymerization may be ready to be formed, given the requisite preconditions. Such preconditions include the splitting of a few water molecules, making the resulting parts available as potential constituents of replicating polymers. They also include sudden, very

---

[1]Gibson, Sheila and Robin. *Homoeopathy for Everyone.* Chapter Nine: 'Does Homoeopathy Work? The Results of Research.' Harmondsworth, Middlesex: Penguin Books, 1987, pp 141-158.

[2]Heintz, E. 'The Physical Effect of Highly Diluted, Potentized Substances' [title translated]. *Die Naturwissenschaften,* 1941, vol IXXX, pp 713-725.

great temperature increases near those water molecules that would then result in the proximate molecules' break-up. The dissolved air and other gases always found in the solvent are known to be compressed suddenly in the abrupt succussion stroke which raises their temperature instantly to several thousand degrees Celsius. The succussion would not only knock the minority of free molecular particles (produced through heat-induced sporadic molecular disintegration) into their constituent place in the nascent polymeric aggregates, but would also knock these newly formed polymers themselves into solute-specific shapes, and then, when they grow to a certain size, these same succussion strokes would also fracture them, all of which processes ensure continued polymer replication. This macromolecular pattern, peculiar (i.e. unavoidably shape-specific) to each homoeopathic drug, is later even capable of replication in the absence of the original solute. It maintains a stable and specific order for the constituent molecules in the total molecular aggregate, but is capable of being destroyed by heat.[1]

In 1974 Mrs Cl. Luu D Vinh presented her doctoral thesis in the Pharmacy Faculty at Montpellier University. It was a study of the physical structure of homoeopathic potencies using a Raman laser, following naturally both the infra-red absorption studies of Heintz and the viscosity studies of Barnard. She demonstrated that any substance introduced by a process of Hahnemannian dynamization into a hydro-alcoholic solvent brings about a new molecular cluster arrangement in that solvent, in fact polymerization. She was also able to show certain stereotypical deformations in the alcohol itself. In her conclusion she stated:

> 'The intensity of Raman spectres of homoeopathic potencies of the same Hahnemannian deconcentration is specific to the basic substance's material. The spectral study concerned potencies of the same kind but of different "heights" [meaning deconcentrations] ranging from 1CH to 30CH and beyond'.

It has been shown that this clustering, this physico-chemical force field, is destroyed by heating it, by passing ultrasound through it, and by certain other types of irradiation.[2] Subsequently this study was continued by Mrs Luu D Vinh and others under the aegis of Mlle Bardet, Professor of Industrial Physics at the Faculty of Pharmacy in Montpellier. In fact it was all undertaken in Prof Bardet's laboratory. The results of a selection of more recent research in this area of homoeopathy is given under 'Potentizing Methods' below. Although

[1] a) Barnard, G P. 'Microdose Paradox: a New Concept'. *Journal of the American Institute of Homoeopathy*, 1965, vol LVIII, pp 205-212.

b) Barnard, G P, and James H Stephenson. 'Microdose Paradox: a New Biophysical Concept'. *Journal of the American Institute of Homoeopathy*, 1967, vol LX, pp 277-286.

c) Barnard, G P, and James H Stephenson. 'Fresh Evidence for a Biophysical Field'. *Journal of the American Institute of Homoeopathy*, 1969, vol LXII, pp 73-85.

[2] a) Luu D Vinh, Cl. 'Les dilutions homéopathiques: Contrôle et étude par spectrographie Raman-laser'. Thèse de Doctorat en Pharmacie, Faculté de Montpellier, 1974/06/03.

b) Luu D Vinh, Cl, and J Boiron. 'Contribution to the Study of the Physical Structure of Homoeopathic Dilutions by the Raman-laser Effect' (this is in English). Sainte-Foy-Les-Lyon: Editions Boiron, 1976.

it seems very probable that the giant molecular clusters peculiar to each stimulating drug are directly linked to the empirically observed curative effects of homoeopathic medicines, this has not yet been conclusively established.

The final question to be determined would be whether the polymeric structure peculiar to each of the remedies in potency has a corresponding receptor system in the living organism that selectively either responds to, or remains insensitive to, such homoeopathic potencies (investigative work in this area is touched on under 'Physiological Response in Homoeotherapeutics, Mechanism of'). If this proves to be so, then Hahnemann was not only a pioneer in polymer chemistry, but also had the genius to recognize the significance of his discovery. (See 'Altered Receptivity in Disease', 'Dose Repetition', 'Drug Preparation', 'Drug Strength', 'Homoeopathic Laws, Postulates and Precepts' 4, 5, 6, 7, 10 and 11, 'Physiological Response in Homoeotherapeutics, Mechanism of', 'Potentization', 'Potentizing Methods' and 'Solvation Structures'.)

Potentiation

In medicinal therapeutics, a degree of synergism that is greater than additive.

Potentization

Dynamization; imparting (along serial dilutions) the pharmacological message of the original substance (i.e. creating a template of the active principle) by means of trituration or succussion. It describes the process of modification of medicines as invented by Hahnemann. It is characterized by the following four distinguishing features:

a) It is a purely mechanical and mathematico-physical process.
b) The procedure involves neither uncertain, unreliable nor immeasurable factors.
c) The resultant product is stable and can readily be maintained that way.
d) The process is theoretically illimitable, though it becomes laboriously time-consuming in the higher range of potencies.

(See 'Drug Preparation', 'Energy', 'Potency', 'Potentizing Methods', 'Solvation Structures', 'Succussion', 'Trituration' and 'Vitalism'.)

Potentizing Methods

The technique used by homoeopathic pharmacists and dispensing practitioners for the preparation, potentization (dynamization) and dispensing of drugs as laid down with precision in Hahnemann's *Chronic Diseases, Materia Medica Pura,* the *Organon* and the major homoeopathic pharmacopoeial texts, which are:

Dispensatorium homoeopathicum, 1825 (Carl W Caspari produced this prototype of homoeopathic pharmacopoeias; later, under the penmanship of Franz Hartmann (1796-1853) it became part of the fourth edition of the *Organon* in 1829 and was translated into French in 1832)

Der homöopathische Codex, 1831 (by Georg Adolf Weber; preface was written by Hahnemann himself and was published by Friedrich Vieweg Press, Brunswick, Westphalia; translated into French in 1854)

Pharmacopoeia homoeopathica, 1834 (by Harvey Foster Quin (1799-1878), which was the forerunner of the *BHP.*

New Homoeopathic Pharmacopoeia, 1841 (by Georg Heinrich Gottlieb Jahr: remained the profession's standard reference work for a long time, and is still viewed as the ultimate source of reference today; was translated into English in 1845; the second edition appeared in 1853, while the third edition appeared in 1862; in the later years he published the pharmacopoeia in collaboration with M Catellan)

The British Homoeopathic Pharmacopoeia, 1870 (published by the British Homoeopathic Medical Association in London, UK; the BHP was later re-edited in 1876 and again in 1882)

Pharmacopoeia homoeopathica polyglottica, 1872 (for an international scientific medical movement there was a need for a multi-lingual pharmacopoeia; this publication filled this need; English rendering by Leopold Suess-Hahnemann; French rendering by Alphonse Noack; it was produced by Willmar Schwabe of Leipzig, Germany; it was followed by successive editions, the last of which appeared in 1958; in 1978 this became the *Homöopathische Arzneibuch* [HAB], the German Pharmacopoeia [see below])

The Pharmacopoeia of the American Institute of Homoeopathy, 1897 (re-edited several times; the standard reference work was the 1928 edition; the last supplement dates from 1964; in more recent times the official reference work in the USA appears under the name *Homoeopathic Pharmacopoeia of the United States)*

Pharmacopée francaise homéopathique [French Homoeopathic Pharmacopoeia], 1893 (by H Ecalle, L Delpech and A Peuvrier; the second edition appeared in 1898)

Codex medicamentarius homoeopathicus neerlandensis, 1913 (official Homoeopathic Codex of the Netherlands; never re-issued subsequently)

Codex medicamentarius chilensis III, 1941 (official Chilean Pharmacopoeial Codex, which included a supplement for homoeopathic drugs)

Farmacopea Nacional de los Estados Unidos Mexicanos II [Mexican Pharmacopoeia], 1952 (and two successive pharmacopoeias include homoeopathic drugs)

Farmatechnica Homeopathica (Prof D S de Gonzalez Lanuse published this as an ever up-datable manual for Argentina; this became the model for France's *Homéopathie − Pharmacotechnie et Monographies des Médicaments Courants* published in stages, beginning 1975, by the Syndicat des Pharmacies et Laboratoires Homéopathiques)

Pharmacopée francaise [French Pharmacopoeia], 1965 (this edition is the standard reference work, which includes an entire homoeopathic section)

Indian Homoeopathic Pharmacopoeia, 1971 (published in two volumes by the Ministry of Health, Government of India)

Farmacopeia Homeopatica Brasileira [Brazilian Homoeopathic Pharmacopoeia], 1977 (published by the Government of the United States of Brazil)

Homöopathisches Arzneibuch [German Homoeopathic Pharmacopoeia], 1978 (abbreviated as HAB, is the successor to the Pharmacopoeia homoeopathica polyglottica [see above] published 1872 by Willmar Schwabe, Leipzig, Germany; translated into English 1990 and published by the British Homoeopathic Association, 27a Devonshire Street, London W1N 1RJ, UK)

European Homoeopathic Pharmacopoeia is currently in preparation.

Preparation and Dispensing of Drugs

There are two forms of preparation of the basic drug in homoeopathic pharmacy:

(i) mother tinctures or solutions; and (ii) triturations.

i) The former may be dispensed
   a) with aqua destillata (distilled water),
   b) with lactose (sugar of milk),
   c) as tincture-triturations,
   d) in impregnated cones, globules, granules or pillules (mother tinctures only, but not solutions)
   e) in impregnated tablets (mother tinctures only, but not solutions).

ii) The latter may be dispensed
   a) singly (i.e. without mixing with any other vehicle)
   b) in the form of tablets (called tablet-triturates).

ad i) Method for dispensing mother tinctures or solutions:
   a) with aqua destillata: The number of drops required is poured into a new clean phial; aqua destillata is added to the medicine in the proportions either 5ml, 10ml or 15ml to a drop according to the prescription. (Should aqua destillata be unavailable, boiled water, cooled and filtered, may be used.)
   b) with lactose: The number of drops are poured on a measured quantity of lactose in the proportion of 50mg, 100mg or 250mg according to prescription. Lactose may not be impregnated with medicines prepared with dilute alcohol or distilled water, as the lactose will be partially dissolved thereby.
   c) as tincture-triturations: These are triturated preparations made of lactose saturated with the mother tincture of the desired drug. They are convenient for dispensing lower potencies and mother tinctures of vegetable drugs. The preparation: to make the first potency of the tincture-trituration (TT or tinc-trit) 10ml of the desired mother tincture and 10g of lactose are used.

   The lactose together with the mortar are warmed moderately, then the tincture and the lactose are gently mixed and triturated for one hour, by which time the menstruum will have been completely volatilized. A stable and perfectly dry substance is obtained. This is labelled '[name of drug] tinc-trit (or TT) 1DH'.

The 2DH potency and all succeeding tincture-triturations are prepared by adding one part of the preceding tinc-trit to 9 parts of lactose and triturating for one hour.

d) with cones, globules, granules, pillules and pellets: These are placed in a bottle and the requisite remedy is poured over them in sufficient quantity to moisten each one thoroughly. The bottle is corked and allowed sufficient time for complete saturation. The bottle is then grasped firmly and moved rapidly in a circular motion, first perpendicular then horizontal. Following this the phial is kept in an inverted position for a few minutes. Thereupon the cork is loosened a little, and the liquid that may have collected within the neck of the bottle is allowed to drain out. The phial may be left inverted on a clean, white piece of blotting paper until the globules cease to cling together. Once perfectly dry these are ready for dispensing. If carefully prepared, kept well corked and correctly stored, they retain their effectiveness for years.

This process is not to be used with attenuations prepared either with aqua destillata or dilute alcohol, as the globules, etc., melt due to the solvent effect of the water contained in these dilutions.

e) with tablets: An easy, economical and accurate method of dispensing drugs in a compact, palatable and readily assimilable from: One drop of the mother tincture of the desired drug on each 50mg tablet (two drops on a 100mg tablet) – and the tablet is ready for administration.

ad ii) Method for dispensing triturations:

a) Triturations: These are generally dispensed without being mixed with any other vehicle. Perfectly clean, non-chlorinated new paper, about 6cm x 10cm, is folded into self-sealing packet-envelopes, about 2cm x 4cm, each to hold 50mg of the drug trituration.

b) Tablet-triturates: These serve as an effective, cohesive and protective excipient of the drug. Liquid drugs are triturated with lactose, in given proportions, for not less than two hours till the whole is thoroughly comminuted; this trituration is then made into a paste with alcohol and moulded into tablets. When the alcohol evaporates the partially dissolved lactose rapidly re-crystallizes and is ready for administration. The tablet-triturate (tab-trit) is allowed to dissolve perlingually or in 5ml of filtered or spring water, then taken per os.

Potentization

Dynamization, meaning the same thing (note: in French, though, the word 'dynamisation' means succussion, rather than potentization), is a physical process through which latent curative powers of medicines are aroused into activity, though these may have been inevident in their crude states. By this process quantitative deconcentration of drug substance occurs as qualitative increment takes place. This process of preparing medicine was introduced by Hahnemann in the fifth edition of the *Organon,* in 1831.

Attributes which distinguish the changes medicines have undergone once potentized:

a) Quantitative (chemical) reduction linked to qualitative increment of therapeutic (reactive) property.
b) Physical solubility (even of medicines, like metals, believed to have been insoluble [see 'Colloid']).
c) Physiological assimilability and bioavailability.
d) Altered therapeutic activity (suppression of primary [direct], and enhancement of secondary [reactive] effect of drugs.

Many important properties of the drug are observed only after dynamization (potentization). For example, salt (NaCl) and Lycopodium clavatum and sand (Silica) become important medicines only after potentization. They become effective in their dynamized form, but remain latent in their crude form.

How Do Homoeopathic Medicines Act?

Hahnemann himself had asked the same question and gave the answer that his process involved much more than mere mixing of medicine with a diluent, saying that 'by the succussion and trituration there ensues not only the most intimate mixture, but at the same time – and this is the most important circumstance – there ensues such a great and hitherto unknown and undreamt of change, by the development and liberation of the dynamic powers of the medicinal substance so treated, as to excite astonishment'.[1] In paragraph 269 of the *Organon* he says much the same thing in greater detail. This discovery was made through his customary genial intuition. Hahnemann, though he found evidence that consistently corroborated the medicinal effectiveness circumstantially, could not clearly substantiate that pharmacological effectiveness.

Recent scientific investigations, however, have made it possible to advance Hahnemann's hypothesis in a more concrete way: it is postulated that a specific arrangement must take form, triggered by the molecules of the basic substance, involving those of the solvent, i.e. of the water-ethanol vehicle. A shape-specific polymerization is now thought to occur in the liquid vehicle, leaving an impress that is, in fact, a clustering of the water molecules different for each drug, formed into long chains of water polymers, initiated through the succussion. A great deal of work has been carried out in the attempt to verify this hypothesis. A selection of it is described under the entry for 'Potency'. So-called Raman-laser studies were carried out, virtually without interruption for about a decade from 1974, on a research project into the physical structure of homoeopathic potencies by Mrs Luu D Vinh in the laboratory of the Professor

---

[1] Hahnemann, Christian Friedrich Samuel. *The Lesser Writings of Samuel Hahnemann.* Collected and translated by R E Dudgeon. New York: Radde, 1852, pp 728-729.

of Industrial Physics, Mlle L Bardet, at the faculty of pharmacy in Montpellier.

It was shown conclusively that any substance introduced with the Hahnemannian dynamization process into a hydro-alcoholic solvent brings about – in that solvent – a new molecular cluster arrangement peculiar to itself (e.g. the homoeopathic base drug). One is also able to show certain stereophysical deformations in the alcohol itself on such occasions. There is reason to believe that these intermolecular and intramolecular complementary influences, formations and clusters are responsible for the changes which Hahnemannian potencies undergo, and seemingly for the therapeutic action of homoeopathic medicines as well, and current research is aimed at conclusively establishing this last link in the chain of scientific evidence which couples Hahnemannian potentization to therapeutic effectiveness. This clustering, this specific polymerization, is destroyed by heating the potencies certainly beyond 120 degrees Celsius, or through direct exposure to ultrasound, and to other irradiations, when the potencies can be shown to have become medicinally inert and no longer show the peaks on the infra-red absorption spectra of succussed solutions (pioneered by Heintz – see 'Potency'). Such experiments show convincingly that homoeopathic drug activity does indeed depend on its physical structure created by succussion or trituration.

Experimental Evidence (first part; second part at end of this entry)

Two other examples of investigations in the area of physics are reported:[1]

a) A team led by a senior researcher of France's CNRS investigated the physical properties of Hahnemannian 'dilutions' by studying the effects due to certain such 'dilutions' on sensitized crystallizations of copper chloride.

b) Two studies on MNR (nuclear magnetic resonance) were in progress with one team at the University of Lyons, the other at Rome University covering very delicate experimental work. This would follow on the nuclear magnetic-spin resonance studies of 1966.[2]

One example of investigations in the area of the pharmacology of the infinitesimal is reported:

c) The seven year work (from 1980) by the team under Prof Cazin in Lille, on the kinetics of the elimination of arsenic is now an experimental model in homoeopathy. After approach-work lasting two years to research the best protocol (choice of best animal species, optimal age of animals, most suitable elapsed time between subintoxation and the homoeopathic treatment, etc.), it was possible to highlight very clearly the action of Hahnemannian 'dilutions', given as a once-only dose, on the reduction of the blood concentration of

[1] Boiron, Jean. 'Une année de recherches biopharmacologiques'. Under section 'Recherche et homéopathie', *Homéopathie*, 1988, vol I, pp 13-18.

[2] Smith, R B, and G W Boericke. 'Modern Instrumentation for the Evaluation of Homoeopathic Drug Structure'. *Journal of the American Institute of Homoeopathy*, 1966, vol LIX, pp 263-280.

arsenic as well as its simultaneous faecal elimination. The merits of this model are that it is fairly rapid (total time is 60 hours) and that it enabled the investigators to test sequentially the whole gamut of dynamizations (potencies) from 5CH through to 30CH (French upper legal limit) on sufficiently large numbers of animals. The model has been shown to be reliable and reproducible, yielding statistically significant results, as well as being manipulable as a mathematical model. It permits the study of different parameters that intervene in potency manufacture. Comparisons have been made between decimal and centesimal scales of deconcentration; different succussion rates and/or associated rest periods; the effects of diverse temperatures; and selected routes of absorption. All results, without a single exception, showed all potencies (dynamizations) to be active, though unequally so. It was, in fact, established that Arsenicum album 7CH and 14DH were consistently the most active biologically. Three other parameters were systematically examined:

i)   statistical significance [Snedcor and Student tests <0.1%];
ii) reproducibility [66 repetitions of the experiment on groups of animals consistently produced positive results – in not one single case was there a negative result];
iii) succussions [identical deconcentrations, like 7CH and 14DH, where one would have been succussed twice as often relative to the other, showed no significant difference in biological effectiveness. The distilled water, as placebo, was also divided into succussed and non-succussed, producing results that were indistinguishable from one another, strengthening the above polymerization-template hypothesis].

Classes of Dynamization (Potencies)

The object of homoeopathic pharmacy is so to prepare each substance that the whole of its reaction-eliciting virtues should be retained in a suitable form. The resulting product, the base drug, is called mother tincture, mother solution, or mother trituration, as the case may be. With homoeopathic dilute alcohol (see 'Alcohol'), or aqua destillata, the mother tincture or solution may be divided (deconcentrated) and further subdivided. A mother trituration may be divided by triturating it with sugar of milk (lactose). These divisions and further subdivisions of a substance (liquid or solid) are attenuations that, if succussed at the intervals, are called potencies or dynamizations; it is quite inappropriate to refer to the liquid versions of potencies as 'dilutions', because they are more than just that.

In dynamizing (potentizing) three scales are used:
(i)   decimal;
(ii) centesimal;
(iii) quinquagenimillesimal (often written as 50-millesimal).

ad (i) The decimal scale, introduced by Constantin Hering, is based on the principle that the first potency should contain one tenth part of the homoeopathic base drug and each succeeding potency should contain one-tenth part of the one immediately preceding. The decimal potency is denoted by suffixing D (sometimes the Roman digit 'x' for 'decem' [ten] is used instead) to the numerals denoting the deconcentration stage of the drug: as Apis mellifica 2D, or 3D, denote the first and second decimal deconcentrations of the homoeopathically prepared base drug of Apis mellifica. (Note: In preparing the homoeopathic mother tincture, or the base solution of a drug, the quantity of the original drug and the vehicle would be proportioned [with only few exceptions, listed under 'Mother Tincture'] in such a manner that it already represents one-tenth of the original succus.)

ad (ii) The centesimal scale, introduced by Hahnemann, is based on the principle that the first potency should contain one hundredth of the base drug and each succeeding potency should contain one-hundredth part of the one immediately preceding. The centesimal scale is denoted by suffixing C after the numerals denoting the deconcentration stage of the drug: as Apis mellifica 3C, or 6C, denote the third and sixth centesimal deconcentrations of the homoeopathically prepared base drug of Apis mellifica.

ad (iii) The quinquagenimillesimal (50-millesimal) scale is discussed in detail in the next section.

The Mechanics of Dynamization
(i) Instructions for the preparation of liquid potencies:
a) Decimal scale: Take a round phial of about 30ml capacity, perfectly clean and new, fit a good new cork into it; mark the potency of the drug 2D preceded by its name on the cork. Remove cork from the phial. Consult the pharmacopoeia under the drug to be dynamized and follow any special directions given.

Pour the exact proportion of the base drug (where Θ=1D already, with few exceptions) into the phial, and then add the liquid vehicle required, taking care that about one quarter of the phial remains empty for succussion. Fit the marked cork back into the phial. Grasp the phial in the right hand with the thumb held firmly over the cork, and shake it with ten vigorous downward strokes of the arm, and to succuss the mixture let each stroke terminate in a jerk when striking the closed right hand against the open palm of the left hand.

The 2D potency is now ready. Mark the name of the drug with 2D around the phial too. For all succeeding potencies add to one part of the preceding dynamization 9 parts of the vehicle then shake and succuss as before.

b) Centesimal scale: Take a round phial of about 30ml capacity, perfectly clean and new, fit a good new cork into it; mark the potency of the drug 1C preceded by its name on the cork. Remove the cork from the phial. Pour the exact proportion of the drug into the phial, having consulted the pharmacopoeia for any special directions. Add the liquid vehicle as required, taking care that about one quarter of the phial remains empty. Fit the cork marked 1C back into the phial. Grasp the phial in the right hand and proceed to succuss as described under the section for 'Decimal scale' above. Mark 1C around the phial itself also. In making the succeeding dynamizations, mix 1 part of the preceding potency to 99 parts of the vehicle, and succuss each time as directed above.

c) **Quinquagenimillesimal (50-millesimal) scale:** This was introduced in the sixth edition of the *Organon* (section 270), which was only published seventy-eight years after Hahnemann's death. Potency on this scale is denoted by 0/1, 0/2, 0/5, 0/10, etc. and generically referred to as the 'LM potencies' (on account of the Roman digits for 50 and 1000). Pierre Schmidt of Geneva speaks very highly of it both in the *British Homoeopathic Journal* (July/October, 1954) and later in the *Journal of the American Institute of Homoeopathy* (December/January, 1955-6).

The salient features of the stages of its preparation are condensed here:

Dry powder trituration of the base drug – for three attenuations on the centesimal scale, i.e. up to the 3C potency, having taken the drug deconcentration then to 1 : 1000000 or:

$$\frac{1}{10^6}$$

The next operation, converting the dry 3C trituration into liquid form, is on the 500th scale, yielding for all practical purposes, the 'LM mother tincture' which may be regarded as approximately 4C, with its drug deconcentration at:

$$\frac{1}{5 \times 10^8}$$

The liquid stage of the potency progression is then made from the solution, in the normal 4C to 5C procedure on the centesimal scale. The deconcentration here becomes equivalent to a little more than 5C, at:

$$\frac{1}{5 \times 10^{10}}$$

Considering that the base drug deconcentration of what may be termed this '1C potency of the LM', its name becomes clear as it may be said to be conveying the 50000th (fifty thousandth) part of the 3C trituration, from which it may be seen as issuing on the quinquagenimillesimal (50-millesimal) scale, albeit through two different stages on two different scales. It may also be viewed as 1 quingentesimal (= 5-centesimal) and 1 centesimal, thus:

$$\frac{1}{500} \times \frac{1}{100} = \frac{1}{5000}$$

All subsequent potencies are prepared on the 50000th scale, i.e. quinquageni-millesimal (50-millesimal) scale. The procedure for this is: a poppy seed-sized 'globule 10', or granule, (500 of which are capable of absorbing a drop of alcohol) is saturated with the potency at hand and it is then crushed and dissolved in 100 drops of alcohol fortis, giving the forward drug strength for each ascending 'LM dynamization' as:

$$\frac{1}{500} \times \frac{1}{100} = \frac{1}{5000}$$

i.e. on the quinquagenimillesimal scale.

It follows, therefore, that the chemical proportion of medicine to menstruum, or deconcentrating medium, is 1 : 50000 in each potency stage, instead of 1 : 100, as on the centesimal scale. This is so, because each poppy seed-sized 'globule 10' of a subsequent potency conveys the 50000th part of a same-sized globule of the preceding potency, since 50000 poppy-sized globules could be saturated with the medicine thus subsequently prepared.

The mathematical calculations to exemplify the deconcentrations:

    i)   At the point where the 3C has just become the 'LM mother tincture': as stated above =

$$\frac{1}{5 \times 10^8}$$

    ii)   At the next stage of one further centesimal potentization:

$$\frac{1}{5 \times 10^8} \times \frac{1}{100}$$

$$= \frac{1}{5 \times 10^8 \times 10^2} = \frac{1}{5 \times 10^{10}}$$

$$= \frac{1}{5} \times \frac{1}{10^{10}} = \frac{1}{5} \text{ of 10D} = \frac{1}{5} \text{ of 5C.}$$

    iii)   All potencies above this are on the regular quinquagenimillesimal (50-millesimal) scale, expressible as:

$$\frac{1}{50000} = \frac{1}{5 \times 10000} = \frac{1}{5 \times 10^4}$$

    iv)   Therefore, the comparative calculations for the higher potencies are arrived at as given in the two examples hereunder:

    1)   The 0/6 potency is approximately equivalent to 34D or 17C, thus:

$$\frac{1}{5 \times 10^{10}} \times \frac{(1)^5}{(5 \times 10^4)} \text{ (there being five subsequent stages)}$$

$$= \frac{1}{5 \times 10^{10}} \times \frac{1}{5^5 \times 10^{20}}$$

$$= \frac{1}{5^6 \times 10^{30}}$$

Now, as 5^6 is a little in excess of 10000, it may be expressed in powers of 10 as 10^4 (approx.)

Hence:

$$= \frac{1}{10^4 \times 10^{30}} = \frac{1}{10^{34}}$$

$$= 34D \text{ or } 17C \text{ (approximately).}$$

(Note: For the 0/6 potency there are 5 stages after the point which is reached in subsection (ii) above; likewise for 0/12 11 stages are to be taken into account.)

2) The 0/12 potency is approximately equivalent to a 62D or 31C, thus:

$$\frac{1}{5 \times 10^{10}} \times \frac{(1)^{11}}{(5 \times 10^4)}$$

$$= \frac{1}{5 \times 10^{10}} \times \frac{1}{5^{11} \times 10^{44}}$$

$$= \frac{1}{5^{12} \times 10^{54}}$$

Now, as 5^{12} expressed in powers of 10 can be stated as 10^8 (approximately):

$$= \frac{1}{10^8 \times 10^{54}} = \frac{1}{10^{62}}$$

$$= 62D \text{ or } 31C \text{ (approximately).}$$

In summary, the preparation of the mother tincture according to this scale:

The time required for the preparation of the LM mother tincture with lactose is about three hours of trituration on the centesimal scale to the deconcentration of 10^{-6}. To convert it into a liquid potency, the trituration is dissolved in 500 drops of a mixture of one part alcohol to four parts aqua destillata. So, the base drug deconcentration in this scale is:

$$\frac{1}{5 \times 10^8}$$

The potentization procedure under this scale, then: In a suitable phial, one drop of LM mother tincture to 100 drops of alcohol fortis. About one quarter of the phial is to remain empty. One hundred strokes of uniform force are applied, ending in the succussive jerk.

The 0/1 potency will then have been produced, with the base drug deconcentration at:

$$\frac{1}{5 \times 10^{10}}$$

Poppy seed-sized 'globules 10' are moistened with it and spread quickly on a piece of clean, non-chlorinated blotting paper to dry. These impregnated globules are to be kept in a well corked phial marked 0/1. Since five hundred such globules are able to absorb with each becoming saturated by just one drop of alcohol fortis, it follows that one such poppy-sized 'globule 10' represents one five-hundredth deconcentration. To obtain the 0/2 potency one 'globule 10' prepared as above is placed in a new glass phial and dissolved in a drop of aqua destillata. Then 100 drops of alcohol fortis are added and 100 succussions are given to this. Then 'globules 10' are medicated with this potency as for the previous dynamization. Every succeeding potency is prepared in this manner, each containing a 50000th part of the preceding one: (1/500 x 1/100). (See P Barthel 'Das Vermächtnis Hahnemanns – die fünfzigtausender Potenzen', *Allgemeine Homöopathische Zeitung,* Mar/Apr 1990, vol CCXXXV(2), pp 47-61; and A C Dutta, 'Fifty Millesimal Potency in the light of the Micro-Isotopic Concept', *Hahnemann Homoeop Sandesh,* Aug 1989, vol XIII(8), pp 177-180.)

ii) Instructions for the preparation of triturated potencies:

The process of trituration should be carried out in a warm and dry atmosphere and all utensils must be perfectly clean. Wash the mortar with water, wipe it dry, and burn a little alcohol in it. Do this for each subsequent trituration stage, to obviate the Korsakoff effect (see below). Hard substances, as a general rule, are triturated more easily than soft substances: Zincum metallicum and Iridium metallicum (the hardest substances to be triturated in homoeopathic pharmacy) produce finer particles than, say, Graphites, Mercurius or Plumbum metallicum. In triturating the last-mentioned one ought to use the pestle very softly; and in making the first trituration of Mercurius, Graphites or Plumbum metallicum, one should double the time. When triturating Ferrum metallicum, the moisture must be removed by warming up the mortar at frequent intervals. Argentum nitricum and hygroscopic salts (e.g. Calcarea chlorinata or Kali carbonicum) cannot be kept well in trituration.

a) **Decimal scale:** There are three stages in the process of trituration:

Take 66.6mg of the crude drug to be triturated in a wedgewood mortar. Add to it 200mg of lactose and mix these well with a horn spatula (About 10 minutes). With a wedgewood pestle triturate this mixture vigorously (for 6 minutes) applying a steady circular motion. The grinding pressure should be hard: scrape (3 minutes) all the particles off the mortar and the pestle with the horn spatula. Stir the mixture with the spatula (for 1 minute). The first stage is now complete (in 20 minutes).

Add another 200mg of lactose to the triturated material and again mix well with the spatula. With the pestle the mixture is to be triturated thoroughly (for 6 minutes) by a steady circular movement. The grinding pressure should be hard; scrape (3 minutes) all the particles off the mortar and the pestle with the spatula; and stir the mixture (for 1 minute). Again triturate the mixture with the pestle (for 6 minutes) as before, scrape (3 minutes) all the particles off the mortar and the pestle with the spatula; and stir the mixture (for 1 minute). The second stage of the process is now complete (20 minutes).

Add another 200mg of lactose to the triturated product and proceed as before. The third stage of the process is now complete (20 minutes). The entire trituration is now complete (one hour's duration). Bottle it in a clean and dry glass phial, corked and labelled 1D after the name of the medicine.

To make the 2D trit. take 66.6mg (or its multiple) of the 1D trit., and carefully proceed through the three stages of the process as before, and so on for all the succeeding triturations.

b) Centesimal scale: There are three stages in the process of trituration:

Take 66.6 mg of the crude drug to be triturated in a wedgewood mortar. Add 2.2g of lactose and mix these well with a horn spatula. Triturate the mixture thoroughly with a wedgewood pestle (6 minutes) by a steady circular movement. The grinding pressure should be hard. Scrape (3 minutes) all the particles off the mortar and the pestle with the spatula. Stir the mixture (for 1 minute). Again triturate the mixture with the pestle (for 6 minutes) as before. Scrape (3 minutes) all the particles off the mortar and the pestle with the spatula. Stir the mixture again (for 1 minute). The first stage of the process is now complete (in 20 minutes).

Add another 2.2g of lactose to the triturated material and mix well with the spatula. With the pestle triturate the mixture (for 6 minutes) thoroughly by a steady circular movement. The grinding pressure should be hard. Scrape (3 minutes) all the particles off the mortar and the pestle. Stir the mixture (for 1 minute). Again triturate the mixture (6 minutes) as before. Scrape (3 minutes) again as before. Stir the mixture (1 minute) as before. The second stage of the process is now complete (in 20 minutes).

Add another 2.2g of lactose to the triturated product and proceed as before. The third stage of the process is thus complete (another 20 minutes).

The entire trituration required is now complete (in 1 hour). Bottle it in a clean, dry glass phial, corked and labelled 1C preceded by the name of the medicine.

To make the 2C trit., take 66.6mg (or its multiple) of the first trit. and carefully proceed through the stages of the process as before; and so on for all succeeding triturations.

(Note: If one moistens the lactose with a little alcohol one can substantially reduce the tedious 'stirring' and 'scraping' so that the trituration proceeds with much greater facility.)

(iii) Instructions for converting triturations into liquid potencies:

The triturations are taken up to the 6D trituration first, at which level they will have become soluble in a liquid vehicle (see 'Colloid'). Then the undermentioned instructions are followed:

Take a round phial of 30ml, clean and new, fit a new cork into it, mark the name of the drug to be processed on it, followed by 8D or 4C. Remove cork and introduce 66.6mg of the 6D trituration of the drug, adding 3.3ml aqua destillata, which is dissolved by agitation. Then add 3.3ml of dilute alcohol (refer to this entry) and then succuss the phial ten times. Ensure that the phial is only about two-thirds full. The 8D or 4C potency is now ready.

Whichever is applicable is to be marked on the phial. (Note: One cannot prepare a 7D potency, on the decimal scale, from one part trituration in the 6D potency with nine parts of dilute alcohol.)

a) **Decimal Scale:** Prepare the 9D dynamization by adding one part of the 8D potency to nine parts of dilute alcohol, succussing it ten times. All succeeding attenuations are prepared by adding one part of the preceding potency to nine parts of dilute alcohol and succussing it ten times at every stage.

b) **Centesimal Scale:** Add 99 parts of dilute alcohol to one part of the 4C dynamization, succussing ten times, to make the 5C potency. All succeeding attenuations are prepared by adding one part of the preceding dynamization to 99 parts of dilute alcohol and succussing it ten times at every stage.

The Specifications Relating to Potentization Methods

Essential to the understanding of the homoeopathic potentizing (dynamizing) process, and to the subsequent employment of the products of such a process, is an explanation of the different methods that are used in preparing homoeopathic drugs since Hahnemann first introduced the dynamized homoeopathic attenuation (deconcentration). The variations in the method of drug processing result in homoeopathic medicinal strengths which differ from each other, depending on the method used.

Hahnemann personally prepared most of the medicines which he prescribed to his patients. Whenever he had medicinally provoked a reaction, he monitored it, using his exceptional gift of observation. In this way he was progressively able to improve his method of processing drugs. During his entire medical career, which was long, he patiently sought to perfect his method in an endeavour to afford his patients the quickest cure with the least possible aggravation.

He stipulates in 1819, in the second edition of the *Organon:*

'Homoeopathic remedies must be administered in much smaller doses than is customary in ordinary practice, in fact, in as minute a dose as possible. Since the medicine precisely affects only those parts of the body already affected by the disease, only a little strength is required to supersede the latter.'

In amplification, Jahr states in the 1853 edition of his *Pharmacopoeia:*

'In the beginning Hahnemann was content to make a centesimal attenuation, but noting that these preparations still acted in a manner that was too drastic, he soon went further and prepared a second and third centesimal attenuation. Hahnemann still found these too active, and he progressively increased. Later, he decided to increase the number of attenuations as high as the 30th for many of his remedies.'

Hahnemann's primary motivation clearly was to reduce the quantity of the substance he administered as a remedy. To that end he introduced the lactose base (milk sugar) for triturations and dilute alcohol for liquid deconcentrations. He was obviously surprised at the medicinal activity displayed by the higher attenuations which he used and concluded that the explanation for this activity was inherent in the mode of preparation which, according to him, infused his remedies with a new quality and power, as the following quotations show:[1]

'How can small doses of such very attenuated medicine as homoeopathy employs still possess great power? . . . The answer to this is, that in the preparation of the homoeopathic medicinal attenuations, a small portion of medicine is not merely added to an enormous quantity of non-medicinal fluid, or only slightly mingled with it, . . . but by the prolonged succussion or trituration, there ensues not only the most intimate mixture, but at the same time – and this is the most important circumstance – there ensues such a great, and hitherto unknown and undreamt of change, by the development and liberation of the dynamic powers of the medicinal substance so treated, as to excite astonishment.'

'In the homoeopathic pharmaceutical operations . . . , as only a small quantity of the attenuating fluid is taken at a time (one drop of medicinal tincture shaken up with only 100 drops of alcohol), there ensues a union and equal distribution in a few seconds.'

Hahnemann was conscious of the necessity to proceed in measured stages, using a limited amount of the diluent-vehicle at each stage, as the only way to achieve this effect, and may have even dimly realized that it was the water that was important to the carrying of the homoeopathic pharmacological message:

'Were we to attempt to impregnate . . . e.g. a hogshead [= 240 litres] of water with one drop of medicine, no conceivable stirring, were it ever so prolonged, would succeed in distributing this drop uniformly throughout the whole mass – not to mention that the constant internal change and chemical decomposition of the component parts of the water continually going on, would overwhelm and annihilate the medicinal power of a drop of plant tincture.'

If stress is often laid on two aspects of homoeopathic drug processing, namely 'quantity' of the substance and 'medicinal quality' of the end product, it is because these two reciprocal aspects have formed the basis of all possible discussions about homoeopathic medications. Moreover, different techniques used in potentization are known to affect 'quantity', and therefore also 'quality', differently. Hahnemann's method of drug processing was first set out in pharmacopoeial form in Carl W Caspari's *Homoeopathic Dispensatory*.

To make potencies of any substance, the exact number of empty phials (or small bottles) is first selected which will be required in accordance with the

[1] Hahnemann, Christian Friedrich Samuel. Preamble to volume VI of *Materia Medica Pura*. Dresden: Arnold, Second edition, 1827, translated by R E Dudgeon 1880, reprinted Calcutta: M Battacharyya & Co, 1952, vol II, pp 43-44.

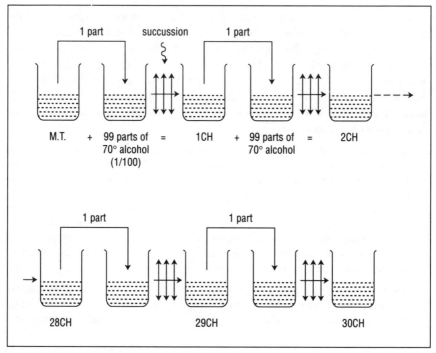

Figure 1: Centesimal Hahnemannian Method, using Separate Phials

number of the potency to be made. Each phial is marked with the name of the substance and numbered, and then placed in numerical order. Ninety-nine drops of dilute alcohol are introduced into each phial. One drop of the mother tincture (solution) is added to phial no 1, it is succussed, and allowed to rest for about three minutes. Then one drop from phial no 1 is added to phial no 2, succussed, and allowed to rest as previously described. This process is repeated up to the envisaged potency, always ensuring that the drop taken out of one phial is instilled into the very next higher number and into no other. A separate, dedicated sterilized dropper is used for each dynamization. The symbol H, after the potency scale, as in 6CH or 30CH, denotes this, the Hahnemannian, method of potentization (dynamization). Figure 1 schematically represents this process.

In 1832 General von Korsakoff, a Russian passionately interested in homoeopathy, devised what he considered as a simplification of Hahnemann's lengthy dynamization procedure. He sent details of the amended potentization process to Johann Ernst Stapf who published it in the second issue of the *Archiv für die homöopathische Heilkunst* in 1832. Von Korsakoff advocated the use of only one bottle to obtain the desired potency, surmising that probably sufficient liquid would adhere to the inner surface of the phial in which the first deconcentration had been made, to provide for the one drop required to prepare the next; and so on for each subsequent stage. The symbol to denote

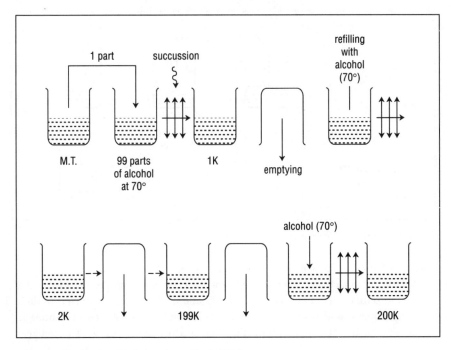

Figure 2: Korsakovian Method, using a Single Phial

this method of dynamization is K, appearing generally on its own, though signifying CK.

When consulted on this, Hahnemann did not give a negative opinion. On the contrary, he considered that 'the eminent von Korsakoff's process might be as sensible as it was useful'. This pronouncement coming from Hahnemann may seem surprising, since his uncompromising attitude towards any deviation brought to his notice is well documented. The only possible explanation is that he did not see any difference between the preparations obtained by using either of these two methods. This was the case for all homoeopathic practitioners and pharmacists until 1926, when A Berne conclusively established the considerable extent of difference in their respective rates of deconcentrations.

Prior to the production of this evidence the misbelief existed that the two methods of dynamization (potentization) were equivalent. From the earliest times this had led to the mixing of these two processes in the making of the same series of potencies. As early as 1845, and again in 1853, Georg Heinrich Gottlieb Jahr, in his pharmacopoeia, and still later Jahr and M. Catellan, in 1862, noted that 'for the attenuations which one did not want to preserve, one could empty the contents of the bottle containing a specific attenuation and fill it again with 100 drops of hydro-alcohol, in order to obtain, after 100 successions, the succeeding attenuation'. He continues, 'if one wants the 30th, any of the intermediate attenuations could be made in this manner'. That was

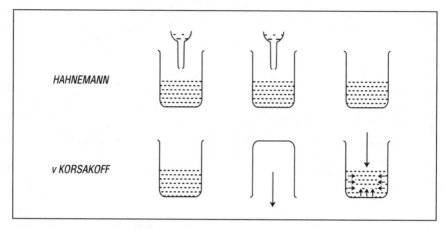

Figure 3: Comparative Illustration of the Two Methods

mixing of the two processes, Hahnemann's and von Korsakoff's.

Weber, in *Der homöopathische Codex* (French translation) published in 1854, did not fall into this error. However, in 1892, Ecalle, Delpech and Peuvrier, in their pharmacopoeia, had reverted to the process which mixes the two methods in succession in the course of preparing one and the same series of potencies.

International Distribution of Scales and Methods

In the francophone area only the centesimal scale is used, except for some very low dynamizations (3DH and 6DH). In the English-speaking countries the centesimal scale is predominantly used, whereas in the German-speaking area the decimal scale is almost exclusively used. The quinquagenimillesimal scale (LM potencies) is used in all parts of the world, though relatively seldom.

Hahnemann's multiple-phial method is the only method permitted by French law, where potencies are always referred to with precision as CH (=centesimal/Hahnemannian). Similarly the HAB, the German Homoeopathic Pharmacopoeia, does not recognize the Korsakovian method, but only the Hahnemannian. In the UK the Korsakovian method is also not used by homoeopathic pharmacists below the 1M potency. On the other hand, von Korsakoff's single-phial method is used commercially in Belgium for all potencies. Furthermore the Korsakovian method is universally used whenever a practitioner has to prepare an auto-isopathic or tautopathic agent in potency for a particular patient (see 'Isopathy').

An additional method of potency preparation, restricted to one country only (USA), according to Hamish Boyd,[1] is by drug deconcentration of 1 in 1000 parts between succussions; that range is also called 'M' potencies. This is confusing as the 1000CH and 1000K potencies are elsewhere referred to as 1M,

[1] Boyd, H. *Introduction to Homoeopathic Medicine* Beaconsfield: Beaconsfield Publishers Ltd, 1981, p 51.

and the difference in mathematical terms is enormous, in that the former 1M represents a deconcentration of 10^{-3}, whereas the latter 1M stands for a deconcentration of 10^{-1999}.

The Korsakovian method commends itself on account of its efficiency and economy. The Hahnemannian method, however, provides for the best and most clearly defined standardization between laboratories. One could, obviously, also standardize the Korsakovian method of dynamization, but that would require a minutely detailed prescription for the mode of preparation. This the French, for instance, considered impractical. So they simply outlawed the method, not least because it would introduce the danger of a variable factor into their extensive experimental work. There are many aspects of the Korsakovian method which demonstrably affect its exactness. Some of these are:

a) The size, shape and internal smoothness of the phials (or small flasks).
b) The material of which the phials are made.
c) The solubility of original drug substance.
d) The surface tension of the original drug substance.
e) The greater or lesser tendency of the substance to adhere to the phial's edge, and whether or not the phial's outer edge is lipped.
f) The temperature in the laboratory.
g) The haphazard differences due, perhaps, to the arm action of the one doing the actual pouring out of the contents (e.g. does every glass of wine that has been drunk empty and left to stand always have the same amount [just one drop?] gathering at the bottom?).

The error factors inherent in Korsakovian potencies have been experimentally ascertained by the use of radioactive material (isotopes) in comparative dynamization (potentization) processes. Taking the view that the number of potentizing steps, namely the number of events involving succussion, is more important in the homoeopathic pharmaceutical process than the ratio of medicinal agent to vehicle, has become untenable since the evidence of Cazin's work mentioned in this entry earlier, under Experimental Evidence, at c)(iii). It has been established experimentally that in terms of the residual quantity of the original material:

- a 30K potency is approximately equivalent to a 5CH;
- a 200K potency is approximately equivalent to a 7CH;
- a Korsakovian 1M (1000K) is, surprisingly, approximately equivalent to a 9CH.

Dr Burdick, of New York, who had eminent scientific qualifications, was able to show as early as 1877, by calculation and microscopic investigation, that the potency Dr Swan marketed as MM (i.e. thousand thousandth, or one millionth), 'cannot exceed the tenth centesimal of Hahnemann, and is liable to be much lower'.[1] Elsewhere it was cruelly suggested by an unnamed person

[1] Burdick, P in the *Hahnemannian Monthly*, November, 1877.

at about that time, that the reason why the very high potencies, which are always made by some process that is quite illegitimate in strict Hahnemannian terms, have been found to be so efficacious is that they are really much lower attenuations than their adopters had believed they were employing. Furthermore, as will be shown later, the standard high (centesimal scale) potencies of 1M, 5M, 10M, etc. are not subject to the process of true dynamization at all. It must be pointed out that for one person to prepare, say, a Belladonna 10M through successive stages of true Hahnemannian potentization, would take 1667 hours of labour, which is ten weeks (70 days), working 24 hours each day.

General von Korsakoff merely wanted to simplify the method of preparation of the potencies and economize on the number of phials used. He worked manually. Yet little by little, some of those who used his method started to go beyond the limit set by Hahnemann, the 30th centesimal. Convinced that succussion alone potentiated the medicinal effect, the thinking was 'the more often succussed, the greater the medicinal effectiveness' . . . ad infinitum. Potentization went up to the 100th and later even to the 200th centesimal potency, but the manufacturers unfortunately also became secretive about their method of preparation. In 1853, that is only ten years after Hahnemann's death, Jahr and Catellan wrote, 'for some years there has also been much suspicion as to the so-called high attenuations, that is to say, from the 100th to the 1000th and even the 10000th and 40000th. We merely wish to mention that much mystery still surrounds the method of preparation used in obtaining these attenuations by Jenichen, first propagator of these preparations. It is more than probable that their numbering corresponds not to the dilutions, but more or less to the number of succussions which were used in the preparation of each' (see 'Nomenclature, Discrepancies in'). Later Hughes said Jenichen was purported to have produced the 60000th centesimal potency, by simply succussing 'an ordinary attenuation without further dilution – ten of such shakes being reckoned as producing a potency one step higher in the scale'.[1] R E Dudgeon remarked that fortunately Jenichen shot himself when he reached that potency or there would be no telling what heights he might have reached.[2] It was mainly in the USA that the use of these extremely high attenuations increased extensively, particularly of those prepared by Drs M Swan and B Fincke. In the UK it was Dr Thomas Skinner (1825-1906) who actively propagated very high potencies. In homoeopathic literature mention is made of 1000th, 10000th, one hundred-thousandth, and even the millionth deconcentration.

It is sobering to read what James Tyler Kent wrote to a colleague about the high potentizing methods of Swan, Fincke and Skinner (the letter is reproduced in the catalogue of Boericke and Tafel): 'I know in detail how the

[1] Hughes, Richard. *A Manual of Pharmacodynamics*. Sixth edition, London: Leath and Ross, 1893, p 104.
[2] Dudgeon, R E. *Theory and Practice of Homoeopathy*. London: Leath and Ross, 1854, p 355.

Skinner potencies are made. One weighs a dry phial and after making the potency and pouring it out one re-weighs the phial and finds that a hundredth part remains inside. This is always exactly one hundredth part. The Skinner system is the only high potency apparatus (dynamizator) that makes exact potencies. The potencies of Fincke are of totally unknown origin. The potencies of Swan are a fraud of the highest degree and I have thrown them all away after I saw how he prepared them'.[1]

There rests a heavy obligation upon the manufacturer of homoeopathic pharmaceuticals to make available to the prescriber/user only homoeopathic medicines which have had all stages of the manufacturing process fully verified, so that they are known to be

safe,

true to required mensuration,

conforming exactly with pharmacopoeial standards,

uncontaminated, and

properly succussed at each stage of deconcentration, thereby processed to carry
   the exact pharmacological message.

For the prescriber of homoeopathic potencies, the following information is of relevance.

At Boericke and Tafel, Philadelphia, the largest manufacturers in the USA:

They manufacture about 1500 remedies from the 1C to the 30C according to
   the Hahnemannian process.

They also manufacture from the 30C upward a number of remedies up to 200,
   500 and 1000, prepared by hand in alcohol, with 12 successions at each
   stage, according to von Korsakoff's method.

The 1000th thus obtained is then used as a base for the preparation of the
   10000th and 100000th potencies, using the 'Skinner dynamizator', where
   the single bottle is automatically emptied and filled under pressure with tap-
   water (the point has been made that the tap-water of today and that of
   Kent's day, a hundred years ago, are two very dissimilar things).

At Ehrhart and Karl, Chicago, another very large manufacturer in the USA, approximately the same sequence is followed:

From 1C to 30C they use the Hahnemannian process.

From 30C upward, manual preparation of the 200th, 500th and 1000th, exactly
   as above stated.

From the 1000th up to 10000, 500000 and 100000th with filtered tap-water
   using the Kent dynamizator (this was the model Skinner improved,
   mechanically).

From the 100000th of Kent up to the 500 thousandth and 1 millionth of
   Allen, the dilutions are prepared by the Skinner continuous fluxion
   method.

[1]Boericke and Tafel. 'Catalogue 1938: Physicians' Price List and Therapeutic Handbook', p 26.

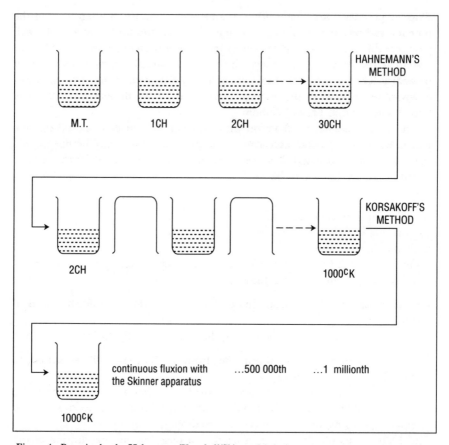

Figure 4: Potencies by the Hahnemann/Korsakoff/Skinner Method

These are the only two laboratories which still supply certain pharmacies in the USA, South America, India, South Africa, New Zealand, Australia and the UK.

The Skinner continuous fluxion method comprises of running a continual flow of tap-water through a glass tube equipped with an overflow control system above a level of 5ml, causing a progressive 'washing away' of the original potency contained at the bottom of the tube, whilst maintaining a continuous agitation during the complete operation. When one litre of water has thus run its course, the remaining 5ml at the bottom of the tube corresponds to the 200th (i.e. 5ml x 200 = 1000ml or one litre). With this method it takes 75 hours and 180 litres of tap-water to have run through to manufacture a CM potency from a 10M.

The homoeopathic pharmacist, Kurt Hochstetter, made a personal inspection tour of all the homoeopathic pharmaceutical manufacturing plants in South America, the USA, France, Germany and the UK. Afterwards he made the following pertinent comment regarding the very high potencies, for which there continues to exist a fair demand from a large section of homoeopaths internationally: [1]

'In the sixth edition of the 'Organon' Hahnemann described the method for preparing LM potencies. It is regrettable that this edition was not published in 1843, as was intended, because the manner in which LM potencies are made would have precluded the manufacture of the very high potencies which became the fashion in the USA' [author's translation].

The situation in France is very different. Until 1953 Korsakovian potencies accounted for more than 65% of French homoeopathic prescriptions. A number of laboratories and specialized pharmacies there used mechanical potentizers to prepare these dynamizations. It had been Antoine Nebel (Snr), who having returned from visiting Dr Thomas Skinner in London, set about having a model produced by a Swiss engineer, Mr Perdrizat. Soon the Drs Leon Vannier and Rene Baudry obtained the same Swiss machine. Some years later Dr Jean Jarricot of Lyon improved considerably on the method, and produced several succussive dynamizators. It is interesting to note that, contrary to the usage in the rest of the world (where potencies are kept on the shelf for long periods of time), all French pharmacists always manufactured their Korsakovian potencies starting from the mother tincture (or the first liquid potency of insoluble substances [see 'Colloid']). The general potencies used were 6, 12, 30, 200 and M. These attenuations were only produced by the Korsakovian method, where many molecules of the original drug substance can still be found even in an M potency. This means they were totally different from the similarly numbered US dynamizations, which are produced by a mixture of three methods, as described. The first codification of homoeopathic preparations in France was published in the form of a decree by the Minister of Public Health in the *Journal officiel de la République Francaise* on 21st December 1948. Yet homoeopathic medicine only became official when it was included in the eighth edition of the French Pharmacopoeia in 1965, was made refundable through the Securité Sociale, and homoeopathic pharmacy was taught to all pharmacy students throughout the country. By that time the Korsakovian method and all potencies above 30CH, except one or two proprietaries, such as 'Oscillococcinum 200', had been outlawed.

A growing section of homoeopaths would like to see implemented what Hahnemann had obviously wanted, the employment of the quinquagenimillesimal scale (for the LM potencies) by those who much prefer the highest ranges of potency in homoeopathy. This section of homoeopaths considers it doubtful that Hahnemann would have agreed to the process of continuous fluxion for the preparation of his highest potencies, particularly with tap-water. They feel that Hahnemann had tirelessly pursued his research into ideal methods for producing a medicine which was both very active and very gentle. In 1842 he wrote to his publisher, thereby making public the results

[1] Hochstetter, Kurt. 'Survey of Homoeopathic High Potencies' [author's translation of the title from the German], *Allgemeine homöopathische Zeitung*, 1978, no.2.

of his quest. He had defined the procedure for the preparation of the LM potencies – also called the 'granule potencies' – and he had wished to reveal it in 1843, together with his other modifications, in the sixth edition of the *Organon*. He died at the age of 88 without having seen it published. It was only in 1921 that this edition was finally published in German. By this time the other methods for producing the highest dynamizations had long been established, and had unwarrantedly assumed the mantle of Hahnemannian legitimacy. Today, probably due to long-established habits, such non-Hahnemannian potencies (produced by continuous fluxion, etc.) are far more widely employed than Hahnemann's own LM potencies. Figure 5 graphically illustrates the method recommended by him in the posthumously published sixth edition of the Organon.

The principal difference between Hahnemannian and Korsakovian potencies concerns the deconcentration of the basic substance. The most important factor is that the Hahnemannian process, as established experimentally through the tagged isotopes, curiously produces a faster

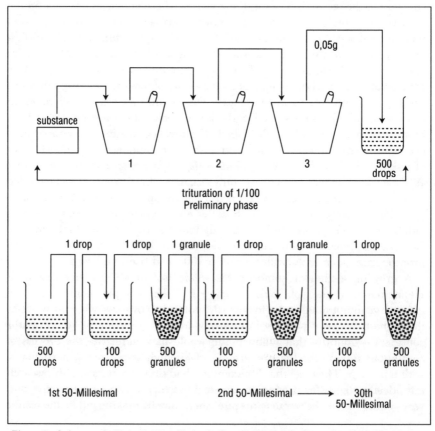

Figure 5: Quinquagenimillesimal (50-millesimal) Granule Method for Preparing 'LM Potencies'

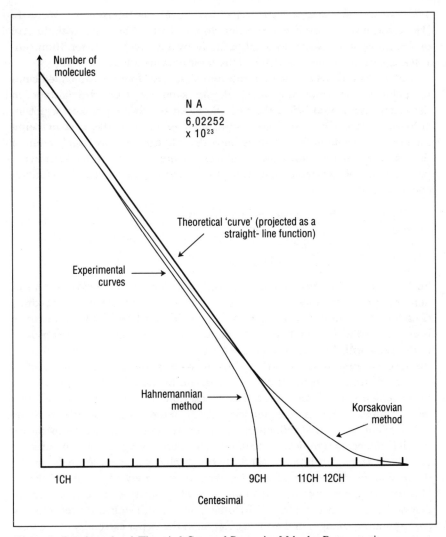

Figure 6: Experimental and Theoretical Curves of Progressive Molecular Deconcentrations

deconcentration than theoretically perceived, whereas the Korsakovian process will allow for a much slower deconcentration after the fifth centesimal attenuation and only permit an asymptotic-curve approach toward the zero number of molecules. Figure 6 portrays this visually.

Experimental Evidence (Second part)

In 1983 the Deutsche Homöopathie-Union [DHU][1] published

[1] Deutsche Homöopathie-Union, Wissenschaftliche Abteilung, Postfach 410280, D-7500 Karlsruhe 41, Germany.

Wirkungsnachweis homöopathischer Arzneien durch thermographische Messungen [Demonstration of the Effectiveness of Homoeopathic Medicines with the Aid of Thermographic Mensurations], a study by Prof Arno Rost of Tübingen, FRG, begun in September 1977. This is summarized here.

Any medicine ought to be both safe and effective. Homoeopathic medicines in potency are generally accepted as safe, as they are always in deconcentrations well below the toxic doses known to pharmacology. Yet on account of this same fact, they were often accused in the past of being ineffective placebos at best. The perhaps absurd, though grave, implication of this, namely that homoeopaths had consistently, and possibly knowingly, purveyed ineffective medication for the last two centuries, had to be irrefutably countered:

a) with a repeatable clinical method that was
b) statistically significant, as well as
c) placebo-controlled, and
d) in the form of a double-blind trial.

Such a trial would, once and for all, need to demonstrate the effectiveness of homoeopathic medicines, particularly in deconcentrations beyond Avogadro's (Loschmidt's) number. The experimental model developed by Rost has since been repeated with a number of other homoeopathic agents, but was originally undertaken with Veratrum album, which has a significant reactive effect on the circulatory system according to the materia medica. The work of E Schwamm[1] and others was used as the basis for the points of thermoregulation measurements on man. As a homoiothermic organism, man has two temperatures. One is the nucleic (core) temperature, which remains independent of external influences; the other is the body's shell temperature which is subject to significant fluctuations. The unvarying nucleic temperature can be measured on humans (and at comparable points on animals) at the depression in the centre of the forehead immediately above the glabella. Changes in the circulatory function have empirically been established by Schwamm, and since confirmed by others, as most prominently reflected by corresponding changes in thermoregulation at the upper extremity of the nose between the two orbits, namely the radix nasi. Because of its constancy the glabella temperature is taken as the reference temperature in thermography. In individuals with a healthy circulatory system the radix nasi temperature equals the glabella reference temperature. Whenever the former temperature registers below the reference temperature, a circulatory instability or insufficiency is invariably ascertainable by standard cardiological investigations. It was considered that if a defective circulatory system produced a lowering of the radix nasi temperature, then a homoeopathic agent that is said to stimulate a reactive correction affecting the circulatory system ought quickly to bring that temperature up to reference level.

[1]Schwamm, E. 'Thermoregulation und Thermodiagnostik'. *Physikalische Medizin und Rehabilitation*, 1968, vol IX, pp 130-138.

Ambient temperature was stabilized and all the normal precautions affecting probands, experimenters and equipment (contact temperature gauge 'Erti HTM 534' accurate to 1/20 degree Celsius) were observed. Temperature measurements occurred at one minute intervals, preceded by three pre-medication mensurations. One minute after the administration of Veratrum album 3D there consistently was in the radix nasi temperature reading a measurable approximation to, and two minutes after an equalization with, the reference temperature. Exactly the same results were obtained with Veratrum album 12D. Since Avogadro's (Loschmidt's) number is at 23D, this experiment was continued with Veratrum album 30D, which is an ultra-molecular (infinitesimal) deconcentration. The results were again exactly as for the 3D and the 12D dynamizations. To establish whether the dilute alcohol in the Veratrum album drops administered was perhaps responsible for this favourable effect, exactly this potentized alcohol, though unmedicated, was administered after the third pre-medication measurement, after which a further three measurements were taken, followed by the ultra-molecular Veratrum album 30D. The result was that one minute after the administration of the unmedicated potentized dilute alcohol the radix nasi temperature dropped still further (deterioration also occurred with placebo controls). However, three minutes after the introduction of the Veratrum album 30D into such 'alcoholized' probands there again was an equalization with the reference temperatures. Identical probands were given different potencies (i.e. 3D, 12D or 30D) on different days, always with favourable results. Probands without any problems in their circulatory system, who, of course, showed identical readings at the two temperature measuring points, were also given Veratrum album and no change in the readings followed. Where stress was put on the circulatory system of such healthy probands, by having them inhale the tobacco smoke of one cigarette, the two equal temperature readings moved apart, with the radix nasi dropping below the reference reading; to be equalized again in about 2.5 minutes after the administration of Veratrum album 30D.

It is to be emphasized that these experiments yielded statistically significant results. They all, in fact, produced the same results, except when the circulatory defect involved severe arterial hypertension, to which condition, at any event, Veratrum album is not homoeopathic. Here another indicated homoeopathic drug in a 30D potency once again produced the above results. By means of these experiments, which are clinically exact, readily reproducible and conclusive, the effectiveness of homoeopathic remedies in the ultra-molecular potency range have been experimentally proven on human beings. This was done in a manner analogous to the way homoeopathic drugs undergo pathogenetic experimentation (provings).

Two rather useful text-books on the subject of dynamization procedures are:

Hilfsbuch für Apotheker zum Potenzieren und Taxieren homöopathischer und biochemischer Arzneimittel, 2nd edition, by Alfred Reder, Ulm – Donau: Karl F Haug Verlag, 1958, 55 pp.

A Treatise on Homoeopathic Pharmacy (for Diploma and Degree Students) [prescribed by Calcutta University for BMS degree course students], by N K Banerjee and N Sinha, Calcutta: Dr (Mrs) Kamala Banerjee, 1980 (2nd edition), 182 pp.

(See 'Drug Preparation', 'Drug Strength', 'Hempel, Charles Julius (1811-1879)', 'Potency', 'Potentization', 'Solvation Structures', 'Succussion' and 'Trituration'.)

Poultice

Cataplasm; a soft mass of absorbent materials moistened by homoeopathically medicated fluids, usually applied warm to the surface to be treated. It exerts a soothing and at the same time homoeopathically counter-stimulant effect upon underlying tissues and their skin cover.

Pox

Eruption, first papular then pustular, occurring in the drug pathogenesis of Antimonium tartaricum, just as in smallpox and cowpox.

Precautions With Homoeopathic Drugs

See 'Homoeopathic Practice'.

Precipitating Factors

See 'Aetiotropism'.

Precipitation

Process by which a solution or liquid suspension forces a solute that had previously been held in a liquid vehicle to be eliminated as an accretion of itself, re-forming as solid matter out of solution. Analogous to, but not to be confused with, this solid-from-liquid process is the liquid-from-gases process, known as condensation, which is used in distillation.

Pregnancy

Gravidity; gestation; state of a female from conception to delivery. Unlike many phytopharmaca and almost all orthodox medicines, homoeopathic medicines in potency are quite safe to administer during pregnancy. All the normal criteria apply in selecting a like-drug for a gravida. In addition to 'euthenic (nosode) treatment' as a prophylactic for the growing foetus, the mother will need to have nutrients available for the offspring. Therefore, the homoeopath will advise her on a diet, with a probable emphasis on foods mentioned below. This is generally preferred in homoeopathy to the prescription of a quantity of mineral and vitamin tablets.

a) Iron: found in black pudding, liver and offal;

b) Folic acid: found in leafy green vegetables & liver;

c) Calcium: found in legumes, sardines and almonds;

d) Vit. A: found in fish liver oils, cream, beet greens, spinach, broccoli and carrots;

e) Vit. C (helps with iron, amino acid & calcium absorption): found in green peppers, guavas, citrus, blackcurrants, rose hips, strawberries & acerola cherries;

f) Vit. D: found in sunlight on the skin, fish liver oils and leafy green vegetables.

Special Note: Care must be taken with the micronutrient vitamin A, which is also present in liver and some offal, since it can sometimes cause hereditable miasmatic defects in the offspring if consumed in ponderal doses during gestation by the mother.

Some homoeopathic medicines that often suggest themselves during pregnancy are:

Bryonia alba: Constipated with dry, hard stool with perhaps a slight headache;

(Cephaelis) Ipecacuanha: Uninterrupted nausea that is not relieved by vomiting, diarrhoea, and sharp cramplike attacks of abdominal pains near the navel;

Nux vomica: Often feeling that some stool is left behind, after defaecation, and sour eructation, indigestion or heartburn, with nausea that is relieved by vomiting;

Pulsatilla nigricans: Weepiness, mood swings, comforting sought, absence of thirst, nausea with very little vomiting; improvement from fresh air;

Sepia officinalis: Heaviness, sluggishness, ineffectual defaecatory urgings, nausea aggravated by thought or smell of food, though eating may ameliorate the nausea, sinking sensation in solar plexus, milky water brought up, indifference to children, parents, family in general and her husband.

Two works of reference on the subject are:

Repertory of Pregnancy, Parturition and Puerperium by Alberto Soler-Medina (Heidelberg: Karl F Haug Verlag, 1989, 79 pages).

Homöopathie in Frauenheilkunde und Geburtshilfe By Erwin Schlüren (Heidelberg: Karl F Haug Verlag, 1980, 211 pages); it is conveniently divided into ten thumb-indexed sections.

(See 'Antenatal Homoeopathy', 'Euthenic (Nosode) Treatment', 'Gynaecology' and 'Obstetrics and Homoeopathy'.)

Preparation of Homoeopathic Medicines

See 'Drug Preparation' and 'Potentizing Methods'.

Prescribing

Giving directions, either in a written formula or orally, for the preparation, dispensing and administration of any remedy to be used in homoeopathic treatment.

Two basic rules are considered by the homoeopath when prescribing. These are:

i) A prescription can only be made on those signs and symptoms which have their counterparts, or close semblances, in the materia medica. The only exceptions would be certain prescriptions based on some isopathic considerations, or some very rare instances (terminal illness, emergencies), when enantiopathic treatment may be advisable.

ii) A prescription is to be aimed at the functional, dynamic process, rather than at any tangible lesion or gross pathological product.

There are five different ways in which a homoeopathic remedy (in any standard form) may be prescribed:

1 Sequentially, with potency unaltered – a single remedy in an unchanging potency is all that is given (the simillimum); as presenting symptoms change so this remedy may be withdrawn and replaced by another single remedy with constant potency, but only after a full re-assessment of the disease picture.

2 Sequentially, with potency variation – same as in 1) above, but the potency may be increased or decreased, once or several times, as considered advisable.

3 Concurrently and sequentially – as in drainage, where a deep-acting remedy is administered as in 1) above, along with two or more other pathological remedies that may be changed as the objective and subjective symptom totality changes.

4 Concurrently, or in combination – three or four remedies are administered together, or prescribed in a previously prepared combination such as 'M.A.P.' (a combination of three potentized fungi – see this entry), or 'ABC 30CH' (= Aconitum napellus 30CH + [Atropa] Belladonna 30CH + [Matricaria] Chamomilla 30CH, as dispensed by the Royal London Homoeopathic Hospital for many childhood ills).

5 Alternately – two (or three, or four) remedies are administered in alternation, with a fixed mandatory time interval (from 15 minutes to many hours) between the application of each different remedy.

(See 'Dosage', Dose' and 'Dose Repetition'.)

Prescription Errors

The inappropriate homoeopathic remedy generally fails to elicit any response in the patient. Since there are no side-effects, no direct harm can have been inflicted medicinally. However, there are rare occasions when there is a patient who happens to be particularly sensitive to the remedy given, which may produce a very active response (in itself, no danger, nor really homoeopathically undesirable, but anxiety-inducing for the patient). Such a remedy may just be bringing to the surface previously suppressed symptoms. The effects of such a remedy are easily antidoted by its opposite (listed in the materia medica) or, in many instances, by Sulphur 6CH, three times daily until the reaction subsides. (See 'Antidote' and 'Miasma'.)

Press

See 'Utensils of Homoeopathic Pharmacy'.

Prevention

Disordered functions, organic changes or other objective symptoms are preceded by a subjective alteration in the patient's mind, intellect or emotions. Homoeopathic prevention consists in treating according to the subjective sensations in order to forestall the changes in structure and function occurring. Other aspects of prevention are discussed under 'Euthenic (Nosode) Treatment', 'Foods as Health Problems', 'Immunization and Homoeopathy' and 'Isopathy'. (See also 'Homoeopathic Laws, Postulates and Precepts' 12 and 13(a) & (b).)

Primacy

The state of being foremost in significance, as constitutional propensity is taken to be in relation to environmental influence.

Probabiliorism

The philosophical principle according to which that side on which the evidence preponderates is held to be more probably right and, therefore, ought to be followed. (To obviate any misconception it must be distinguished from the very different philosophical theory of probabilism which holds that there is no absolutely certain knowledge, but that there may just be enough grounds for belief in the pursuit of one's practical life.) Probabilis, -e, is the Latin adjective for credible, likely, commendable, or that which may be proved or believed; probabilior is the second degree of comparison of that adjective; hence, more credible, more likely, etc. Since Empirical Medicine (of which homoeopathy is taken to be the ultimate scientific development) relies on practical experience as a guide to practice, and forms its opinions 'a posteriori', it is philosophically strongly inclined toward this philosophical principle. Historically this is seen to have been true as well. By contrast, Rationalist Medicine adopted determinism instead. Examples of the two philosophical guiding principles as applied are juxtaposed below in just three randomly chosen areas of science, though similar comparisons could validly be made for every area of science:

Probabilioristic influence and its effects	Deterministic influences and its effects

Ecology

Ecologists look very closely at equations that entomologists use to describe population fluctuations, finding that these show an unbelievable variety of dynamical patterns of behaviour, a diversity much richer than ever could have been assumed under determinism. Ecologists do not artificially distinguish between 'environmental distractions' and a 'constant signal', believing this deterministic custom leads inevitably to incorrect population forecasts.	Ecologists tacitly assume that the effects regulating the population density of an insect species, without other factors intervening, would maintain a population at a steady level, and that irregularities in fluctuations are due to unforeseen ups and downs in so many environmental influences. Analyses of population dynamics attempt to extract a constant signal from the overlay of environmental distractions.

Astronomy

Astronomers believe that at least some satellites and a few planets may be distinctly non-spherical, their rotation asynchronous, their orbit irregular, have their spin axis not fixed, or two orbits may have a resonant relationship, this and other imponderables leading to repeated destabilizing configurations, all of which produces instability, making complete predictability illusory.	Astronomers believe in the absolute immutability of the orbits of the planets and their satellites in this solar system, making it completely predictable.

Chemistry

Ilya Prigogine, the Nobel laureate from Brussels, Belgium demonstrated in 1968 that so very many chemical reactions happen in conditions far from thermodynamic equilibrium and that, as held by probabiliorism, there is much oscillation and chaos in inorganic chemistry, putting severe limits to predictability in chemical dynamics.	Chemists believe that the course of a chemical reaction is always predictable under conditions of thermodynamic equilibrium, where the reaction's products have lower energy than the starting materials.

Uncertainty in the predictions of quantum mechanics are not seen in probabiliorism as indefiniteness or arbitrariness of the laws of nature. Probabiliorism's hallmark is its open recognition that nature is so constituted that too close a specification of certain parameters cannot be achieved by any realizable process of measurement. The science of Empirical Medicine is based on this too, and its flowering, homoeopathy, has incorporated the concepts of contingency and particularity into its scientific therapeutics. (See 'Determinism', 'Empirical Medicine', 'Hahnemann, Christian Friedrich Samuel (1755-1843)', 'Heuristic Thinking', 'Philosophical Premise of Homoeopathy', 'Rationalist Medicine' and 'Science'.)

Processing of Homoeopathic Drugs

See 'Drug Preparation' and 'Potentizing Methods'.

Prognosis

Forecast of the probable course and/or outcome of a disease process in a particular patient.

(See also 'Diagnosis'.)

Proof Spirit

A mixture of water and alcohol (ethanol) that contains a standard proportion of the latter. In the UK and most of the (former) British Commonwealth countries proof spirit must have, at 10.5 degrees Celsius, twelve-thirteenths of the weight of an equal volume of distilled water. At 15.5 degrees Celsius this mixture contains 49.3% by weight, and 57.1% by volume, of alcohol. In the USA proof spirit must contain 50% by volume of alcohol, having a specific gravity of 0.7939 at 15.5 degrees Celsius. Water-ethanol mixtures that have a greater alcoholic strength are said to be 'over-proof' and those having less are described as 'under-proof'. (See 'Alcohol'.)

Prophylactic Treatment

Therapeutic intervention to prevent disease. (See 'Bowel Nosodes', 'Epidemiology', 'Euthenic (Nosode) Treatment', 'Immunization and Homoeopathy', 'Isopathy', 'Miasma' and 'Prevention'.)

Proto-History of Homoeopathy

See 'Philosophical Premise of Homoeopathy'.

Proto-History of Isopathy

See 'Isopathy'.

Protoplasm

Living matter; the material of which plant and animal tissues are formed. Functional protoplasm, referred to as kinetoplasm, however, denotes the chromophil substance in nerve cells that is only present when these begin to perform their proper function, and also refers to the most contractile part of the cell. Totipotential protoplasm is the phrase used to describe living matter with the least noticeable structural differentiation but with a greatest potential capability for self-differentiation, being capable of development into a complete organ or embryo, meaning that all cell organs are formable by it.

Prover

Proband (see 'Pathogenetic Experiment').

Proving

See 'Pathogenetic Experiment'.

Provitamin

Precursor substance convertible into a vitamin. (See 'Vitamin'.)

Pseudo-Psora

See 'Miasma'.

Pseudo-Psoric Miasma

See 'Miasma'.

Psionic Medicine

System of medicine aiming to get at the fundamental causes of disease by esoteric means; devised by George Laurence, an English surgeon, who was joined in 1968 by a number of others, all from an orthodox medical background. Yet, it is as foreign to orthodox medicine as parapsychology is to behaviourism. Psionic Medicine employs radiaesthesia, dowsing and similar techniques as diagnostic and healing aids, to harness a higher level of intuition or 'aetheric force', attempting by such means to determine acquired or inherited influences affecting the patient. With regard to the latter source of influence, Psionic Medicine has adopted the Hahnemannian concept of miasmata, placing particular emphasis on the luetic and the tuberculinic miasmata and their hereditability. It also postulates the unitary concept of disease, which homoeopathy favours. A group of not more than fifty, worldwide, make up the Psionic Medical Society. Their members maintain that Psionic Medicine is an extension of Hahnemannian homoeopathy, though there is no obvious historical evidence for this. Notwithstanding this, Psionic Medicine would seem to have an obvious affinity with bio-resonance therapy. (See 'Bio-resonance Therapy', 'Disease' and 'Miasma'.)

Psora

See 'Miasma'.

Psoric Miasma

See 'Miasma'.

Psychodynamics in Homoeopathy

See 'Mental Disease, Homoeopathic Assessment of'.

Psychological Commitment in Homoeopathic Practice

See 'Commitment to Homoeopathy'.

Psychotherapy

Treatment of mental and emotional disease conditions in patients through the medium of communication (whether verbal or non-verbal) rather than by, or as a complement to, the dynamically equilibrating treatment of homoeopathy. Some of the many variations in psychotherapeutic input are categorized by their descriptive labels listed here: anaclitic; autonomous; communal; contractual; directive; existential; family; group; heteronomous; hypnotic; intensive; nondirective; psychoanalytic (Adlerian, Freudian, Jungian); psychosynthetic; social; suggestive; supportive; and transactional. There is another form, orthomolecular psychotherapy, which is the only form where the therapeutic communication is augmented by a dietary attempt to correct suspected nutritional deficiencies of the normal chemical constituents of the patient's central nervous system. (For brief historical comment on homoeopathy's pioneering contributions to psychology as a natural science, refer to 'Raue, Carl Gottlieb (1820-1896)'.)

Q

Quackery

Charlatanry. From the perspective of the user of this word, it describes a false claim to competence in the medical discipline taken as authentic. From homoeopathy's viewpoint, it indicates fraud through claims to cure disease without adequate knowledge of scientific homoeopathy, or by employing inappropriate procedures, secret nostrums, ineffectual therapeutic or diagnostic machines, and similar pretensions.

Quantity and Quality in Homoeopathic Medication

The well-known apologist for homoeopathy of the first half of the twentieth century, Charles Edwin Wheeler (1868-1946), had the following to say on this subject in his lecture delivered on the 8th October 1937 in the Great Hall, British Medical Association, Tavistock House, London:

> 'It is well known that different drugs in poisonous doses affect human bodies with characteristic differences. Each has its own symptom picture, as well defined as that of any natural disease. When these drug symptom pictures are known in detail, it is rare indeed to find a case of disease that does not resemble one or other of them. The one that has the closest likeness, the simillimum, is the drug which the homoeopathist looks for and uses. An obvious corollary to this doctrine is that drugs must be systematically tested on human beings in order to elicit their symptom complexes. A less obvious corollary is that the similar remedy is best given in a small dose. . . . Many – most homoeopathists use very small, actually infinitesimal, doses but the principle of homoeopathy is applicable with any range of dosage. Hahnemann tested it and confirmed his belief in it for ten years with doses not far removed from those of ordinary practice and no scholar needs reminding that homoeopathic does not mean infinitesimally small.'[1]

The discovery by Hahnemann, though, of the biphasic action of medicines actually makes the situation more complicated than Wheeler's presentation might lead one to assume. Hahnemann discovered that any medicine provokes two more or less opposite effects, in succession, in any one person, whether patient or prover. The primary symptoms are those due to the coercive, immediate drug action proper, the secondary symptoms (quasi opposing the primaries) represent the corrective reaction by the organism to that coercive onslaught. To some extent these two effects are a function of the size of the dose administered.[2]

[1] Wheeler, Charles Edwin. *A Hundred Years of Homoeopathy*, London: The British Homoeopathic Association, 1937, p 4.
[2] Coulter, Harris Livermore. In his *Homoeopathic Science and Modern Medicine*, Berkeley, Ca: North Atlantic Books, 1981, he discusses the issues surrounding the biphasal action of medicines against their full scientific and historical background in chapter 4, pp 34-42.

It fell to Georg H G Jahr (1800-1875) to discover that patient susceptibility to a drug conforms to the rule that the clearer and more positively any finer, or peculiar, or even any characteristic symptoms of a remedy are evident in a patient the higher the degree of receptivity that may be anticipated to that medicine, and, hence, the higher the potency of choice is likely to be. Jahr further observed that while there is no change in a drug's homoeopathicity as it is taken from crude substance, through the low potencies, beyond Avogadro's number, to the high potencies, there is a subtle change along the way. It is not in the drug's strength or weakness, it is in the development of the drug's peculiarities (away from the commoner symptoms) as it rises in the scale of dynamizations. (See 'Homoeopathic Laws, Postulates and Precepts', particularly sections 2 to 11, and 'Jahr, Georg Heinrich Gottlieb (1800-1875)'.)

Quantum

General term for the indivisible unit of any form of physical energy (e.g. the unit of electro-magnetic radiation energy, the photon, the magnitude of which depends on frequency only; similarly: graviton, magnon, phonon, and roton, some of which are hypothetical units). More popularly it refers to an interval on a measuring scale, the fractions of which are considered irrelevant.

Quantum Physics and Homoeopathy

See 'Eclipse of Homoeopathy (1920-1965)' and 'Epistemological Assumptions in Homoeopathy', sections 1 and 2.

Quarantine

Restriction placed on the movements of individuals, or the imposition of isolation on them, associated with a case of communicable disease; location or period of detention (previously 40 days) of ships, or imported animals or fomites, coming from infected, or suspect, ports. (See 'Verdi, Dr Tullio Suzzara (1829-1902)'.)

Quarin, Dr Joseph Baron von (1733-1814)

Hahnemann's most influential teacher. In the area that was to become unified Germany about a century later, Leipzig University was the most famous and the most frequented medical school at the time Hahnemann was a student there (1775-1777). Yet it could offer him no more than scholastic book-knowledge of medicine, as it lacked any clinical or hospital facilities to provide any hands-on medical experience to students.

Hahnemann resolved to continue his studies at the University of Vienna, as there was the Leopoldstädter Hospital run by the Brothers of Mercy, where its Medical School (founded 1365) provided a large measure of clinical experience to students (Gerhard van Swieten, as director of Vienna's Medical Faculty from 1749 to 1753, had revolutionized the teaching of medicine by introducing the novel concept of holding lectures at the side of the sick-bed). This Medical School was subsequently under the direction of Dr Quarin, then forty-four years old, who was the physician-in-ordinary to the Empress Maria Theresa, and later also to the Emperor Joseph II. Quarin, in the prime of life, personally produced the plans for the General Hospital of Vienna (built in 1784), which was far ahead of its time, with an attached maternity home, a nursing home for foundlings, and a separate lunatic asylum (the 'Narrenturm'). This has remained in service for more then two centuries since, and was for a long time unsurpassed in size and excellence anywhere in Europe.

It was intellectually a very fertile environment for Hahnemann. Some of the famous men directly or indirectly associated with Quarin's Vienna General Hospital were: the great anatomist Karl Baron von Rokitansky (1804-1878); the naturopath who originated the modern hydrotherapy later adopted by the hospital ('genius of the cold waters') Vinzenz Priessnitz (1799-1851); the clinician who perfected auscultatory percussion Joseph Skoda (1805-1881); the forerunner of modern psychiatry Ernst Baron von Feuchtersleben (1806-1849); the early dermatologist Ferdinand Ritter von Hebra (1816-1880); and the pioneering gynaecologist, Ignaz Philipp Semmelweis (1818-1865), who, in the 1840s, long before Joseph, Lord Lister's antisepsis and Robert Koch's bacteria, had empirically discovered that the contagion of puerperal fever was carried by the hands of doctors and students from the dissected cadavers to the genitalia of parturients and who, therefore, introduced compulsory hand-washing with a chloride solution in the hospital; this met with implacable opposition. After many years of campaigning in Vienna, the foremost German obstetrician came to Austria to conduct a personal survey of comparative results between the death rates ascribable either to 'no hand-washing' or to 'hand-washing with the chloride solution'. Although the death rate was 27% for the former and only 0.23% for the latter, he said he 'could see nothing' in it, and suggested people should not wash their hands to excess, and that in puerperal fever more purging and blood-letting was far more effective and certainly safer.[1] Finally in 1865, with his mind clouded in the fullness of despair, Semmelweis felt he had to prove it conclusively to the unbelieving world at large through infecting a scratch on his own finger, which 'proof' consequently cost him his life.

Hahnemann, whose unusual intellectual potential Quarin recognized immediately, became the latter's protegé. Although he was a Protestant, he was given preferential treatment at the teaching hospital run by the Catholic Order of the Brothers of Mercy. Quarin, the medical director of the hospital and six times elected Rector of Vienna University, treated the student

[1] Glasscheib, H S. *The March of Medicine*, translated from the German. London: Macdonald & Co (Publishers) Ltd, 1963, p 105.

Hahnemann almost as a friend and certainly as an intellectual equal. He took him on his rounds in the hospital, even to his private patients (i.e. the nobility) and he also allowed him to assist him in his private practice. This happened neither before nor has it since to any other student. He did this knowing quite well that the Saxon pupil could not pay him a single Kreuzer. All other students always had to pay full tuition fees at the hospital. In this way Hahnemann acquired the fullest and best of practical medical education of the time, which was entirely missed by those colleagues he was destined to come across in later life who had taken their degree in nothing but sterile medical dogma at Leipzig, or at other universities like it, without acquiring any clinical experience.

By August 1777 Hahnemann's meagre savings of 68 Gulden with which he had come to Vienna had been consumed by the cost of lodgings and general living expenses. The attentive Dr von Quarin seemed to sense the problem straight away, since exactly then he procured for Hahnemann the well-paid job of becoming assistant to Samuel von Bruckenthal (curiously, also a native Saxon and a Protestant). This man was the Imperial-Royal Austro-Hungarian Governor of Transylvania. Hahnemann was to put order in the Governor's very extensive library and in his numismatic collection, while at the same time – though not yet fully qualified – he was to act, as indeed he did, as family physician. Quarin's high esteem of Hahnemann can be gauged against this extraordinary fact.

On the protracted journey to their destination which was Hermannstadt in Transylvania (now Sibiu, Rumania) they traversed Raab (now Györ, Hungary), Komorn (also Gomorrn, now split into Komarno in Czechoslovakia and Komarom in Hungary), Maria-Theresiopel (now Subotica, Yugoslavia), Temeschwar (now Timisoara, Rumania) and Karlsburg (now Alba Iulia, Rumania), areas in most of which quartan fever was then extremely common. This gave Hahnemann the authority, based on first-hand medical knowledge in this field, to enable him, thirteen years later, to make his momentous contradiction of Cullen's views on Cinchona in the translation (in 1790) of *A Treatise on the Materia Medica*. (See also 'Hahnemann, Christian Friedrich Samuel (1755-1843)'.)

Questionnaires

Printed questionnaires occasionally given to patients prior to the homoeopathic consultation generally rely on direct, either/or questions (e.g. the presence or the absence of symptoms). Their value is greatly diminished through inherent defects. Questionnaires cannot encompass all possible ailments; they fail to distinguish between the significant symptom and those that are less so; they cannot identify the degree of emphasis given to a symptom by the patient, nor its subtler relationship to other problems. In the standard history-taking it is the homoeopath who interprets and decides on the weighting to be given to a symptom, based on his judgement of the patient's personality, mode of expression, physical symptoms and many other factors. Though the questionnaire saves time, it creates misleading distortions. Skilled homoeopathic history taking, when the patient is first encouraged to describe his problem in his own words and thereupon freely questioned, cannot be replaced in this way. (See 'Diagnosis'.)

Quicksilver

Mercury; important metallic remedy.

Quin, Frederick Foster Hervey (1799-1878)

Outstanding English homoeopath who, later in his life, was openly revered by the French as Hahnemann's greatest successor. The measure of that intense reverence can be gauged from the following. The Gallic Homoeopathic Society gave Hahnemann a festive reception on his arrival in Paris in 1835. He and his wife were driven to the Society's assembly in two magnificent coaches and the white-haired Hahnemann was installed in the presidential chair by Dr Leon Simon, Master of the Council, after the following short speech by the Society's Chairman, Dr Pierre Dufresne:

> 'Hear, Gentlemen, hear, all ye inhabitants of Paris, what the philosopher wrote when he so well described your customs and institutions: "When will there come a noble and far-seeing man, who will re-open the temple of old Aesculapius, who will smash to pieces the dangerous instruments, will close the apothecaries' shops and destroy this hypothetical medicine with all its remedies and fastings? What friend of man will preach in the end a new science of healing, since the old one is killing mankind and depopulating districts and countries?" Behold! There is the man! He is presiding over your Society. His name impresses me to silence. He is supreme above all praise.'[1]

The Society then elected Hahnemann as Honorary President for life and he was always to take that seat of honour, whenever he could attend at meetings, with the further proviso that in his absence, his seat must always remain unoccupied. After Hahnemann's death this same honour was bestowed upon Quin, the English homoeopath so fervently admired by the French. What extraordinary quality did Quin possess to evoke such endearment?

Quin, a graduate from Edinburgh in 1820 (his thesis was on arsenic), is said to have been the grandson of the famous Earl-Bishop of Bristol, Frederick August Hervey. He was a talented linguist, apparently speaking French better than his native English. While he was resident and practising medicine in Naples among the British community there, he attended, together with the Comte des Guidi from France, the clinic at the Ospedale della Trinita run by

[1] Haehl, Richard. *Samuel Hahnemann: His Life and Work*. 2 vols, London: Homoeopathic Publishing Co, 1922, vol I, pp 232-233.

Romani and de Horatiis, demonstrating the new scientific method in medicine. That was early in 1826. Quin's attention had, however, already been drawn to homoeopathy earlier by Dr Georg Necker, who from 1825 onward had kept him regularly supplied with writings on the subject. Quin had to acknowledge that, over a period of years, all those patients who had turned from orthodox treatment to homoeopathy consistently achieved better results. He finally decided that the new therapeutic system deserved serious investigation. After attending the clinic his favourable impression was further strengthened. He then resolved to go to Leipzig to make an in-depth study of homoeopathy. Before setting out, however, he studied the new scientific system privately at a prodigious rate, putting in nine uninterrupted hours every day. He managed to master the new theory and many of the ramifications of its application. He spent a little time in Venice, Trieste and Vienna on the way to Leipzig, arriving at his destination in July 1826. After the Leipzig lecture course he visited Johan Ernst Stapf (1788-1860) in Naumburg an der Saale, Prussia, followed by a ten-day stay with Samuel Hahnemann himself in Coethen, Duchy of Anhalt. After all this the careful Quin was at least intellectually convinced that the new system of medicine had absolute scientific merit. Yet the event that is regarded as the precise time of his total conversion to the new method occurred in 1831, when he was touring through Austria, and was struck down in Tischnowitz, Moravia, by the Asiatic Cholera epidemic then raging across Europe. He was there cured homoeopathically (see 'Cholera Epidemics'), which then utterly convinced him of the evident value of Hahnemann's medical method.

He returned to London in 1832 and set up in homoeopathic practice at 19 King Street. All medical opinion was immediately ranged against him. His success in treatment was such that he became well known. He came under personal attack from medical journals, which called his qualification into question. The animosity that his successes aroused reached such a pitch that the Censors of the Royal College of Physicians challenged Quin by notice imputing he was practising illegally in the London area. Quin decided to ignore this harassment. He responded to the more menacing follow-up notice, simply and with dignity, saying he had not replied to the first, since he did not think the situation applied to himself. Thereupon the matter was dropped. It was Quin's way always to return vindictive scorn with good-natured humour. During his long homoeopathic career this very charming man was always very scrupulous, never giving any ground for complaint. His high social qualities, good connections and his undoubted homoeopathic ability, his abundant enthusiasm and energy, coupled with his extensive general knowledge made him the best advocate of the new medical system in the conservative British environment. He gradually gathered colleagues around himself and twelve years later (in 1844), with seven like-minded homoeopaths he founded the British Homoeopathic Society. This continued to meet monthly from the date of its formation. Quin was constantly re-elected to its presidency until his death. From 1852 to 1864 Quin, assisted by Drs Leadham and Russell, provided lecture courses at the London Homoeopathic Hospital, which courses later (finally in 1877, at the instance and by the efforts of Dr Bayes) became the London School of Homoeopathy (now the Faculty).

It was due to Quin's insistence and his vision that the homoeopathic dispensary of his close friend Paul Curie ultimately became the spot where the London Homoeopathic Hospital was constructed in 1850. Undoubtedly it was the high regard in which members of the Curie family were held in France that contributed to Quin's being seen in a favourable light by the French homoeopaths. But it was certainly the tact, sagacity, truthfulness and total devotion to the homoeopathic cause that earned this charming man their admiration in the fullness in which it was expressed. (See also 'History of Homoeopathy before 1900', section on United Kingdom.)

Quincke's Oedema

Giant urticaria. (See 'Emergencies – Homoeopathic Treatment', section Angioneurotic Oedema.)

Quinquagenimillesimal Scale of Dynamization

Fifty millesimal potency; LM potency scale; 50-milles dynamization; the only high potency devised by Hahnemann. (See 'Potentizing Methods'.)

R

Racemose

● **In a bunch.**

Found in the Latin form, 'racemosa', as part of various medicines in the homoeopathic materia medica. Epithet used of flowers or seeds, of plant growth, of cluster of berries or fruits, of compound glands: when in the form of a raceme, which is a cluster resembling a bunch of grapes or currants.

Rademacher, Johann Gottfried (1772-1850)

Although he was a virtual contemporary of Hahnemann, whose junior he was by only seventeen years, this physician was one of the more noteworthy proponents in the true Empirical tradition of pre-Hahnemannian medicine. Following in the line of Paracelsus and, to a lesser extent, Sydenham, he practised during his entire life in Goch, Rhineland, Western Prussia (a mere two kilometres from the Netherlands border). At the age of sixty-nine years (1841) this very able clinician published his accumulated, mature therapeutic observations in two volumes (over 800 pages each) in Berlin under the rather cumbersome title:

Rechtfertigung der von den Gelehrten misskannten, verstandesrechten Erfahrungsheillehre der alten scheidekünstigen Geheimärzte (Justification of the Empiric Medical Practice of the Alchemistic Physicians of old, Misjudged by the Learned, though Perfectly Rational).

Soon it was simply referred to as 'Rademacher's "Erfahrungsheillehre" (Rademacher's 'Medical Tenets Derived from Practical Experience"). This man's vast store of practical medical experience contained in the two massive German volumes, caused a stir in medical circles. The publication went through four editions in the short space of five years, and influenced homoeopathic thinking to some extent for several generations. For instance, the prolific homoeopathic writer James Compton Burnett (1840-1901) dedicated his *Diseases of the Liver,* published in 1890, 'To the Memory of Rademacher, the Resuscitator of Paracelsic Organopathy', although he knew quite well that Rademacher denied the homoeopathic law of similars. The *Erfahrungsheillehre* was substantially abridged and translated into English by A A Ramseyer of Salt Lake City, Utah, USA in 1909. Due to a recent moderate revival of interest in the concept of organ correspondences, his work is once again available under the title *Rademacher's Universal and Organ Remedies* (New Delhi: World Homoeopathic Links, reprint 1980, 104 pages). (See 'Organotherapy' and 'Philosophical Premise of Homoeopathy' under Philippus Aureolus Paracelsus and Thomas Sydenham.)

Radaesthesia

See 'Psionic Medicine'.

Radiant State of Matter, Theory of

In the 1860s the equations of the Scottish physicist James Clerk Maxwell (1831-1879) led him to the unified electromagnetic field theory which elucidated the interaction between electromagnetic waves and matter and enabled electricity, magnetism and light to be brought within a broad mathematical framework. He also introduced the concept of fields, which the German-born scientist and mathematician Albert Einstein (1879-1955) later (in 1905) established to be non-material in nature.

Electromagnetic radiation describes the emission and propagation of energy from a source; it includes long (radio) waves, heat rays, the light spectrum, röntgen ('x-') rays and (hard) gamma-rays. In accordance with Maxwell's electromagnetic theory, all charged particles (electrons, protons, photons) when accelerated by application of electric fields emit (or absorb) electromagnetic radiation. According to the German physicist Max Planck (1858-1947) this radiation exists in the form of photons. This means that accelerated protons or electrons emit or absorb photons. In Maxwell's theory one charged particle attracts or repels another charged particle by first producing an electromagnetic field in the surrounding space, which in turn acts on the second charged particle.

The next landmark in elementary-particle physics' development was the product of the work of both the English mathematical physicist Paul Adrien Maurice Dirac (1902-1984) and the Austrian mathematical physicist Erwin Schrödinger (1887-1961), Nobel laureates both, which began in 1926 with the latter's discovery of the field equations which enabled most atomic properties to be calculated. Dirac, on the other hand, showed (from 1928) that all particles in nature exist in pairs; that to every particle there is a corresponding antiparticle of the same mass and spin but opposite charge. The proton's opposite became the antiproton, the electron's the positron. Dirac also showed that under suitable circumstances, a photon can 'materialize' into a pair of particles, consisting of an electron and a positron, or a proton and an antiproton; conversely an electron and a positron could, on collision, annihilate one another and both disappear, while surplus energy would appear in the form of photons – the stuff radiation consists of. Photons (electromagnetic waves), electrons, neutrinos, muons (discovered later) were all found to possess zero 'intrinsic' rest mass. The familiar Newtonian distinction between matter and energy had been completely obliterated and by then (up to about 1935) matter was taken to be in a 'radiant state'.[1]

---

[1]Close, Stuart. *The Genius of Homoeopathy: Lectures and Essays on Homoeopathic Philosophy* New York: Boericke and Tafel, 1924, pp 218-219.

Yet long before this, in the second half of the nineteenth century, the French homoeopath, Dr Ozanam, had already postulated the theory of the radiant state of matter to explain a variety of natural phenomena involving material, biological and other modifications

1) clearly produced by radiant energy, as in phototropism, photoperiodism, photosynthesis, radioanaphylaxis, or the heritable genetic changes in plants and animals brought on by ultra-violet or other radiation; and

2) those which are linked to the reactive effects observable in biophysics, as in the dynamics of blood flow, the electrical occurrences involved in nerve conduction and cardiac stimulation, the changes in osmosis, surface tensions, membrane potentials, and the altered organic response evident in biological functions, both to luminescence and to the pathogenetic action of the infinitesimal quantities of poison secreted by bacterial and other micro-organisms.

Up to about 1935 this explanation was occasionally invoked by apologists for homoeopathy to explain the mechanics of the homoeopathic effect, and concepts such as resonance or the physics of the infinitesimal. Yet some homoeopaths had thought the premise to be uncomfortably close to the position of the Rationalist tradition in medicine which derives its models for understanding disease from sciences outside of itself. That is why this argument has sometimes been deprecated as self-defeating by some homoeopaths. It must be pointed out, however, that such misgivings are unfounded in that this 'essentialistic' philosophical position could never have led either to 'a priori' diagnoses or to the determining of any therapeutic decision in homoeopathy.

The real defect in this theory is, simply, that it was philosophically 'essentialistic', offering, as it did, a final overall unconfirmed explanation, namely that everything can be said to be ultimately reducible to an electro-magnetic energy field. This was shown to be untenable from 1935 by the Japanese physicist (and Nobel laureate of 1949) Hideki Yukawa (born 1907) who predicted the existence of mesons and pointed out consequent inconsistencies in the 'radiant state of matter' theory. In 1947 Cecil F Powell actually discovered these mesons: unstable sub-atomic particles that were found to have a resting mass, which may be electrically charged or may be neutral. They were found to obey the law of conservation of parity and were certainly not merely an electromagnetic wave phenomenon. (See also Dr Ozanam in the section headed France in 'History of Homoeopathy before 1900', 'Laws of Nature', 'Rationalist Medicine' and 'Science and Homoeopathy' regarding 'essentialism' as a philosophical concept.)

Radionics

● **Machine-assisted disease divining.**

Non-homoeopathic method whereby the patient's problem is to be diagnosed using a dowsing technique, frequently assisted by a radionic machine. The medicine or treatment may also be decided by means of dowsing, and the drug might then be 'broadcast' to the patient with the aid of a radionic machine.

Radionics uses the dowsing methods with any medicine – orthodox pharmaceuticals, vitamin or mineral supplements, phytopharmaca ('herbals'), homoeopathic remedies, auto-isopathics, or any other. Occasionally remedy simulation is also done with the aid of a radionic machine whereby a targeted inert vehicle is to be transsubstantiated into the requisite medicinal agent. (See 'Bio-Resonance Therapy' and 'Remedy Simulation'.)

Raeside, John Robertson (1926-1971)

Scottish homoeopath and scientist, born and educated in Glasgow, who, throughout his life, admitted to a slight attraction to Rudolph Steiner's tenets as contained in Anthroposophical Medicine. He was first to become assistant to Dr Blackie at the Royal London Homoeopathic, Hospital. Later he became pre-eminent in homoeopathic research, where he undertook the provings of (pathogenetic experiments with) new remedies and reprovings of older ones. Details of publication of his major provings are:

Hirudo medicinalis *Brit Hom J,* 1964
Hydrophis cyanocinctus *Brit Hom J,* 1956
Lophophytum leandri *Brit Hom J,* 1969
Luffa operculata *Zeitschr f klassische Homöopathie,* 1965
Mandragora officinarum *Brit Hom J,* 1966
Mimosa pudica *Brit Hom J,* 1971
Penicillinum *Brit Hom J,* 1962
Selenium *Brit Hom J,* 1961
Tellurium *Allgemeine homöopathische Zeitung,* 1969
Triosteum perfoliatum *Brit Hom J,* 1960
Venus mercenaria *Brit Hom J,* 1962

He was tragically killed on Sunday, 18th June 1972 in British European Airways' Trident air disaster en route to the Brussels Congress of the Liga Medicorum Homoeopathica Internationalis. Also killed were the following who accompanied him:

Frederick W Adams, former Secretary and Registrar of the Pharmaceutical Society of Great Britain;
Dudley Wootton Everitt, homoeopathic pharmacist;
Miss E S Hawthorn, Matron of the Glasgow Homoeopathic Hospital;
and nine other homoeopaths:
Isabel Mackay Campbell
Marjorie Golomb
Sergei William Kadleigh
Ludi Marylone Kandalla
Kawther Teresa Kandalla
Joan Natalie Mackover
Mary Young McArthur Stevenson

Elizabeth Somerville Stewart
Thomas Fergus Stewart.

Ranking the Parallels in Symptom Complexes of Disease to Drug

See 'Disease and Drug Action in Homoeopathic Congruity'.

Rationalist Medicine

More correctly: the Rationalist tradition in medicine; derives its models for understanding disease and for determining therapy from systems, disciplines, sciences and paradigms outside of itself, even though these constantly change with time. Historically it has always represented the deterministic mainstream of Orthodox Medicine. Causal assumptions derived from elaborations in other sciences always form the 'a priori' basis in diagnosis, which, in turn, leads to determining therapeutics. By its adherents this is seen as scientific medicine. (See 'Determinism', 'Diagnosis', 'Empirical Medicine', 'Hahnemann, Christian Friedrich Samuel (1755-1843)', 'Philosophical Premise of Homoeopathy', 'Probabiliorism' and 'Vitalism'.)

Raue, Carl Gottlieb (1820-1896)

German homoeopath who became professor of Special Pathology and Therapeutics at the Hahnemann Medical College of Philadelphia, USA, and one of the three co-editors of Constantin Hering's *Guiding Symptoms of Our Materia Medica* upon the author's death in 1880. Some of his major writings are:
  Special Pathology and Diagnostics with Therapeutic Hints 1868
  Subjective and Objective Symptoms 1868
  Record of Homoeopathic Literature 1870-75
  A Memorial of Constantin Hering 1884
However, this man's eminence springs from his pioneering work in the area of psychology, where he was far ahead of his time. He published:
  Mental Symptoms in 1870
  Elements of Psychology in 1871
  Psychology as a Natural Science in 1889.
At that time psychology was still essentially a speculative philosophical discipline, which did not seek to verify its assertions experimentally. Only in 1879, well after Raue's first two books, did Wilhelm Wundt found the world's first laboratory for psychological research at the University of Leipzig, Saxony, Germany. Raue's psychological theories were grounded in homoeopathy's vitalism and as such characterized by the assumption of a non-material agency (dynamis) underlying vital phenomena. Yet as a man with an enquiring, scientific mind, he is said to have favoured phenomenological experimentation (at the Hahnemann Medical College) and to have viewed perceptual, mental

and behavioural processes as wholes and to have been treating them as such. He argued that it was not the task of science to fractionate experiences, stimuli, emotions, or the like, but always to see them together as a unique unitary group-relationship, just as the individual psychological patient does. He was effectively half a century, or more, ahead of: Kurt Lewin's 'Field Theory' (1919), Kurt Goldstein's 'Organismic Theory of Human Nature' (1939) and A H Maslow's 'Hierarchical Theory of Human Motivation' (1954) – some of the acknowledged landmarks of scientific advancement in the 'Gestalt' School of psychology.

Reactivity

The property, or process, of responding homoeopathically, chemically, physically, dynamically or in any other manner to a remedial impulse, an antidotal stimulant, or simply to an irritant, incentive, excitant, and the like.

Reappearance of (Suppressed) Symptoms

See 'Externalization of Disease', 'Relapse' and 'Response to Therapy, Deficient or Superabundant'.

Receptivity

See 'Altered Receptivity in Disease'.

Reciprocal Action, Law of

See the Law of Stimuli under 'Homoeopathic Laws, Postulates and Precepts', section 5 and the Law of Bioenergetic Drug Action in the same entry, section 2.

Recoveries Mistaken for Cures

See 'Remission, Spontaneous'.

Reductionism

The philosophical doctrine, closely allied with the mechanistic theory and atomism, in terms of which it is maintained that human behaviour can ultimately be reduced to the behaviour of inanimate matter, within the laws of nature. In biology the term stands for the tacit belief that all the phenomena of life's abundance can ultimately be understood in terms of physics and chemistry alone. The formula for setting up causal dependence through reductionism is an integral part of the Rationalist tradition of medicine and, therefore, of orthodox medicine whose motto remains 'tolle causam' (seek out the cause). In orthodox medicine the process of reducing disease in a patient to the simpler or clearer terms of its apparent cause validates therapy. Without this reductionist process no effective therapy is deemed to be possible within the paradigm of orthodox medicine. That is the deterministic position. In the Empirical tradition of medicine, which culminated in homoeopathy, the probabilioristic position is represented on this point, which states:

'It is seldom, if ever, between a consequent and a single antecedent that this invariable sequence subsists. It is usually between the consequent and the sum of several antecedents; the concurrence of all of them being requisite to produce, that is, to be certain of being followed by, the consequent. . . . The real cause is the whole of [such] antecedents, and we have no right, philosophically speaking, to give the name of the cause to one of them, exclusively of the others.'[1]

(See also 'Atomism', 'Determinism', 'Eclipse of Homoeopathy (1920-1965)', 'Holism', 'Laws of Nature', 'Probabiliorism' and 'Vitalism'.)

Reflexology

● **Foot (or hand) massage therapy and the science of untrained physiological reactions.**

The study of innate stereotypical responses to stimuli (called reflexes). The word was coined by the Russian, Dr Wladimir M von Bechterew (1857-1927), to express the thesis, later adopted as a keystone in Behaviourist psychology, that in principle all behaviour can be explained through the relayed working-together of relatively complex reflex arcs.[2] The distinctness of reflexes had been recognized in orthodox medicine as early as 1833,[3] but it was Osteopathy later in that century which defined a reflex arc as a functional unit of the central nervous system, the components of which include: afferent nerve fibres, sensory receptors, CNS reflex centres, efferent fibres, and effector organs; it is a mechanism that enables very quick, dynamic adjustment to the environment, where many combinations and degrees of complexity are possible. The autonomic reflexes regulate visceral functions automatically.[4]

However, reflexology (better would be 'reflex therapy') also describes what some would call a naturopathic therapeutic approach, and that a fair number of homoeopaths will accept as complementary. Its method, briefly, is the applying of pressure or suction at particular points, principally on the feet or hands, that is designed to stimulate healing processes in corresponding parts of the patient's body. It was introduced into Western Empirical medicine by

[1] Close, Stuart. *The Genius of Homoeopathy: Lectures and Essays on Homoeopathic Philosophy* New York: Boericke and Tafel, 1924, pp 267-268.
[2] Popper, Sir Karl R, and Sir John C Eccles. *Das Ich und sein Gehirn* Munich: R Piper GmbH & Co KG, 1987, p 174.
[3] Hall, H. 'On the Reflex Functions of the Medulla Oblongata and Medulla Spinalis' *Philosophical Transactions of The Royal Society,* London, 1833, pp 635-665.
[4] Hoag, J Marshall, Wilbur V Cole and Spencer G Bradford. *Osteopathic Medicine* St Louis: McGraw-Hill Book Co Inc, 1969, pp 87 & 88.

the otorhinolaryngologist William Fitzgerald in the USA, who found that by applying pressure to a certain area of the foot he was able to anaesthetize the ear, enabling him to perform minor ear surgery.

The reflex effect was evident. Occasionally, therefore, reflexology has been caricatured as an apocryphal form of specialized osteopathy, whereas at other times it is said to be a step-child of acupuncture, in that it is a form of acupressure. With Pratt's Method of orificial surgery it has even been named as a relation to surgery. There can be no doubt that this is an ancient form of treatment; both hand and foot reflexology are vividly depicted on an Egyptian wall-painting (dated around 2330 BC) in the tomb of the akhmahor (highest in rank after the pharaoh) in a funerary monument at Saqqara. Massage of pressure points in the feet was, moreover, a part of Chinese medicine at even an earlier time, and is also known to certain tribes in Africa and to some Amerindian nations. (See also 'Surgery', concerning Orificial Surgery.)

Regulation-Thermography

Diagnostic dermatic contact calorimetry. Skin surface temperature measurements (at Head's zones, for instance), taken with quick-response electronic thermometers before and after a low-temperature stimulus to the organism, register its homoeothermic regulatory response. This yields measurements that may permit of a variety of diagnostic conclusions. This process, which is considered to be compatible with clinical procedure by a number of homoeopaths, and which is considered to be particularly valuable in locating foci (see 'Focus'), has been extensively developed by Prof Arno Rost (born 1919) of Tübingen, Würtemberg, Germany. Valuable experimental work for homoeopathy was undertaken by Prof Arno Rost using regulation-thermography (see 'Potentizing Methods', under Experimental Evidence [Second Part]).

Relapse

● **A falling-back into illness, making the homoeopath perhaps look anew at the treatment approach used.**

Recurrence of disease after convalescence has begun. This may induce the homoeopath to modify the existing therapeutic programme, which may lead to the appraisal of the patient in line with the following seven considerations:

1 Is the patient undergoing a 'proving' of the particular remedy? If so, the medicine may be discontinued and the problem quickly disappears.
2 Is the patient experiencing what is described in the second part of the corollary of Hering's Rule of Disease Metastasis, viz. 'cure occurs from within outwards'? If so, the appearance of the symptoms is quasi-symbolic and will pass quickly enough without intervention; if not, a new deep-acting

remedy which also takes the new symptoms into account may have to be found and given.

3 Is there perhaps a miasma that has been overlooked? If so, the constitutional, or other, remedy may need to be replaced by the appropriate antimiasmatic drug.

4 Are there environmental or nutritional factors that were not eliminated? If so, they must be identified and, if possible, removed, with the remedial therapy remaining unaltered.

5 Was the prescription choice determined by the 'particulars' more than by the 'generals'? If so, this might need to be reversed and a fresh medicine chosen.

6 Was the drug right, but the level of dynamization perhaps wrong? If so, a different potency may be introduced.

7 Were there resistant peripheral (pathological) changes of long standing in a chronic disease, which have recurred because they now almost have a life of their own? If so, pathological prescriptions for each of these may be considered.

Relationship of Indicated Drug to Organic Need

See 'Altered Receptivity in Disease', 'Constitutional Type' section on Experimental Evidence, 'Heterostasis', 'Homoeopathy' and 'Homoeosis'.

Relative Density

See 'Specific Gravity'.

Relaxation Therapy

Naturopathic approach, complementary to homoeopathy, that strives to achieve abatement of intensity or vigour, a diminution of strictness or of energy dissipation, a physical slackening of fibres, ligaments or joints, and a turning away of the mind from severe application, as well as its release from ordinary tensions or exceptional cares. It is often aided by involving mesmerism (suggestion, hypnosis). (See 'Mesmerism' and 'Naturopath'.)

Remedial Effect, Evidence of

The effects of a medicine are evident from changes in the symptoms of the patient. Such changes may include:

i) production of new symptoms;
ii) disappearance of symptoms;
iii) aggravation of symptoms;
iv) amelioration of symptoms;
v) alteration in direction and order of symptoms.

(Implications inherent in each of these changes determines the further course of therapeutic action. These implications are discussed under 'Aggravation', 'Disease and Drug Action in Homoeopathic Congruity', 'Dose Repetition', 'Externalization of Disease', 'Homoeopathic Practice', 'Relapse' and 'Response to Therapy, Deficient or Superabundant'.)

Remedy Abbreviation and Numeric Identification Attempts

Despite the lack of uniformity in remedy abbreviations, there have been shortened forms for the names of medicines in general use in homoeopathy from the earliest times. Common sense made their interpretation obvious in most cases. In the English-speaking area, the abbreviations suggested by John Henry Clarke in 1904 (in his *Clinical Repertory to the Dictionary of Materia Medica*, pages 3-27) seem to have remained in general, albeit non-formalized, use. With the 1974 issue of the *US Homoeopathic Dispensatory and List of Drugs* published in the Compendium of Homoeotherapeutics (Addendum to the Homoeopathic Pharmacopoeia of the US) by the American Institute of Homoeopathy, a little fewer than 2000 homoeopathic drugs were each allocated a standardized four-letter abbreviation as well as a four-digit code number for identification in information technology (computerization). This was described as a 'partial list of eligible drugs' (page 11), but, nonetheless, it covered most of the frequently used medicines. Yet this, like other similar attempts at standardized abbreviations in homoeopathy, does not seem to have found general acceptance.

Remedy Picture
See 'Drug Picture'.

Remedy Simulation
The non-homoeopathic process that is occasionally carried out with the aid of a radionic machine whereby an inert vehicle is 'transsubstantiated' into the desired actual medicinal agent. (See 'Bio-Resonance Therapy' and 'Radionics'.)

Remission, Spontaneous
● **The natural subsiding of illness without help from outside the body.**

Abatement of the symptoms of disease not ascribable to therapeutic intervention; 'vis medicatrix naturae' in action. This is the effect that homoeopathic treatment purposefully aims to achieve. To distinguish homoeopathic medicinal cures from unaided recoveries, homoeopathy stipulates the following two requirements of cure:[1]

---

[1]Close, Stuart. *The Genius of Homoeopathy: Lectures and Essays on Homoeopathic Philosophy* New York: Boericke and Tafel, 1924, p 130.

1) It shall be the result of the clear application of the definite principles of scientific therapeutics, whether accidental or intentional.

2) The therapeutic application of the medicine must be (capable of being) individualized, generally to the needs of the individual patient, less frequently to a particular miasma or genus epidemicus.

Repertorization

See 'Repertory'.

Repertory

From the Latin 'reperio, -ire, repperi, -tum' meaning to find out, obtain, devise or procure; in its widest sense in homoeopathy it denotes an indexed catalogue of cross-references to medicines and/or their homoeopathic applications. Such listings are useful for the study of drug comparisons, and may be referenced from different points of departure, such as John Henry Clarke's *A Clinical Repertory to the Dictionary of Materia Medica* (358 pages, Bradford, North Devon: Health Science Press, 1979). This has five such distinct sections:

1 The Clinical Repertory – listing affections in which the referred-to remedies have been found most frequently indicated in practice;
2 The Repertory of Causation – listing causes subsequent to which the appended medicines have been noted to be curative in a diversity of conditions so produced;
3 The Repertory of Temperaments, Dispositions, States and Constitutions – listing descriptions of types of person that have been observed to respond particularly well to certain homoeopathic drugs;
4 The Repertory of Clinical Relationships – listing each drug's therapeutic congenerousness or otherwise under the following eight headings:
   a) complementary remedies;
   b) drug follows well;
   c) medicine is followed well by;
   d) compatible remedies;
   e) incompatible remedies;
   f) medicine antidotes;
   g) drug is antidoted by;
   h) remedy's duration of action.
5 The Repertory of Natural Relationships – listing the place in the natural order of any remedy in question, readily permitting, for instance, the location of the nearest botanical (or mineral, or zoological) relation of any plant (or mineral, or animal) remedy.

In its more usual, though narrower, sense in homoeopathy the word 'repertory' describes the reference book that schematically indexes the symptoms sought to be located in the materia medica. These symptoms are classified in a logically structured way, and related to each appropriate medicine, offering around each general or particular symptom and its modalities one, or a clutch of, potentially suitable remedies. A patient is said to have been 'repertorized' when the total symptom complex has been matched against the listings in such a repertory and the drug that best parallels the majority of the symptoms has been identified.

Clemens Maria Franz Baron von Boenninghausen (1785-1864) and Georg Heinrich Gottlieb Jahr (1800-1875) are both credited, independent of one another, to have pioneered the homoeopathic repertory in 1833. Apart from those already mentioned, the following five symptom repertories are widely in current use:

Synthetisches Repertorium (3 vols), Horst Barthel and Will Klunker, Heidelberg: Karl F Haug Verlag GmbH, 1974;

Repertory of the More Characteristic Symptoms of the Materia Medica, Constantin Lippe, reprint Calcutta: M Bhattacharyya & Co Pvt Ltd, 1972, 438 pages;

Repertory of the Homoeopathic Materia Medica, James Tyler Kent, reprint Calcutta: Roy Publishing House, 1971, 1465 pages;

Homöopathie, Band 6: Symptomenverzeichnis, Mathias Dorcsi, Heidelberg: Karl F Haug Verlag GmbH, Second Edition, 1982, 457 pages.

A Synoptic Key of the Materia Medica, Cyrus M Boger, Fourth Edition, Lebanon, Pennsylvania: Sowers Publishing Co, 1931, 350 pages

Perforated mechanographic card repertories, that may be used either manually or machine-assisted, have been published by George Broussalian of Grenoble, France in 1969 and by Rudolph Fleury of Berne, Switzerland in 1979. Much earlier in the twentieth century Boger and Leers had each produced a punched-card repertorization technique, which is still in use by a few homoeopaths here and there. The latter has, until recently, constantly added new cards thereby greatly enhancing the quality of his system. In 1978 Ramanlal P Patel published his 'Handbook of Autovisual Homoeopathic Repertory (an Apparatus) Based on Dr Hahnemann's Unpublished Work' to accompany a patented 'visual strip-repertory' derived from Hahnemann's habit of pasting handwritten strips for symptoms into his own repertory, extant in the Hahnemann Archives, Stuttgart, Germany (published Kottayam, Kerala: Sai Homoeopathic Book Corp, 1978, 144 pages). Since about 1980 computer-assisted repertorization is now feasible either by means of a dial-up system to communicate with a database stored on a mainframe, or, more simply, off a diskette or hard disk.

The most frequently used therapeutic (clinical) repertories are:

Clinical Repertory and Therapeutic Index, Oscar E Boericke, reprint Calcutta: Roy Publishing House, 1969, 328 pages (also incorporated into William Boericke's ninth edition of his *Materia Medica*, Philadelphia: Boericke & Tafel Inc, 1927).

Homoeopathic Vade Mecum, Edwin Harris Ruddock, reprint New Delhi: Ashoka Publishing, 1972).

Diverse specializations in repertory compilation exist. They may have an organ, a systemic function, an authority, modalities, or any other point of special focus, e.g.:

Complete Repertory to the Homoeopathic Materia Medica – for Diseases of the Eye, Edward W Berridge, originally published 1873, reprint New Delhi: B Jain Publishers, 1972, 335 pages;

A Concise Repertory of Aggravations and Ameliorations, P Sivaraman, New Delhi: B Jain Publishing Co,1980, 320 pages;

Index & Repertory to the Homoeopathic Drug Pictures of Dr M L Tyler, N W Jollyman, Saffron Walden, Essex: The C W Daniel Co Ltd, 1988, 224 pages.

Unabridged Dictionary of the Sensations 'As If', James William Ward, originally published 1934, 2 vols, in three parts, reprint New Delhi: B Jain Publishing Co, ca 1978, 1638 pages.

Repertory of Pregnancy, Parturition and Puerperium, Alberto Soler-Medina, Heidelberg: Karl F Haug Verlag, 1989, 79 pages.

Repetition of Homoeopathic Drugs

See 'Dose Repetition', 'Exhaustion' and 'Homoeopathic Practice'.

Repulsion and Attraction

Two forces operative in physics, and said to be observable in psychology, where 'the like' repel and 'the unlike' attract each other in an inverse ratio of the physical proximity between the two. Homoeopathy's pharmacodynamic reliability is grounded in the observed antagonistic effect between 'the like' disease and drug action. Its pharmacological trustworthiness has been widely, though perhaps analogously, ascribed to the judicious employment of the force of repulsion. (See Law of Stimuli under 'Homoeopathic Laws, Postulates and Precepts', section 5 and Law of Bioenergetic Drug Action, same entry, section 2.)

Research in Homoeopathy

See 'Experimental Research in Homoeopathy'.

Resin

Rosin; exudate from or secretion of a variety of plants that becomes an amorphous, brittle, and sometimes translucent, glassy material when hardened. [The term 'colophony' is not its precise synonym, since that refers only to the residue after distilling the oil of turpentine from the oleoresin obtained from various species of Pinaceae.] Resins are used to prepare a group of plant sarcodes (see entry under 'Isopathy') comprising homoeopathic medicines with greatly diverse drug pictures, such as Abies nigra, Angophora lanceolata (Kino australensis), Balsamum peruvianum, Balsamum tolutanum

(Myroxylon balsamum), (Styrax) Benzoin [or Acidum Benzoicum, obtained from Gum Benzoin, as distinct from Benzoin oderiferum, where tincture is made of the resin-filled twigs], (Laurus) Camphora, Copaiva officinalis, Euphorbia heterodoxa, Euphorbium officinarum (Euphorbia resinifera), Gambogia (Garcinia morella), Guaiacum officinale, Myristica sebifera, Myrrha (Commiphora molmol), Opium, Pinus lambertiana, Podophyllum peltatum, Populus candicans, Propolis and (Convolvulus) Scammonium. Most in this remedy group tend to be used pathotropically, exercising a pronounced protective function through the reaction they evoke, though some, like Opium and Podophyllum peltatum, are very deep-acting. Furthermore, certain top-ranking medicines are produced in homoeopathic pharmacy among those where the resinous secretion is a significant part of the starting material. The succi are obtained from some interesting plants, as in:

Drosera rotundifolia (tincture is made of the active fresh plant, whose leaves are covered with odd, resin-sticky hairs curving in towards the centre; when the resinous juice sparkles colourfully in the sunlight it fatally attracts insects which are then trapped on it with other hairs soon bending over the insect and the resin breaking down the proteins in the insect's body)

Eucalyptus globulus (a.k.a. Blue Gum; tincture is made of the fresh sickle-shaped leaves, that are covered with a layer of wax and the main constituent (about 70%) of which is cineole (formerly eucalyptol)

Grindelia robusta and Grindelia squarrosa (the terminal heads of yellow flowers are covered with a viscid balsamic secretion, due to which they are also referred to as 'Gum plants'; tincture is made from leaves and flowers)

Humulus lupulus (tincture made of small resinous granules covering the scales of what is commonly known as hops and was introduced into beer as a preservative by the Germans during the Thirty Years' War)

Jalapa officinalis (Exogonium purga, Ipomoea purga) (trituration of root, the tubercles of which contain more than 10% jalap resin)

Piper methysticum (tincture made of the fresh root which when ground with a pestle produces a cloudy, milky-resinous mash rich in lactones, collectively known as kava-pyrones)

Populus candicans (tincture is made of the resinous buds)

Silphium laciniatum (a.k.a. Turpentine weed, Rosin-wood, Pilot-weed, Compass plant, and Polar plant; tincture is made of the fresh plant, the stem of which exudes an abundance of resin as two of its vernacular names indicate; the other common names testify to the fact that its leaves, at first, present their faces uniformly north and south, although later, when the leaves become heavy, that polarity ceases to be evident)

Thuja occidentalis (Alphonse Teste (1814-1888) already remarked on the 'resinous callosities of the stems and leaves of Thuja occ.' and Douglas Gibson (1888-1977) in his *Studies of Homoeopathic Remedies* says a 'transparent oil with a strong odour and a slightly acrid taste' is obtainable from these; the tincture is made of its fresh green twigs).

In the study mentioned under 'Mother Tincture', Experimental Evidence, the homoeopathic mother tinctures made from resinous preparations were amongst the most potent agents tested for preventive and inhibiting effects on the pathogenic action of microbial organisms.

Resistance, Dynamic

● **The protective-corrective response shown by all living things to anything that affects them.**

Vital (dynamic) resistance is the defensive reaction of a living organism to any noxious stimuli, elements, organisms, disease-producing agents, or to toxins in general, in conformity with the urge to self-preservation, inherent in all organic life. In that sense then, disease is resistance by the dynamis. Disease, a costly and painful struggle, manifested by symptoms, expresses that vital reaction, that dynamic resistance, of the living organism to the inroads of some injurious agent or influence. Disease is a somato-psychic process, not a pathological end product. In other words, a neoplastic tumour is not the disease, but the entire host body's battle to overcome it, which very occasionally even ends in spontaneous remission, certainly is.

Resonance

The acoustic quality of reinforcing, or the prolongation, of sound by reflection, or by synchronous or harmonic reverberation. By logical extension, such quality or prolongation in any oscillating, regularly impulsed or vibrating system. Some of the more specific meanings are given below.

In auscultation: The hollow character and the intensification of sound obtained over a cavity.

In physics: The inherent frequency of any oscillating system, as in nuclear magnetic resonance, electron spin resonance, etc.

In chemistry: The ordered manner in which electrons are distributed among the atoms in compounds which are planar and symmetrical, especially those with (alternating) conjugated double bonds, where it is evidence of increased stability and lowered energy content.

In homoeopathy: When medication is homoeopathic to a reversible condition it is in resonance with the diseased organism's deepest response and a vital reaction occurs, manifested by external changes in the symptom pattern, an increase in available energy and a stimulation of the recuperative processes, liberating fixed areas of immobility, stress or dysfunction, beginning with the most recent, outer layers of stasis or dyscrasia. (See 'Homoeosis'.)

Response to Therapy, Deficient or Superabundant

● **Cases where there is either too much or too little reaction to treatment.**

Depleted energy reserves perhaps in old age or after a long taxing illness, or an organic obstruction requiring surgical correction, or diminished susceptibility may each produce a deficient, or failed, reaction to a well-indicated homoeopathic medicine. For patients with a low vital energy, Hahnemann's great disciple C M F von Boenninghausen (1785-1864) recommended that one of the following six drugs be prescribed, as usual, according to the presenting homoeopathic symptom image overall:

Carbo vegetabilis
(Prunus) Laurocerasus
Moschus moschiferus
Opium
Sulphur
Thuja occidentalis.

If a miasma is suspected, corresponding miasmatic remedies, or appropriate nosodes (Lueticum, Psorinum, Medorrhinum, one of the Tuberculinums, or Scirrhinum) may be prescribed by the attending homoeopath.

An excessive response shows itself in a severe aggravation, occurring most frequently after any steroidal suppression of symptoms when the homoeopathic medicine suddenly releases them, setting off a so-called 'homoeopathic rebound'. However, enantiopathic phytotherapy or palliative orthodox medication of long duration may set up the same preconditions, with the same 'homoeopathic rebound' effect unavoidably taking place. Such a superabundant response does not reflect inaccurate homoeopathic prescribing, but the powerful start of a buoyant homoeopathic reactive state, possibly after years of ineffectual suppression. It may also indicate a state of general hypersensitivity, where the patient seems to suffer an aggravation from every remedy without corresponding improvement. For severe responses in such cases C M F von Boenninghausen recommended the following eleven medicines to be prescribed, similarly, to fit the overall homoeopathic symptom picture:

(Narthex) Asafoetida
Asarum europaeum
(Matricaria) Chamomilla
Coffea tosta
Cinchona officinalis
Ignatia amara
Nux vomica
Pulsatilla nigricans
Sulphur
Teucrium marum
Valeriana officinalis.

Baron von Boenninghausen's corrective intercurrent prescription method described here has proved itself in the course of more than a century.

Rest

Repose; quiet. A rhythmic life-style with regular habits and few routinely performed, undemanding tasks might be recommended to the patient by the homoeopath, when complete rest would be impractical. Avoidance of all excesses, such as stimulants or depressants, heavy meals, highly spiced foods, noxious influences such as from the tobacco habit, will be urged by the homoeopath during the course of treatment.

Retardation

Slowing up of movement or development; most often applied to the mental development of a child, whose mentality is considered clearly below normal. Perhaps not an entirely satisfactory description when applied to the level of children with an intelligence quotient of below 70 (considered the upper limit of feeblemindedness), but which could not be labelled as definitely defective. Common problems that predispose to this state of subnormality which the homoeopath will attempt to identify include vitamin, protein, mineral, or hormone deficiencies, family violence, diet and nutritional factors, foetal distress or other deleterious intrauterine episodes, food hypersensitivities, accidental injuries, infections, birth traumata, chronic diseases, and any inherited miasmata. Leon Vannier's *Difficult and Backward Children* is a good reference work on the homoeopathic treatment required for such patients (translated from the French, Calcutta: Hahnemann Publishing Co Pvt Ltd, 1978 [sixth edition], 117 pages). (Refer also to 'Emotional and Intellectual Reactive States and Some "Mentals" '.)

Reversal of Primary Direction of Drug Response

See 'Homoeopathic Laws, Postulates and Precepts', section 5.

Ross, Andrew Christie Gordon (1904-1982)

Scottish homoeopath, born in Glasgow and educated at its Academy and the University of St Andrews, who until the age of twenty-nine years followed a commercial career, when he switched to homoeopathy. He joined his brother and brother-in-law in their practice in 1940 and carried it on after their deaths until he retired to St Andrews in 1965. He was also an author and playwright, but was especially prolific in his homoeopathic articles: more than two hundred of them are reported to have appeared in various journals. His best known book is:

Homoeopathic Green Medicine (Wellingborough: Thorsons, 1978) which is a comparison between the homoeopathic and orthodox-medical approaches to the healing powers in plants, weeds and trees.

Thomas Douglas Ross (1902-1964), brother of the above, was superintendent and later consultant at the Glasgow Homoeopathic Hospital. He was a musician and, like his brother, a writer.

Ross, Thomas Douglas (1902-1964)

See 'Ross, Andrew Christie Gordon (1904-1982)'.

Royal, George (1853-1926)

US homoeopath from Des Moines, Iowa, who was professor of Homoeopathic Materia Medica and Therapeutics at the State University of Iowa for fully thirty years. He had also been president and chairman of the Council of Medical Education of the American Institute of Homoeopathy. Both his sons, Malcolm Allen and Paul Ambrose, became graduates of the College of Homoeopathic Medicine of the State University of Iowa. His major writings comprise:

Text-Book of Materia Medica (1918)
Text-Book of Homoeopathic Theory and Practice of Medicine (1923)

Rubric

Title or heading of a particular section of a book; in homoeopathy, of a repertory or of the materia medica.

Ruddock, Edwin Harris (1822-1865)

Scottish homoeopath, who qualified from Edinburgh University and was trained at Guy's Hospital and at St Bartholomew's Hospital. He was the original editor of the *Homoeopathic World*, a semi-popular monthly journal. (Its editors that followed him were Drs Shuldham, Burnett and Clarke, in that order.) Among his major homoeopathic literary accomplishments are:

A Ladies' Manual of Home Treatment
Pocket Manual of Homoeopathic Veterinary Medicine
Stepping Stones to Homoeopathy and Health
Consumption and Tuberculosis of the Lungs
Diseases of Infants and Children

His most important work, however, which is still much in demand today, one and a quarter centuries later remains his:

Homoeopathic Vade Mecum (revised by J C Nixon; 922 pages).

Rule of Drug Non-Repetition During Treatment

See 'Homoeopathic Laws, Postulates and Precepts', section 8.

Rule of Drug Non-Repetition in Provings

See 'Homoeopathic Laws, Postulates and Precepts', section 9.

Rule of Least Action in Posology

See 'Homoeopathic Laws, Postulates and Precepts', section 6.

Rule on Direction of Cure

See 'Homoeopathic Laws, Postulates and Precepts', section 14.

Rules of Potencies in Provings

See 'Homoeopathic Laws, Postulates and Precepts', section 10.

Ryoduraku

System of acupuncture, considered by many as complementary to homoeopathy, developed in the 1950s by the Japanese Yoschio Nakatani, somewhat similar to that originated by Reinhold Voll in the FRG (and briefly explained under 'Bio-Electronic Regulatory Medicine').

S

Saccharum Lactis

Sugar of milk; lactose; $C_{12}H_{22}O_{11}$ 'H_2O; usually in powder form (see also 'Colloid' and 'Vehicle'). Homoeopathic uses:

1   preparation of trituration from insoluble base substances;
2   serial potentization (dynamized triturations);
3   administration as a (near-)placebo (see following paragraph);
4   vehicle for dispensing medicines (after its impregnation by them).

Pathogenetic experimentation has established that no substance is absolutely inert when undergoing a proving, and the less so once dynamized. Clinical usage has fully confirmed this observation. Hence, there can be no such thing as an absolute placebo. The employment of Saccharum lactis in placebo-controlled clinical trials is because homoeopathy regards it as a near-placebo and evaluates results accordingly. (See 'Epistemological Assumptions in Homoeopathy', section 6 Placebo-Nocebo, 'Isopathy', section 2 Sarcode (ii) of animal, or human, origin, and 'Potentizing Methods'.)

Safety of Mother Tinctures, Solutions and Low Potencies

See 'Mother Tincture'.

Sanitation

Implementation of measures in the environment conducive to health, and tending to prevent particular miasmatic effects. (See 'Miasma' and 'Verdi, Tullio Suzzara (1829-1902)'.)

Saponin

General term for what is found in a large number of plants, being non-nitrogenous glycosides which are soap-like in that they will make suds when strongly agitated in an aqueous solution. Saponins can hold resins or fats in suspension in water. Homoeopathy, unlike orthodox pharmacy or, to a lesser extent, phytotherapy, accords saponins separated from the plants in which they occur no more special attention than it does alkaloids, and for the same reasons (see 'Alkaloid').

Sarcode

Term originally applied to the substance of which animal and vegetable tissues are formed, in the proposed third kingdom of living things, the so-called protista (embracing the protozoa and protophyta), according to Ernst H Haeckel (German naturalist, 1834-1919). However, the prevalent meaning refers to a homoeopathically prepared remedy made from a preparation of healthy animal tissue and/or secretion(s) with its own full distinct drug picture, without which it would merely be an 'organotherapeutic preparation'. However, preparations of poisonous animals (e.g. Erythrinum, Sanguisuga officinalis) are not included under the category of the sarcode as these are simply considered to be standard homoeopathic medicinal material, quite like any other. Homoeopathy recognizes two separate categories of sarcodes, and a further one of sarcode-derivatives (these are fully described under 'Isopathy'). (See also 'Nosode' and 'Sarcode-Derivative'.)

Sarcode-Derivative

Homoeopathic preparation made from a substance itself derived from healthy animal tissue an: /or secretion(s) with its own full distinct drug picture. This slightly arbitrary subcategory of the sarcode (it includes remedies like Cholesterinum, Pepsinum, Sepia officinalis and Urea) also covers all potentized ophio-toxins (venomous secretions of snakes) as well as all other comparable remedies based on animal secretions (e.g. of porcupines, insects, arachnids, molluscs and other sea-dwellers, such as echinodermata and coelenterata). (See 'Isopathy' and 'Sarcode'.)

Saturation

State of being united in complete solution with another substance to its full capacity, when no more of the same can be accommodated at the same temperature. (See 'Solute', 'Solution', 'Solvation Structure' and 'Solvent'.)

Scales and Balances

See 'Utensils of Homoeopathic Pharmacy'.

Schmidt, Pierre (1894-1987)

A francophone Swiss homoeopath of considerable eminence who graduated from Geneva University. He was profoundly impressed as a young man when his father's life-long enteritis was effectively cured by homoeopathy after all other methods had failed. At the age of 24 he experienced at first hand the benefits of the nosode Influenzinum during the Spanish Influenza epidemic of 1918. For a time he worked at the Royal London Homoeopathic Hospital and became acquainted with John Henry Clarke (1853-1931) and Sir John Weir (1879-1971). After that he went to Philadelphia, Pennsylvania, USA where he came under the abiding influence of the late James Tyler Kent (1849-1916) and his teaching of prescribing single remedies in very high potencies, absorbing this from Fredericka Gladwin, one of Kent's pupils.

Together with Dr J Thuinzing of the Netherlands he founded the Liga Medicorum Homoeopathica Internationalis in 1925. He translated into French Hahnemann's *Reine Arzneimittellehre* (Materia Medica Pura), *Die chronischen Krankheiten, ihre eigenthümliche Natur und homöopathische Heilung* (The Chronic Diseases, Their Peculiar Nature and Their Homoeopathic Cure), and the sixth edition of the *Organon der rationellen Heilkunde* (Organon of Medicine). He is renowned for his many homoeopathic dissertations on its mateiia medica, its philosophy and its clinical effectiveness. At the LMHI bicentenary celebrations of Hahnemann's birth in 1955 he, the League's life-long President of Honour, gave a rousing valedictory address entitled 'The Legacy of Hahnemann'. Many years later he reported with a veterinarian pupil of his quite outstanding results in Foot-and-Mouth disease using an annually prepared nosode of the disease products, along with Acidum nitricum 6CH which was employed pathotropically.

He retired and went to live in Nancy, France. His major work is *Defective Illness* (1980)

In it the universal defect might well appear to be seen by the reader as all illness' unfailing defencelessness against correctly indicated homoeopathic treatment. However, what the title literally refers to is Hahnemann's term 'einseitige Krankheiten' ('one-sided illnesses', in sections 172-175 of the *Organon*), which had been incorrectly translated into French as 'partial illnesses', whereas it signifies lop-sided, catalectic, or inadequate. Hahnemann uses this expression for a disease picture with too few presenting symptoms, not because the illness itself is fragmentary in its effect but, rather, because such an illness, though still involving the whole individual, does not show itself completely. Schmidt's own full examination of this problem in homoeopathic drug diagnosis is published in *The Wholistic Practitioner*, Winter (June) 1990, vol VII, no 1, pp 12-58.

Schüssler, Wilhelm Heinrich (1821-1898)

Originator of Biochemic Therapy and the so-called tissue salts. He was born in Zwischenalm, Grand Duchy Oldenburg, where he spent his youth. He studied in Berlin, Paris and Giessen. At the university of the last-mentioned city he ultimately graduated in medicine. He then went to Austria-Hungary to do three terms of post-doctoral studies at Prague university. After that he also took up the study of homoeopathy. Subsequent to his examination by the Collegium Medicum of Oldenburg in 1857 he received his licence to practise there which, right from the beginning, he did as a homoeopath.

He was inspired by the work of Prof Moleschott (Austrian physiologist, at

Rome University) and Rudolph Ludwig Karl Virchow (German pathologist [1821-1902], at the Friedrich-Wilhelm Institut, Berlin) who together propounded the hypothesis of 'cellular pathology', which attempted to explain all disease in terms of alterations in cells, making the cell the fundamental unit in pathology, to be studied intensely if insight into states of illness was to be gained. This theory was in opposition to the then dominant 'humoralist pathology' of the Viennese Karl Baron von Rokitansky, the greatest pathological anatomist of the day. Prof Moleschott said in his work *Kreislauf des Lebens* (The Cycle of Life): 'The structure and vitality of organs are conditioned by the necessary amounts of inorganic constituents. It is owing to this fact that the proper estimation of the relation of the inorganic substances to the various parts of the body . . . promises to Agriculture and to Medicine a brilliant future'.[1] This was at a time when homoeopathy was becoming ever more deeply embroiled in the emotion-charged 'symptomatology versus pathology' debate. Schüssler sided with the low potency prescribing, pro-pathology faction (see 'Hempel, Charles Julius (1811-1879)' for the issues in this debate).

In 1872 he introduced into his clinical practice just such inorganic substances to which Prof Moleschott had made reference – in low dynamizations (usually 6DH). One year later he published *An Abridged Homoeopathic Therapeutics* using the twelve salts that were found in the organism's cells. Later he was to insist, though, that his Biochemic System of Medicine was quite distinct from homoeopathy. In the 25th edition, published shortly before his death, he even denied all previous connexion with homoeopathy. This defection roughly in the direction of orthodox medicine is in line with what has happened since to a great many homoeopaths who also tried unsuccessfully to make pathology the centre-piece of homoeopathy. Nonetheless, after his demise his twelve tissue salts were gradually re-absorbed into mainstream homoeopathy. Thus homoeopathy was to reclaim that which had been rightfully hers, as seven of his twelve Biochemic Remedies (the tissue salts) had had normal provings done and, in most cases, they had been a permanent part of the materia medica for several decades[2] before he arrogated them into his System of Biochemistry. (See 'Biochemic Therapy', 'Mineral Remedies' and 'Tissue Salts'.)

Schulz Law

Arndt-Schulz law; the law of stimuli formulated by Prof Hugo Schulz and Dr H R Arndt. (See 'Homoeopathic Laws, Postulates and Precepts', section 5.)

[1] Schüssler, Wilhelm Heinrich. *An Abridged Therapy Manual for the Biochemical Treatment of Disease*, Philadelphia: Boericke & Tafel, 1898, quoted in the Preface, p 17.
[2] Calcarea fluorica was originally proved in 1874
Calcarea phosphorica was originally proved in 1834
Calcarea sulphurica was originally proved in 1847
Kali muriaticum was originally proved in 1832
Natrum muriaticum was originally proved in 1828
Natrum sulphuricum was originally proved in 1832
Silica was originally proved in 1828.

Science

Natural philosophy; the study of either a connected body of demonstrated truths or of observed facts systematically classified; cognizance acquired through trustworthy methods of investigation for the discovery of new truths colligated under the laws of nature. The object of all scientific endeavour is the ever greater approximation to the overall truth behind reality. The term 'Science' has now often come to be used as an abbreviation for 'Natural and Physical Science'.

'Speculative Science' is the branch of science which suggests hypotheses and theories and develops rigorous, critical tests for subsequent coherent colligation within the existing body of science (always open to subsequent 'falsifiability' or refutation). (See 'Laws of Nature' and 'Probabiliorism'.)

Science and Homoeopathy

Homoeopathy is sometimes described by its detractors as an unscientific medical system, because it is said to proceed from an entirely rigid dogmatic base. That is tantamount to the system being condemned for wrongly believing it to operate in pre-ordained scientific sterility, taken to flow from its assumed acceptance of the philosophical fallacy of 'essentialism' as its scientific premise.

The idea of man's tacit knowing, his intuitive comprehension of essence (i.e. by means of essentialistic interpretation arriving at an ultimate, so to say, infallible, explanation) was elevated to full conceptual respectability by Edmund Husserl (1859-1938), the Austrian philosopher who founded 'constitutive phenomenology' (from which 'existentialism' ultimately emerged in the 1930s). Since then Sir Karl R Popper (born 1902), the philosopher of science, has lucidly distinguished the method of the 'conjectural explanation' from that of the said 'ultimate explanation' and shown them to be diametrically opposed to one another.[1]

The first-mentioned is called the speculative method, by which a hypothesis is initially postulated and then tested by probing the consequences of its underlying suppositions. This is considered to be the true scientific method which seeks to answer the question 'Why is . . .?'. This, in turn, leads on to experimental research that tests the germane hypotheses for their veracity. Every conjectural explanation when tested can throw up new problems.

The second method is that of the intuitive grasping of the inherent essence or nature of whatever is at issue, seeking, as it does, to answer the question 'What is . . .?' resulting in a definition of essence, which attempts to provide the ultimate explanation, the final infallible answer that brooks no further explanation. An example of essentialism in science is the unified field theory in physics, which remains as yet an unverified attempt to link the properties

---

[1] Popper, Sir Karl R and Sir John C Eccles. *Das Ich und sein Gehirn,* Munich: R Piper GmbH & Co KG, sixth edition, 1987, pp 215-220.

of all fields (electric, gravitational, magnetic and nuclear) into a unified system, it being the inferred 'ultimate explanation' (see also 'Radiant State of Matter, Theory of').

However, as all the hypotheses of homoeopathy are constantly being tested for their veracity in the continuing scientific program of experiments described under 'Experimental Research in Homoeopathy' it is incorrect to ascribe the error of essentialism to homoeopathy. The success of the high calibre of homoeopathy's experimental work has, inter alia, provided clear evidence of the biological effectiveness of Hahnemannian deconcentrations, despite the absence therefrom of any molecular trace of the basic (original) substance. This momentous evidence has confronted a section of the scientific community with an intricate paradigmatic problem of considerable dimensions, because homoeopathy has thereby successfully challenged certain existing standards, previously taken to be axiomatic by that section in scientific circles. (See 'Radiant State of Matter, Theory of'.)

Science of Therapeutics

See 'Therapeutic Science'.

Scientific Evidence in Support of Homoeopathy

See 'Clinical Trials', 'Epistemological Assumptions in Homoeopathy', particularly section 1, and 'Experimental Research in Homoeopathy'.

Scientific Paradigm

Ideate framework that is shared by members of a scientific community, according to which phenomena are seen and interpreted; a world-view that provides models of acceptable ways in which problems can be understood by such a community. Homoeopathy is a world-view that provides such a model.

Scientific Principles of Homoeopathy

See 'Epistemological Assumptions in Homoeopathy', 'Hahnemann, Christian Friedrich Samuel (1755-1843)', 'Laws of Nature', 'Philosophical Premise of Homoeopathy' and 'Science and Homoeopathy'.

Seasonal Variations in Drug Pictures

A number of medicines have a more pronounced effect at certain times of the year. For example, Sabadilla officinarum has been shown to have a powerful effect on intermittent fever in Spring, while Pulsatilla nigricans will be at its most effective against nocturnal enuresis in Autumn. It is noteworthy that this last-mentioned remedy produced in its pathogenetic experiments aggravation of toothache when sitting or when lying with head low, whether on painful or on painless side, much more particularly from the warmth of the room, and that such conditions in the patient will respond best in Spring (not in Autumn as the enuresis). Consequently it can be very misleading to assign to a homoeopathic drug a fixed seasonal epithet (e.g. speaking of a 'Spring remedy').

Self-Medication

See 'Home Remedy Kits'.

Semi-Pellets

See 'Cones'.

Sequential Development of Drug Action Tabulated

See 'Therapeutic Science'.

Serapion of Alexandria (around 240 BC)

See 'Philosophical Premise of Homoeopathy'.

Serocytotherapy

See 'Isopathy'.

Sesame Oil

See 'Teel Oil'.

Sextus Empiricus (around 200 AD)

See 'Philosophical Premise of Homoeopathy'.

Shamanism and Magic

● **In the craft of witch-doctors appears to lie the origin, at least in part, of all forms of medical practice.**

In these are found the primitive roots of healing. For an insightful perspective on their present-day relation to both homoeopathic and orthodox medical practice refer to *Planet Medicine – from Stone Age Shamanism to Post-Industrial Healing* by Richard Grossinger (Henley-on Thames: Routledge & Kegan Paul Ltd, 1982 [436 pages]).

Shiatsu

See 'Acupuncture'.

Side Effects in Homoeopathy

Homoeopathic aggravation, which is the intensification of symptoms during the healing crisis, the re-appearance of past symptoms in reverse order of their previous appearance, or the externalization of disease manifestations, are all beneficial side effects, signalling an approaching cure, to be expected in the course of homoeopathic treatment.

Sieves

See 'Utensils of Homoeopathic Pharmacy'.

Simillimum

Similimum; the single homoeopathic medicine the drug picture of which most nearly approaches the total symptom complex of the patient, which will certainly cure that patient, if the patient's condition is within reversible limits. (See also 'Contra-Indication against Administering Simillimum' and 'Disease and Drug Action in Homoeopathic Congruity'.)

Simmons, George Henry (1852-1937)

This extraordinary man, who at first was a homoeopath, has the distinction of having adroitly manoeuvred orthodox medicine past seemingly insuperable impediments both within the American Medical Association and outside of it. His genius for political manipulation brought about the twentieth century's most far-reaching changes in medical history. His well-executed machinations certainly elevate him to the position of the single most important man of the century measured in terms of the beneficial effects on the politics and economics of orthodox medicine and its pharmaceutical industry. He has had a correspondingly devastating effect on homoeopathy. Born in England, he migrated to the USA at an early age and in 1882 he graduated from the Hahnemann Medical College of Chicago, Illinois. For a number of years he successfully practised as a homoeopathic obstetrician in Lincoln, Nebraska. His allegiance to homoeopathy in the early 1880s was not in question, as may be seen from a letter he wrote to an orthodox medical journal[1] wherein he reproves the orthodox medical profession for constantly consulting with homoeopaths, despite the fact that their code of ethics (contrary to that of the homoeopaths) made such communications illicit. In 1892, after he had

---

[1] Simmons, George Henry. Letter in *Medical Brief*, 1883, vol XI, pp 168 to 169.

radically altered his medical views and turned his back on homoeopathy, he obtained an orthodox medical degree from the Rush Medical College of Chicago and very soon became secretary of the (orthodox) State Medical Society and also of the (orthodox) Western Surgical and Gynaecological Society. Furthermore he launched the *Western Medical Review* which, from its inception, presented a very marked anti-homoeopathic slant. He was clearly imbued with the fervour that generally characterizes converts. When the Board of Trustees of the American Medical Association cast about for a suitable individual for the position of secretary in 1899, Simmons was selected to fill the vacancy and was also made editor of the *Journal of the American Medical Association*. From 1899 he thus held the post of General Secretary and General Manager of the AMA up to 1911 but he remained editor of the Journal for a full twenty-five years.

Background – Up To The Time When Simmons Took Office

[All statistical information and the source references in this section are derived from the very instructive, thoroughly researched and unique philosophico-historical work by Harris Livermore Coulter, Ph.D. as detailed in footnote 2 below. That vast work is well worth consulting.]

In April 1844 the American Institute of Homoeopathy [AIH] had been formed with Constantin Hering as its first president. To counterpoise this perceived new threat to orthodox medicine, the American Medical Association [AMA] was constituted two years later, in May 1846. During the following year, in 1847, the AMA laid down a binding Code of Ethics that proscribed for orthodox practitioners the promoting of, attesting to, and/or dispensing of 'patent or secret medicines'.

Up to 1876 there had been only two categories of drug manufacturers of relevance to orthodox physicians and pharmacists: (i) The makers of patent medicines or nostrums (trade-marked and/or patented compounds of secret ingredients, with copyrighted names, generally glowingly advertised as specifics for one or usually many disease conditions); and (ii) the so-called 'ethical' drug manufacturers (producers of identified medicinal substances, advertised [almost] solely to the orthodox medical profession). For more than half a century the AMA sharply denounced all patent medicines as possibly involving either fraudulent or dangerous quackery, both incompatible with the AMA Code of Ethics that prohibited an orthodox medical practitioner from prescribing (i), but permitted the prescribing of (ii) above.

However, in the last quarter of the nineteenth century a third category of drug manufacturer appeared and quickly proliferated massively, throwing the AMA into a quandary: (iii) The makers of proprietary medicines (identical to the patent medicines in all respects, except that the ingredients would either be publicized or be at least confidentially disclosed to an adjudicating party, like the editor of a journal, before running an advertisement for that particular 'proprietary' drug). All the old, formerly 'ethical' companies immediately jumped on that bandwagon too.

The approximately 2700 'proprietaries' on the market in 1880 increased almost fifteenfold to 39000 in the next twenty-seven years.[1] By then the AMA estimated that about 70% of prescriptions in New York City were for 'proprietaries'[2] and in up to 47% of prescriptions examined in a survey the prescribing orthodox physician called for remedies of unknown composition.[3] It must be remembered that the first half of the nineteenth century had been the period of so-called 'heroic dosage' when it was routine orthodox practice to administer extremely large amounts of strong mineral medicines to patients, usually many on top of one another, or compounded together, frequently with catastrophic results. The 'proprietaries' now seemed to offer hope of a therapeutic approach that stood a better chance of competing against the resounding success of homoeopathy. However, orthodox medical ethics were in complete turmoil over the 'proprietaries' issue when Simmons took office.

Certainly, the 'proprietaries' were still classified as patent medicines by the AMA (since they were, in fact, patented, copyrighted or similarly protected) and, as such, to their practitioners unequivocally proscribed. Yet the orthodox practitioners found them to be irresistible. Apart from the reason given earlier, they were popular with orthodox physicians because they spared them the tedium of acquiring pharmacological competence that the writing of prescriptions for formulae of compounded 'simples' inevitably presupposed. Instead it would simply be reduced to the relative effortlessness of memorizing the names of a series of specific 'proprietaries' and prescribing them for the disease-names of the patients as listed in the manufacturers' pamphlets. As Coulter, the medical historian, so aptly says in his intellectually wide-ranging and well-documented overview of the period (work mentioned in footnotes 2ff), this proscription was most frequently observed in the breach. As a consequence, the compounding of medicines became centralized with the manufacturers. There developed a pervasive lack of pharmacological knowledge in both the orthodox physicians and the pharmacists concerning the effects of these new compounds. Even the teaching of pharmacology and pharmacognosy at the orthodox medical schools began to be neglected more and more significantly.

On the one hand, pharmacists were relieved at being unburdened of the need to compound prescriptions by having instead only to hand out sugar-coated 'proprietary' pills or syrups, on the other, they were being squeezed economically by the emerging 'drug stores' who sold patent medicines and 'proprietaries' direct to the public together with a miscellany of fancy goods, ice cream, soda pop, tobacconist's requisites, toiletries, sweets and toys. The pharmacists sought to redress the situation by beginning to counter-prescribe

---

[1] Coulter, Harris Livermore. *Divided Legacy: A History of The Schism in Medical Thought* 3 volumes, Washington DC: Wehawken Book Company, 1973, Vol III *Science and Ethics in American Medicine: 1800–1914*, p 404; quoting Kremers and Urdang, *History of Pharmacy* (3rd edition, Philadelphia: J B Lippincott, 1963), p 285.

[2] Ibid., p 411, quoting *Journal of the AMA*, 1906, vol XLVI, p 718.

[3] Ibid., p 411, quoting *Journal of the AMA*, 1908, vol L, p 959.

on a massive scale, thus affecting the patient-flow to orthodox physicians.

A further knock-on effect of the omnipresence of 'proprietaries' was that there was a sharp decline in the ability by orthodox practitioners to adjust their therapeutic method to the individual patient's needs. In other words, the approach of the orthodox practitioner became stultified. Yet both the orthodox physicians and pharmacists went along with the convenient trend of (counter-) prescribing the lucrative 'proprietaries'.

Meanwhile the manufacturers' direct advertising to the public meant that the public no longer needed the orthodox physician, or, at most, only for the first prescription. Thereby more patients were deflected from the orthodox physicians, to the pharmacists and drug stores.

By 1900 most orthodox physicians were struggling financially to survive, and many simply did not, whereas most homoeopaths were becoming affluent by diligently serving a large and growing patient group with professional dignity. Many hard-pressed orthodox practitioners accepted fees for writing spurious or exaggerated testimonials extolling the benefits of 'proprietaries', the AMA's proscriptive Code of Ethics notwithstanding. These texts were then used in the very promotional campaigns that would take yet more custom from them and their colleagues.

The reason for the apparent support of the 'proprietaries' by the orthodox medical journals was that half the journals were financially subsidized by the manufacturers of 'proprietaries', and many of the remaining, previously independent journals had been acquired outright by the manufacturers (with a single manufacturer becoming the sole owner of, perhaps, six such medical journals). This, amongst other things, meant that many impecunious orthodox practitioners were given well-paid positions in medical journalism, while such a journal would then be effectively muzzled. In the advertising contracts that the manufacturers imposed on the medical journals (weak from a vast market over-supply) the journals were forced to 'agree to publish, in addition to the advertisement in its proper place, and without extra compensation, certain advertising matter among its original articles or editorials'.[1] In this way the manufacturers contrived to have a plethora of bogus scientific articles, that were really disguised advertisements, constantly published in apparently respectable medical journals. Coulter states: 'About 250 medical journals were published at the turn of the century, and only one was supported by the profession alone. All the rest, including the Journal of the American Medical Association, the New York Medical Record, and the American Journal of the Medical Sciences were supported by 'questionable advertisements'.[2]

The Homoeopaths' Concurrent Situation

The homoeopaths were thoroughly vexed by what was happening to their

[1] Ibid., p 420, quoting P Maxwell Foshay, editor of the *Cleveland Medical Journal* in the *Journal of the AMA*, 1900, vol XXXIV, pp 1041-1043.
[2] Ibid., p 415, quoting various sources.

opposition, as can be seen from this sample excerpt quoted by Coulter from the Southern Journal of Homoeopathy:

> 'Who more than these self-same Pharisees are now suborned by . . . nostrum-vending corporations to furnish the knowledge necessary for the preparation of villainous quackish compounds for gulling, robbing, and even poisoning people. Nearly every compound and patent medicine on the market is based upon a prescription furnished by some Old-School practitioner who "stands in" with the manufacturer and shares his ill-gotten gains . . . Take up the medical journals of the day and scan their pages. Who interleaves their would-be-Gospel expounders with advertisements for sordid gain more greedily than they do? Who more than they, in their publisher's departments, mislead their fellows with paid puffs, oftentimes false and quackish in the extreme . . . "Everything goes, for gold" is the motto of many an Old-School journal which preaches purity and holiness and orthodoxy . . . , but which at the same time practices quackery and fraud, pure and simple, for dollars which proprietors of secret nostrums pay into the till. O consistency, thou art a jewel, and a rare one indeed in orthodox medical circles.'[1]

The fact that in any homoeopath the functions of physician and pharmacist are fused aroused lasting antagonism in both the manufacturers and the dispensers of medicines, whose livelihood appeared threatened by this element in homoeopathy. Moreover, protectionist laws that prohibited physicians from dispensing their own medicines had been abolished earlier (as a result of homoeopathic political pressure) fuelling the pharmacists' on-going resentment directed against homoeopaths who were seen as the main beneficiaries of this abolition.

Whereas in the orthodox medical schools the teaching of pharmacology of the 'singles' had declined very substantially, the materia medica syllabus in the homoeopathic colleges and university departments had become voluminous. During the 1880s and 1890s many state legislatures had instituted licensing examinations for physicians, which compelled orthodox practitioners to co-operate with homoeopaths, first in obtaining passage of the legislation and then in consultations during the assessing of levels of qualification of candidates. This was in conflict with the AMA's Code of Ethics which prohibited all such consultations with non-orthodox physicians. The problem no longer existed for the homoeopaths, as the AIH had already declared itself open to non-homoeopathic physicians (at its annual meeting in 1870).

In 1900 the homoeopaths were a comfortable ratio of 1 to 5333 persons in the USA, totalling just under 15000 homoeopaths in all,[2] whereas the orthodox practitioners were a meagre 1 to every 767 in the population, with orthodox practitioners totalling just over 104000.[3] That is a ratio of one homoeopath to every seven orthodox practitioners, which had remained approximately

---

[1] Ibid., p 412, quoting *Southern Journal of Homoeopathy*, N.S., 1888, vol I, p 32.

[2] Ibid., p 439 [15000 is an estimate by Coulter]; in 1894 the AIH gave the number of homoeopaths to be at around 14000: *Transactions of the AIH*, 1894, vol XLVII, p 131.

[3] Ibid., in footnote 147, referring to p 439, quoting *Journal of the AMA*, 1901, vol XXXVII, p 838.

constant since 1871. [At that time Tullio Suzzara Verdi (1829-1902) (see entry under this name) wrote to US President Grant informing him that the number of homoeopaths in the USA was then around 6000. In the same year the AMA estimated the number of orthodox practitioners in the USA to stand at about 39000].[1]

Around 1900 the homoeopaths of the USA controlled 112 hospitals (offering a total of 11421 beds), 34 sanatoria or nursing homes, a large number of maternity homes, 62 orphanages and geriatric homes, 149 dispensaries, and 16 mental hospitals. Some of the best endowed hospitals and institutions were in homoeopathic hands at that time. Yet there were serious weaknesses in three areas in the seemingly vibrant homoeopathic camp:

i) The affluence and the high personal esteem in which each was generally held by the community, made the rank and file homoeopath thoroughly complacent and unfortunately rather unconcerned about the activities of the AIH.

ii) The deep desire for the removal of all professional ostracisms that attended the maintenance of the distinct homoeopathic identity by a physician. (For an explicit statement of this yearning, see the quotation by Richard Hughes given under 'History of Homoeopathy before 1900', section United Kingdom, under Hughes' philosophical approach, point 5.)

iii) The irreconcilable division that racked the conceptual fundamentals of homoeopathy in the unresolved 'symptomatology-pathology' dispute that had gone on for four decades. (See 'Hempel, Charles Julius (1811-1879)' and 'Pathology' for a discussion of the issues involved.)

The 'symptomatology-pathology' dispute was particularly acute inside the twenty-two homoeopathic medical schools, where the feud split the professors and lecturers into two contradictory factions: the departments of pharmacology, therapeutics, materia medica and miasmatics were usually on the one side, and anatomy, chemistry, physiology and pathology on the other. The open antagonism on the hallowed precincts of homoeopathy's very propagation so seriously disturbed the students that in 1901 they submitted a complaint to the AIH asking that the contradictory teaching in the several chairs be, in some measure, tempered by the establishment of a Chair of Applied Homoeopathic Therapeutics (which should recommend remedial practice measures not at variance with the laws of Homoeopathy).

The Accomplishments of Simmons
In his obituary one reads:

Unquestionably he was the greatest figure in his generation in the American Medical Association and the profession which it represents.[2]

Simmons identified the AMA's and the profession's problems as:

[1] Ibid., p 293, footnote b.
[2] Ibid., p 420, quoting *Journal of the AMA*, 1937, vol CIX, p 807.

a) Chronic lack of funds in the AMA's coffers.

b) Threatened domination by the pharmaceutical industry.

c) Comparative excellence of a competing homoeopathic profession.

d) Oversupply of graduates from orthodox medical schools.

He tackled all these with aplomb.

Its Journal was always the AMA's chief source of income and under his editorship the number of subscribers to it increased more than sixfold, from 13078 (1900) to 80297 (1924), which helped to improve the AMA's financial position accordingly.

In eight consecutive issues of the AMA's Journal during 1900 Simmons published a series of articles entitled 'Relations of Pharmacy to the Medical Profession' probing into most facets of the 'proprietaries' dilemma that had bedevilled the AMA for almost a quarter of a century. These articles were summarized, still in 1900, in an editorial of that Journal. Clearly Simmons felt that orthodox medicine's future lay in the expedience of dropping the AMA's official animosity toward the 'proprietaries' and to forge a quasi-symbiotic alliance with the pharmaceutical industry. Quite brilliantly, Simmons had mapped out in 1900 the policy that the AMA was, in fact, to adopt and pursue from 1903 onward:

i) It ought to be a matter of irrelevancy to the AMA whether or not a process, a pharmaceutical composition, or a name were protected by trade mark, copyright, patent, or the like.

ii) Quite to the contrary, it needed to be acknowledged that a manufacturer had a right to claim protection when he had devised something of value to the orthodox medical profession, or to the public.

iii) Medicinal preparations, the composition of which is kept secret, should be denied all orthodox medical patronage.

iv) Advertisements for 'proprietaries' or patent medicines that do not accord with the stipulation of such full disclosure would have to be eliminated from the pages of medical journals on expiration of the then existing contracts.

During 1900, too, the (orthodox) US Pharmacopoeial Convention began the reform process to which Simmons was pointing when it decided to accept into the orthodox US Pharmacopoeia the patented synthetic chemicals that had been flooding into the USA from Germany since before 1890. These chemicals were known by their registered trade names and included Acetopyrin, Antifebrin (or Acetanilid), Antipyrin, Benzopyrin, Bromopyrin, Exalgin, Formopyrin, Kairin, Phenazon and Salipyrin.

Then, in 1903, the AMA promulgated a new Code of Ethics, which simply omitted the word 'patent'. Its revised proscription read that orthodox physicians might not 'dispense or promote the use of secret medicines'. This made advertising quite respectable by 'proprietary' and patent medicine manufacturers, provided a pro forma list of ingredients was supplied. A blind eye was initially turned to the fact that such lists were drawn up in a manner that made the duplication of the medicine impossible in almost all instances. In other words the listings were *de facto* unverifiable and only served the *de jure* purpose of legitimizing an existing unwholesome situation. The manufacturers were delighted because their products had finally been granted proper recognition. The orthodox physicians were relieved because their prescriptions would no longer be illicit. Gradually the independent medical journals could shake off the hated 'shot-gun contracts' they had been forced to enter into with the manufacturers.

Having won the first skirmish, Simmons quickly moved to a forward position for the next battle with the pharmaceutical industry. He again first announced his plans in the Journal of the AMA in 1905. He then executed them by having the AMA establish its own Council on Pharmacy and Chemistry with a mandate to distinguish the good 'proprietaries' from inferior ones, since it was evident that the provision of incomplete formulae did not allow for the verification of manufacturers' claims. Through this new Council a standard was to be set for all medicines that were not accepted into the orthodox US Pharmacopoeia. The stated aim was that the orthodox physician might obtain a true, not merely a pro forma knowledge of the medicines he was prescribing. The AMA was to issue what became the 'New and Non-Official Remedies' listing for all 'proprietaries' and similar medicines that conformed to the set standards. Despite efficacy claims contained in labelling, packaging and package-inserts being henceforward prohibited, this stricture did not, unfortunately, cover advertising in medical journals nor to literature distributed to orthodox physicians. This meant physicians were still being fed information the manufacturers liked them to believe, rather than genuine, independently established knowledge. Moreover, when the formulae of 'proprietaries' were scrutinized by the Council only active substances and the motivating grounds for their combination in one formula were looked into and not, for instance, the vehicles, preservatives, colourings or flavourings. All the same, these less than stringent standards together with the prospect of orthodox patronage easily induced most manufacturers of 'proprietaries' to agree to 'full' disclosure and to submit their products to the Council's scrutiny. The manufacturers were then also persuaded to make the obligatory purchase of space in the 'New and Non-Official Remedies', which turned the exercise into a very profitable one for the AMA.

But the resourceful Simmons' stratagem was really aimed at the longer-term future. He had contrived to place the manufacturers and their products firmly in the hands of the AMA's new Council for their standards to be applied gradually ever more stringently, while they were continually helping to swell further the AMA's coffers. Although the ratio of orthodox practitioner to population number remained about 1:700, a large number of orthodox physicians were eventually employed in one or other way for drug manufacturers' research, etc., which the tighter standards later necessitated ever more compellingly. As a direct consequence of this, the remaining number actually engaged in patient care declined to a more comfortable ratio of about

1:1800. Also by tying the orthodox medical profession to the drug industry Simmons assured a constant source of funds for the profession from advertising, research and/or educational grants, etc., while at the same time having tamed the pharmaceutical industry.

Simmons had been active in another area too. Soon after Simmons took office, he also had a Committee on Organization established in the AMA, with himself as its secretary. Soon (by 1901) this committee had drafted a new AMA constitution and a corresponding set of bylaws, the adoption of which reduced the number of representatives in the AMA's House of Delegates, its legislative arm, to less than ten percent of the previously very unwieldy body that had comprised one and a half thousand representatives. This made the legislative body much more manageable for the General Secretary's purposes. A testimony of Simmons' political far-sightedness is that he skilfully managed to suppress in the bylaws the requirement that the constituent State Societies of the AMA would have to subscribe to the AMA's Code of Ethics, which, in its so-called 'ban on consultation' clause, still prohibited all professional contact between orthodox physicians and homoeopaths. Besides, the membership requirement for the constitutions of County Societies (the subsidiaries of State Societies) was radically liberalized to read:

'every reputable and legally qualified physician who is practising or who will agree to practise non-sectarian medicine shall be entitled to membership'.[1]

The wily Simmons, whose slogan was 'A united profession in the United States', had decided to replace the AMA's fifty-year old policy of confrontation with homoeopathy as a medical system by one of conciliatory assimilation of individual homoeopaths. He, the ex-homoeopath, knew precisely how strong the yearning for scientific integration was amongst homoeopaths, and how weakened the AIH had actually become from both the apathy arising from the prosperity of individual homoeopaths and the effects of the internecine 'symptomatology-pathology' feud. The change in this membership requirement was an expedient ploy to have State and County Societies admit the affluent homoeopathic physicians (again bringing in new funds), which, soon enough, would force the AMA's House of Delegates to reappraise the 'consultation clause', which had almost attained the status of the AMA's sacred cow. In 1902 the Journal of the AMA stated that this policy had been a success in that a considerable number of homoeopaths had joined the orthodox medical societies. The inducement to homoeopaths was conciliatory in the sense that the homoeopath who joined an orthodox medical society would, in theory, be quite free to continue to practise according to the Similia Principle for as long as he so wished to do, but he was no longer permitted to attach the epithet 'homoeopath' to himself, nor could he proselytize for homoeopathy. In fact, all other sectarian epithets, like Eclectic, allopath and hydropath, were also banished from orthodox medical jargon at the same time, allowing the former allopaths seemingly to occupy the central ground of scientific

---

[1] Ibid., p 428, quoting *Journal of the AMA*, 1902, vol XXXIX, pp 314-316, 1158.

impartiality. But in practice it was different, as so many reported in both the homoeopathic and the orthodox medical press. For example:

'In consultation with Old-School practitioners all goes placidly until you speak of homoeopathic methods. Immediately you lose caste. In place of interest being aroused towards you, or that which you represent, all is a silence. Their approval lasts as long as you acquiesce in their methods'.[1]

Simmons was also behind the following developments in the AMA concerned with medical education. In 1902 the Committee on Medical Education was formed, out of which emerged (in 1904) the AMA's Council on Medical Education, with a mandate for upgrading all US medical schools. It set down a table of criteria against which the colleges would be rated. It brazenly put about its claim that since the AMA was now admitting homoeopaths to membership it was representative of the whole medical profession, and thereby enabled to pass judgement on orthodox as well as homoeopathic and other medical schools. During 1907 all medical schools were visited by AMA representatives and graded. The results was that firstly the homoeopathic, Eclectic and physio-medical colleges denied the AMA's proper competence in law to such an evaluation and secondly many orthodox medical schools had serious complaints intrinsic to the issue of the actual grading methods employed. Furthermore, the homoeopaths could point to an AMA survey of medical licensing examination results showing a greater failure rate (for the 1900 to 1905 period) by orthodox medical graduates when compared with that of the homoeopaths in 'basic science' subjects.

But Simmons' Council on Medical Education was not to be outsmarted. It suggested calling in an objective outsider, and then quickly proceeded to ask the prestigious Carnegie Endowment for the Advancement of Teaching to lend its support. This was an astute manoeuvre: since none of the medical schools would want to fall foul of Carnegie Endowment's fund allocation program, they might all be expected to try to present a liberated facade. As a result the AMA's Nathan Colwell was joined by Carnegie Endowment's Abraham Flexner in 1909 and 1910 in making a survey of all US medical schools. This survey is known as the 'Flexner Report', although Colwell admittedly provided far more guidance in this survey than its name would suggest.

The criteria employed by Colwell and Flexner against which all US medical schools were assessed were established only from within orthodox medicine's philosophical paradigm, embedded in the Rationalist tradition. For example, the following would count against homoeopathic medical schools: 'excessive' allotment of time to pharmacology, toxicology, organic chemistry and materia medica in the homoeopathic curriculum; 'too little' emphasis on non-homoeopathic subjects like inorganic chemistry and pathology; perceived 'inadequacy' of laboratory science instruction and/or laboratory facilities; the 'shorter' number of hours spent in the lecture rooms of homoeopathic colleges, because the homoeopaths did much bed-side teaching; finally, no value was

---

[1] Ibid., p 437, quoting *Homoeopathic Recorder*, 1910, vol XXV, p 425.

attached to the homoeopathic research area of controlled pathogenetic experimentation undertaken at some schools.

The State examining boards accepted the findings of the Flexner Report and the AMA's continuing evaluation of the medical schools, with the result that all candidates (even the most successful) from medical schools with a low rating were simply debarred from the licensing examinations. Such lowly-rated medical schools were forced to close. The cynical truth is that this helped, in some measure, to reduce the oversupply of medical graduates, as Simmons had wanted.

In an attempt to adjust to the continuing imposition by the AMA of criteria foreign to homoeopathy, the 'basic science' departments of the homoeopathic medical schools came to be controlled by non-homoeopaths. They, swept along by the prevailing current of mechanistic philosophy, soon heaped ridicule – in front of students – upon the homoeopathic departments of materia medica, medicine, miasmatics and pharmacology. The homoeopathic professors were pressured into joining the orthodox medical societies by which, *ipso facto*, they emasculated themselves. They then reserved homoeopathic treatment for their families and some selected patients, but otherwise did not advocate or practise it. Since they were not allowed to proselytize, they then taught what someone has called 'dilute orthodoxy'. Their courses were soon converted into unredeemed orthodox medical courses.

Within ten years of the publication of the Flexner Report 15 of the 22 homoeopathic medical schools were no more and about fifteen years after that the remainder had disappeared or become orthodox. That, of course, helped to reduce still further the oversupply of medical graduates. Without centres for tertiary education there were no more homoeopathic practitioners turned out and the patients, though they did not like it, looked elsewhere. Because the AIH did not have a man to match the dedicated, agile mind and political acumen of the AMA's Simmons, whose towering political genius loomed behind all these stunning developments, the USA, and such countries as emulated this development there, paid an enormous scientific forfeit in the twentieth century.

That forfeit was homoeopathy.

(See 'Eclipse of Homoeopathy (1920-1965)', 'Epistemological Assumptions in Homoeopathy', 'Hempel, Charles Julius (1811-1879)', 'History of Homoeopathy before 1900' sections on UK and USA, 'Pathology' and 'Philosophical Premise of Homoeopathy'.)

Simpson, Sir James Young (1811-1870)

Scottish Professor of Obstetrics first at St Andrews University, Fife, later at Edinburgh University, who first used chloroform as an anaesthetic, both in labour and in surgery. He designed an obstetrical forceps now named after him. This teacher and later a close friend of the homoeopaths John Drysdale and Thomas Skinner was undoubtedly one of the leading lights among surgeons of the nineteenth century. In 1847 Simpson read his first paper on chloroform anaesthesia to the Medico-Chirurgical Society of Edinburgh which met with a storm of antagonism. This was gradually subdued and in 1857, the year in which Skinner (1825-1906) graduated, Simpson's triumph was total. The enthusiasm of Skinner, the homoeopath, for chloroform anaesthesia was such that he invented an inhaler (known as Skinner's mask) and a drip-feed bottle (known as Skinner's dropper-flask). Although Simpson never became a homoeopath, he learned from his friends Drysdale and Skinner the value of giving only one medicine at one time, which resulted in his inveighing against poly-pharmacy ever fashionable in orthodox prescribing.

Single Remedy

For the homoeopath who practises in the classical tradition it is a *sine qua non* that, in order to match an appropriate drug to a particular disease picture, only one medicine can ever be truly homoeopathic to the presenting illness at any one time. Therefore, single remedies (and not combinations thereof) should be administered to patients. This is so since the remedies were proved singly and not as mixtures, and combinations of remedies may well present reactive effects which are different from their constituting medicines individually. When one single remedy should prove to be inadequate in any particular case, the homoeopaths Sheila and Robin Gibson advise as follows: 'Where more than one remedy is required they can be given in sequence, one at a time, a certain length of time apart – one every ten minutes, for example, or one every half hour. Administering the remedies in this way allows the body to process each remedy individually, a situation analogous to presenting a computer with only one program at a time'.[1]

It is, however, true that there is a section of 'homoeopaths' (perhaps more correctly called 'prescribing naturopaths') who, in fact, do use remedies in combination, and who report good clinical results with this method, even when subjected to controlled clinical trials. (See 'Classical Homoeopathy', 'Clinical Trials' and 'Combinations of Homoeopathic Drugs'.)

Skin Disorders

See 'Eczema', 'Epistemological Assumptions in Homoeopathy', section 1 (where dermatitis medicamentosa is discussed in some detail), 'Externally Applied Homoeopathic Drugs' and 'Externalization of Disease'.

Skinner, Thomas (1825-1906)

Scottish homoeopath who graduated from St Andrews University in 1857. He was a late convert to the new scientific method in medicine to which at first

---

[1] Gibson, Sheila and Robin. *Homoeopathy for Everyone*, Harmondsworth: Penguin Books Ltd, 1987, p 75.

he was antagonistic. He had moved to Liverpool, Lancashire, England where for three years he was incapacitated as he suffered from intractable insomnia, severe dyspepsia and constipation. No treatment seemed to help him at all until the homoeopath E W Berridge prescribed Sulphur in a high potency for him. Dame Margery Blackie in her book *The Patient, Not the Cure* (London: Macdonald and Jane's, 1982, pp 157 & 158) says, '. . . its effect was a revelation to Dr Skinner. He said, "I shall never forget the marvellous change which the first dose effected in a few weeks, especially the rolling-away, as it were, of a dense and heavy cloud from my mind". He was cured of his constipation and acid dyspepsia, sleeplessness, deficient assimilation and debility and restored to a life of usefulness and vigour.'

Skinner invented an inhaler (known as Skinner's mask) and a drip-feed bottle (known as Skinner's dropper-flask) for chloroform anaesthesia about which he was enthusiastic. He conducted a few pathogenetic experiments (provings) for homoeopathy, for instance in 1893 on Melitagrinum (squamosa of eczema capitis), which nosode has since been shown to be clinically effective in milk crust (crusta lactea). For homoeopathic pharmacy he devised the 'Skinner Continuous Fluxion Apparatus' which is still used by Boericke and Tafel, Philadelphia, Pennsylvania, USA in the manufacture of very high dynamizations (above 1000CK). (For a description of the functioning of the Skinner apparatus see entry under 'Potentizing Methods', section entitled International Distribution of Scales and Methods).

Toward the end of the nineteenth century Skinner became a member of the Dining Club that also comprised John Henry Clarke, Robert Cooper and James Compton Burnett. Skinner, who had already won the gold medal for merit in obstetrics and gynaecology at St Andrews University, retained a life-long interest in that area of homoeopathy and his major work is *Homoeopathy and Gynaecology* (1878).

Soft Paraffin

See 'Vaselinum Flavum'.

Solute

The dissolved substance in a solution.

Solution

Method for the solving of a problem; answer to a significant question; resolution of disease by crisis; more commonly, in homoeopathy, it refers to tinctures, or the homogenous state of a liquid, resulting from the incorporation of extraneous substance(s), not of biological origin, whether liquid, gaseous or solid. (See 'Dose' and 'Mother Tincture'.)

Solvation Structures

Are taken to be produced in homoeopathy by successive 'consolidations' and 'adaptations' of the original molecular clathrate-like structure of the solvent, shaken into drug-specific shapes by the mechanical stimulus (succussion or trituration) accompanying each stage of dilution in potentization (refer to 'Potency' for experimental evidence). As all biological reactions are shape-specific, it is of considerable significance that the potentization processes should result in solvation structures of a diversity of drug-specific shapes in the diluent of the homoeopathic medicines.

In 1977 the Austrian homoeopath Gerhard Resch of the Institut für wissenschaftliche Homöopathie, Mariahilferstrasse 74b, A-1070 Vienna published the intricate results of his highly technical pioneering work in this significant field, done in part with Dr Viktor Gutmann, professor of chemistry. He presented this comprehensive thesis at the XXXIInd International Homoeopathic Congress, held from 5th to 11th October 1977 in New Delhi, India, under the auspices of the Liga Medicorum Homoeopathica Internationalis.[1] He challenged the then widely accepted view in physics that particles dissolved in water or in hydro-ethanol mixtures rearrange the molecules of the solvent only in their immediate vicinity, allowing the solvated solutes to be considered as mobile units within a continuum of a nearly undisturbed medium. The following summarized evidence in physics refuting this seemingly over-simplified model is part of that presented by him:

a) Micelle formation of polyethylene-oxide derivatives shows hydration numbers up to 200 water-molecules and hence a long range distribution of hydration structure.

b) In a 1 molar aluminium sulphate solution nearly all water molecules are engaged in the hydration structure.

c) Calculations based on the oversimplified model show that only after the addition of six layers of water molecules is the limiting bond energy attained in successive water molecules if arranged in a hypothetical chain beginning from an alkali metal ion.

d) Exceptionally long range structural stabilization has been inferred from the rheological properties of an aqueous solution of the copper salt of cetyl-phenyl-ether-sulphonic acid, which retains elastic properties even in a 0.002% solution, corresponding to a solute concentration of 2.10^{-6} mol/litre. Thus it contains about 25 million water molecules per solute molecule, or more than 100 water layers arranged around every solute molecule.

e) Water will dissolve quartz-glass if it is contained in capillary tubes of silica of a diameter up to 4 micrometres (formerly microns), corresponding to 14800 water layers from surface to surface. Given that the glass dissolution process sets in up to that diameter, it follows that up to 7400 layers of water are involved.

[1] Resch, Gerhard. *Transactions of the XXXII International Homoeopathic Congress held under the auspices of the LMHI Geneva:* Vigyan Bhawan, New Delhi, India, 5th-11th October, 1977, pp 113-116.

He pointed out that analogous structural features were evident elsewhere too. For example, the structural features involved in growing successive layers of SiO_2 on an aluminium-silicate surface showed that its effects were completely lost to the Al-O bonds only once twenty SiO_2 layers had been added.

He directed attention to the fact that the exigent pressures for the reorganization of the solvent's structural pattern resulting from the acceptance of a solute are:

1 the co-ordinative effects;
2 the possible polarization effects between solute and surrounding water;
3 the coactive polarization effects between the individual solvation spheres.

(He maintained there were, in principle, no delimitations between a solvation sphere structure and a solution structure.)

He emphasized that liquid water consisting exclusively of water molecules, as believed by many, in fact, did not exist in reality. Water contains hydrogen and hydronium ions (H_3O+) to the extent that 820 water layers are available for each ion. In addition, aqua destillata contains various amounts of carbon dioxide and constitutes a 10^{-3} molar solution of oxygen and nitrogen, corresponding to approximately 44000 water molecules for one gas molecule.

He drew attention to the fact that in the crystalline compounds known as clathrates the dissolved molecules of the recessive component, such as an inert gas (e.g. xenon), are known to be contained within structural holes in which they can rotate freely. In such compounds many of these holes remain empty. He postulated that such structural holes might be expected to be present in the liquid state also. He proposed the concept of liquid water as a highly differentiated 'pseudo macromolecule' containing both hydronium ions and mobile holes, saying that to some extent this description agreed with the so-called flickering cluster model (believed by a few physicist-theoreticians to flicker as frequently as once every tenth of a billionth of a second), where the boundaries between the clusters change, and which could be described in terms of the mobile holes. Furthermore, the cluster model implied the existence of a surface tension within the inner surface area of each of the holes. According to the extended donor-acceptor approach by Viktor Gutmann, each inner surface area is characterized by hydrogen bonds shorter than those of the successive layers. This is supported by nuclear magnetic resonance (NMR) measurements on solutions of hydrocarbons, where an upfield shift is found which denotes a decrease in hydrogen bonding (Engelfeld and Nemethy, 1973.) [NMR can measure the spin of protons; recent studies on twenty-three different homoeopathic medicines and dynamizations showed distinctive readings of sub-atomic activity, though the placebo did not.[1,2] Two more homoeopathic studies on MNR at the University of Lyons and at Rome

[1] Sacks, Adam. 'NMR Spectroscopy of Homoeopathic Remedies', *Journal of Holistic Medicine*, vol V, Autumn/Winter 1983, pp 172-175.

[2] Boericke, G W, and R B Smith. 'Changes Caused by Succussion on NMR Patterns and Bioassay of Bradykinin Triacetate (BKTA) Succussions and Dilution', *Journal of the American Institute of Homoeopathy*, vol LXI, November/December 1968, pp 197-212.

University have been reported since.][1] Further support for the inner surface tensions is provided by thermodynamic data (Cox et al., 1974).

Resch showed that the three-dimensional pattern of collective structures is composed of structural elements that differ slightly from any one spatial layer to another, in that the greatest hydrogen bond lengths are to be found in the regions which are most remote from the inner and outer surface areas. He also showed that the situation is analogous for solutes that have been hydrated in that these break the water structure with the formation of hydration structures involving most ions of the polar solutes, whose molecules, in consequence, are capable of dipole moment and orientation. Hence, Resch considered each solute molecule, or a cluster of these, and each hole as a structure-regulating centre. The sum of the effects of all structure-regulating centres determines the actual structural pattern of the liquid. [Polar substances – like salts, alkalis and acids – ionize into cationic (positively charged) and anionic (negatively charged) components.]

The actual structural pattern was typified by what he decided to call the 'bond-length variation spectrum'. At very short distances between two structure regulating centres the number of water layers is small and, therefore, the bond length relatively short. By increasing the distance the number of water layers increases between the centres and with it the maximum value for the hydrogen bond lengths. By increasing the distance the stated effects become greater and, hence, the number of less differentiated hydrogen bonds is increased; that is to say, the number of molecules assigned to nearly undisturbed water molecules is increased.

Water is anomalous in so many ways. It is one of only four substances which expand upon solidification (the others: Ge, Si and crystalline C), whereas every other substance contracts. It can form nine different forms of ice crystals, depending upon variations in atmospheric pressure, and when water is frozen in a magnetic field the resultant crystal pattern is again altered. Both its boiling point and melting point are much higher than its formula would suggest: at ambient temperatures and pressure it ought not to be a liquid but to be a gas. It becomes a more viscous liquid with decreasing temperature. Resch says, 'Water is a *conditio sine qua non* for any life process' and goes on to compare it to heavy water (D_2O; deuterium oxide) in which most of the hydrogen atoms are deuterium (2H; heavy hydrogen). Heavy water, though it has a higher boiling and freezing point than normal water, otherwise has structural differences that are too small to be detected with accuracy by available methods. Nonetheless, it shows drastically different biological effects to normal water, in that it is retardative and even toxic. Thus biological and (bio)chemical reactions, as well as combinations formed with other substances depend on the way the electrons are arranged in the molecules involved, which will allow for a stable configuration to be achieved. It seems to be the difference in the

[1] Boiron, Jean. 'Une année de recherche biopharmacologique', *Homéopathie*, vol V(1), 1988, pp 13-18.

hydrogen bonds of the two that accounts for the biological difference between water and heavy water.

Resch inferred that increasing inter-centre distance, with increasing dilution, would have to lead to a decreasing variety in hydrogen bond lengths in water. In other words, the number of molecules with the maximum bond length, as in the peak areas, is increased as the inter-centre distance is increased, as their number is decreased, i.e. as the solution becomes more dilute. The more dilute the solution the more uniform the 'bond length variety spectrum' will become and hence the more significant the relative differences within the structural pattern will be.

Ordinary ice formed at standard atmospheric pressure by a normal drop in temperature is known as hexagonal ice. This produces an open lattice structure of hydrogen-bonded molecules of H_2O. That is a three-dimensional honeycomb of empty spaces that run at right angles to, as well as parallel to, the lattice layers of the hexagon-produced furrows. This structure is substantially maintained when ice melts, becoming a liquid made up of a random network of its molecules linked by hydrogen bonds, perhaps strained at times, and even broken, but similar in general structure to the hexagonal ice.

This liquid is seen as a complex random clathrate-like three-dimensional structure, like a kaleidoscopic agglomeration of polymers, constantly re-organizing, in line with gravity, and strain-reducing or other reorganizing effects. Non-polar molecules dissolved in it are seen to be accepted into the holes where they induce adaptive shape-specific polymeric structures around each solute molecule, comparable to a complementary solute-specific cage or mould. This countersunk die is an impress in the water polymer that may be stabilized through a process of succussion (as utilized in homoeopathic dynamizations). Such a repeated succussion process may, moreover, continue to pass on that characteristic shape-encoding to other parts of the solvent, and onward into ultramolecular dilutions thereof, in line with the exigent pressures towards uniformity in bond length and structural patterns. It is probable, therefore, that the information of the original solute (the impregnating basic medicine in homoeopathy) may be transmitted to the solvent (the hydro-alcoholic mixture in homoeopathy) and along ultramolecular dilutions of it by means of succussion.

Resch asked the pertinent question, 'What are the effects of shaking the solution after each dilution step?' He put forward these answers:

a) The mechanical deformation of the holes and hence the changes in the inner surface tension provoke different arrangements in their neighbourhood with consecutive structural and energetic changes.

b) The structure-regulating centres come more proximately under one another's influence, or even intimately into contact with each other, provoking stronger interactions and, therefore, co-operative processes.

c) The incorporation of oxygen molecules in some empty holes of the solution is accompanied by an increase in its thermal stability (although the actual role of this oxygen in homoeopathic medicines is unclear).

A number of other models to explain the structure and properties of water have been put forward by other physicists, though all studies so far have been inconclusive.

(See 'Aqua Destillata', 'Clathrate', 'Drug Strength', 'Drug Preparation', 'Pharmacological Message', 'Physiological Response in Homoeotherapeutics, Mechanism of', 'Potency', 'Potentization', 'Potentizing Methods', 'Science and Homoeopathy', 'Succussion' and 'Trituration'.)

Solvent

Fluid in which a substance is (capable of being) dissolved.

Sound Therapy

Uses audible sound and ultrasound to heal. It is a naturopathic approach that is considered to be complementary to homoeopathy by many. (See 'Naturopath'.)

Sources of Homoeopathic Drug Semiology

Homoeopathy gathers its fund of knowledge about drug actions and medicinally provoked reactions from four sources:

1 pathogenetic experimentation – the provings, which are controlled drug tests on healthy human subjects;
2 data from toxicology and pharmacology – the accidental poisonings of forensic medicine, the 'side-effects' of allopathica, and the teratogenic and other abnormal effects induced by a variety of factors (e.g. radioactivity, pollution, food adulterants, etc.);
3 clinical use – this establishes genuine similarities and verifies curative effect (see 'Guiding Symptoms of the Materia Medica');
4 veterinary use and experimental studies done on animals – many homoeopaths have serious doubts as to the justification for any experiments on animals, feeling that even the so-called humane experiments (in the course of which ensue only subtoxic, painless alterations of an animal's biochemistry) amount to gross abuse; nonetheless data are also gathered daily by veterinary homoeopaths, while actually treating sick animals, where there is no primary intention to do research, and where the suggestive component (placebo-effect) is virtually excluded.

This fund of knowledge, derived from the above four sources, constitutes the essence of the materia medica of homoeopathy. (See 'Materia Medica'.)

Spa

Hydropathic clinic or water-cure establishment in a locality with a spring or springs of special balneotherapeutic properties; naturopathic health resort with at least one mineral spring, the waters of which possess therapeutic properties as a result of being:

borated,
muriated,
silicious, or
sulphated.

The waters may be either (1) alkaline, (2) alkaline-saline, (3) saline or (4) acidic. If they are (5) neutral the waters are said to possess no therapeutic properties and the spa then merely provides hydrotherapy treatment in these waters. So-called hydrothermal treatment, i.e. with naturally heated waters, may be a feature of any such spa. The attending homoeopath will advise a patient on the suitability or otherwise of exposure to reactive effects of identified mineralized spring waters.

Spagyric

Method derived from plant alchemy for preparing tinctures, committed to writing by Johann Rudolf Glauber (1604-1668) in his *Pharmacopoeia Spagyrica* and earlier by Paracelsus (Theophrastus Bombastus von Hohenheim, 1493-1541) in his book *Paragranum*. The manner in which spagyrics differ from non-spagyric mother tinctures is that, according to the principles of alchemy, the spagyric preparation opens the plant, liberating stronger curative powers than standard tincture preparations. Whereas plant residues are normally thrown away after extraction in the preparation of a succus, the spagyric preparations always contain the salts retrieved through calcination and incineration of the plant residue. These are, in large part, water-soluble, having been leached with aqua destillata from the calcined material. The other salts that are insoluble in water are often but not always put aside as alchemically unacceptable terra damnata (damned earth). The salts that go into the preparation are called sal salis (salt of the salts) and are known to have great curative effects, since these were often used on their own.

The Thuringian (German) homoeopath, Carl Friedrich Zimpel (1800-1878) devoted himself intensively to the study of the works of Paracelsus and Glauber. Originally he was an engineer and later he studied medicine, obtaining doctorates in both philosophy and in medicine. This learned man, who was widely travelled, was elected an honorary member of the Mineralogical Society of the University of Jena (Germany). He was also awarded the Gold Medal of Prussia for Science and Art. He began a new production of spagyric medicines, which has survived to this day and is now known as the Müller/Göppingen Chemisch-Pharmazeutische Fabrik in western Germany. This company's special division of Staufen-Pharma, producers of internationally renowned homoeopathic preparations, manufactures homoeopathic spagyric mother tinctures and derivative potencies. Other homoeopathic pharmaceutical laboratories, one of which is in France, are also known to use spagyric mother tinctures from which they run up their homoeopathic dynamizations (potencies). Zimpel himself later established himself in London as a homoeopath (in 1849), but did not play a great political role in the development of homoeopathy in the UK. A current textbook on the subject is *Spagyrische Arzneimittel-Lehre,* Göppingen: Staufen Pharma, 1938 & 1953.

The term 'spagyric' has also been used as a synonym for 'alchemist'.

Spatula

As much a part of the small-scale comminution equipment as are mortars and pestles. The spatula, a broad-bladed scraper, is used to loosen the powdered material that becomes packed on the inner side of the mortar. Many substances will pack easily under the pressure exerted by the pestle and, unless the compacted mass is loosened frequently, work is hampered. Spatulas come in a variety of sizes and materials. The powder spatulas, used in weighing or during trituration, are made of stainless steel and have a balanced handle. The weight of the handle is sufficient to counterpoise the weight of the blade so that when the spatula is put down on a flat surface the blade will not touch that surface. A solid hard-rubber spatula, or a horn spatula, is used with corrosive materials that would react with steel. A spatula used to push a patient's tongue down, or to the side, should, even though sterilized, never thereafter be used in any medicine preparation work. (See 'Utensils of Homoeopathic Pharmacy'.)

Specific

Remedy said always to have a definite curative action in relation to a particular disease state or (set of) symptom(s), as Cinchona officinalis in malarial intermittent fevers, or Mercurius in the secondary stages of syphilis. (See 'Miasma'.)

Specific Disease

See 'Miasma' and 'Specific'.

Specific Gravity

Relative density. Ratio of the mass of a given volume of a substance to the mass of an equal volume of aqua destillata at 4 degrees Celsius.

Spiritus Vini Rectificatus

Alcohol; ethanol; rectified spirit. (See 'Alcohol'.)

Spontaneous Remission

See 'Remission, Spontaneous'.

Spoons

See 'Utensils of Homoeopathic Pharmacy'.

Stahl, Georg Ernst (1660-1734)

See 'Philosophical Premise of Homoeopathy'.

Stapf, Johann Ernst (1788-1860)

Hahnemann's most intimate friend from 1812 to 1835 (Hahnemann's removal to Paris) and beyond that time his regular correspondent right up to 1843 (Hahnemann's death), was born in Naumburg an der Saale and died in Kösen, both in the Electorate of Saxony (now Germany). He studied medicine at Leipzig and in 1814 he graduated, having written a dissertation entitled 'De antagonismo organico'.

In 1812 he had read the *Organon* and Hahnemann's first big work *Fragmenta de viribus* (published 1805). In 1813 he began corresponding with Hahnemann, who soon commissioned him to prove medicines. Little by little he contributed to the provings of Chamomilla matricaria, Rhus toxicodendron, Pulsatilla nigricans, Nux vomica, Cinchona officinalis, Opium, Camphora and Helleborus niger. Over the years he ultimately proved no less than thirty-two homoeopathic medicines. He was a very talented man of unusual accuracy in scientific thought, a gifted clinician, and a man of wide general knowledge and a pleasant disposition. From 1822 to 1839 he published the first scientific homoeopathic journal, the *Archiv für die homöopathische Heilkunst* (from 1836 Gustav Wilhelm Gross, a champion of Isopathy, became co-publisher with him). Stapf, his co-publisher's inclinations notwithstanding, was the first to point out the crucial differences between a homoeopathic nosode (having a defined drug picture established by provings) and an auto-isopathic preparation (where no standard proving is possible). He remained a consistent defender of the 'pure' homoeopathic theory as propounded by Hahnemann, whom he always loyally and openly supported in all the many disputes. He always treated Hahnemann with the deepest respect in his *Archiv* and he became an indispensable pillar of support for the earlier days of the new scientific movement in medicine. On Hahnemann's doctorate jubilee in 1829 he arranged to have published the *Lesser Writings* of homoeopathy's founder he admired so greatly. He was much sought after as a homoeopathic clinician, who believed strongly in the harmful effects of coffee, alcohol and tobacco, in particular. His fame was such that in 1835 he was called to London, England to continue treatment of the Queen of Great Britain which he had begun by letter; thus he became the first of many homoeopaths appointed (down to this day) to the British royal household. He played host to F F H Quin in Naumburg in 1826, where he strengthened Quin's growing conviction of the scientific veracity of homoeopathy. Later he was appointed Medical Councillor for the State of Saxony. His major literary contribution to homoeopathy, apart from the *Archiv,* was that he published the supplements to Hahnemann's *Materia Medica Pura.*

In 1851 von Boenninghausen led him, already deaf with age, the oldest student and friend of the great medical innovator, to hang up the first wreath on the iron railing around the newly erected Hahnemann monument in Leipzig at its unveiling.

Starting Materials

All substances, whether active or 'inactive', or whether they remain unchanged or become altered, that are employed in the preparation of a medicine.

Steiner, Rudolf (1861-1925)

Austrian founder of the philosophical movement of Anthroposophy (= knowledge concerning human attributes) and the dogma of the three-part structure of the social organism, the basis of which he set out in 1894 in *The Philosophy of Freedom.* He was motivated initially as an opponent of Theosophy, and was neither a homoeopath nor an orthodox medical practitioner and came to develop Anthroposophical Medicine (refer to this entry) only later in life. Fifteen months before his demise he founded the School of Spiritual Science (with its Anthroposophical Medical Section, amongst others) at the Goetheanum in Dornach (near Basle), Switzerland for continuing research into the application of his teachings. (See 'Goethe, Johann Wolfgang von (1749-1832)'.)

Stereotypical Disease Condition

See 'Causes of Disease', 'Disease' and 'Miasma'.

Sterilization of Equipment

See 'Cleansing of Utensils and Sterilization'.

Stimulus, Morbific

A pathogenic affect that would tend to arouse a dynamic reactive response (becoming evident as symptoms) if it overwhelms the organism's defence mechanism. Most morbific stimuli, however, do not. They are successfully managed by the organism's life force (dynamis).

Stings (Insect)

See 'Emergencies – Homoeopathic Treatment', section Insect Stings (non-allergenic, including bluebottle- and scorpion-stings, spider- and horsefly-bites) and 'Externally Applied Homoeopathic Drugs', under Acidum aceticum.

Straining

Running off, or percolating, a liquid through a filtering device, with perhaps a little force, to remove insoluble solid particles. Also the making of an effort to the limit of one's capacity, or the act of injuring due to overuse or improper application.

Stress

Burden; strain exerted by a load. Resistance set up by the dynamis as a reaction to a deleterious strain exerted upon the organism, that disturbed its homoeostatic equilibrium. This is too wide a symptom category in the context of homoeopathy, or, rather, it is not a reactive symptom in the strict meaning of that word at all, since an external pressure is actually described by it. Yet occasionally this term is also used for a reactive symptom, for what may be called 'tense nerves'.

Example of syndetic pointers to a homoeopathic medicine where 'tense nerves' are part of the symptom picture:

Neuralgic affections from a fit of anger; drawing pain internally in the region of the right scapula as though the nerves and vessels were made tense – (Citrullus) Colocynthis.

Strong Alcohol

See 'Alcohol'.

Subjective Symptoms

● **Effects of drugs or disease that are discoverable by oneself alone, though they are just as important as those which can be measured by anyone.**

Disease is classified (in homoeopathy) by means of the nominal identification of the illness with the name of the medicine that cures it. For instance, 'a sulphur case' might be an ill patient responsive to treatment with Sulphur, and where the patient's total symptom picture resembles (parts of) that in the materia medica for Sulphur. That means the whole dynamic pattern of the disease response in a patient would have to be considered to arrive at a homoeopathically matching medicine; conversely the full drug picture is checked before matching it to the patient. In both instances so-called subjective symptoms form an important integral part of the semiological complex identifying that particular disease-to-drug parallel. It was Hahnemann's genius that elevated the subjective symptoms to the full status of scientific medical validity.

Succus

Plant juice obtained by expression from fresh plant material.

Succussion

The action of shaking up, or the condition of being shaken up, vigorously of a liquid dilution of a homoeopathic medicine in its phial or bottle, where each stroke ends with a jolt, usually by pounding the hand engaged in the shaking action against the other palm. (See 'Solvation Structures' and 'Trituration'.)

Sugar of Milk

See 'Saccharum Lactis'.

Sulpho-Carbonic Constitution

See 'Constitutional Type'.

Sulphuric Constitution

See 'Constitutional Type'.

Supportive Diet

Since foodstuffs, condiments, drinks and other comestibles all have a reactive effect of their own, this is an indispensable component of effective (i.e. predictable) homoeopathic therapy, quite apart from the attention that must be paid to the nutritional balance of the foods consumed by the patient. In fact, historically all renowned homoeopathic practitioners are known to have placed great emphasis on this aspect of their treatment, as, indeed, Hahnemann had. (See also 'Foods as Health Hazards'; some rudimentary suggestions in regard to this entry are given under 'Homoeopathic Practice'; see also 'Nutritional Equipoise'.)

Suppository

Small, semi-solid plug of either glycerinated gelatin or theobroma oil (as the vehicle) used in homoeopathy as the pharmaceutical means for the introduction of medicine into one of the patient's orifices, other than the oral cavity. The shape given to the small suppositorial mass (e.g. cone-, candle-, spindle-, pencil-, globe- or egg-shaped) varies with its application. For example, vaginal suppositories are generally egg-shaped, ear suppositories cone-shaped, rectal suppositories spindle-shaped, urethral suppositories pencil-shaped.

Suppressive Treatment

Heteropathic therapeutic approach, in the Rationalist tradition of medicine, modelled – nowadays usually subconsciously – on the maxim 'contraria contrariis curentur', whereby a symptom (e.g. an eczema) is often mistaken for the patient's real disease (e.g. an inherited miasmatic hypersensitivity). This sort of treatment aims at holding back, putting down, curtailing or repressing symptomatic responses usually with one or more of the thirty-odd orthodox 'suppressive' classes of drugs listed under 'Hahnemann, Christian Friedrich Samuel (1755-1843)', section entitled The Rationalist Medical Tradition. Such an attempt, either at symptom suppression, or to do something for the body though, in reality, in the body's stead, thwarts or at least confounds its reactive propensities. It may even cause a rebound effect with symptom intensification upon recurrence (e.g. post-steroidal eczema), and produce a more severe (i.e. deeply-seated) form of disease process, the so-called metastasis of disease in accordance with Hering's rule (given under 'Homoeopathic Laws, Postulates and Precepts', section 14).

Historically, this therapeutic approach consciously took its origins in Aristotle's (ca. 384-322 BC) 'principle of contradiction', which is a cardinal part of his Formal Logic ('a thing cannot be and not be at the same time'). It was consistently taught throughout the ages by those who followed the Rationalist philosophical model in medicine. It formed part of Galen's teachings (Claudius Galenus, ca. 129-200 AD), whose prolific medical writings were regarded as almost infallible by 'Rationalist Medicine' until well into the sixteenth century. Since then, until the earlier part of the twentieth century, the principle 'contraria contrariis' has regularly been put forward by apologists for mainstream medicine. Only at this comparatively recent time did orthodox medicine expressly repudiate this, and indeed any, therapeutic law or principle, but it is plain that the 'rule of contraries', though now stripped of its official status, still permeates much of orthodoxy's practical medicinal approach to disease.

The suppression of symptoms is absolutely against homoeopathy's empirical principles, as, for that matter, the suppression of people and opinions is utterly against its own fundamentally libertarian tradition. Homoeopathy does, on specific occasions, make a brief exception: in an overwhelming infection and in intractable pain that is not a true disease-response by the dynamis (say, after an operation) as well as in terminal illness (for details concerning the last-mentioned see 'Contra-Indication against Administering Simillimum'). The authority for such an exception comes, quite uncharacteristically, from Hahnemann himself in note 67 to section 67 of the *Organon:* '. . . in the most urgent cases, where danger . . . allows no time for the action of a homoeopathic remedy . . . it is admissible and judicious, at all events as a preliminary measure, to stimulate the irritability and sensibility (the physical life) with a palliative . . . When this stimulation is effected, the play of the vital organs again goes on in its former . . . manner. It does not follow that a homoeopathic medicine has been ill selected for a case of disease because some of the medicinal symptoms are only antipathic to some of the less important and minor symptoms of disease . . . ; the few opposite symptoms also disappear of themselves after the expiry of the term of action of the medicament, without retarding the cure in the least.' He goes on to warn that his statement should not be interpreted as a licence for mixers who wish to 'justify their convenient employment . . . of other injurious allopathic trash besides, solely for the sake of sparing themselves . . . trouble . . . and . . . conveniently appearing as homoeopathic physicians, without being such.' (See 'Pain Relief Methods in Homoeopathy' and 'Philosophical Premise of Homoeopathy'.)

Surgery

Chirurgery; it attempts to deal correctively with disease, disorders or the results of accidents, if amenable to operative or manual treatment. Examples of such treatment are: reduction of a dislocation or fracture; amputation; restoring injured or diseased parts; dentistry; structural adjustment of osteopathy, naprapathy, bonesetting and chiropractic; physical treatments of podiatry or chiropody; excisively and reconstructively eliminating or reducing congenital malformations or acquired joint deformities; and operative intervention in obstetrics when there is a complicated delivery. Generally, surgery is a complementary form of treatment to homoeopathy as shown in the five points of Woodward's comparative summary:[1]

Surgery deals with the results of disease.	Homoeopathy deals with the causes of disease.
Surgery concentrates on structural lesions.	Homoeopathy concentrates on functional disorders.
Surgery deals with a local lesion and sympathetic disorders arising therefrom.	Homoeopathy deals with a group of functional disorders and a lesion arising therefrom.
Surgery requires diagnosis of the disease entity, regardless of cause.	Homoeopathy requires diagnosis of the causes operating, regardless of the disease entity.
Surgery treats the disease directly by removal of the irritant or lesion.	Homoeopathy treats disease indirectly by arresting the causes operating to produce a lesion.

Surgery is the appropriate form of treatment in many instances, and is practically mandatory in emergencies, as in a perforated stomach ulcer or a

[1]Woodward, A W. *Constitutional Therapeutics*, New Delhi: Jain Publishing Co, 1977, p 12.

complicated fracture of the leg. Yet there are also many situations in which the correctly indicated homoeopathic medicine would effectively help the patient and avert the need for an operation. An example is: the earlier stages of peptic or duodenal ulceration, which, in most cases, heal completely in response to the well-indicated homoeopathic medicines and supportive measures to reduce stress reactions and improve dietary habits.

There are allopathic forms of surgery which homoeopathy rejects outright. These would include: lobotomy (division of nerve tracts in the prefrontal area of the brain for the surgical treatment of pain and emotional disease), or stereoencephalometry (also known as stereotactic surgery, which is used to place destructive lesions in subcortical ganglia or their pathways).

There is a widespread tendency to confound orthodox medicine with surgery. The two are not one and the same. Whereas homoeopathy strongly deprecates the use of orthodox medicinal therapeutics as largely dangerous, it is wholly in support of surgical intervention where indicated.

Among a number of publications that describe the reciprocal relationship between surgery and homoeopathy, a very comprehensive book is *Homoeopathy in Medicine and Surgery* (311 pages) by Edmund Carleton,[1] who for more than forty years practised pure Hahnemannian homoeopathy along with surgery. Other useful publications are: S P Verma's *Practical Handbook of Surgery with Homoeopathic Therapeutics* (554 pages);[2] the *Guide to Surgery* by D P Rastogi and A K Sharma (218 pages);[3] 'A Treatise on Homoeopathic Surgery' by P Elias and R P Patel (136 pages);[4] *Before and After Surgical Operations* by Dean T Smith, professor of Surgery and Clinical Surgery, University of Michigan, Homoeopathic Department, Ann Arbour (264 pages).[5] Recent contributions to the literature are to be found in:

'Injuries and Emergencies' (pp 1-15) and 'Pre- and Post-Operative Treatment' (pp 94-100) of *Homoeopathy in Practice* by Douglas Borland (edited by Kathleen Priestman, Beaconsfield: Beaconsfield Publishers Ltd, 1982); and the 'Table of Pre- and Post-Operative Treatment' (p 194) in *Tutorials on Homoeopathy* by Donald Foubister (Beaconsfield: Beaconsfield Publishers Ltd, 1989).

Homoeopathy has made some notable contributions to the practice of surgery, e.g. Pratt's Method (orificial surgery). E H Pratt, professor of Principles and Practice of Surgery, Chicago Homoeopathic Medical College, developed a therapeutic system based on the observed fact that many morbid conditions are linked to reflexes originating at the anus or other orifices (see

[1] Carleton, Edmund. *Homoeopathy in Medicine and Surgery*, New Delhi: B Jain Publishers, 1982.
[2] Verma, S P. *Practical Handbook of Surgery with Homoeopathic Therapeutics*, New Delhi: B Jain Publishers, 1981.
[3] Rastogi, D P, and A K Sharma. *Guide to Surgery*, New Delhi: Jain Publishing Co, 1977.
[4] Elias, P, and R P Patel. *A Treatise on Homoeopathic Surgery*, Kottayam: Hahnemann Homoeopathic Pharmacy, 1962.
[5] Smith, Dean T. *Before and After Surgical Operations: A Treatise on the Preparations for, and the Care of the Patient after, Operations, Including Homoeopathic Therapeutics*, New Delhi: World Homoeopathic Links, 1980.

also 'Reflexology'). Such morbid conditions were shown to be relieved by dilation or other forms of stimulatory treatment of these body openings. He published his discoveries in 1887.[1] Another lasting contribution was reported by a surgeon, Marcos Jiminez, in the *Homoeopathic Digest* (1978, vol III) of which he was an international editor. He developed a technique akin to sealing punctures in tubeless tyres that reduced hernia repair to an uncomplicated painless procedure, easily and safely performed under local anaesthesia. The procedure relies on the body's auto-regulatory mechanism and upon harnessing the peritoneum's natural tendency to produce adhesions. This tendency is stimulated by the implantation of slivers of solidified gelatin into the fibro-muscular defect. The hernial sac, in fact, is repaired from within, and can resist high internal pressures. The procedure induces the formation of a large fibrotic patch, which adheres firmly to the posterior abdominal wall and seals the defect. After one week there is no pain and examination shows a hard ridge of connective tissue in the treated area, which is slowly absorbed in the course of the following months, leaving only a very strong resistant area. The recurrence rate is virtually zero.

Susceptibility

Capacity, proneness or disposition to be affected. (See 'Adaptiveness', 'Altered Receptivity in Disease', 'Constitutional Type' and 'Idiosyncrasy'.)

Suspension

Dispersion throughout a liquid of a solid in finely divided, undissolved particles of a size large enough to be detected with the aid of a magnifying glass. If the particles are very much smaller and cannot be seen under a microscope, but are still capable of scattering light (Tyndall effect) the liquid is then a colloid, in which the particles will remain dispersed indefinitely. Other meanings are: the hanging from any support; the interruption of any function for a time; or, in surgery, the supportive fixation by an organ to adjacent tissue. (See 'Colloid'.)

Sycosis

See 'Miasma'.

Sycotic Miasma

See 'Miasma'.

[1]Pratt, E H. *Orificial Surgery*, reprint, New Delhi: B Jain Publishers, 1971.

Sydenham, Thomas (1624-1689)

See 'Philosophical Premise of Homoeopathy'.

Symbols

See 'Abbreviations, Symbols, Weights and Measures'.

Sympathicothérapie Nasale

See 'Olfactory Medicines'.

Symptom

● **Change of condition accompanying disease or drug response, that shows the way the patient's body wants to correct what is wrong. It will be supported by homoeopathic treatment.**

Manifestation of (part of) an organism's reactive effort in disease, or as a drug response, being a disturbance either of normal functioning within that organism, or of the harmonious interaction between the body and its environment. The reactive force manifested in a symptom is the response of the vital force to a morbific stimulus whenever this stimulus is stronger than the defence mechanism. That response invariably represents a spurt in the direction of cure, of self-correction, of adjustment or re-alignment, to re-establish harmony both within the organism and externally with the surrounding environment. Hence it is a sign of a curative, and is not itself a morbific, process. It points the way the organism wishes to be taken in coping with the disturbance, to overcome its disease.

The point ought to be made that homoeopathy also regards foods and condiments as capable of eliciting symptoms in individuals, in other words that these have distinct pharmacological properties in the homoeopathic sense. Therefore, which foods are eaten by any person may make a health difference. Moreover, foodstuffs can modify the symptom response of a patient, so that the diligent homoeopath generally scrutinizes diets. A book on the subject is *The Food Pharmacy* by Jean Carper (London: Simon & Schuster Ltd, Positive Paperbacks, 1990, 380 pp; unfortunately its author makes the classic non-homoeopathic error of extrapolating from a series of particular instances to the general, ignoring individual idiosyncrasies [for instance, representative of the general presentation by her, she roundly recommends bran for diverticular disease and haemorrhoids – p 325, though this is known to aggravate these complaints in as many cases as it may, or may not, alleviate]).

Symptoms and signs are used by the homoeopath to be guided in the choice of a truly homoeopathic medicine applicable to the individual patient. That means he chooses the medicine's symptom picture that would evoke the identical symptom picture, though some (or even most) may well be subjective symptoms. In this the peculiar, unexpected, striking, or unaccountable symptoms are taken to be of pre-eminent significance. (See 'Bran', 'Disease and Drug Action in Homoeopathic Congruity' and 'Individualization'.)

Symptom Character Resemblance

See 'Disease and Drug Action in Homoeopathic Congruity'.

Symptom Concentricity of Tinctures and Low Potencies

See 'Therapeutic Science'.

Symptomatology in Homoeopathy, Sources of

See 'Sources of Homoeopathic Drug Semiology'.

Symptoms Better For . . .

See 'Aggravation', section on Aggravation and Amelioration.

Symptoms Worse For . . .

See 'Aggravation', section on Aggravation and Amelioration.

Synchronicity of Symptom Evolution

See 'Disease and Drug Action in Homoeopathic Congruity' and 'Therapeutic Science'.

Syncretisms in Presenting Symptoms

Apparently contradictory symptoms in one patient at the same time are often significant pointers in locating the one well-indicated homoeopathic medicine. An example might be:

'patient is shivering, but likes to have window open',

pointing to Carbo vegetabilis as a remedy to be considered by the homoeopath.

Syndetic Pointers

Outstanding indicators serving to associate, unite or connect; used in this text to focus on examples of homoeopathic concordance between the enormous wealth of signs, symptoms and concomitants at an early stage of drug diagnosis that may orientate the experienced homoeopath's percipient current of attention and lead more swiftly on to a likely remedy.

Syphilinic Miasma

See 'Miasma'.

Syphilis

Lues venera; the chronic luetic miasma. A chronic contagious illness with a myriad of constitutional symptoms involving Treponema pallidum (Spirochaeta pallida). (See 'Miasma'.)

Syrupus

Simple syrup; sucrose ($C_{12}H_{22}O_{11}$) 66.67% w/w in aqua destillata, with a weight per ml of from 1.315 to 1.327g, produced at 90 degrees Celsius. Its specific gravity is 1.33. When the syrup contains a homoeopathic substance, such as Kreosotum or Guaiacol (incidentally, both will inhibit the growth of moulds in syrupus), it is termed a 'medicated syrup'. (See 'Vehicle'.)

T

Tablets and Tabloids

Squat-cylindroid or roller-shaped compactions, each substantially composed of 80% saccharum lactis (sugar of milk) with 20% sucrose. They are relatively soft, their weight generally ranges from 60 to 100 mg, and their diameter is about 10mm with a thickness of around 5mm. Homoeopathic use: solid vehicle for dispensing the medicines with which they would have been impregnated. (See 'Dose', 'Saccharum Lactis' and 'Vehicle'.)

Tabloids

See 'Tablets and Tabloids'.

Tachycardia

Synchopexia; rapid heartbeat, usually over 100 beats per minute. (See 'Emergencies – Homoeopathic Treatment', under this heading.)

Tacit Knowing

See 'Science and Homoeopathy'.

Tampon

Cylindrical or spherical absorbent plug for bodily cavities or orifices that is made of gauze, cotton wool, etc. and used for the control of haemorrhages or the absorption of secretions or the holding in position of displaced organs (e.g. uterus).

Taste, Strange

See 'Mouth, Peculiar Taste in'.

Tautonym

Botanical, zoological or homoeopathic name in which the specific epithet repeats (part of) the generic name as in Ioduratum kali hydriodicum (ioduretted potassium iodide), Kara kara, Kawa kawa (Piper methysticum), Mephitis mephitica putoris or Moschus moschiferus.

Tautopathy

System of isopathic treatment employing a homoeopathized preparation of the very allopathica of which the patient in question had previously received a ponderal, coercive dosage with apparently or suspected injurious results. As the allopathic pharmaceutical substance to be dynamized in this system is the (presumed) exopathic causal agent of the supervening disease, the method is, by definition, isopathic. Yet the method's propagator, Dr Raman Lal P Patel of Kottayam, India, maintains that it is a distinct method and not part of Isopathy, because, he says, Isopathy postulates that 'a disease may be cured or prevented by administering one or more of its own products'.[1] This is, however, not the majority view in homoeopathy about Isopathy (see entry under this). Patel's 100-page book (see footnote 1 below), nonetheless, makes out a good case for using homoeopathized allopathica, whether or not it is to be called 'Tautopathy'. That book was originally published in 1960 (dedicated to Donald Macdonald Foubister) and went through four editions in fifteen years. In it, the adverse reactions to one hundred and fourteen orthodox drugs are briefly recorded and some case histories given. The methods (trituration or dilution/succussion) of tautopathic medicinal preparation are also described in this work. Since then Kailash Narayan Mathur has devoted the entire chapter 24 to 'Tautopathy' in his book *Principles of Prescribing – Collected from Clinical Experiences of Pioneers of Homoeopathy*.[2]

Taxonomy

Study of the theory, procedure and rules of classification of living organisms according to the differences and similarities between them.

Technique

Details of a method of procedure. For example:

Rebreathing technique: a method of inducing hypoxia by rebreathing air with CO_2 replacing oxygen in the air mixture to be breathed.

Teel Oil

Sesame oil; the fixed oil expressed from the seeds of Sesamum indicum. It is pale yellow with a slight pleasant odour and a bland taste. It does not solidify when cooled to 0 degrees Celsius and is slightly soluble in alcohol and miscible with light petroleum. Its weight per ml is 0.916 to 0.919 g. It is sterilized by

[1] Patel, Raman Lal P. *What is Tautopathy?* Kottayam: Hahnemann Homoeopathic Pharmacy, fourth edition, 1975, p 1.
[2] Mathur, Kailash Narayan. *Principles of Prescribing – Collected from Clinical Experiences of Pioneers of Homoeopathy*, New Delhi: B Jain Publishers, 1981, pp 477-485.

heating to 150 degrees Celsius for one hour. Teel oil is more stable than other fixed oils, and has many properties similar to Oleum olivae, and has been used in homoeopathic pharmacy instead of the latter in the preparation of liniments, ointments and soaps. (See 'Oleum Olivae' and 'Vehicle'.)

Teleology

Explains events (particularly in biology) in part by reference to end goals, as, for example, in homoeostasis. (Refer to that entry and to 'Vitalism'.)

Teleonomy

Science of adaptation; study of purposive-seeming behaviour, functions and structural developments, that are viewed as assimilative transformations necessitated, perhaps at least in part, by the exigencies of natural selection. (See 'Epistemological Assumptions in Homoeopathy', section 1 Similarity – as a Concept in Science, and 'Homoeosis' for the assimilative process.)

Teleosis

Purposive development.

Tellurism

Disease-inducing influence emanating from the soil. Hence 'telluric'.

Temperament

The nature peculiar to an individual, expressed in manner of thought and action, and general attitude to life as a constitutional predisposition modified by experience and externalized through expressions of impulse, appetite, desire or emotion. Temperament can profoundly influence, and may itself be influenced by, individual dynamic responses in the disease process.

Temperaments in Humoral Pathology

See 'Humoral Pathology in Prescribing'.

Temperature

Degree of hotness or coldness as measured on various scales with respect to a defined zero value. Values on the Celsius scale accepted as normal in health by homoeopathic veterinary and human medicines are (degrees):

Humans	36.9
Horses	38.1
Cattle, Dogs & Cats	38.6
Pigs	39.2
Goats & Sheep	39.4

(See 'Zero'.)

Template

Framework, pattern or guide for determining the shape of a substance. Term used metaphorically in homoeopathy to indicate the specifying nature in which the pharmacological message (perhaps contained in the profile of an eventual solvation structure) is carried within the medicine. (See 'Solvation Structure'.)

Teratogenicity

See 'Teratology'.

Teratology

Deals with the development, the anatomy and the classification of monsters, as well as the causes for their production. The tragic story of the German pharmaceutical 'Contergan' (alpha-Phthalimidoglutarimide marketed under 35 different proprietary names in pharmaceutical combinations worldwide; under 'Thalidomide' in USA and 'Distaval' in the UK, amongst others) has finally also made teratogenicity a recognized miasmatic hazard in non-homoeopathic circles. What homoeopathy has maintained for two centuries has become generally accepted, namely that hereditable miasmatic defects may result from the ponderal administration of certain coercive drugs. (See 'Miasma'.)

Terminal Illness

See 'Contra-Indication Against Administering Simillimum'.

Terrain: Predisposing to Patient's Resistance or Susceptibility

A basic homoeopathic concept is that the cause of all illness is a multi-factorial milieu, in that disease only becomes possible if a combination of a diversity of preconditions is found to be present. Impaired resistance, increased susceptibility, diminished vital energy, the presence of toxins, parasites or other debilitants, the absence of regular symbiotes, nutritional imbalance, dietary or other abuse, psychogenic strains and/or an inherited miasma are some of the deleterious predisposing factors that may 'weaken the terrain' and conspire to make a patient receptive to infection, inflammation, tumour, abscess formation or similar disease process. Stuart Close explained this very carefully:

'The fatal tendency in . . . medical research to focus attention and effort upon one cause to the exclusion of all others inevitably leads into error and failure. . . . Admitting the existence and presence of the bacilli as one causative factor, we still have to reckon with sanitary, atmospheric and telluric conditions; with economic and social conditions and habits of life; with means and modes of transportation and intercommunication between individuals and communities; with individual physical, mental and emotional states, etc., all of which are essential factors, in some combination, in determining and modifying the susceptibility of individuals to the bacilli; for without some combination of these factors the bacilli are impotent and the disease would never occur. Each of these factors is a cause at least equal in rank with the bacilli, and any successful method of treatment must be able to meet all the conditions arising from any existing combination of the causes. . . . Experience proves that homoeopathy, with a mortality record [for example] in cholera as low as four percent and less, against a record as high as seventy percent under other forms of treatment, is able to meet it. The secret of this success is that homoeopathy does not direct its efforts primarily or solely to the destruction of the proximate physical cause of the disease (the micro-organism), but against the disease itself, that is the morbid vital process as manifested . . . causing a counter action. . . . The power of the bacilli or other infectious agents is always relative and conditional, never absolute, as many are led to believe. The bacilli, therefore, are not the sole cause of the disease, but only one factor in a group or combination of causes or conditions [that have altered the patient's terrain], all of which must exist and act together before the disease can follow.'[1]

(See also 'Causes of Disease'.)

Tessier, Jean-Paul (1811-1862)

The recognized leader of early French homoeopathy, who had been the favourite student of Gabriel Andral, who taught him hygiene and internal pathology, and was soon to become the principal figure of the Paris School. This School of Medicine was led by Tessier's former teacher for about two decades after the demise of Francois Joseph Victor Broussais (1772-1838; proponent of 'physiological medicine'). In 1856 the Anatomical Society unanimously expelled Tessier and three others for publishing scientific reports in homoeopathic journals. In 1858 the journal *L'Union Médicale* published a thoroughly calumnious article, and the homoeopaths, with Tessier in the lead, sued for defamation. Ironically it was Andral's son who was the lawyer who successfully defended *L'Union Médicale* in court. After this episode, however, the acrimonious relationship between homoeopathy and orthodoxy softened a little. Spokesmen for the latter were maintaining, all evidence to the contrary, that homoeopathy's premises were being irreparably undermined by the advances of orthodoxy. In reality it was under Tessier that homoeopathy made

[1]Close, Stuart. *The Genius of Homoeopathy*, New York, Boericke and Tafel, 1924, p 269-270.

great strides forward: several public hospitals, quite some official support, and an ever-growing popularity all fell to homoeopathy. Yet it was Tessier who also seems to have the dubious distinction of having cast the first stone (even before Charles Julius Hempel [1811-1879]) in the baneful symptomatology-pathology feud that was to rack homoeopathy for more than half a century, when he said: 'Hahnemann's theories embody two different hemispheres, his pathology corresponding to his mistakes and his therapy amounting to the truth'.[1]

Teste, Alphonse (1814-1898)

Eminent French homoeopath who undertook a number of original pathogenetic experiments ('provings'). He was considered an authority in homoeopathy, so that John Henry Clarke (1853-1931), for instance, quotes him very frequently in *A Dictionary of Practical Materia Medica* (published 1900). His major works include:

A Practical Manual of Animal Magnetism (1844) [deals with hypnoidal methodology]

The Homoeopathic Materia Medica, Arranged by Systems (1854) [organized by structures that are functionally or anatomically related]

A Homoeopathic Treatise of Diseases of Children (1862)

Testing of Drugs on the Healthy

See 'Pathogenetic Experiment'.

Thalassotherapy

Hydropathic treatment of disease by bathing in the sea, or in sea water, by employing seaweed externally, by residence at the seashore, by a sea voyage, or by some other therapeutic approach utilizing the sea. This is generally compatible with homoeopathy. (See 'Naturopath'.)

Theotherapy

Treatment of disease by religious exercises and/or supplications. (See 'Shamanism and Magic'.)

Therapeutic Science

To approximate its scientific objective, viz. the predictability of curative efficacy, homoeopathy has made its central scientific objectives, jointly:

[1]Haehl, Richard. *Samuel Hahnemann: His Life and Work*. English translation, 2 vols. London: Homoeopathic Publishing Company, 1922, p 295.

1 the observation and study of the action of remedial agents both in health and in disease; and
2 the treating (with the aim of curing) of any disease condition by medication according to a fixed law derived, a posteriori, from this observation and study.

The law is demonstrably effective and in harmony with other observed scientific facts. It is known as the law of equivalents or similars (see 'Epistemological Assumptions in Homoeopathy', section 1 Similarity – as a Concept in Science, and 'Homoeopathic Laws, Postulates and Precepts'). With it homoeopathy took a leap into the scientific practice of medicine, and away from the merely speculative and/or the inconsequentially empirical approaches which characterize all non-homoeopathic medical systems. Through the homoeopathic method medicine at last became a pure self-consistent science of experience, in a way like physics or chemistry. It forged an analytical link between disease and its remedial agents. The homoeopathic therapeutic method is aimed at curing affections of the living organism in which sense-perceptible symptoms exist, and which is always successful when correctly applied and if two conditions are met. These are that adequate integrity of the tissue as well as the reactive bio-energy for recovery must exist, and, further, that the exciting cause(s) of the affections and/or obstacles to cure have been removed or have ceased to operate.

The first step toward the full development of an applied therapeutic science was taken by Georg H G Jahr (1800-1875) when he pointed out the essential difference between the action of the low and high potencies. It is a well known fact that provings of the mother tincture and lowest dynamizations (potencies) of any drug usually produce only the more common and general symptoms of the drug, not very different from other drugs in its class. It is in the provings of the medium potencies, and those beyond, where the special and peculiar character of a drug emerges, the drug's personality, so to speak. Jahr produced geometrical drawings to illustrate this. These consisted of a number of concentric circles, with radii drawn to represent the same drugs in different potencies. In the first, second and third potencies, represented by the innermost circle, similar remedies, such as Arsenicum album, Bryonia alba, Rhus toxicodendron and Sulphur, have a great many symptoms in common. However, the higher one goes in the scale of potentiation the more distant the radii become from one another, with each one moving further away from the next on the circumferences of the ever-larger circles. Thus Jahr represented the stages of higher potentization, as well as the unfolding of ever more distinctly characteristic features of each drug in pathogenetic experimentation (proving). The narcotics (which include [Atropa] Belladonna, Opium and [Datura] Stramonium), for example, in massive and crude (ponderal) doses act in a manner equally stupefying, producing death by paralysis or apoplexy; the so-called drastics cause purging and vomiting, and so forth. Only in the small, potentiated attenuations do the individual characteristic differences of action, that each drug is capable of producing, begin to appear. Jahr says, 'By continual diluting and succussing remedies get neither stronger nor weaker, but their individual peculiarities become more and more developed' and their sphere of action is enlarged quite like his concentric circles illustrated.

Though any disease condition, if within reversible limits, would be curable by any potency of the homoeopathically indicated drug, the process is accelerated by selecting the appropriate potency and dose (see 'Dose Repetition', 'Homoeopathic Laws, Postulates and Precepts' and 'Potency').

Broadly, the two considerations that influence the choice of potency and dose are:

1 Different susceptibility aspects of the patient; and
2 Various developmental aspects of the disease process.

Susceptibility to medicinal action is affected by factors such as age, habits, sex, environment, constitution, temperament, idiosyncrasy, nutritional status, other weaknesses in the individual's 'terrain' and a possible miasma. These are the indicators for the matching homoeopathicity of a drug's particular potency. The rule, in the words of Stuart Close (delivered in his lectures as professor of Homoeopathic Philosophy at the New York Homoeopathic Medical College (1909-1913): 'The more similar the remedy, the more clearly and positively the symptoms of the patient are seen to take on the peculiar and characteristic form of the remedy, the greater the susceptibility to that remedy, and the higher the appropriate potency.' This paraphrases the law of quantity and dose (under 'Homoeopathic Laws, Postulates and Precepts; see also 'Altered Receptivity in Disease' and 'Terrain: Predisposing to Patient's Resistance or Susceptibility').

By contrast, the developmental aspects of a disease process (whether experimental or natural), apart from also influencing the potency choice as already described, may additionally profoundly and repeatedly affect the remedy selection proper. The aspects of a disease process to be considered are: the seat of disease, its nature and intensity, its duration, the stage of disease, previous treatment and the influence of toxic agents, as well as any alterable miasmatic or hereditary factors. Yet, except the last-named, none of these is immutable or static. In fact, the individuality of each disease is such that it often changes into various symptom constellations and it keeps varying these, quite like the altering presentations of a kaleidoscope, and there is no known limit to its variegation in ever-changing symptom-syndromes. An example, taken from the writings of A W Woodward, who for twenty-five years had taught Materia Medica and Clinical Therapeutics at the Chicago Homoeopathic Medical College: He describes 'the development of a Rhus case of typhoid. It was noted that at first the cutaneous and spinal symptoms caused more complaints, then as these abated, there developed higher temperatures, and pulmonary symptoms were most urgent; later, delirium and sopor became more pronounced, and afterward the diarrhoea and enteric symptoms. While these phenomena, respectively, were leading at each stage, other symptoms arising from the organs first involved continued to be present in less degree. Therapeutically considered, did these varying conditions require a change of remedies?' Woodward answers in the affirmative. He goes further, saying that 'another cause for a change of remedy will be found in a change in the character of the symptoms exhibited by the case; though the same functions are involved the indicated remedy no longer operates'.[1]

All this, he felt, urgently demanded the refinement in the scientific method of clinical therapeutics that would make reliable adaptation to a constantly changing individual case possible. This should ideally be by being able to select the remedy that had a drug picture that changed in the same fashion during provings. He realized this meant that the records of provings would have to be carefully looked at to have the extra dimension of the time-sequences covering changes in provers added back into the now 'moving' drug pictures. Woodward did a lot of work on this over many years, poring over original provings at his homoeopathic medical school, while comparing these recorded, artificially induced changes in action of a drug with its counterpart in 'natural' disease, and then the observed effect of that drug on such a changeable disease picture in the homoeopathic hospital of Chicago. For example, he compared certain mild manifestations of typhoids and pneumonias, in which time is required to develop different stages. He would watch one group under what he called 'the expectant method' (where he only gave placebos), then a second group under what he called 'undifferentiated prescribing', and a third group under 'adapted prescribing'. Using the first group's results as his base reference, he found that the second group's results were acting curatively for a limited time only. They then ceased to operate, with the results toward the end tailing off and becoming very similar to group one. Only group three responded successfully in most cases right up to cure.

Woodward then undertook the task of systematically analysing the records of large numbers of pathogenetic experiments (provings), and extracted the variations in symptom response for each remedy in its chronological context. His remarkable contribution to therapeutic science is captured in his synopsis of this huge task. He prepared a table which highlights, at a glance, the distinguishing individuality of each remedy in so far as its time-bound variability is concerned. This, however, for any conscientious prescriber, also delimits each remedy's useful area of application as a therapeutic agent. It is interesting to note that Woodward's massive undertaking clearly confirms Hering's rule on the direction of disease metastasis (See 'Homoeopathic Laws, Postulates and Precepts', section 14): in about two-thirds of the analysed sequences of artificial drug diseases, these begin on the skin or sense organs (the surface) and move to the interior, and in the remaining one-third they begin in the digestive tract (less vital organ) and then move to the mental functions, the spinal, or respiratory, or circulatory systems. In his concept of

---

[1] Woodward, A W. *Constitutional Therapeutics,* originally published around 1892, reprint New Delhi: Jain Publishing Co, 1977, pp 88-90.

homoeopathic pharmacodynamics, Woodward also made provision for two classes of drug in the context of systemic physiology: one acting primarily on the nervous system; the other acting primarily on the humoral system. It needs to be said that this proved to be a very successful scientific development in medicinal therapeutics though it was possibly best suited for a hospital setting, where it was first introduced. Regrettably it was introduced very late in the nineteenth century in the USA, just shortly before the 'Simmons manoeuvres' (see 'Simmons, George Henry (1852-1937)'), which meant that the method had no time to become widely known and accepted before the homoeopathic hospitals began to disappear in all but name.

Pharmacodynamic Homoeopathicity

The sequence of drug action and the group of physiological derangements produced by each medicine are represented by numbers [see key below], as arranged for clinical use by A W Woodward.[1]

Key: No. 1 – Skin and sensorial organs
No. 2 – Digestive
No. 3 – Spinal
No. 4 – Respiratory
No. 5 – Circulatory
No. 6 – Genito-Urinary
No. 7 – Mental functions

Class I
Medicines for morbid conditions associated with irritation of the nervous system and shown by:
a) Severe pain or suffering, unattended by fever.
b) Painful paretic conditions of body or mind, unattended by fever.
c) Secondary fevers along with pain.
d) Secondary spasms or delirium produced by pain.
e) Secondary structural lesions associated with and attended by pain and fever.
These remedies will be useful until the pain is relieved. If a lesion remains, then a complementary medicine from Class II is required.

Class II
Medicines for morbid conditions arising from tissue irritation, shown by:
a) Primary fevers, unattended by pain or suffering.
b) Primary spasms, convulsions, etc, unattended by pain.
c) Primary morbid growths developing without pain.
d) Secondary pains in consequence of structural lesions.
e) Secondary paresis of body or mind from like causes.

If the lesion is removed and the pain remains, then a complementary medicine of Class I is required.

[1]Ibid., pp 548-550.

Class I

Aconitum napellus	12437
(Matricaria) Chamomilla	12473
Cantharis vesicator	12643
Arnica montana	12734
Cocculus indicus	12736
Cyclamen europaeum	12746
Nux vomica	13247
Ignatia amara	13246
Rhus toxicodendron	13472
Rhododendron	13426
Tarentula hispanica	13467
Ranunculus bulbosus	13427
Lilium tigrinum	13642
Gelsemium sempervirens	13724
Hypericum perforatum	13762
Apis mellifica	14236
(Trigonocephalus) Lachesis	14273
Secale cornutum	14326
Crotalus horridus	14327
Hamamelis macrophylla	14367
Naja tripudians	14372
Cactus grandiflorus	14376
Camphora	14732
(Atropa) Belladonna	17342
(Daphne) Mezereum	12346
Graphites	12347
Arsenicum album	21347
Ferrum metallicum	21346
Lycopodium clavatum	21436
Plumbum aceticum	21437
Zincum metallicum	21473
Stannum	21463

Class II

Sulphur	12537
Sepia officinalis	12563
Croton tiglium	12536
Physostigma venenosum	13257
Cicuta virosa	13256
Hyoscyamus niger	13275
Conium maculatum	13562
Veratrum album	13527
Helleborus niger	13526
Acidum salicylicum	13572
Cimicifuga racemosa (Actea racemosa, Macrotys)	13652
Clematis erecta	13756
Sambucus nigra	13752
Cinchona officinalis	15237
Tabacum	15326
Alcohol (Spiritus alcoholisatus, C_2H_5OH)	15327
Cannabis indicus	15367
(Erythroxylon) Coca	15372
Coffea cruda	15376
Glonoiunum	15723
Opium	15732
Calcarea carbonica	12356
Silicea	12357
Thuja occidentalis	12365
Hepar sulphuris careum	12375
Natrum muriaticum	21357
Pulsatilla nigricans	21536
Baptisia tinctoria	21537
Chelidonium majus	21536
Hydrastis canadensis	21567
Acidum carbolicum	21573

Class I		Class II	
Argentum nitricum	21736		
Cuprum aceticum	21743		
Acidum nitricum	21746		
Mercurius solubilis		Aloe socotrina	23165
Hahnemannii	23176	Podophylum peltatum	23167
Mercurius corrosivus	23146	Acidum hydrocyanicum	25371
Helonias dioica	23617	Ammonium carbonicum	25163
Aletris farinosa	23674		
Bryonia alba	23714		
(Citrullus) Colocynthis	23716		
Phosphorus	24137	Kali bichromicum	25136
Terebinthina	24176	Rumex crispus	25137
		Iodium	25163
		Sanguinaria canadensis	25173
		Bromium	25176
(Cephaelis) Ipecacuanha	24316	Antimonium tartaricum	25317

Applied therapeutics, apart from this parameter, aims to approximate as many as feasible of the other seven undermentioned drug-to-disease concordances by means of repertorization:

Constitutional compatibility (see 'Constitutional Type')
Matching of 'mentals'
Concurrence of symptoms and signs
Generic similarity
Causal similarity
Matching of modalities
Likeness in character of abnormal sensations.

Some homoeopaths have played down the predictive exactness of homoeopathy's therapeutic science. Such were its two very articulate apologists, Richard Hughes (1836-1902) and Charles Edwin Wheeler (1868-1946), who both hoped during their entire lives to facilitate a *rapprochement* with orthodox medicine by making homoeopathy more palatable to the rank and file follower of mainstream medicine. To this end they said, for instance, that homoeopathy, far from being a therapeutic science, was no more than a medical art, or a method or rule of practice:

'[It] is a **method** – not a doctrine or a system. It belongs to the art of medicine rather than to its science', says Hughes addressing his students in his lectures on Therapeutics and Materia Medica in London from 1867 to 1878.[1]

'We offer you an addition to your resources not as a supersession of all others

[1] Hughes, Richard. *The Principles and Practice of Homoeopathy*, London: Leath and Ross, 1903, p 1.

than ours. Our heresy then is not a theory, it is a rule of practice. . . . It . . . involves no dogmatic faith, it is a simple rule of practice, applied to a particular sphere of medicine, the treatment of the sick by drugs.' Wheeler speaking in the Great Hall, British Medical Association, Tavistock House, 8th October 1937.[1]

Yet this rule of practice, in fact, is no less than the only scientific medical method, capable of using better medicinal 'agents more precisely indicated'.[2]

(See 'Disease and Drug Action in Homoeopathic Congruity'.)

With a miasmatic component in the patient's condition yet another, and important, factor enters into the drug-to-disease equation (this is discussed under 'Miasma').

(See also 'Altered Receptivity in Disease', 'Disease and Drug Action in Homoeopathic Congruity', 'Homoeopathic Practice', 'Organic Clock' and 'Tissue Affinity'.)

Therapeutics

Practical branch of homoeopathy, or of any other medical discipline, concerned with the treatment proper of disease, whether medicinal (curative, palliative, preventive), suggestive (psychotherapeutic), or somatic (reflexive, physiological, surgical).

Thirtieth Centesimal (30CH): as Hahnemann's Potentization Limit

See 'Potency'.

Time Modalities

Some patients may experience a worsening of symptoms recurrently at particular times. This may provide the homoeopath with one useful indicator for the selection of an appropriate medicine. Some widely recognized times of aggravation, for instance, are:

Arsenicum album: 01h00 to 02h00
Kali carbonicum: 03h00 to 04h00
Lycopodium clavatum: 16h00 to 20h00
(See 'Organic Clock'.)

Tincture

See 'Mother Tincture'.

---

[1]Wheeler, Charles Edwin. *A Hundred Years of Homoeopathy*, London: The British Homoeopathic Association, 1937, pp 5 and 7.
[2]loc cit, p 5.

Tissue

Collection of cells or fibres forming one of the structures composing an organism.

Tissue Affinity

The materia medica, among the many pathogenetic effects described therein, also contains affinities of medicines with particular tissues, systems or organs. Examples are:

Aesculus hippocastanum: congested venous tissue
Arnica montana: injured tissue
(Atropa) Belladonna: central nervous system
Cantharis vesicator: urinary system and genitalia
Chelidonium majus: gallbladder and liver
Hypericum perforatum: nerves
Iodium: thyroid gland
Ruta graveolens: periosteum
Rhus toxicodendron: locomotor system
Sepia officinalis: female organs, excluding breasts

Tissue Salts

A group of twelve homoeopathic medicines that are frequently and popularly used in self-medication. The term is due to the unconfirmed claim made by Wilhelm Heinrich Schüssler (1821-1898) that they function as cellular nutrients. In fact, they are homoeopathic remedies in low potency (usually 6DH). Homoeopaths normally select one of them when a pathological remedy is required, to be frequently repeated. They are:

Calcarea fluorata;[1] Calcarea phosphorica;[2] Calcarea sulphurica;[3] Ferrum phosphoricum;[4] Kali muriaticum;[5] Kali phosphoricum;[6] Kali sulphuricum;[7] Magnesia phosphorica;[8] Natrum muriaticum;[9] Natrum phosphoricum;[10] Natrum sulphuricum;[11] Silicea.[12]

[1] Schüessler's 'bone salt'.
[2] Schüssler's 'anti-psoric'.
[3] Originally Schüssler's 'connective-tissue salt', but discarded by him in the last edition of his *Biochemic Therapy* because it is not an actual constituent of the tissues; he distributed its functions between Natrum phosphoricum and Silicea.
[4] To be distinguished from Ferrum phosphoricum hydricum. In Schüssler's *Biochemic Theory* this is the 'salt of painless irritability of fibre', and also corresponds to disturbed states of circulation, inflammation and anaemia.
[5] Schüssler's 'fibrinotrophic salt'.
[6] According to Schüssler this is present in the cells of brain, nerves, muscles, blood (corpuscles and plasma), and intercellular fluids.
[7] Schüssler states that this, in reciprocal action with iron, effects the transfer of the inhaled oxygen to all the cells, and is present in all ferruginous cells. *(Footnotes cont. overleaf)*

(See also 'Biochemic Therapy', 'Mineral Remedies' and 'Schüssler, Wilhelm Heinrich (1821-1898)'.)

Tongue Conditions

The well-being, or otherwise, and general appearance of the tongue have universally been regarded as an indicator of the overall state of an individual's health. For this reason the homoeopath will examine a patient's tongue to assist in gauging the current state of curative response. There are, however, aspects that the homoeopath would also consider while looking at the patient's tongue. Of these the following may be some:

The 'baked tongue': dry, dark and dehydrated – points to the possibility of an acute miasma febris typhodes (typhoid fever).

The 'beet tongue': intensely red, usually painful and looks shiny – may indicate a nutritional deficiency, pellagra (niacin and, perhaps, riboflavin deficiency).

The 'black tongue': has yellowish-brown and blackish patches, occasionally with elongation of the papillae – possibly there is a fungus (Aspergillus niger) on the tongue.

The 'furred tongue': has a whitish layer on its upper surface – may be associated with indigestion or fever.

The 'hobnail tongue': shows wartlike changes in the papillae – points to miasma luetica (syphilis).

The 'magenta tongue': swollen with a purplish-red colour and flattened papillae – points to nutritional deficiency (riboflavin deficiency).

The 'strawberry tongue': a strong pink with a whitish coat over it through which the enlarged papillae project – points to the possibility of an acute miasma scarlatina (scarlet fever).

In such cases the homoeopath would first wish to remove the nutritional deficiency, or perhaps prescribe Borax veneta 3DH for the fungus, or choose

[8] According to Schüssler this is present in blood corpuscles, muscles, brain, spinal marrow, nerves and teeth; it is Schüssler's 'anti-spasmodic salt'.

[9] Schüssler's 'hygroscopic salt', meaning it attracts water into the cells and the intercellular fluid, and brings about hydraemia.

[10] Schüssler's 'gaseous exchange salt', saying that through it lactic acid is decomposed into carbonic acid and water, it then binds itself to the carbonic acid and with a blood corpuscle is thus conveyed to the lungs where it is liberated and exhaled as carbon dioxide in exchange for the oxygen which is absorbed by the iron of the blood corpuscles.

[11] Discovered by Johann Rudolf Glauber (1604-1668) in 1658 and named Sal mirabile; it has been renamed Sal glauberi ('Glauber Salts') in his honour; it is the chief ingredient of Carlsbad and other spa waters; von Grauvogl studied it and found in it the typical constitutional remedy for the 'hydrogenoid constitution'. Schüssler said, 'The action of Natrum sulphuricum is contrary to that of Natrum muriaticum. Though both attract water, Nat mur puts it to use in the organism, whereas Nat sulph secures its elimination from the organism. Nat mur aids cellular multiplication, while Nat sulph withdraws water from the superannuated leucocytes, and thus causes their destruction.'

[12] Schüssler's 'salt for suppurative processes' and for diseases of the bone, caries and necrosis.

remedies specific to the miasma, as the respective case may be. The following medicines may be considered with the corresponding indications:

Acidum fluoricum: Leucoplakic tongue; with epitheliomatous nodule; gummatous ulcers on tongue in miasma luetica (syphilis)

Acidum muriaticum: Darkened, thick tongue; mouth, tongue and fauces covered with greyish-white coat; blistered and burning; indurations; recurring ulcers

Acidum nitricum: Sore, blistered tongue; with halitosis; sublingual ulcer in whooping-cough

Acidum oxalicum: Dry, burning, swollen, red; or with thick white coating, ulcers on gums, loss of taste, unquenchable thirst, nausea, aphthes; tongue and fauces whitened

Aconitum napellus: Tongue numb, burning, dry, red or white furred

Aeschulus hippocastanum: White or yellow tongue

Alumen: Tongue dry, burning, sour sensation, worse at the tip

Antimonium crudum: Thick, milky coat; dirty tongue in children

Antimonium tartaricum: Red in streaks, dry in middle; thinly coated white with ruddy papillae and raw edges; or bilious brown fur, dry tongue

Apis mellifica: Acute oedema of tongue

Argentum nitricum: With white patches on tongue

Arnica montana: Tongue bitten in an accident or a convulsion

Arsenicum album: Red tip, silvery – sometimes brown – coat with red streak down the middle; burning as if covered in stinging vesicles

Arum triphyllum: Cracked, bleeding and painful; root of tongue and palate feel sore

Aurum metallicum: There are hard nodules in tongue

Bacillinum: Pippy, strawberry-like tongue

(Atropa) Belladonna: Tongue cracked, dry, parched; papillae deep red, swollen

Baptisia tinctoria: Swollen, thick, white-coated or yellowish-white; thick fur with baked appearance in the middle

Baryta carbonica: (see below)

Bryonia alba: Thick white coat

Cantharis vesicator: If inflammation arises from a scald or burn on the tongue

Carbo animalis: Blisters; burning at tip; rawness of mouth

Causticum: Tongue paralysed; white at both sides, red in the middle

(Gonolobus) Condurango: Painful pustules on the tip or in left side of tongue

(Solanum) Dulcamara: Tongue stiff, swollen, seems paralyzed; cannot be protruded

Fragaria vesca: Pippy, strawberry-like tongue; and macroglossia

Gelsemium sempervirens: Can hardly speak; tongue feels very thick

Gymnocladus canadensis: Bluish-white coating on tongue

Hydrastis canadensis: Tongue, large and indented as if scalded or raw;

yellow coat on dark red tongue with raised papillae; broad yellow stripe

Kali cyanatum: Painful in right side of tongue

Lycopodium clavatum: Prominent papillae; white coat; yellow blisters; burning; ulcers under the tongue

Mercurius corrosivus: Coat is red with blackish parts; much coated; moist; edges red

Mercurius solubilis hahnemanni: Swollen, thickly coated, white, indented tongue

Mercurius vivus: Great swelling and protrusion, subacute inflammation of bucal mucosa, sweat taste, thick yellow mucous coat or black, with red edges, pale, offensive, tremulous

(Daphne) Mezereum: Swollen, red tongue; prominent papillae on white background; burning sensation down to the stomach

Natrum muriaticum: Blisters with burning; white or yellow coat; mapped tongue

Nux moschata: (see below)

Nux vomica: White; clean at tip; yellow behind

Phosphorus: Dry tongue, with dark brown coating

Pulsatilla nigricans: Dry in morning; tongue broad; covered with tenacious mucus as if with a membrane

Rananculus sceleratus: Desquamation and rhagades on tongue

Rhus toxicodendron: Tongue red at apex

Rhus venenata: Cracked down centre, covered with little vesicles; distress at the root of the tongue

Sulphur: Thick, dirty yellow fur

Taraxacuim dens-leonis: Skin of tongue peeling off; mapped tongue

Examples of syndetic pointers to two homoeopathic medicines:

Sudden panic attack at or around 08h00, as though the circulation had stopped
  with tingling in the whole body, extending to the patient's tongue – Baryta
  carbonica
Patient cannot talk, as if it were difficult to move the tongue – Nux moschata

Tonic

Invigorating; a remedy that enhances enfeebled functions and promotes well-being. Except in so far as nutritional equipoise may be re-established through supplementation when required, this is tautological within the homoeopathic concept. John Henry Clarke (1853-1931) summed the position up:

'. . . the very common habit of taking a "tonic" – no matter what – . . . is not merely ridiculous, it is pernicious. Medicines in general only have a strengthening action when there is a lack of strength in the patient; and the same strengthening medicine is not suitable for every kind of debility. The best "tonic" in any case is that medicine which has produced in the healthy a similar kind of weakness to that experienced by the patient.'[1]

[1]Clarke, John Henry. *The Prescriber: A Dictionary of the New Therapeutics,* ninth edition, Rustington: Health Science Press, 1972, 344-345.

Toothache

Odontalgia; pain in a tooth or teeth with involvement of the periodontal membrane or the pulp, sometimes associated with trauma, caries or gum inflammation. John Henry Clarke's detailed 'Repertory of Remedies for Toothache' is probably the best source reference for effective homoeopathic treatment (pages 347 to 360 of *The Prescriber: A Dictionary of the New Therapeutics*, Rustington: Health Science Press, ninth edition, 1972). (See also 'Douche', section Toothache and Gums, as well as 'Pain Relief Methods in Homoeopathy'.)

Topical Treatment

Aesculus hippocastanum, Arnica montana, Balsamum peruvianum, Calendula officinalis, Echinacea angustifolia, Hamamelis virginica, Hydrastis canadensis, Hypericum perforatum and Tamus communis are the better known homoeopathic medicines that seem to act well in topical treatment. Homoeopathy is not greatly in the habit of using its medicines in this way, except if it be for external distress or injuries, which do not amount to what may be called a full disease condition. In such cases local applications may be the appropriate homoeopathic measure. (See 'Externally Applied Homoeopathic Drugs'.)

Totality of Signs and Symptoms

Hahnemann (in section 7 of the *Organon*) states that the totality of symptoms points to the curative medicine, because that totality, that holistic aggregate, is the image which outwardly reflects the internal disease process and the corrective reaction of the dynamis thereto. In any assessment of the totality of symptoms and signs the homoeopath ought to cover the majority of the patient's signs and symptoms (including such non-verbal things as mannerisms, gait, effects of grief, body-odour, choice of clothes, facial expressions, and the like) and find a corresponding drug picture. In this image-to-image comparison, which, in fact, is the homoeopathic diagnosis, only odd, isolated symptoms may be ignored. (See 'Disease and Drug Action in Homoeopathic Congruity', 'Pathology' and 'Unity of Symptoms, Pathological'.)

Toxicological Theory of Disease

Stuart Close expounded this essentialistic theory.[1] It runs as follows: Life is defined as 'a continuous adjustment of internal to external relations'. The definition of disease is amplified: 'Disease is a morbid dynamical disturbance of the vital force caused by some morbific agent actually or

[1] Close, Stuart. *The Genius of Homoeopathy: Lectures and Essays on Homoeopathic Philosophy* New York: Boericke and Tafel, 1924, pp 105-111.

relatively external to the organism'. From that point of view all diseases may be regarded as intoxations. Close maintains that all drugs act by virtue of their specific toxic properties; all bacterial disease is primarily intoxation or toxaemia. He says, 'Pathologists agree that all pathogenic micro-organisms produce their effects in the living body by means of the specific poisons which they secrete while living, or generate after death. Diseases arising from physical injury or mechanical violence are toxaemias resulting from chemical changes in the injured tissues' bringing about 'inhibition of normal functioning, which leads to degenerative changes and the formation of toxins' and can be explained as 'chemico-toxic' effects. He goes on: 'Disease arising from chemical agents, aside from the direct physical injury or destruction of tissue as by corrosive poisons, are poisonings of the organism. Disease resulting from mental . . . trauma occurs as a result of the toxic chemical . . . changes that take place in the fluids and tissues of the body through the medium of the nervous system'. He postulates: 'If all diseases are the result of some form or degree of poisoning, then in the last analysis all curative treatment is antidotal treatment'. Since 'dynamical antidotes, in their crude state, are themselves poisons of varying degrees of power', what Boenninghausen had said applies (according to Close): 'Medicines producing similar symptoms are related to each other and are mutually antidotal in proportion to the degree of their symptom-similarity'. Hence 'similia similibus curentur'. Close sums up by saying, 'One fundamental principle underlies all – the law of reciprocal action or equivalence. The law of chemical affinity and definite proportions; the law of . . . dynamical affinity; the law of assimilation [see 'Homoeosis']; the law of antidotes or the repulsion of similars (upon which is based the theory of cure) are all phases of the universal law of mutual action, which governs every action that occurs in the universe'.

In 1952 Hans-Heinrich Reckeweg overhauled this theory, by describing what he called homotoxicosis as a subnormal state of health due to a toxic burden arising from poor elimination of accumulated, potentially poisonous, by-products of both endogenous and exogenous origin. (See 'Disease', 'Homotoxicosis' and 'Science and Homoeopathy'.)

Trace Element

One of a number of elements required in very small amounts (a few milligrams or much less per day) and present in minuscule quantities in living organisms. These 'micronutrients' are essential for proper metabolic function. They include chromium, cobalt, copper, iodine, iron, manganese, molybdenum, selenium, silicon and zinc. They are indispensable for the production of important compounds, in the manufacture of enzymes, insulin, cyanocobalamin (vitamin B12), thyroid hormone, etc.. By contrast, calcium, chlorine, magnesium, phosphorus, potassium, sodium and sulphur are referred to as the 'macro-minerals', because these are the bulk elements involved largely in structural functions in an organism.

Trituration

One of the processes of homoeopathic drug preparation. It is the act of prolonged grinding with a pestle in a mortar (or a similar mechanical procedure) to reduce a homoeopathic drug to a fine powder while amalgamating it thoroughly with Saccharum lactis (sugar of milk) by rubbing the two together under the pestle in the mortar. (See 'Drug Preparation', 'Potentizing Methods', 'Solvation Structures' and 'Succussion'.)

Trivial Name

Name of a homoeopathic medicine giving no clue as to either structure or systematic classification in the natural order of the starting material, as would its generic name. Examples are Gunpowder (for the rather cumbersome 'Nitrum cum Sulphuri Praecipitati et Carboni'), Jalapa (for 'Ipomoea purga'), Glonoinum (for 'Nitroglycerinum'), or Jaborandi (for 'Pilocarpus pinnatifolius'). Trivial names are not necessarily synonymous with vernacular names – for instance, the vernacular name for Jalapa is 'Jalap', and for Glonoinum it is 'Nitro-glycerine'.

Tropism

An orienting response to physical, biochemical and/or dynamic agencies within organisms. (See also 'Aetiotropism', 'Functiotropism', 'Organotropism' and 'Pathotropism'.)

Tuberculinism

See 'Miasma'.

Tyler, Sir Henry James (1827-1908)

This Englishman's contribution to homoeopathy was as the benefactor to the London Homoeopathic Hospital. He created the annual Tyler Scholarship in the UK for homoeopathic studies in the USA. Douglas M Borland, Sir John Weir, and very probably Margaret L Tyler (his own daughter) were some of the homoeopaths who travelled to the USA on the Tyler Scholarship.

Tyler, Margaret L (1875-1943)

Sir Henry's daughter was an inspiring lecturer who worked for more than four decades at the London Homoeopathic Hospital, where she ran a clinic for mentally handicapped children on Monday mornings. She worked closely with the NSPCC and often achieved astonishing results with such maltreated children. She used the following five remedies quite regularly:

Baryta carbonica for the heavy, dull, slow child with enlarged lymph nodes and a tendency to have sore throats; **Capsicum annuum** for the homesick, retarded child; **Medorrhinum** for a child with Down's syndrome; **Tuberculinum bovinum** for the spoilt, resentful child with a mental slowness, followed by **(Delphinium) Staphisagria** for the extremely resentful and very touchy child.

In her 1916 eulogy of James Tyler Kent (1849-1916), Margaret Tyler expressed her regret never to have heard him lecture. This author received the assurance from one of Sir John Weir's former patients that she did, in fact, travel to St Louis, but that Kent was absent at the time so that she did not actually hear him lecture. This patient was well informed in other respects, so the story seems plausible, the more so as Sir John had known Margaret Tyler well. They had co-authored *Repertorizing* in 1912.

For some time she lectured at the Missionary School of Homoeopathic Medicine which is linked to the Royal London Homoeopathic Hospital.

Her major publications include:

Repertorizing (with Sir John Weir) (1912)

A Study of Kent's Repertory (1914)

Drosera (1927)

Homoeopathic Drug Pictures (1942)

Index and Repertory [to the preceding] was produced by N W Jollyman (1988)

Pointers to the Common Remedies (not given) (originally as nine separate booklets; later published in one bound volume [337 pages; New Delhi: B Jain Publishers])

Initial Lectures to the Missionary School of Medicine; Some Drug Pictures; Acute Conditions (years not given)

Type

Individual specimen upon which the description of a homogeneous group, or in taxonomy of a new species or genus, may be based. In psychology: a major classification of traits the characteristics of which may typify an individual in terms of personality theory. In criminology: a class of offender the criminal pattern and modus operandi of whom would indicate to the behavioural scientist information about that person's social grouping and personality. In humoral pathology: refer to that entry. In homoeopathy: a class of individual/patient having a pattern of characteristics in common – physical, mental and morphological – that allows identification with a matching drug picture. The aspects that might be indicative to the homoeopath could include: direction of interests, kind of imagery preferred and nature of ideas communicated, temperament, body build, relationship to order, openness to change, unusual extensions of thought, control of bodily motions or lack thereof, creativeness, humour, strength of volition, antagonisms, possessive relations and affections, morals and religious interests, as well as any number of physical attributes. (See 'Constitutional Type', 'Disease and Drug Action in Homoeopathic Congruity', 'Drug Picture', 'Epistemological Assumptions in Homoeopathy', section 4, 'Morphology' and 'Taxonomy'.)

U

Ullman, Dana

Successfully canvasses the cause of homoeopathy in the USA now for many years. Holder of a master's degree in public health from University College Berkeley, USA, he has written some 50 articles that have appeared in respected publications (including orthodox medical journals). He is the founder and current president of the Foundation for Homeopathic Education and Research, and has edited *Monograph on Homeopathic Research*, volumes I and II. His other major literary works to date include:

Everybody's Guide to Homeopathic Medicines (co-authored with Stephen Cummings; awarded the Medical Self-Care Book Award)

San Francisco Foundation's 'Health Report' (by which he changed the funding priorities of the San Francisco Foundation, for whom he authored it)

Homeopathy: Medicine for the 21st Century (Berkeley, Ca: North Atlantic Books, 1988, 295 pages).

Ultramolecular Dynamization

See 'Avogadro's Number', 'Epistemological Assumptions in Homoeopathy', section 5, and 'Potency'.

Ultrasonic Potency Destruction

High-intensity ultrasonic waves can produce a dispersion of one medium in another, e.g. mercury in water. Similarly it is known that such ultrasonic waves can destroy homoeopathic dynamizations that are exposed to them. This may happen inadvertently (possibly when ultrasound is used during physiotherapy, dental surgery, certain types of scanning, etc.).

Ultrasound Therapy

See 'Sound Therapy', 'Naturopath' and 'Ultrasonic Potency Destruction'.

Ultra-Violet Irradiation

See 'Actinotherapy' and 'Naturopath'.

Uncertainty Principle

Formulated in 1927 by the German physicist and Nobel laureate Werner Karl

Heisenberg (1901-1976), postulates that as consciousness is part of the measurement in natural science and of the reality within which it is embedded, it must make that scientific reality (as understood in the West for four centuries) unavoidably indeterminate. Indeterminism was seen henceforth as inherent in physical nature, though this has been resisted fiercely by many outside of homoeopathy. (See 'Probabiliorism', 'Science and Homoeopathy' and 'Uniformity of Nature'.)

Unconscious

Insensible; not having the characteristic of (full) awareness. 'The unconscious' (with the definite article) can be understood as the aggregate of dynamic elements constituting that segment of a personality of which the subject is entirely, or perhaps largely, unaware. It covers primordial urges, repressed memories, desires and aversions, fears and fixations, etc. (partially) concealed from normal thought processes.

Uncture

Greasy ointment.

Understanding

Comprehension; apprehension of meaning conveyed by symbols, words or phenomena. Also used as a general term covering functions which involve perceptual and/or conceptual assimilation processes such as would involve the engagement of memory, the marshalling of thought currents by classification systems, the attainment of recognition, the solving of problems and, ultimately, the forming of opinions. For each of these affects, the similarity principle is the undisputed ultimate component that is indispensable for their coherent development, as is discussed under 'Epistemological Assumptions in Homoeopathy', section 1: Similarity – as a Concept in Science.

Ungentum Flavum

Yellow ointment; yellow beeswax 5 to Vaselinum flavum 95, makes a good vehicle for, say, Chrysarobinum ointment (pathotropic to psoriasis). (See 'Vehicle'.)

Unified Field Theory

See 'Science and Homoeopathy'.

Uniformity of Nature

Principle, taken to apply to natural phenomena, setting out that with the same antecedents exactly the same consequences will always follow. (See also 'Determinism', 'Probabiliorism' and 'Uncertainty Principle'.)

Unilateral

Referring to, or involving, only one side of the body. Just as some patients present with all their ailments on one side only, so, likewise, some homoeopathic drugs pick out either the right or the left side of the body for the presentation of their symptoms. Margaret L Tyler (1875-1943) comments in her *Homoeopathic Drug Pictures* (Rustington: Health Science Press, 1970, p 104): 'Black type drugs that are very especially left-sided are Arg n, Asaf, Asar, Caps, Cina, Clem, Croc, Euphorb, Graph, Kre, Lach, Oleand, Phos, Selen, Sep, Stann. The very especially right-sided remedies in black type, are given as Ars, Aur, Bapt, Bell, Bor, Canth, Lyc, Puls, Ran b, Sars, Sec, Sul ac.'

This term bears no relation to Hahnemann's 'einseitige Krankheiten' ('one-sided diseases') of sections 172-175 of The *Organon*, discussed under 'Schmidt, Pierre (1894-1987)'.

Unitary Disease Concept

See 'Disease'.

United States' Food, Drug and Cosmetic Act of 1938

This well-known piece of original legislation was introduced and assiduously piloted in its slow and tortuous five-year passage to the US statute books by the homoeopath Royal Copeland, who was a US senator. It is thought that the extreme stresses caused by arduously battling this Act through a reluctant legislature for five uninterrupted years caused the exhaustion to which his death has been ascribed. He had been propelled by his dedication to the moral imperatives he saw underpinning this Act and died only a few days after it was finally adopted by the US Congress. (See 'Coulter, Harris Livermore' and 'Medico-Legal'.)

Unity of Symptoms, Pathological

The disease picture consists of the pathological unity of symptoms, revealing the matching remedy to the homoeopath. (See 'Disease and Drug Action in Homoeopathic Congruity', 'Drug Picture', 'Pathology' and 'Totality of Signs and Symptoms'.)

Urinalysis

Examination of the urine for constituents, such as protein, glucose, ketones (aceto-acetic acid), nitrites, blood, bilirubin, urobilinogen, leucocytes, uric acid, chloride, calcium oxalate and calcium phosphate.

Urination

Passing of urine; micturition. Changes in urination patterns may point the homoeopath toward considering certain remedies.

Urinometry

Determination of the relative density (formerly 'specific gravity') and sometimes also the pH, indican and redox levels of urine.

Uromancy

● **Urine divining.**

In the early eighteenth century it was customary for many physicians of the Rationalist tradition in Europe to presage not only a patient's disease and its prognosis but for some also to reveal other circumstances (whether or not the patient was a virgin, pregnant, had a spouse, and the like) from the divination of the urine belonging to that person. The celebrated Dutch physician and philosopher Hermann Boerhaave (1668-1738) made a speciality of diagnosis from the urine. As a source of external causal knowledge (pathology) by which orthodox therapeutics might take its direction, it was displaced in the nineteenth century by vivisection and autopsy.

Current medical histories report that Boerhaave was a medical innovator, revived clinical instruction, lectured on diseases of the eye, made chemistry a popular subject, was the first to expound the principles of medical thermometry, and advocated post mortem examinations. Yet curiously, this Dutch physician's uromancy[1] is generally not reported in these medical history books, even though he explicitly deplored the urinary soothsaying about non-disease matters in which many fellow physicians indulged, which should have made it less objectionable to the historians. This neglect probably occurs because such books have as their main purpose – indeed they have always had – the re-interpretation of the past in the light of the particular medical orthodoxy of the present. That which is compatible with today's view of mainstream 'medical progress' is featured, but whatever is discommodious is often expurgated or will receive no more than scant comment. This tendency

[1] Boerhaave, Hermann. *Elements of Chemistry* (translation by Timothy Dallowe) two volumes in one, London: Pemberton publisher, 1735, VI, pp 216-220 and 235-236.

toward selective narration is not the prerogative of orthodox medicine's chroniclers: the historians of science all too often appear to do the same. It is, for instance, not generally reported that during his entire life Sir Isaac Newton had been steeped in, if not obsessed by, the occult sciences, particularly by alchemy.[1] It is not widely realized that the 'enlightened' eighteenth century 'cleaned Newton up' for public viewing[2] and an almost unbroken line of thoroughly sanitized versions of that great man has been paraded before the world ever since.

Homoeopaths have learnt to allow for such a Rationalist bias in most medical history books. (For a historical overview of medicine in both the Rationalist and the Empirical traditions see 'Hahnemann, Christian Friedrich Samuel (1755-1843)'.)

Urticaria

Hives; nettlerash. (See 'Allergy' and 'Emergencies – Homoeopathic Treatment' under Angioneurotic Oedema.)

Usage, Clinical

● **The use of homoeopathic medicines over and over again in disease conditions has established the way these work their cures.**

This is not to be confused with 'Clinical Trial' (refer to this entry). Clinical usage confirms what the law of similars (equivalents) indicates. Clinical usage is the source of accumulated knowledge derived from untold millions of homoeopathic medicinal prescriptions over fifty, a hundred, one hundred and fifty, or even two hundred years, depending when the remedy was introduced into the homoeopathic materia medica. The cumulative experience from clinical usage in other settings such as allopathic practice, ethnopharmacy, phytotherapy, etc. has the same confirmatory function of the law of similars.

As an empirical science homoeopathy relies heavily on the well ordered registration of experience – and of its ready retrievability by the homoeopath. In a number of ways the computer has become an indispensable and very powerful tool for homoeopathy. It has helped to make homoeopathy much more effective by making repertorization very much more wide-ranging, yet simpler. The computer can now effortlessly be a competence-extending tool for the homoeopath by offering quick and precise access into the tangled plethora of what is contained in many volumes of homoeopathy's materia medica. If properly used it must add precision to homoeopathy in its clinical application. Moreover, Peter Fisher and R A van Haselen have pressed the computer into

[1] Dobbs, B J T. *The Foundation of Newton's Alchemy*, Cambridge: Cambridge University Press, 1975, pp 13-14.
[2] (i) Manuel, Frank E. *A Portrait of Isaac Newton*, Cambridge: Harvard University Press, 1968; and (ii) Kubrin, David. Essay in *The Analytic Spirit*, Harry Woolf, ed., Ithaka, NY: Cornell University Press, 1981.

service in another application, i.e. in the field of homoeopathy's own clinical usage.[1] They have devised a computerized homoeopathic data collection, storage and retrieval method. The information storage promises to provide a tremendous reservoir of homoeopathic post-prescription experience which can be 'scanned' for patterns within the context of the homoeopathic methodology, thereby introducing further progressive refinement into its systematic application.

It seems likely that homoeopathy may, at some stage in the near future, test hypotheses and investigate postulates in focused and controlled trials upon the firmer foundation offered by the computer-extracted statistical significance that may have been opaquely embedded in systematized computer registrations of post-prescription experience. This could certainly point the way out of the impasse due to individualization that has, in the past, so often thwarted homoeopathic trials. (See also 'Homoeopathic Ethnopharmacology', 'Homoeopathized Allopathica', 'Individualization', 'Isopathy', section Homoeopathized Allopathica, 'Materia Medica', 'Miasma' and 'Sources of Homoeopathic Drug Semiology'.)

Ustus

Latin past participle of 'uro; urere; ussi; ustum', to burn. Means calcined, burnt or roasted, as of constituent(s) employed in spagyric preparations, including certain homoeopathic mother tinctures. (See 'Mother Tincture' and 'Spagyric'.)

Utensils of Homoeopathic Pharmacy

The instruments in use in a standardly equipped homoeopathic pharmaceutical laboratory are:

Mortars and pestles
of polished steel for pulverizing hard substances, such as seeds;
of porcelain with unglazed surfaces for crushing soft substances, such as charcoal or fresh plant material;
of glass for triturating mercurial preparations
Spoons and spatulas
of horn, bone, chromed steel, porcelain or of another inert material; the latter are required for trituration, and in the preparation of ointments, the weighing of powder, etc., while the former are used for handling sugar and for similar purposes

---

[1] van Haselen, R A, and Peter Fisher. 'Analysing Homoeopathic Prescribing Using the READ Classification and Information Technology', *British Homoeopathic Journal*, 1990, vol LXXIX, pp 74-81.

Sieves

    of silk, animal hair or wire; the latter two are used for ordinary purposes and coarser substances, while silk sieves are used for powders or in connexion with manufacture of tinctures or triturations; sieves used for sugar of milk may not be used for any other purpose

Measuring glasses

    a few properly graduated measuring cylinders, made of glass, are required; no dynamized drugs should be measured in these and strict rules for their cleansing apply if they are used interchangeably for the holding of various crude medicinal substances

Presses

    for expressing juice (succus) from medicinal plants, or as a filter after maceration or percolation (see 'Expression')

Funnels

    of glass or porcelain only (no metallic funnels)

Chopping board & knife

    the board is made of hard wood, free of knots and knot-holes, and the knife is made of stainless steel; these are required to cut the fresh medicinal plants, leaves, shoots, pods, roots, barks and flowers into small pieces

Balances (two types)

    a chemical balance for weighing, to a high degree of accuracy, the small amounts of material sometimes dealt with;

    a physical balance for weighing larger quantities when strict accuracy is not essential: with three types of pan scales:

        brass pan scales for general use,

        glass pan scales for corrosive or moist substances, and

        horn pan scales for sugar of milk, for poisons, etc.

Dessicators

    for removing moisture from substances, each of which is an air-tight glass vessel with a lid that seals hermetically on to the upper greased rim; around its middle there is a contracture upon which a perforated sheet of zinc is placed, as a shelf which separates the upper from the lower half; drying agents like fused calcium chloride or concentrated sulphuric acid are placed at the bottom to keep the air inside the dessicator dry; the substance to be dried is kept on a triangle formed by clay pipes

Hot-air oven

    for drying and heating up to almost 100 degrees Celsius: it is a double-walled copper vessel with a door and a movable perforated shelf; the hollow space between the two walls is partially filled with water from an opening at the top; this is kept boiling with a burner from below filling the upper space of the hollow with steam; the substance is dried by placing it on the shelf inside the oven where there is a constant temperature of nearly 100 degrees Celsius

Evaporator

    a still made of suitable inert material, designed to evaporate moisture or solvents to obtain the concentrate

Thermometer

to measure temperature of substances during various stages of preparation

Hydrometer

to measure relative density (formerly known as 'specific gravity') of a liquid

Microscope & magnifying glass

for the examination of minute (particles of) substances

An assortment of other instruments

Bunsen burner; glass retort; timer; tripod stand; beakers; flasks; tongs; tweezers; pans; test tubes; bottles and matching corks; percolator; pipettes; burettes; filter stand.

Additional instruments in a modern fully equipped aseptic homoeo-pharmaceutical laboratory might comprise these:

Glassware for extractions, macerations, triturations, reflux and distillation procedures, etc.; electrical heating mantles; separating funnels; Buchner funnels; suction pumps; thin layer chromatographic materials, UV light station with photographic facilities for TLC[1] plate recording, UV spectrographs with standard storage facilities and printer link, AA spectrograph facilities, gas chromatograph; laminar flow units for medicine preparation; autoclaves; globulus, granule, tabloid and tablet making equipment; trituration moulds; suppository, pessary and bougie moulds; automatic metered dispensing pipettes; ball mill; ribbon blender; vacuum chamber; tablet/pill disintegration/dissolution equipment; hardness tester; incubators; plating facility; potency bank; mother tincture storage facility; infusion pots; magnetic stirrers; pH, redox and conductivity meters; polaroid facilities for microscopes; refractometers; titration flasks for specific quantitative, qualitative and analytical procedures (organic and inorganic); herbarium; viscometer; polarimeter; ampoule filling and sealing equipment; micropore filtration units for auto-isopathic, nosode, sarcode and potentized allergen preparations; high speed particle impact disintegration mill; comminuter; tincture presses; mechanized dynamizators (potentizers) 5ml to 30ml capacity; korsakovian automatic attenuator; mechanized mortars and pestles; capsule filler; globulus and granule impregnation turning banks; sterile and particle free compressed air supply; pill pans and sieves; vacuum pumps; hot blowers for pill pans; stainless steel pill whisks and drying pans; drying oven with vacuum facilities; cream and ointment preparation vats; tube filling equipment; tube sealing equipment; tablet counter; electronic balances; stainless steel maceration vats with sealing lids; water still; de-ionizer; gloved sterile unit and biological preparation unit; powder folders; porcelain/glass ointment slabs; small triple roll mill; and particle counter for air monitoring.

---

[1]TLC = Thin-layer chromatography/ic: in this compounds are separated by a suitable solvent (mixture) on a thin layer of adsorbent material coated on to a glass plate; the method is rapid and excellent separations can be obtained thereby.

V

Vaccination

Inoculation in the skin with the live cowpox (vaccinia) virus as a prophylaxis against smallpox; and by logical extension, in orthodox medicine now, more or less inaccurately, also the injection of an attenuated or killed microbial culture to cure, or as a prophylaxis against, illness associated with that same micro-organism. The orthodox concept underlying the original meaning is quasi-homoeopathic, but that underlying the second is Isopathic. Homoeopathy has no 'vaccination' in the current orthodox sense. Moreover, its nosodes have not undergone thorough clinical evaluations yet, though historical evidence seems to suggest their long-term, miasmatically beneficial, prophylactic effects. (See 'Burnett, James Compton (1840-1901)', 'Hering, Constantin (1800-1880)', 'Immunization and Homoeopathy' and 'Isopathy'.)

Vaccinosis

Disease triggered by vaccination. This concept was originated in the mid-1890s by the homoeopath James Compton Burnett. It is an incontrovertible fact that the appearance of serious disabilities such as asthma, rheumatoid arthritis or eczema, and some other insidious low-grade disorders are often initiated by immunization, though this is denied by many orthodox medical practitioners. Despite his disturbing discovery, J Compton Burnett was not an anti-vaccination campaigner. He believed, as Hahnemann had (refer *Organon*, sections 46 and 47), that vaccination was a clear demonstration of the Law of Similars. (See 'Burnett, James Compton (1840-1901)' and 'Miasma'.)

Van Gogh, Vincent (1853-1890)

Eccentric Dutch painter, who was the first of the great Expressionists and is probably now the best known among them, whose paintings fetched staggering prices at art auctions in the decade from 1980. The picture that was sold for the then record price of £49 million sterling in May 1990, through the New York branch of the art auctioneers Christie's, was van Gogh's renowned portrait of his friend and confidant, the French homoeopath Paul-Ferdinand Gachet. He painted this and another portrait of Gachet with 'the heartbroken expression of our times' at Auvers-sur-Oise, France. They are his last masterpieces before he shot himself on 27th July 1890. His last lesser canvases, in fact, depicted endless wheatfields under hot and troubled skies through which he compellingly expresses 'sadness and extreme loneliness'.

The homoeopath Gachet was an accomplished painter himself who had exhibited his own work at the Salon des Indépendants. He had other painters like Jean Baptiste Camille Corot (1796-1875) and Honoré Victorin Daumier (1808-1879) as patients, as well as being the patron of, and a friend to, a number of famous Impressionists like Camille Pissaro (1830-1903), Pierre Auguste Renoir (1841-1919) and the Post-Impressionist Paul Cézanne (1839-1906). He allowed his artist-patients, who were usually short of cash, to pay him with paintings instead of collecting fees from them. Thus, Renoir came to give him a portrait of one of his models in lieu of fees for having treated her for tuberculosis. (See also 'David, Pierre Jean (also David d'Angers) (1788-1856)', 'Goethe, Johann Wolfgang von (1749-1832)' and 'Well-Wishers and Supporters of Homoeopathy'.)

Vaselinum Album

See 'Vaselinum Flavum'.

Vaselinum Flavum

Yellow petroleum jelly; by-product of the petroleum industry, also known as yellow soft paraffin (in some areas of the world; moreover, only in the UK was 'Vaseline' registered as a trade-mark, elsewhere this is a generic term used in pharmacopoeias). Once bleached, it becomes Vaselinum album, or white petroleum jelly, or white soft paraffin. Its melting point ranges from 38 to 56 degrees Celsius. It is tasteless and odourless, has a soft consistency and is insoluble in water. On open wounds it retards epithelialization and granulations, and therefore slows down healing a little, but it is an excellent lubricant, provides a barrier where necessary and makes a good vehicle for medicinal ointments.

Veganism and Vegetarianism

The first of these is avoidance of all animal products, including milk and eggs; the second is abstention from all meat, poultry, fish and non-herbal seafood. The differences, in the concentrations of stomach acids, in the gastric enzymes and in dentition between carnivorous animals and man, make it apparent that the latter is not adequately adapted to a diet exclusively or predominantly consisting of flesh-products. However, the presence of canines in man's dentition, some point out, would seem to indicate that birds and small animals were, indeed, part of the normal diet of this species to which it would have been homoeotically adjusted, and which certainly would have provided adequate vitamin B12 intake. Two problems that may arise from both the vegan and vegetarian diets are:

(i) vitamin B12 deficiency; and

(ii) zinc deficiency – due to phytates binding this trace element, thus impeding its absorption.

B12 is obtainable, to some limited extent, from milk products, while yeast and sprouted grains counteract the said effects of phytates. Some vegans may, therefore, still require B12 supplementation. Generally there is no reason why such diets may not be adopted by the patients of homoeopaths. Vegan or vegetarian patients ought not to be given homoeopathic medicines of animal origin, without their prior consent.

Remarkably, several homoeopathic drug pictures include the unwelcome, though painless, sensation of animals in the epigastrium or abdomen, e.g. Cannabis sativa, Chelidonium majus, Crocus sativus, Podophyllum peltatum and Thuja occidentalis, while another, (Trigonocephalus) Lachesis, can produce a mental and perceptual identification with animals. (See 'Dietary Therapy', 'Foods as Health Problems', 'Homoeosis', 'Nutritional Equipoise' and 'Vitamin'.)

Vehicle

● **In homoeopathic pharmacy, the medium which carries the effective medicinal agent.**

A neutral substance which, in homoeopathic pharmacy, has practically no medicinal or therapeutic property of its own, intended to convey the dynamic powers of a drug safely to the organism to be treated. It is used to hold the active principle of a medicine. A vehicle must be stable, that is have 'keeping qualities', which means it will not readily undergo any change or decomposition, yet act both as solvent and as preservative. A water-ethanol (hydro-alcoholic) mixture is frequently the most suitable liquid solvent. Acids as well as some metals and chemicals, when mixed with alcohol, will produce chemical reactions, in such cases distilled water becomes the most suitable vehicle. In a few instances glycerinum is the vehicle of choice (mother tinctures and lower potencies of Apis mellifica, Tarentula cubensis and Naja tripudians, for instance; also for the preservation of certain ophiotoxins, like Crotalus cascavella, Crotalus horridus and Elaps corallinus).

By the use of a solid vehicle, chemicals, metals, and some animal substances and certain other drugs are dynamized (potentized) as powders (see 'Colloids'). Saccharum lactis (sugar of milk), in accordance with pharmacopoeial specifications, is the most frequently used neutral solid vehicle.

The uses of vehicles are: preparation of mother tinctures, solutions, triturations, potencies, the preparation of internal medicines (e.g. suppositories) and external applications. Where apposite, vehicles must be comestible, unobtrusive to the palate, resorbable, etc.

Some of the less frequently used liquid vehicles include: Oleum olivae, teel oil (sesame oil) and syrupus; infrequently used semi-liquid vehicles comprise vaselinum album and flavum, bees' wax, lanolin, glycerinated gelatin and cetaceum (spermaceti).

Venesection

Bloodletting from a vein. (See 'Hahnemann, Christian Friedrich Samuel (1755-1843)' section The Rationalist Medical Tradition, when bloodletting was at the height of its fashion, ca. 1810-ca. 1870.)

Verdi, Tullio Suzzara (1829-1902)

This remarkable homoeopath displayed a rather rare combination of dedicated professional thoroughness along with extraordinary political agility. These qualities made his the career of a distinguished public figure, ultimately setting an example of a homoeopath's consummate competence in public health issues while establishing homoeopathy's reliability in epidemiological emergencies.

Highlights of his Life

Verdi came to the USA when he was forced to leave his native Italy after participating in an unsuccessful uprising at Novara in 1848. Upon graduating as a homoeopathic physician in 1856 from the Hahnemann College in Philadelphia, he married advantageously and settled in Washington. Through his marriage he had access to the capital city's social life and his practice as a gynaecologist and obstetrician meant he gained influence with politicians through their wives and daughters.

While two rival orthodox medical societies were pillorying each other and vying for the granting of a charter by the US Senate in 1869, Verdi profited from this 'allopathic' split and applied to Congress for a charter for the Washington Homoeopathic Medical Society. His bill was passed by both houses unanimously in April 1870, whereas the 'allopathic issue' was never voted on.

When the American Medical Association manipulated the Federal Commissioner of Pensions to coerce him into allowing only 'allopathic' pension examiners to be employed by the Federal Government, and as a direct consequence nineteen homoeopaths were dismissed, Verdi used his influence very effectively with the press, and a chorus of editorials in favour of the homoeopaths followed. Verdi also wrote to President Grant on this matter, which resulted in a cabinet meeting on the following day when the name of the successor to the responsible Federal Commissioner of Pensions was summarily sent to the Senate for confirmation. A fortnight later that Federal Commissioner of Pensions was surprised to have been so suddenly replaced. The dismissed homoeopaths were restored to their positions without delay.

Verdi strongly championed the cause of blacks and women in medicine, who, at that time, were both still virtually excluded from all orthodox medical societies and their medical schools in the entire USA. He asked the governor of the District of Columbia to be included, as a matter of moral solidarity, as one of the incorporators of a projected orthodox National Medical University, because it was to be open to blacks also. When the other ('allopathic') sponsors of the university rejected Verdi's request, the governor himself resigned as director in protest and Verdi efficiently orchestrated a petitions campaign by quietly urging homoeopathic constituents far and wide to prepare petitions. This resulted in his receiving 140 different ones. He 'separated them by states, and every day, for three weeks', he 'sent petitions to some Senator or Representative', so that 'the claims of homoeopathy were read in Congress' daily 'and put on their Journal'.[1] This induced the orthodox physicians, by most of whom the homoeopaths were generally viewed as radical abolitionists, to end any support they had ever given to the project, suspecting it to be the homoeopaths' Trojan Horse. In this manner Verdi contrived to have this 'allopathic' university project aborted.

In 1871 Verdi became Health Officer of the District of Columbia Board of Health, whereupon he established homoeopathic dispensaries and strictly enforced the smallpox vaccination law. Two years later he investigated the more advanced sanitary laws of cities in Austria, England, France, Germany and Italy during a trip through Europe for that purpose. On his return he published a very thorough report.

In 1875 he was elected president of this Board of Health, to which position he was subsequently re-elected.

In the wake of the Yellow Fever epidemic of 1878 the US Surgeon-General appointed a medical commission with a mandate to look into the causes of the Yellow Fever outbreak and its future prevention. Only orthodox practitioners served on this commission. To forestall a one-sided finding, Verdi appointed another medical Yellow Fever commission, composed of eleven homoeopathic physicians, including himself, with a somewhat wider mandate: in addition to the causes, and prevention, of Yellow Fever, it was also to look at its successful homoeopathic cure. After visiting all the principal towns, Verdi's commission put together a report from verifiable sources under rigorous public and press scrutiny which showed that those who had been treated homoeopathically had a much lower mortality rate: 5.6% in New Orleans and 7.7% for the entire remaining South. By contrast, the 'allopathic' Yellow Fever commission had to report an overall mortality rate of never less than 16%, but often in the twenties. These figures made a profound impression on the US Congress. Whereas the orthodox commission recommended nothing other than a rigid quarantine, believing that Yellow Fever was a contagion brought in on ships, Verdi's commission decided that Yellow Fever was caused by a specific germ which had to be both indigenous and imported and thus could not be prevented by quarantine alone. It recommended the setting up of a permanent sanitary commission, drainage of the cities, the burning of refuse, flushing of streets, and the like, and it merely suggested the discriminating use of quarantines; it found that Yellow Fever had three distinct phases and that specific homoeopathic medicines were effective in each, depending on the corresponding homoeopathic indications (see 'Therapeutic Science').

[1] *Transactions of the American Institute of Homoeopathy*, vol XXIV, 1871, 100.

The remedies most frequently employed successfully in that epidemic had been:

Aconitum napellus; Arsenicum album; (Atropa) Belladonna; Carbo vegetabilis; Crotalus horridus; (Trigonocephalus) Lachesis; Phosphorus.

The low potencies had been employed predominantly, though some homoeopaths were reported to have gone up to the 30DH potencies.

The homoeopathic results were well received by Congress and the recommendations of the homoeopathic commission were to be acted upon by the National Board of Health which, as the report had proposed, was duly brought into existence in April 1879. Congress elevated Verdi to this Board on which he subsequently served and where he finally ended his distinguished public career.[1,2]

Vermifuge

Promotes the expulsion of worms and other non-microbian, non-viral parasites from the intestines. To be acceptable to homoeopathy it may not coercively affect the host organism.

Veterinary Homoeopathy

● **Treatment of sick animals by means of homoeopathy. The constant flow of information and experience derived from this adds to the completeness of the homoeopathic materia medica.**

A strong and continuous tradition of veterinary homoeopathy has spread throughout the world since the days of Hahnemann. In the library of the University of Leipzig there is a paper written by Hahnemann entitled 'Homoeopathic Medicine of Household Animals'. In it he called for veterinarians to take up homoeopathy. Johan Joseph Wilhelm Lux (1776-1849), at the time of Berlin's Civil Veterinary University, introduced homoeopathic treatment for animals in 1823 with immediate success. Lux later published the veterinary review *Zooaiasis*. He contributed markedly to the diffusion of both veterinary and human homoeopathy, to the point at one time of almost causing a schism in veterinary as well as human homoeopathy with his headlong pursuit of Isopathy (see this entry). Notwithstanding this, nosodes – soon to become indispensable to homoeopathy – were popularized through the impetus of his Isopathic movement.

Of the veterinary homoeopathic text-books that have been published a few of the leading English-medium publications are:

Homoeopathic Veterinarian F E Günther (German orig)

[1] *Transactions of the American Institute of Homoeopathy*. 'An Obituary of Dr T S Verdi', vol LIX, 1903, 730-731.
[2] Coulter, Harris Livermore. *Divided Legacy: a History of the Schism in Medical Thought*, Washington: Wehawken Book Company, 1973, vol III, 290-304.

The Hand-book to Veterinary Homoeopathy John Rush
Homoeopathy in Veterinary Practice J Sutcliffe Harndall
Pocket Manual of Homoeopathic Veterinary Medicine Edward Harris Ruddock
Homoeopathy in Veterinary Practice K J Biddis
The Treatment of Horses by Homoeopathy G Macleod
The Treatment of Goats by Homoeopathy G Macleod
The Treatment of Cattle by Homoeopathy G Macleod
The Treatment of Dogs by Homoeopathy K Sheppard
The Treatment of Cats by Homoeopathy K Sheppard
Veterinary Materia Medica and Clinical Repertory with Materia Medica of the Nosodes
G Macleod

Experimental Evidence

See 'Epidemiology' and 'Schmidt, Pierre (1894–1987)' for details of an annually prepared nosode in combination with Acidum nitricum 6CH in successfully arresting foot-and-mouth disease. Double blind trials, to demonstrate the differentiated action of Caulophyllum 30DH in farrowing sows as well as to establish the curative effect of Lophophytum leandri (Flor de Piedra) in acetonaemia in cattle, were undertaken and published.[1] Many controlled animals studies have successfully demonstrated the efficacy of homoeopathic medicines on animals.[2] A good many of these are succinctly described by Harris L Coulter.[3] There are also zoological experiments that have been reported by David Taylor Reilly:[4] Dr Endle's experiments in an Austrian university zoological institute demonstrating that

> 'the onset of metamorphosis from tadpole to toad in healthy specimens of Bufeo bufo could be induced earlier by tri-iodothyronine in a 30DH homoeopathic dilution. No pretreatment, no illness model, no individualized prescribing, . . . the dilution, proven molecule-free by gas chromatography, tested blind . . . against water'.[5]

The Frenchman, Bernard Poitevin's two experiments:
1) With Apis mellifica reducing uv erythema in guinea pigs; and
2) The activation of mouse macrophages with Silica.

[1]Wolter, Hans. 'Wirksamkeitsnachweis von Caulophyllum D30 bei der Wehenschwäche des Schweines' and 'Die Wirksamkeit von Flor de Piedra D3 bei der Azetonaemie des Rindviehs'. *Beweisbare Homöopathie*, Heidelberg: K H Gebhardt Herausgeber, 1980.
[2]Wurmser, Lise. 'Die Entwicklung der homöopathischen Forschung'. Deutsche Homöopathische Union's special off-print.
[3]Coulter, Harris Livermore. *Homoeopathic Science and Modern Medicine: The Physics of Healing with Microdoses*, Berkeley, California: North Atlantic Books, 1981, PP 90-91.
[4]Reilly, David Taylor. 'Zentrum zur Dokumentation für Naturheilverfahren e V – Homöopathie im Brennpunkt: Hazy Reflections from Essen' [report on the Homoeopathic Scientific Conference held there 14th-15th October 1989], *Complementary Medical Research*, May 1990, vol IV, no 2, pp 51-53.
[5]loc cit, p 52. [Details are obtainable from: Zentrum zur Dokumentation für Naturheilverfahren e V, Hufelandstrasse 56, D-4300 Essen 1, Germany.]

(See also 'Animal Experiments', 'Clinical Trials' and 'Physiological Responses in Homoeotherapeutics, Mechanism of'.)

Vicarious Menstruation

See 'Xenomenia'.

Visualization Therapy

See 'Naturopath'.

Vital Dynamics, Science of

See 'Vitalism'.

Vital Factor and/or Vital Force

'Elan vital', or the momentum of life, of philosopher Henri Louis Bergson (1859-1941); the 'Lebenskraft' of Hahnemann (see 'Dynamis', 'Laws of Nature' and 'Vitalism').

Vitalism

● **Theory holding that underlying all vital phenomena there is a life-giving, life-preserving, life-directing and integrating force in every living organism.**

The philosophical and biological theory, consonant with, and supportive of, homoeopathy's epistemological assumptions, that living organisms are truly dynamic, in the sense of being vital (i.e. animated or alive). It sees life not merely as 'the state of existence characterized by active metabolism'[1] but as the potential to exercise functional activities (usually more than one of these in concert with others) that are designed to further the continuance of an organism's autarkic existence. Such autonomic activities include reproduction, regeneration, independent nutritional sustainment, awareness (on some level), imparting motion independently (even plants send roots after water and can turn to the light), evincing the curative impulse, and in every other way being an open, non-isolated operative system of systems.

Vitalists often view life – cosmologically – as the fifth dimension, which cannot ever be fully explained in terms of the next lower, the fourth (length, breadth, depth [thickness], and time); quite like any dimension that cannot

---

[1] *Stedman's Medical Dictionary*, XXIInd edition, Baltimore: The Williams & Wilkins Co, 1973, p 702, 'life' – the fourth entry – other entries were less helpful or tautological ['vitality; the essential condition of being alive; or existence of animals and plants'].

ever be fully explained in terms of any lower dimensions. The most recent celebrated exponent of the theory of vitalism and the life force was the French philosopher Henri Louis Bergson (1859-1941), who received the Nobel Prize for Literature (1927) and became a member of l'Académie Francaise (1941). He is the author of *Matter and Memory* (1896) and *Creative Evolution* (1907).

Within the parameter of the biological sciences, vitalism is regarded by many as the only acceptable theoretical foundation. The Second Law of Thermodynamics established in 1850 by Rudolf Julius Emmanuel Clausius (1822-1888) states that heat can never pass spontaneously from a colder to a hotter body; that a temperature difference can never appear spontaneously in a body originally at uniform temperature; and, in more general terms, that there is a spontaneous tendency towards the highest degree of randomness, or a striving towards so-called maximum 'entropy'. Because of this Second Law of Thermodynamics, biological evolution is generally considered as a challenge to natural science. According to this law, 'any system or heterogeneous compound is inexorably destined to progressive decomposition, its potential energy gradually being transformed into heat, inevitably resulting in thermodynamic death, which is the state of thermal equilibrium known as entropy. It is for this reason that vitalism postulates an autarkic, dynamic, creative principle as a necessary explanation for life and evolution'[P Meier]. [1]

Hahnemann took the vital force to be the fountainhead of all the phenomena of life, the sphere in which the disease process, the primary derangement, takes its origin, and in which medicines induce the fundamental reaction, because that is also where the curative impulse begins. He stated that the 'materies morbi' and the organic changes are secondary products, or effects, of disease. Medicines can provoke chemical or mechanical effects, but these can just as readily be produced in a test-tube on non-living material. 'The exclusively vital reactions they set up in the crucible of the organism belong to another sphere: they correspond with the beginnings of disease, like them are revealed by altered sensations and functions, like them are to be characterized as "dynamic". [2]

Vitalism is neutral on the issue of experimental studies, and certainly presents no obstruction to these continuing investigations in homoeopathy. It is, quite obviously, incompatible with the physicalistic theory which holds that living organisms are ultimately inanimate and essentially mechanical, and that all scientific propositions, including those about mental activity, are expressible only in the terminology of the physical sciences. Sir John C Eccles (born 1903), the distinguished Australian neurophysiologist and 1963 Nobel laureate (for pioneering work on nerve cell mechanisms in the spinal cord), expounds his version of Vitalism in *Evolution of the Brain: Creation of the Self* (London: Routledge, 1989, 298 pages). He postulates a mental-event-field (comparable to the

[1] Meier, P. 'La Veda de la Médecine – 3eme partie; Hypothèses et Perspectives', *De Natura Rerum*, March 1990, vol IV(1), p 42.

[2] Hughes, Richard. *The Principles and Practice of Homoeopathy*, London: Leath & Ross, 1902, p 31.

probability fields in quantum physics) that influences the probability of nerve cell communications by increasing the release of synaptic vesicles, containing the molecules carrying information.

Vitalism is a form of holism that is even reluctant to accept the purely chemico-mechanistic assumption that the systems studied by physicists and chemists are fully inanimate and essentially mechanical. It has, however, not made a definite pronouncement in that last-mentioned, disputed area. Vitalism maintains that organisms are made up of parts (e.g. tissues) which – seen in the direction (perspective) of ever-larger macrostructures – themselves compose other parts (e.g. organs) which then are grouped into still larger entities (namely systems). Yet these tissues – viewed in the opposing direction of ever-diminishing microstructures – are made up of cells, which in turn are constituted by still smaller entities. In other words the body is not a mere agglomerate of molecules or atoms, but a cohesively controlled whole, that is centrally steered, maintained and held together as a concert of organic components and psychic functions nesting in each other, supporting one another, compensating for one another, if need be, and consistently displaying exquisite harmony of purpose. The steering entity, the dynamis, has many synonyms: life principle, vital force, Aristotle called it entelecheia (entelechy), others called it organismic field, immanent organizing principle, and nisus formativus (formative impulse), or just the vital factor. They all infer holistic purposiveness, an entative power that animates the body, as evidenced in the said autarkic faculties of regeneration, regulation and of others, as well as of the curative impulse of any living organism, so effectively utilized by homoeopathy. This entative power has laws of its own to which all phenomena of health and disease necessarily defer.

Central concepts here are *vis medicatrix naturae* (the healing power of nature), homoeosis (assimilation), and homoeostasis. The last-named describes the reactive tendency of any living system to maintain or preserve itself, to return to *status quo* if disturbed. A homoeostatic system is steady-state, which if the need exists, will respond to the correct homoeopathic stimulus and seek to optimize the variables within it. Homoeopathy fully exploits this economical reactive, corrective propensity of the dynamis that Vitalism recognized as 'that which differentiates a living portion of organic tissue from dead or non-living matter'.[1]

All disciplines of the Empirical tradition in medicine recognize this and adopt a biocentric (life-centred) approach to therapeutics. Of them all, homoeopathy most consistently so.

'Dynamic' and 'dynamization' are cognate with 'dynamis', from which they are derived, carrying some of the latter's meaning with them.

'In fact,' Stuart Close says, 'homoeopathy might well be defined as the Science of Vital Dynamics'.[2] (See 'Dynamis', 'Energy', 'Homoeopathic Laws,

[1] *The Shorter Oxford English Dictionary*, two volumes, third edition, Oxford: The Clarendon Press, 1969, vol I, p 1138, 'life' I.b.

[2] Close, Stuart. *The Genius of Homoeopathy*, New York: Boericke & Tafel, 1924, p 39.

Postulates and Precepts', 'Homoeosis', 'Epistemological Assumptions in Homoeopathy' and 'Homoeostasis'.)

Vitamin

Nutritional factor; one of a number of micronutrients, i.e. more precisely substances found in minuscule quantities in nutrients, necessary for proper metabolic functioning. The term, originally spelt vitamine, was coined in 1912 by the Polish biochemist Casimir Funk (1884-1967). He joined 'vita' (life) to 'amine', since he initially believed these substances to be amines [generic name for the compound ammonias in which one or more atoms of hydrogen are replaced by alcohol or other base-radicals].

A prolonged lack of a vitamin in the diet generally causes deficiency symptoms. Conversely, substantial supplementation (outside homoeotic resonance, i.e. above the 'balanced assimilative level') may induce a toxicity state. It must be stressed that dosage required to produce toxicity is highly variable from one patient to the next. Correct assimilative balance must be individually assessed, as only approximations are given below, because deficiencies or excesses ought to be corrected by the homoeopath as a prerequisite for an individual patient's health. So-called mega-vitamin therapy is considered to be a coercive, and therefore a non-homoeopathic, approach. (See 'Foods as Health Problems', 'Homoeosis', 'Naturopath' and 'Nutritional Equipoise'.)

Vitamin A	any fat-soluble beta-ionone derivative, such as retinol, retinal and retinoic acid; the balanced human assimilative dietary level is 5000IU for a male and 4000IU for a female, for these collectively
A1	retinol
A2	dehydroretinol
Provitamin A	water-soluble carotenoids and beta-carotene

Specific vital factors identified with vitamin A:
- growth and repair of tissue, skin, mucous membranes and linings of gastro-intestinal tract;
- maintenance of proper night vision;
- synthesis of ribonucleic acid;
- receptor of free-radical oxygen.

Vitamin B	originally considered as one, later shown to be a group of water-soluble substances (refer to B subentries below).
B1	thiamin hydrochloride; the balanced human assimilative dietary level is 1.4 mg for a male and 1.0 mg for a female.
B2	riboflavin (which at one time was referred to as vitamin G); the balanced human assimilative dietary level is 1.6 mg for a male and 1.2 mg for a female

Vitamin B3   niacin (nicotinic acid) and the related niacinamide
                (nicotinamide); the balanced human assimilative dietary
                level is 18 mg for a male and 13 mg for a female.

         B4   once erroneously believed to be a vitamin, but found to be
                a purine (adenine).

         B5   pantothenic acid; the balanced human assimilative dietary
                level is 4-7 mg.

         B6   pyridoxine and the related pyridoxamine and pyridoxal;
                the balanced human assimilative dietary level is 2.2 mg for
                a male and 2.0 mg for a female.

B10 & B11   each was once taken to be a separate vitamin, but both
                were found to be identical with folacin (refer to subentry
                for vitamin M below).

        B12   cyanocobalamin (cobinamide cyanide phosphate); the
                balanced human assimilative dietary level is 3 mcg.

B Complex   collective term for vitamins B2, B3, B5, B6, B12, H, M,
                choline, inositol and para-aminobenzoic acid in
                combination.

        B13   orotic acid (6-carboxyuracil); usually   these 3 are
                taken as calcium orotate or zinc   dismissed by
                orotate, for which the balanced human   some authorities
                assimilative dietary levels are 800 mg   as without any
                and 15 mg respectively.   merit what-
                                                                 ever, while B17
        B15   pangamic acid; the balanced human   is considered
                assimilative dietary level is 2 mg.   simply as
                                                                 dangerous
        B17   nitrilosides (amygdalin, laetrile) the   cyanide and
                balanced human assimilative dietary   benzaldehyde
                level has not been established, but may   and as such:
                be ca. 0.1 g

**'Laetrile' (B17) is unacceptable to many homoeopaths, the more so since
it does not share with the other B vitamins either common source
distribution (brewer's yeast), their functional relationships, or even their
close association in animal and vegetable tissues.**

Choline	Synonymous: amanitine, bilineurine, bursine, fagine, gossypine, luridine, sincaline and vidine; the balanced human assimilative dietary level has not been established, but may be around 500 mg.	these 3 are part of the B Complex group of vitamins; no alphanumerical codes have been allocated to any; PABA can be toxic to the liver, heart and kidneys, suddenly; with nausea, vomiting, hence:
Inositol	hexahydroxycyclohexane; the balanced human assimilative dietary level has not been established, but may be around 500 mg.	
	Para-aminobenzoic acid, also known as 'PABA'; the balanced human assimilative dietary level has not been established, but may be around 10 mg.	

Para-aminobenzoic acid is unacceptable to some homoeopaths.

Specific vital factors identified with vitamin B (excl B17):
- provision of energy to the body by converting carbohydrates into glucose and in the metabolizing of proteins and fats;
- enabling of healthy functioning of nervous system; maintenance of muscle tone in the gastro-intestinal tract and the health of the liver and other cells.

Vitamin C	Ascrobic acid, a water-soluble nutrient; the balanced human assimilative dietary level is 60 mg.

Specific vital factors identified with vitamin C:
- maintenance of collagen, the intercellular cement in the connective tissue;
- facilitating the metabolism of some amino acids (phenylalanine and tyrosine);
- protection of the following vitamins against oxidation: A, B1, B2, B5, E and M, and converts the last-named from the inactive form (folic acid) into the active (folinic acid);
- production of cortisol by the adrenal glands.

Vitamin D	originally considered as one, later shown to be a group of, fat-soluble substances that have the same effect as the sun's rays in promoting the proper utilization of calcium and phosphorus in body, i.e. calciferol, ergosterol, viosterol and others (refer to D subentries below); the balanced human assimilative dietary level for these collectively is 200IU.
D1	a lumisterol-ergocalciferol mixture

> D2   ergocalciferol
>
> D3   cholecalciferol
>
> D4   22,23-dihydroergocalciferol (activated 22,23-dihydroergosterol)
>
> D5   irradiated 7-dehydrositosterol

Specific vital factors identified with vitamin D:

> ● promotion of bones and tooth formation and regular heart action by enabling absorption of calcium from the intestinal tract, as well as the breakdown and assimilation of phosphorus;

Vitamin E   any fat-soluble tocopherol compound, of which seven forms exist: alpha-, beta-, delta-, eta-, gamma-, epsilon, and zeta-tocopherol, and of tocol and tocotrienol; the balanced human assimilative dietary level is 15IU for a male and 12IU for a female, for these collectively.

> E2   fat-soluble tocoquinone-10 (2,3,5,trimethyl-6-decaprenyl-1, 4-benzoquinone), for which the balanced human assimilative dietary level has not been established.

Specific vital factors identified with vitamin E:

> ● protection of the following vitamins against oxidation: A, B group and C, as well as of the unsaturated fatty acids;
> ● facilitation of cellular respiration (especially of cardiac and skeletal cells);
> ● prevention of elevated scar formation.

Vitamin F   any of the following essential unsaturated fatty acids: arachidonic, linoleic and linolenic acid.

Specific vital factors identified with vitamin F:

> ● transportation of oxygen;
> ● maintenance of resilience of all cells and of normal glandular activity (particularly adrenal and thyroid);
> ● breakdown of cholesterol deposits on arterial walls.

Vitamin G   obsolete term for vitamin B2 (riboflavin).

Vitamin H   biotin, a water-soluble nutrient that is occasionally listed as belonging to the B group of vitamins where it is given by name without an alpha-numerical code; the balanced human assimilative dietary level is 50-200 mcg.

Specific vital factors identified with vitamin H:

> ● assistance, as a co-enzyme, in producing fatty acids, and in the oxidation of fatty acids and carbo-hydrates; in the utilization of protein and vitamins B5, B12 and M.

Vitamin K any of the fat-soluble multiprenylmenaquinone compounds (refer to K subentries below); the balanced human assimilative dietary level is 70-140 mcg, for these collectively.

K1 phylloquinone

K2 menaquinone-6

K3 menadione; menaquinone

K4 menadiol (diacetate or diphosphate)

K5 synkamin (4-amino-2-methyl-1-naphthol hydrochloride)

K6 2-methyl-1,4-naphthalenediamine (toxicity state is easily brought on with this variant)

K7 4-amino-3-methyl-1-naphthol

Specific vital factors identified with vitamin K:
- formation of prothrombin;
- phosphorylation in glycogen conversion;
- assumed promotion of longevity.

Vitamin L nutritional factors of uncertain constitution required for normal lactation (see L subentries below).

L1 lactation factor, derived from liver

L2 lactation factor, derived from yeast

Specific vital factors identified with vitamin L:
- promotion of lactation.

Vitamin M folacin; folic acid (pteroylglutamic acids with oligoglutamic acid conjugates as different forms of folate are collectively known as folic acid), a water-soluble nutrient that is occasionally listed as belonging to the B group of vitamins where it is given by name without an alpha-numerical code, or listed erroneously as either B10 or B11; the balanced human assimilative dietary level is 400 mcg.

Specific vital factors identified with vitamin M:
- in its co-enzyme function with vitamins B12 and C, the breakdown and utilization of proteins;
- carbon-carrier in the formation of haeme (iron-containing protein in haemoglobin);
- for formation of nucleic acid, in the processes of reproduction and growth in all body cells;
- stimulation of the appetite and an aid to liver performance.

Vitamin P bioflavonoids, naturally occurring water-soluble flavone or coumarin derivatives, particularly: citrin, esculin, hesperidin, quercetin and rutin; the balanced human assimilative dietary level has not been established.

Specific vital factors identified with vitamin P:
- adjuvant in absorption and utilization of vitamin C;
- regulation of permeability, and strength, of capillaries;
- protection against susceptibility to opportunist infections.

Vitamin T　　torutilin, an extract of raw sesame butter, torula yeast, egg yolks, or certain insects that feed on the fat of fungi and yeast; the balanced human assimilative dietary level has not been established.

Specific vital factors identified with vitamin T:
- formation of blood platelets.

Vitamin U　　thought to be an amino acid (methionine) derivative and perhaps not a true vitamin, derived from raw cabbage juice; the balanced human assimilative dietary level has not been established.

Specific vital factors identified with vitamin U:
- promotion of healing process (particularly of ulcers).

A source of valuable information on the subject of vitamins is Melvyn R Werbach's *Nutritional Influences on Illness* (Wellingborough: Thorsons Publishers Ltd, 1989, 512 pages).

Vithoulkas, George

A civil engineer from Johannesburg, RSA who in the early 1960s became a homoeopath by studying at homoeopathic medical colleges in Bombay, Calcutta and Madras, India. Together with Irene Bachas, a Greek homoeopathic physician (since deceased), he set up the School for Homoeopathic Medicine and the Centre for Homoeopathic Medicine in Athens which has more than 20 homoeopathic physicians in attendance and is said to treat thousands of patients annually. Vithoulkas, whose base is on the Greek island of Alonissos, spent the two decades from 1970 travelling as homoeopathy's impassioned, articulate crusader to many major cities of the world lecturing, conducting seminars, addressing conferences, and indefatigably bringing homoeopathy to the attention of the general public and creating an awareness of this scientific medical system in the entrenched, institutionalized orthodox medical establishment. He follows in the tradition of James Tyler Kent (1849-1916), whose concepts he has revitalized and substantially developed with consummate logic. His profound works include:

　　Homoeopathy: Medicine of the New Man (Wellingborough: Thorsons Publishing Group; was translated into many major languages)

　　The Science of Homoeopathy (Wellingborough: Thorsons Publishing Group, 1986).

Vivisection

Originally any experimental surgery on a living animal, later extended to mean any form of experiment on animals. (See 'Animal Experiments'.)

Vix Medicatrix Naturae

The healing power of nature (see 'Hahnemann, Christian Friedrich Samuel (1755-1843)', 'Philosophical Premise of Homoeopathy' and 'Vitalism').

W

Warm-Blooded

Homoeothermous; descriptive of animals which have a core temperature constantly maintained at a point above the environmental temperature of which it is independent.

Examples of syndetic pointers to two homoeopathic medicines involving sensations of warmth in the patient or prover:

Sensation as of general warmth with itching of the skin over the whole body – Codeinum

Pulsations, tingling, thrills and a peculiar sensation as of warmth flowing through the body, extending from above downward – Glonoinum

(See 'Organic Clock', 'Regulation-Thermography' and 'Temperature'.)

Wart

Verruca; defined area of hypertrophy of papillae in the corium. The appearance of crops of warts may be a signs of the classical chronic miasma of excess, the sycotic miasma, that is marked by condylomata and where proliferative mucosal and skin changes may take place. For this the Hahnemannian specific remedy is Thuja occidentalis. A wart, or crops thereof, feature in the drug pictures of a number of homoeopathic medicines, a few of which are:

Acidum nitricum: itching, pricking, large jagged, pendunculated, cauliflower-like, bleeds easily, on upper lip

Antimonium tartaricum: wart(s) on glans penis

Calcarea carbonica: horny, inflamed, itching, numerous, small, stinging and ulcerating warts

Causticum: many very small ones soft at base horny on surface; warts on arms, hands, eyelids and face

Ferrum picricum: multiple, pendunculated, lupoid warts

Kali muriaticum: warts on hands; locally: 3DH, as much as would lie on a small coin, in 15ml of water

Natrum muriaticum: wart(s) on the palm

Sepia officinalis: warts on prepuce margin; on the body; large, hard and black warts

Thuja occidentalis: in the miasma of sycosis; locally: Θ to be painted on morning and night.

Examples of syndetic pointers to three further homoeopathic medicines:

The patient who tends to suffer from the terrors of anticipation and who has
wartlike excrescences in the throat that feel like pointed bodies when
swallowing – Argentum nitricum

The surface of the eye feels as though studded with warts in the patient whose
lachrymal discharge is irritating, though the nasal discharge is not –
Euphrasia officinalis

For the patient who is hypersensitive to cold, to touch and to pain, whose warts
become inflamed and stinging as though ulceration would set in – Hepar
sulphuris calcareum

Wash

See 'Colonic Irrigation', 'Douche', 'Lotion' and 'Miasma', under Bad
Hygiene.

In the case of a compulsive ritual that involves or resembles a repetitive
action like that of washing, the following syndetic pointers to one homoeopathic
medicine might come to mind:

At time the patient acts as though s/he were washing, or counting money, or
as if s/he were drinking something – (Atropa) Belladonna

Water

Hydrogen oxide (H_2O); colourless, odourless, tasteless, transparent liquid,
with a freezing point at 0 degrees and a boiling point at 100 degrees Celsius,
containing associated molecules H_3O_2, H_6O_3, etc., which on electrolysis yield
two volumes of hydrogen to one of oxygen. It forms a large proportion of the
earth's surface, precipitates out of the air in the form of rain, and occurs
superabundantly in all living organisms, combines with many salts as water
of crystallization, is an important component in the vehicles used in
homoeopathic pharmacy, and is taken to carry the pharmaceutical
homoeotherapeutic message in solvation structures. (See also 'Alcohol', 'Drug
Preparation', 'Pharmacological Message', 'Physiological Response in
Homoeoptherapeutics, Mechanism of', 'Potency', 'Potentizing Methods',
'Solvation Structures', 'Vehicle' and 'Water of Crystallization'.)

Water-Ethanol Mixture

Hydro-ethanol mixture (see 'Alcohol' and 'Vehicle').

Water of Crystallization

Certain salts while crystallizing out of aqueous solution yield crystals, each
molecule of which is found to be in combination with a definite number of
molecules of water. The particular crystalline shape of those compounds so

formed, is dependent entirely upon those molecules of water and their arrangement which unites them with the salt molecules as an essential part of that crystal's constitution, e.g. $CuSO_4{}^{\prime}5H_2O$ (Cuprum sulphuricum). This proclivity is relevant to homoeopathy in that the molecular linking is already present before crystallizing out of aqueous solution and, in fact, is there as soon as a crystal is dissolved in water. Whether the association is with the aqueous part of either the homoeopathic hydro-ethanol solution or the water molecules present in the lactose used in homoeopathic trituration, is of no consequence to the so-called solvation structures that result and could be carried onward into ultra-molecular (sub-physiological) deconcentrations thereof. (See 'Solvation Structures'.)

Water Polymer

See 'Solvation Structure'.

Wave Function

Mathematical equation representing time and space variables in amplitude for a wave system, used largely in connexion with the Schrödinger equation for particle waves. (See 'Laws of Nature' and 'Radiant State of Matter, Theory of'.)

Wax

Myricyl (melissyl) ester of palmitic acid ($C_{30}H_{61}O{}^{\prime}CO{}^{\prime}C_{15}H_{31}$) and free cerotic acid ($C_{25}H_{51}{}^{\prime}CO{}^{\prime}OH$) with other homologues secreted by bees in a ventral abdominal pouch, as cera flava (yellow beeswax) or cera alba (beeswax bleached by exposure to moisture, air or light) is a plastic solid with a faint characteristic waxy odour and a melting point between 62 and 65 degrees Celsius. It is a component of many cerates and some ointments used in homoeopathy. Some other chemical or plant waxes not used in homoeopathy are cable wax, candelilla wax, cera coperniciae (carnaubia wax, caranda wax or Brazil wax), coccus pela (Chinese wax or coccus ceriferus) and Japan wax (mixture of two vegetable waxes). Ear wax is known as cerumen which, if copiously produced, will cause intermittent loss of hearing, for which either Causticum perlingually or Levisticum officinalis as ear drops could be homoeopathic.

Weakness

See 'Exhaustion'.

Weather Modalities

See 'Modalities'.

Weights

See 'Abbreviations, Symbols, Weights and Measures', page 15 – 17.

Weir, Sir John (1879-1971)

Eminent Scottish homoeopath appointed to the queen of Norway and to the British royal family. He qualified in 1906 in Glasgow, where he came under the influence of Robert Gibson Miller. A patient with abscesses, which had not responded to various orthodox treatments, was treated by the latter with such signal success that Gibson-Miller was adopted by Weir as his mentor. In 1908 he went to Chicago where he studied under John Henry Allen (Professor of Miasmatics and Diseases of the Skin) and James Tyler Kent at the Hering Medical College. He returned to the London Homoeopathic Hospital in 1910. He was a formidable exponent of the single dose and of the concept of non-interference with any homoeopathic aggravation. From 1911 he gave the Compton-Burnett lectures on the Principles and Practice of Homoeopathy.

In 1923 he became President of the Faculty of Homoeopathy. He wrote numerous tracts and articles, which are lucid and well argued, with a refreshing directness in addressing problems. For example, it was he, together with Margaret L Tyler (1875-1943), who introduced the concept of the 'eliminating symptoms' in repertorization. This is described on pages 1436 to 1438 of *Kent's Repertory* (reprint of sixth US edition, Calcutta: Roy Publishing House, 1971). The method is an ingenious labour-saving device reducing the number of contending homoeopathic medicines to be repertorized by about half.

Another Glaswegian homoeopath, Douglas Ross, said of Sir John, on the occasion of the latter's fifty years at the Royal London Homoeopathic Hospital, 'No one has a better grasp of essentials and a quicker eye for detail – and all controlled by his strong Scottish common sense.' A good example of this are the words he chose to end his address to the Liverpool Medical Students' Debating Society in March, 1940: 'I suppose not one of us has approached homoeopathy otherwise than with doubt and mistrust; but facts have been too strong for us.'

His major written work includes:

Repertorizing (with Margaret L Tyler) 1912
Hahnemann on Homoeopathic Philosophy (not given)
The Science and Art of Homoeopathy 1927
Problems of Homoeopathic Education 1929
Homoeopathy: An Explanation of its Principles 1932
Samuel Hahnemann and His Influence on Medical Thought 1934
Homoeopathy, a Science of Drug Therapy 1940.

Well-Wishers and Supporters of Homoeopathy

Among the respected personalities who have openly endorsed homoeopathy are to be found the following, most of whom are listed by Dana Ullman's 'Homoeopathy: Medicine of the 21st Century':[1]

Louisa May Alcott, US author – a favourite among children, with books like *Little Women* published in 1868 (1832-1888)

Pierre Jean David (d'Angers) [see entry] (1788-1856)

Charles (John Huffam) Dickens, novelist of renown, famous for vivid comic characterizations within serious social satire – wrote *Oliver Twist, Nicholas Nickleby, A Christmas Carol, David Copperfield, Hard Times, Great Expectations* and others (1812-1870)

Benjamin Disraeli, Earl of Beaconsfield, British statesman; exercised great influence on Conservative political theories; became prime minister in 1868 and 1874-1880; purchased Suez Canal shares for UK; scored diplomatic triumph at the Congress of Berlin (1804-1881)

William Lloyd Garrison, outstanding US anti-slavery campaigner (1805-1879)

Johann Wolfgang von Goethe [see entry] (1749-1832)

Horace Greeley, founded *New York Tribune,* was a powerful political writer, became candidate for the US presidency in 1872 (1811-1872)

Nathaniel Hawthorne, novelist – author of *The Scarlet Letter* and *The Blithedale Romance* (1804-1864)

Henry James, novelist and younger brother of William James – US born, later naturalized British subject; wrote *The Bostonians* and other enduring works (1843-1916)

William James, great psychologist and philosopher, brother of novelist Henry James (1842-1910)

Henry Wadsworth Longfellow, poet – author of *Hiawatha* and *The Wreck of the Hesperus* (1807-1882)

Yehudi Menuhin, great violinist – a remarkable child prodigy who remained a life-long virtuoso (born 1916)

Pope St Pius X, born Giuseppe Sarto, a man of boundless pastoral zeal, charity and piety, as well as a charming manner, directness and indefatigability, who strenuously tried to prevent the outbreak of World War I; was canonized in 1954 (1835-1914)

John Davison Rockefeller, richest man in the world, donated $750 million to education and charity (1839-1937)

Royal Family of the UK since 1835 when Ernst Stapf was appointed the first homoeopathic physician to the royal household

Karl Philipp Prince Schwarzenberg – Austrian Field Marshal and General Officer commanding the victorious allied armies against Napoleon I in the decisive 'Battle of Nations' at Leipzig (October 1813) (1771-1820)

[1] Ullman, Dana. *Homeopathy: Medicine for the 21st Century,* Berkeley, Ca: North Atlantic Books, 1988, pp 40-42, 51, lists most of these personalities.

William Henry Seward, statesman – governor of New York for two terms; twice elected to US Senate on his anti-slavery stand; in 1861 became President Lincoln's secretary of state who adroitly avoided European intervention in the US Civil War and French expansionism into Mexico; in President Andrew Johnson's cabinet he successfully urged for the annexation of Hawaii and the Danish West Indies, and proposed the purchase of Alaska from the Russian Empire (which was done in 1867, hence the taunt 'Seward's Folly') (1801-1872)

Harriet Elizabeth Beecher Stowe, author of *Uncle Tom's Cabin* (1811-1896)

William Makepeace Thackeray, English novelist – author of *Vanity Fair*; his *Yellowplush Papers* and *The Book of Snobs* [republished from *Punch* magazine] were admired and widely read; his lectures in the USA on 'The Four Georges' were pungently powerful (1811-1863)

Mark Twain (real name: Samuel Langhorne Clemens), journalist, humorist and novelist, who wrote *Tom Sawyer* and *Huckleberry Finn* (1835-1910)

Vincent van Gogh [see entry] (1853-1890)

Daniel Webster, US statesman, lawyer and orator, with enormous influence on constitutional ideas and practice, twice secretary of state, negotiated the Ashburton treaty in 1842 that settled the Maine/Canada (Quebec, New Brunswick) boundary (1782-1852)

William Butler Yeats, Irish lyric poet and dramatist – awarded Nobel Prize in Literature in 1923; member of the senate of Eire 1922-1928; founded Abbey Theatre, Dublin (1865-1939)

Wesselhöft, Conrad (1843-1904)

Son of the homoeopath with whom Constantin Hering founded the North American Academy for Homoeopathic Healing in 1835 in Allentown (53 km north of Philadelphia, Pennsylvania). Himself a homoeopath of some note, he was on Jabez P Dake's consultative US editorial committee (together with H R Arndt and A C Cowperthwaite) for the Anglo-American *Cyclopaedia of Drug Pathogenesy* (4 vols, published from 1886 to 1891). His other major written contributions to homoeopathy include:

The Cause of Contention between the Old and the New 1872
Translated 5th ed. of *The Organon* into English 1876
The Method of Our Work 1880
Plea for a Standard of the Attenuated Dosage 1881
Is the Homoeopathy of Hahnemann the Homoeopathy of Today? 1883
The Law of Similars 1883
How to Study the Materia Medica 1887

Wheeler, Charles Edwin (1868-1946)

This Australian was not only a consummate homoeopath of immense stature and persuasive power. He was also an innovative scientist (see 'Opsonic

Index'), an outstanding linguist (as well as English, his command of German and Italian was exceptional), a playwright of note (the lively *Fools or Knaves* is his work), a poet (he translated Dante's *Divina Commedia* in terza rima, where he showed great mastery of that difficult form), but he also had a fine, generous nature that delighted in sharing his great intellectual gifts and lending a helping hand to anyone who wanted assistance. In a number of ways he could be compared to the poet and craftsman William Morris (1834-1896) before him, because he too hated nineteenth century ugliness, had an unshakable belief in human equality, and in freedom and happiness for all. It was also his conviction that the homoeopathic model would inevitably come to be accepted universally as the scientific framework for medical practice. The central theme of this great exponent of homoeopathy was that health was simply the balanced life.

He was born in Adelaide, South Australia, where he completed his schooling. He studied medicine at Leipzig, Germany and at the medical school of St Bartholomew's Hospital, London, UK, where he gained his MB and BS degrees with first class honours in 1892, carrying off the gold medal for Forensic Medicine. He proceeded to MD a year later. In 1895 he married Miss Ethel Arundel, who later acted at the Court Theatre. He was in general practice at first, but then he became resident medical officer at Nordrach Sanatorium (for chest complaints, in which he had an interest). The pioneering work by Almroth Wright on immunity fascinated him and he entered into the study of immunity with a relish that was never to leave him during his entire professional career in homoeopathy.

He was a founder of the Stage Society, and a close associate of Granville Barker and the celebrated venture of the Court Theatre, which introduced John Edward Masefield (poet laureate) and John Galsworthy's originality and forcefulness to the London public, and thoroughly propagated George Bernard Shaw.

In 1904 he became resident medical officer of the London Homoeopathic Hospital. In 1906 he became assistant physician, then physician in 1914, and was consulting physician from 1928. He was Honeyman-Gillespie lecturer in Materia Medica and Therapeutics from 1908 onward. From 1910 to 1917 he was editor of *Homoeopathic World*. In 1936 he was elected president of the Liga Medicorum Homoeopathica Internationalis. A year before his death he became president of the British Faculty of Homoeopathy. His major homoeopathic publications include a translation of the *Organon*, and, with Edward Bach, of the *Chronic Diseases*. In 1937 he published *A Hundred Years of Homoeopathy* through the British Homoeopathic Association; in this he shows his depth of wisdom. But his most outstanding work remains *An Introduction to the Principles and Practice of Homoeopathy* (with the assistance of Francis H Bodman and J Douglas Kenyon). This went into its third edition by 1948, two years after his death, and has retained its freshness and readership appeal right up to the present time (published Rustington: Health Science Press, 379 pages).

In his obituary 'An Appreciation of Charles Edwin Wheeler' the motto ascribed to this man is: 'Pondus meum Amor meus' (my consistency, my passion) and a colleague, Dr F B Julian, proposed the following epitaph for this charming and wise man: 'Nihil humanum alienum est mihi' (nothing human is foreign to me).

Wholism

See 'Holism'.

Whooping Cough

Pertussis. (See 'Immunization and Homoeopathy', 'Miasma', section Chronic Iatrogenic Miasmata, and 'Vaccination'.)

Wind

The symptom 'flatus' may be meant; if, on the other hand, a weather modality is being referred to, see 'Modality'.

Witch-Doctor

Practitioner of traditional medicine among the tribes of Africa in particular, who as a magician-healer has the dual function of curing disease and counteracting witchcraft by magic art, which two activities are really inseparable from one another. (See 'Shamanism and Magic'.)

Woodward's Comparative Summary on Surgery

See 'Surgery'.

Woodward's Homoeopathic Pharmacodynamics

See 'Therapeutic Science'.

Wool Fat

See 'Adeps Lanae'.

Workplace, Health Hazards in the

See 'Miasma', under occupational hazards.

World Health Organization and Homoeopathy

In 1975 the WHO began advocating the deprofessionalization of primary health care, seeing this as the most important single step in substantially elevating national health levels.[1] Then at the International Conference on Primary Health Care held at Alma-Ata, Kazakh SSR, USSR in 1977 the policy guidelines on primary health care were established for the WHO. It was to further a worldwide movement of barefoot doctors (lay practitioners or feldschers) as community health workers to bring low cost public health and first-line treatment to rural areas, villages and outlying towns and it was to abandon the use of expensive (hence, often, insufficiently supplied), sophisticated and inappropriate (dumped) medicines dispensed by highly-paid specialists to the privileged few.[2] Thereupon in 1977 the WHO officially laid down in a document the programme it would follow in pursuit of this.[3] The WHO's journal *World Health Forum* published an article in 1983 in which this assessment appears concerning homoeopathic treatments being made available in the above context:

> 'Homoeopathic treatment seems well suited for use in rural areas where the infrastructure, equipment, and drugs needed for conventional medicine cannot be provided.'[4]

Worms

In zoology: imprecise term applied both to elongated invertebrates with no appendages, and to immature forms of some insects (mealworm, cutworm, wireworm), and even to millipedes.

In homoeopathy: helminthism; denoting the condition of having intestinal vermiform parasites. A taeniafuge method is discussed under 'Causes of Disease', section 2 External Provocations of Disease (under Mechanical Causes). Prof William Boericke in *Pocket Manual of Homoeopathic Materia Medica* (Philadelphia, Pa: Boericke & Runyon, ninth edition, 1927, pp 191-192) describes treatment for patients with hookworm. John Henry Clarke in *The Prescriber: A Dictionary of the New Therapeutics* (Rustington: Health Science Press, ninth edition, 1972, pp 377-381) describes in great detail homoeopathic treatment for patients with all known varieties of helminth.

Vermifuge treatment, to be acceptable to homoeopathy, may not coercively affect the host organism.

[1] Newell, Kenneth W., ed., *Health by the People,* Geneva: World Health Organization, 1975.
[2] Joint Report by WHO and UNICEF, 'Primary Health Care', on the International Conference on Primary Health Care at Alma-Ata, USSR, 1977, Geneva: World Health Organization, 1978.
[3] World Health Organization, 'The Promotion of Traditional Medicine', Geneva: World Health Organization, Technical Report Series No.622, 1978.
[4] Kishore, Jugal. *Homoeopathy: The Indian Experience,* World Health Forum, vol III, 1983, p 107.

Wound

Transcutaneous traumatism to any body tissue usually caused by mechanical violence, although cutaneous lesions caused by offensive substances or that have appeared as an ulcerative process are also sometimes imprecisely referred to as such. (See 'Emergencies – Homoeopathic Treatment', section Wounds (lacerated; incised; punctured; poisoned), as well as the section Toxic Spills and Leaks, sub-section Chemical Burns and 'Externally Applied Homoeopathic Drugs'.)

X

Xanth-, Xantho-

Prefix meaning yellow or yellowish.

Xenomenia

Vicarious menstrual bleeding; 'representative' menorrhoea from any surface (e.g. navel, urinary tract, cracked nipples, etc.) other than the mucous membrane of the uterine cavity, occurring regularly when the normal menstruation should take place, which, however, is suppressed at the time.

Xerostomia

Asialism; abnormally dry mouth. This is occasionally part of a reactive response by the organism to coercive drugging with orthodox pharmaceuticals.

X-Rays

Röntgen rays, discovered in 1895 in Würzburg, Bavaria, Germany by the physicist, Professor Wilhelm Conrad Röntgen (1845-1923), for which he became the 1901 Nobel laureate for physics; are used in allopathic radiation therapy; are also used by osteopaths, chiropractors and orthodox medical practitioners, as well as engineers and others, in internal radiographic examination procedures where electromagnetic radiation from a vacuum tube, elicited by targeting a stream of electrons (from a heated cathode) on to an anode, either records the varying degrees of radio-opaqueness of the interposed (part of the) patient or object on photosensitive film, or merely projects this as a picture on a screen. These rays can produce radiation damage in organisms from substantive and even minor exposure and can cause serious (occasionally heredotransmissible) miasmatic illness (see 'Miasma'). Anaemia, burns, cataract, dermatitis, sicca syndrome, alopecia, cancer and necrosis are some of the effects of radiation damage. As such, these rays, in the form of irradiated ethanol, have undergone pathogenetic experimentation (provings): originally by Bernhardt Fincke (1897, published in *Proceedings of the International Hahnemannian Association*) and repeated by W B Griggs (1952, published in *Homoeopathic Recorder*).

Y

Yeast

Saccharomyces; a true fungus with a unicellular growth form, capable of producing fermentation at suitable temperatures in malt, fruit juices, doughs, and most things containing any form of starch or sugar other than lactose. For some patients a yeast- and mould-free diet may be prescribed along with the homoeopathic remedy. Moreover, yeast is occasionally used for in-vitro testing of homoeopathic medicines. For example by Michael Jenkins and Raynor Jones, which showed that Pulsatilla nigricans in different dynamizations up to 13CH caused increased growth of yeast and of wheat seedlings as compared to the effects on such organisms by aqua destillata.[1]

Yellow Fever

Acute miasma that may, at times, reach epidemic proportions. It presents as a hepatitis, characterized clinically by fever, jaundice, reduced pulse rate, facial congestion, albuminuria, frequently haematemesis, and nearly always with haemorrhages. A group B arbovirus is associated with the tropical form, although the so-called urban form is thought by some to be connected with Aedes aegypti. (See 'Epidemiology', 'Miasma' and 'Verdi, Tullio Suzzara (1829-1902)'. In the last-mentioned entry will be found the seven homoeopathic medicines that were most frequently successful in the 1878 Yellow Fever epidemic in southern USA. Apart from the remedies there listed, Arsenicum album, Bryonia alba, Cadmium, Cadmium sulphuratum and Camphora (Rubini's) have since each been found to be effective in treating this miasma (that has about a ten percent fatality rate when left untreated.)

Examples of syndetic pointers to two homoeopathic medicines for the third stage of Yellow Fever:

Haemorrhages, violent headache, great heaviness in limbs and trembling body – Carbo vegetabilis

Oozing of blood from every orifice and even from pores of skin, vomiting of bile and blood, yellow skin – Crotalus horridus

Yellow Ointment

See 'Unguentum Flavum'.

[1] Jones, Raynor L, and Michael D Jenkins. 'Comparison of Wheat and Yeast as In Vitro Models for Investigating Homoeopathic Medicines', *British Homoeopathic Journal*, vol LXXII, 1983, pp 143-147

Yin and Yang

In Taoist philosophy, and in Oriental Medicine under Taoist influence, two polar principles or forces which correspond approximately to negative and positive, female and male, night and day, hot and cold, solid and hollow, sedating and tonifying, humid and dry, deficiency and excess, and such similar dual contrapositions that permeate all things.

Yoga

A Hindu system of philosophy, and practice of asceticism, that posits a bioenergetic force like homoeopathy's dynamis, called prana. Other than this it has no real link to homoeopathy, although its physical and mental exercises are compatible with it.

Z

Zero

Nil; cypher or figure nought, denoting nothingness. In calorimetry and thermometry, the point (digit) from which measurements are expressed as a numerical distance on a scale, above or below it. On the Celsius and Réaumur scales it indicates the freezing point of aqua destillata at sea level (273.15K); this is the same as the melting point of ice. On the Fahrenheit scale, however, it represents the degree of coldness produced from mixing salt and ice, which is 32 degrees below the freezing (melting) point. The lowest temperature at which the molecular motion, which signifies heat, is assumed to have ceased altogether is calculated to be -273.15 degrees Celsius, which is generally referred to as 'absolute zero' or zero degrees Kelvin. The 'absolute zero' on other thermometry scales is: Réaumur -218.5; Fahrenheit -459.6; and likewise zero on the Rankine scale.

'Centigrade scale' is now synonymous with 'Celsius scale', although originally (in 1742) the zero on that scale was marked at the boiling-point of water and 100 at the freezing-point by the Swedish astronomer Anders Celsius. This was inverted by Strömer in 1750. Some believe, however, that the Celsius scale, which is the international practical temperature scale standard, was first used by another Swede, the botanist and naturalist Carl von Linné (Linnaeus). A scale still in common domestic use in the Teutonic countries was established by René de Réaumur in 1731 (freezing-point 0, boiling-point 80 degrees) and a scale still in common domestic use in Anglo-Saxon countries was proposed by Gabriel Fahrenheit in 1724 (freezing-point 32, boiling-point 212 degrees). In the nineteenth century the Scottish physicist William Rankine proposed another absolute scale of temperature still used in the engineering profession in English-speaking countries. This is the Rankine scale in which the 'absolute zero' (-459.6 degrees Fahrenheit, taken to be -460 for practical purposes) is marked as zero and the Fahrenheit scale is used above that point, so that 'degrees Fahrenheit' $+ 460 =$ 'degrees Rankine'. At the Eighth Conference on Weights and Measures (1933) thirty-one countries unanimously adopted a precisely re-defined Celsius scale based on a thermodynamic principle first set out by William Thomson (later Lord Kelvin) in 1848. Fixed Celsius temperature points were laid down, in addition to the freezing- and boiling-points of pure water, namely the boiling-points of oxygen (-182.79) and of sulphur ($+444.60$), and the freezing-points of silver ($+960.50$) and of gold ($+1063.00$). The temperature interval on the so-called Kelvin thermodynamic scale of temperature which begins at 'absolute zero' corresponds with that of the Celsius scale but is expressed in 'Kelvins'.

In homoeopathy, as in all medical disciplines, the Celsius scale officially applies since 1960, along with all the other metric SI units of measurement (in terms of the agreed Système International d'Unites). If older works are referred to, it may help to be reminded that a degree Fahrenheit is 5/9 of a degree Celsius and 4/9 of a degree Réaumur, and that a degree Réaumur is equal to 1.25 degrees Celsius and 2.25 degrees Fahrenheit. Formulae applicable for conversions from one scale to another:

R to C:
    R degrees x 5, divide by 4

C to R:
    C degrees x 4, divide by 5

R to F:
    R degrees x 9, divide by 4
    add 32 [above zero degrees R]
       or subtract 32 [below −14.22 degrees R]
       or subtract from 32 [between −14.22 & zero degrees R]

F to R:
    F degrees subtract 32 [above 32 degrees F]
       add 32 [below zero degrees F]
       subtract from 32 [between zero & 32 degrees F]
    then each x 4, divide by 9

C to F:
    C degrees x 9, divide by 5, add 32 [above zero degrees C]
       or subtract 32 [below −17.77 degrees C]
       or subtract from 32 [between −17.77 & zero degrees C]

F to C:
    F degrees subtract 32 [above 32 degrees F]
       add 32 [below zero degrees F]
       subtract from 32 [between zero & 32 degrees F]
    then each x 5, divide by 9

Zimpel, Carl Friedrich (1800-1878)

See 'Spagyric'.

Zone Therapy

See 'Naturopath'.

Zoological Institutes, Experimental Homoeopathic Research at

See 'Veterinary Homoeopathy'.

Zoology

Science of animal life in all its relations.

Zymosis

Fermentation; also the morbid process, previously taken by orthodox medicine to be analogous to fermentation and causing, or constituting, an acute miasma (or 'infectious disease', in the current orthodox idiom). Sometimes incorrectly taken to be synonymous with 'enzymosis', which describes (bio)chemical reactions in organic matter associated with the effect(s) of one or more enzyme(s).

Thorsons Guide to Medical Herbalism

David Hoffman B.Sc., M.N.I.M.H

Herbalism is a truly ancient and worldwide practice. The Egyptians, ancient Britons and native Indonesian tribes all used herbs for healing purposes and today we still utilize their therapeutic properties. *Thorsons Guide to Medical Herbalism* is a complete introduction to this fascinating field. It provides an extensive grounding for anyone interested in developing their herbal skills whether a beginner or more experienced practitioner.

Topics include:

- the nature of herbs and the making of infusions, decoctions, oils and ointments

- the actions of herbs, from emollient to laxative, anti-inflammatory to stimulant

- an A-Z of herbal treatments divided according to the main bodily systems – lymphatic, respiratory, digestive, urinary etc – and their effect on ailments

- the cultivation, harvesting, drying and storing of herbs

- the history of the use of modern herbalism, in China, North America and the Western world

This commonsense guide gives you all the practical information you need to make use of this highly-respected and effective therapeutic system.

Nutrition and Mental Health
An orthomolecular approach to balancing body chemistry
Dr Carl C. Pfeiffer
Edited by **Patrick Holford B.Sc.**

Dr Carl C Pfeiffer was one of the world's foremost figures in nutritional research, and in this pioneering book he poses a radical alternative to prevailing treatment of mental illness by drug therapy.

Dr Pfeiffer spent most of his life researching the connections between nutrition and mental illness, and showed clearly that a proper biochemical balance within the body is the key to maintaining good physical as well as mental health.

His nutritional therapies enjoyed unprecedented success in treating many psychological disorders, from anxiety and depression to phobias and schizophrenia. Here, his revolutionary orthomolecular approach – supplying the body's cells with the right amount of nutrients – is clearly and carefully set out, with particular emphasis on histamine and blood sugar levels, as well as levels of B_6, zinc and copper.

Originally published in 1987 as *Mental Illness and Schizophrenia* it points the way forward in the treatment of mental illness, away from drugs and towards orthomolecular therapy – the medicine of the future.

Shiatsu
The complete guide
Chris Jarmey and Gabriel Mojay

Here is a thorough and comprehensive study guide for Shiatsu students, and a definitive reference work for the practitioner. At the same time it serves as an easy-to-follow guide to Shiatsu for those with an interest in complementary medicine and personal growth.

The book is divided into four sections:

- the essentials necessary for the applications of Shiatsu

- a comprehensive account of the theory and practice of Shiatsu

- traditional Oriental Diagnosis and how Shiatsu fits in

- an explanation of the Five Elements, ascribing to each element a particular energetic and mental focus to directly influence treatment

Chris Jarmey is the Principal of the European Shiatsu School and sits on the Core Group and Examining Board of the Shiatsu Society. He is also the Medical Liaison Officer and correspondent for the Society.

Gabriel Mojay is a Director of Studies in Oriental Medicine for the European Shiatsu School, is an assistant Director of the Institute of Traditional Herbal Medicine and Aromatherapy. He has a private practice in Shiatsu, acupuncture, medical herbalism and aromatherapy.

Palpatory Literacy
Learning to assess musculoskeletal dysfunction by touch
Leon Chaitow N.D., D.O

For manipulative therapists, palpatory literacy – knowing exactly how to interpret what is felt with the hands – is fundamental to good diagnosis and treatment. Practitioners should be able accurately and swiftly to assess the state of a wide range of physiological and pathological conditions and parameters, relating not only to the tissue with which they are in touch, but to others associated with these, often lying at great depth.

The primary aim of this authoritative textbook by internationally renowned osteopath Leon Chaitow is to help practitioners to feel and sense the state of particular tissues; individual therapists can then interpret this information within the framework of their own discipline.

Comprehensive and detailed, *Palpatory Literacy* comprises descriptions of various forms of palpation, and highlights the different ways they can be achieved. Combined with this are numerous exercises to help the development of perceptive exploratory skills.

Homoeopathic Medicine
A doctor's guide to remedies for common ailments
Dr Trevor Smith

Written by a doctor for use by the family, this accessible and practical guide to basic homoeopathy is an invaluable home reference source.

There are five distinct sections, each dealing with the common ailments and first-aid problems associated with the different age groups – childhood, adolescence, adulthood, middle age and the elderly.

As well as general information on each section, along with typical case histories, each ailment, including its causes and symptoms, is defined, and a range of alternative homoeopathic medicines is given with characteristics, so that the specific remedy for your condition can be chosen. In this way the exact remedy for the particular person is more easily found.

Homoeopathic Medicine includes a list of twenty basic homoeopathic medicines for the family medicine chest.

'A most stimulating and practical ready reference.' — Nursing Times

Flower Remedies to the Rescue
The healing vision of Dr Edward Bach
Gregory Vlamis

Most widely known of all the remedies of Dr Edward Bach is the Rescue Remedy – a combination of five of the Bach flowers: impatiens, clematis, rock rose, cherry plum and Star of Bethlehem.

This emergency first-aid remedy has been found to be outstanding in its ability to reduce stress and to stabilize emotional upset during traumatic situations. Its effective use in everyday emergencies is the main subject of this book, but Gregory Vlamis also gives a unique insight into Dr Bach's philosophy of health and the visions he had of the ideal hospital of the future.

Included are many case histories which tell how physicians and other health care professionals (including vets) – as well as members of the general public – have used the Bach Rescue Remedy, often with amazing results.